Health Vis

For Churchill Livingstone:

Editorial Director, Health Professions: Mary Law
Project Development Manager: Katrina Mather
Project Manager: Jane Shanks
Design Direction: George Ajayi

Health Visiting
Specialist and Higher Level Practice

Edited by

Anne Robotham MEd BA RGN ONC DipN(Lond) RHV CertEd(FE) HVT CPT FPCert
Principal Lecturer in Community Health
University of Wolverhampton, UK

Doreen Sheldrake BSc RGN RHV CPT
Health Visitor and Community Practice Teacher
Southern Birmingham Community NHS Trust, UK

Foreword by

Professor Jane Robinson FRCN MA PhD MIPD RGN ONC RHV HVT CertEd
Emeritus Professor, University of Nottingham
Editor, Journal of Advanced Nursing, UK

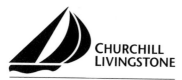
CHURCHILL
LIVINGSTONE

EDINBURGH LONDON NEW YORK PHILADELPHIA ST LOUIS SYDNEY TORONTO 2000

CHURCHILL LIVINGSTONE
An imprint of Harcourt Publishers Limited

© Harcourt Publishers Limited 2000

◢◢ is a registered trademark of Harcourt Publishers Limited

First published 2000
 Reprinted 2001 (twice)

ISBN 0 443 06203 X

British Library Cataloguing in Publication Data
A catalogue record for this book is available from the British
Library

Library of Congress Cataloging in Publication Data
A catalog record for this book is available from the Library
of Congress

Note
Medical knowledge is constantly changing. As new
information becomes available, changes in treatment,
procedures, equipment and the use of drugs become
necessary. The editors, contributors and the publishers have,
as far as it is possible, taken care to ensure that the
information given in this text is accurate and up to date.
However, readers are strongly advised to confirm that the
information, especially with regard to drug usage, complies
with the latest legislation and standards of practice.

Printed in China by RDC Group Limited
P/03

Contents

Contributors

Pat Alexander BSc(Hons) RHV CPT(HV) SCM
RGN FPCert DipCounselling & Interpersonal Skills
DipAromatherapy DipYoga DipFrench
Health Visitor/Community Practice Teacher,
Nuffield House Clinical, Harlow, UK

Karen Reeves Attwood PGD RGN BA(Hons) RHV
Health Visitor, The Wand Medical Centre,
Southern Birmingham Community NHS Trust,
UK

Ros Carnwell PhD BA MA RGN RHV CPT CertEd(FE)
Reader in Primary Care Nursing, Centre for
Health Practice Research and Development,
University of Wolverhampton, UK

Randa Charles BSc(Hons) RGN RM RHV CPT
Health Visitor/Community Practice Teacher,
North Staffordshire Combined Healthcare NHS
Trust, UK

Iain Coleman BSc PhD CBiol MIBiol
Principal Lecturer in Physiology and
Pharmacology, Biomedical Sciences Division,
School of Health Sciences, University of
Wolverhampton, UK

Joanne Davis MMedSci MA RGN RHV
Health Visitor for Travellers, Balsall Heath
Health Centre, Southern Birmingham
Community Health NHS Trust, Birmingham,
UK

Jane DeVille-Almond SRN SCM HV BA(Hons)
Public Health Nurse/Practice Nurse,
Wolverhampton, UK

Janice Frost BSc(Hons) RGN SCM CPT FPCert
Health Visitor/Community Practice Teacher.
North Staffordshire Combined Healthcare NHS
Trust, UK

Jean Glynn MSc BA RHV SRN CPT FPCert
Health Visitor/Community Practice Teacher/
Travelling Families Health Visitor, North
Staffordshire Combined Healthcare NHS Trust,
UK

Shobha Gogna BA MA RGN RM RHV DipOphthalmics
DipCounselling CertTeaching
Health Visitor/Community Practice Teacher,
Wolverhampton Health Care NHS Trust, UK

Tejinder Hari BA(Hons) RGN RM RHV CPT Cert
Counselling (Relate)
Health Visitor/Community Practice Teacher,
South Warwickshire Combined Care NHS Trust,
Leamington Spa, Warwickshire, UK

Jane Harvey MA RN RSCN RHV Family Planning Cert,
C&G-7307 CertEd ObsCert CPT
Nursing Development Officer and Clinical
Supervision Project Nurse, Southern Birmingham
Community Health NHS Trust, UK

Helen Hoult SRN SCM FETC BSc(Hons)
Specialist Health Visitor Traveller Families, Red
Hill Street Health Centre, Wolverhampton, UK

Joy Jeffrey MPH RN RM RHV CPT DipCommunity
Nursing Studies FPCert
Health Visitor/Community Practice Teacher,
Sandwell Healthcare NHS Trust, UK

Joan Leach BSc(Hons) RGN RHV
Health Visitor/Community Practice
Teacher/Accident & Emergency Liaison Health
Visitor, North Staffordshire Combined
Healthcare NHS Trust, UK

Jane McKears MSc BA RGN RHV CPT
Child Protection Adviser, Solihull Healthcare
NHS Trust, UK

Anne Plant BSc(Hons) RGN RM RHV
Health Visitor/Community Practice Teacher,
North Staffordshire Combined Healthcare NHS
Trust, UK

Jane Powell BSc(Hons) MSc
Senior Lecturer in Health Economics, School of
Health Sciences, University of Wolverhampton,
UK

Margaret Reynolds BSc(Hons) RGN RHV CPT
Health Visitor/Community Practice Teacher/
Child Protection Adviser (Health), Dudley
Priority Health NHS Trust, UK

Anne Robotham MEd BA RGN ONC DipN(Lond)
RHV CertEd(FE) HVT CPT FPCert
Principal Lecturer in Community Health,
School of Health Sciences, University of
Wolverhampton, UK

Jan Rose MA CertEd(FE) OHNC RHV RGN
Visiting Lecturer, School of Health Sciences,
University of Wolverhampton, UK

Doreen Sheldrake BSc RGN RHV CPT
Health Visitor/Community Practice Teacher,
Southern Birmingham Community NHS Trust,
UK

Judith Shuttleworth BSc
Information Services Manager, Walsall
Community Health Trust, UK

Ruth Wain MSoc Sci BA(Hons) CertEd
Director, Centre for Health Practice Research
and Development, University of
Wolverhampton, UK

Foreword

The publication of *Health Visiting: Specialist and Higher Level Practice* is timely for several reasons. First, coming as one of the first books on the subject of health visiting in the new millenium, it follows in an important historical tradition. When I began to research into health visiting in the second half of the 1970s I believed initially, and incorrectly, that little study had been carried out historically on the discipline of health visiting. I could not have been more mistaken. The differences of principle that have always underpinned different approaches to welfare and health care provision in Britain have also given rise to vociferous debates concerning the nature of health visiting, and to studies on its nature and function. At the beginning of the twentieth century, the very different conclusions of the Majority and Minority Reports of the Commissioners on the 1909 Poor Law (Webb B & S 1909, Bosanquet 1909) led to fierce arguments over how health care should be provided. Failure to reconcile these views led to the ultimate shape that health services would take throughout the twentieth century, with proactive primary health promotion frequently taking second or third place to the provision of reactive, secondary and tertiary health services. Studies concerning the efficacy of health visiting were considered crucial and began in the early years of the century, largely conducted by the then highly influential Medical Officers of Health, or as government reports. Increasingly carried out by individual health visitors, studies of health visiting have continued to

a greater or lesser extent throughout the succeeding years (Robinson 1982, Elkan et al 2000).

That health visitors themselves should write authoritative, evidence based studies would probably not have occurred to many people in the early 1900s. However, Margaret Llewellyn Davies (1915, 1978), a female sanitary officer and a graduate of Girton College Cambridge, as first General Secretary of the Women's Cooperative Guild, gathered together in *Maternity: Letters from Working Women*, women's own accounts of their experiences of childbirth endured in grinding poverty. Llewellyn Davies' book was to prove enormously influential with government in the development of maternal and child health services following the First World War. Thus Robotham and Sheldrake follow in very distinguished footsteps.

Health Visiting: Specialist and Higher Level Practice is timely for contemporary policy reasons too. After almost two decades of health and social policy that strongly featured the role of the individual in self help and self care, government policies are now in place that encourage mutual community initiatives, are committed to the reduction of inequalities in health, that emphasise the role of primary health care in the design and purchase of health services, and that recognise families' frequent need for skilled help in parenting. These policies demand that the professionals charged with their implementation are highly skilled in a broad range of competencies. These include: health needs assessment, sensitivity to individual and group differences, child development and child protection, the application and evaluation of the most up to date knowledge in the biological, pharmacological, social and psychological fields, and the legal aspects of practice, including personal accountability and responsibility. Faced with such a challenging if daunting prospect, health visitors will welcome the excellent resource that Robotham and Sheldrake's book provides.

Finally, *Health Visiting: Specialist and Higher Level Practice* is timely because it is rooted entirely in *practice*. The beginning of the twenty first century is perhaps characterised above all by consumer rejection of forms of knowledge and practice that hide behind professional rhetoric, or theoretical jargon. The wide availability of sources with which consumers can confirm or reject professional advice, means that practitioners have to reflect on, and re-evaluate constantly, their own practice and its consequences. That virtually every chapter in this book is written by individuals with their feet still firmly rooted in health visiting practice is one of its greatest strengths. The accumulated knowledge is enriched from this direct experience. This is not to say that theory does not have a place – far from it. But theory for health visiting practice has to be developed and tested in the crucible of empirical research and experience. The contributing authors to *Health Visiting: Specialist and Higher Level Practice* bring this resource in abundance to their work. Health visitors, their students and others, will find this a comprehensible and practical text when developing their own higher level and specialist practice.

Professor Jane Robinson

REFERENCES

Bosanquet H 1909 The Poor Law Report of 1909. Macmillan and Co, London
Elkan R, Kendrick D, Hewitt M et al 2000 The effectiveness of domiciliary visiting: a systematic review of international studies and a selective review of the British literature. Health Technology Assessment Report (in press)
Llewellyn Davies M (ed) 1915 Maternity: Letters from Working Women. Virago, London (reprinted 1978)
Robinson J 1982 An Evaluation of Health Visiting. ENB/CETHV, London
Webb B & S 1909 Minority Report of the Poor Law Commission. London

Preface

The seed was sown for this book during the latter half of the 1990s when the Conservative Government was coming to the end of a long period in office and political commentators were voicing opinions that, in relation to the NHS, the government was running out of ideas. Labour came into office in 1997 and the pace of change was breathless, although much of the change was building on new ideas that had emerged from the White Paper *Choice and Opportunity, Primary Care: The Future* (Department of Health 1996a). Germination of the book has taken place with Labour in office, the millennium rapidly approaching and Primary Care Groups finally leading the way in determining the delivery of health care within the community and general practice.

The Editors make no apology for focusing this book on health visiting because that is what it is about. However, it is acknowledged that health visiting is founded on skills that can be practised in nursing, midwifery, social work, health promotion, medicine, counselling, care and friendship, politics, community development and other fields. Thus, these skills are not unique to health visiting. It is the combination of such skills that makes health visiting the profession it is. Little mention is made of the intervention of other disciplines because the book is written for health visitors and their skills include working with a range of other professionals for the benefit of the client, family and community. Much of the material in this book is equally beneficial to other professionals and we hope that they will find the book useful for their practice or for reference.

Anne Robotham
Doreen Sheldrake
Wolverhampton and Birmingham 1999

Editors' note

Following devolution in Scotland we feel that it is necessary to point out that there are corresponding Scottish white/green papers where some English/UK ones are mentioned. Where we have mentioned *The new NHS – modern, dependable* (DoH 1997a) the equivalent Scottish document is *Designed to care: renewing the National Health Service in Scotland* (Scottish Office 1997); where we have mentioned *Our healthier nation: a contract for health* (DoH 1998a) the equivalent Scottish document is *Towards a healthier Scotland* (Scottish Office 1999).

Acknowledgements

The Editors wish to acknowledge with grateful thanks the following:

All the authors for their time and commitment to this volume; Stella Webb for reading countless drafts of material and making invaluable suggestions for improvement.

Introduction

It is against the shifting background of major change historically and recently in the NHS that this book has been planned, and on a very positive note health visiting now has the opportunity to move forward in education, organisation and management. A glance at the contents list will yield a series of topic areas that bear a somewhat tenuous relationship to each other, and yet they exemplify the diversity of health visiting and can all be incorporated into the fields of public, community and family health. The first chapter explores in depth some of the major debates that health visitors have struggled with. Where health visitors are based leads the discussion into organisation and the medical or social model of health, and this inevitably moves the discussion into management. Should health visitors be part of integrated nursing teams, what part does skill mix play, and how is the effectiveness of health visiting measured? Finally, and most importantly of all, what form should health visitor education take in the reorganised structures to determine quality and standards in the delivery of practice and education within the profession?

The second chapter focuses on the public health role of health visitors and explores issues about what constitutes the public health role. In recent years health visiting has moved away from public health, and an understanding of what part epidemiology has to play in health need is an important issue. In an age where information is freely available it is still necessary to ask obvious questions in relation to the validity and reliability of available data, and to recognise that epidemiology plays only one part in multi-causal public health needs. Public health has clearly moved on from hygiene and sanitation but the principles that underlay these issues are the same as the principles underlying the effects of the modern age of over-use of antibiotics, the development of alternative fuel sources, genetic modification and increasing technology with its use and abuse.

The part that health visiting has to play is also increasingly sophisticated and a knowledge base that allows flexible and rapid movement between cause and effect is essential to good health visiting practice.

Awareness and knowledge within the population, facilitation of travel and the movement of family members across continents is a challenge to health visiting, as is the adaptation of practice to support a multicultural society.

Critical to advancing practice is the need to recognise how to use information from a technological viewpoint and as a means of measurement of need and evaluation of effectiveness of intervention. Audit has shown that there is much to criticise in the way in which health visiting has recorded its interventions and determined its practice boundaries. Information is not just about data and statistics but about communication as a skill in effective advice, support and education in evidence-based practice. In the light of these comments Chapter 3 focuses on health informatics and its use in medical care and social need particularly highlighting the important part that risk assessment plays in clinical governance. Clinical governance is also about the effective use of resources and health informatics has been shown to be a much under-used resource which should be crucial to higher level health visiting practice.

Chapter 4 explores the use of models in health visiting practice, recognising that health visiting practice is so dichotomous that there will never be one all-encompassing model. Carnwell argues that for health visiting to be practised to its fullest extent then models for use in public health and health promotion should structure health visiting work. In working with individuals and families then models used in the mental health field may be modified from their nursing origins to fit more comfortably into health visiting. It is necessary to focus more consistently on models of public health and Beattie's framework allows health visiting to use a mechanism which may be easier to evaluate in terms of effectiveness when broken down into its constituent parts. It is essential that health visitors focus on the development of models of public health because they, of all the community health care workers, have the dimension within their education to account for health using Beattie's biopathological model, ecological model, biographical model and communitarian model. Carnwell's discussions of these approaches area model of critical analysis which is outstanding for its clarity and depth and are to be commended to health visitor readers.

In writing about an alternative approach to health visitor education, Robotham (1998) was challenged about the need for health visiting skills, and that to use these effectively in domiciliary visiting was more important than developing a public health curriculum. To identify skills in health visiting the ambivalence of health visiting becomes very obvious, and thus the skills extend across a continuum of individual counselling and intervention type work; through surveillance and modified social policing; on to the capacity to seize opportunistic situations for health promotion and illness prevention teaching; and finally to community development and motivation. It is hardly surprising that most health visitors would question their own abilities to be either skilled or successful in all these situations, but they do have the means to balance the work in a team approach which allows diversification to suit particular skills.

Chapter 5 seeks to capture some of these skills and commences with an approach to modifying nursing skills for use in health visiting. The skills and art of health visiting in the most common settings are then explored with the ways in which the skills are used in relation to the principles of health visiting. The use of psychological skills within health visiting supports and exemplifies the way in which it may be possible to evaluate the dialogue between health visitor and client and thus contribute to the measurement of health visiting effectiveness.

Chapter 6 follows on from the skills approach by examining, from various perspectives, health visiting knowledge and action in practice. The growth of the use of reflective processes in professional healthcare practice has enabled health visitors to critically examine the content and dynamics of professional thinking in practice, and in so doing to capture much of the critical thought of practice using reflective approaches. Critical thinking, critical analysis of and in practice and critical reflection have allowed health visitors to articulate practice more clearly and to develop a greater rigour in evidence-based practice. Continually developing critical thinking has enabled health visitors to use concept mapping as a useful tool both in teaching the art of practice, and also in understanding a new methodology for analysing the client perspective. This is particularly useful in those specialist areas of practice where a new approach to the structure of practice can be identified by concept analysis through mapping.

This approach can be carried further by examining in particular one or two examples of focused roles in health visiting practice, and Chapter 7 has brought together the work of two health visitors who are practising from very different approaches. Jane McKears has considerable experience as a lead health visitor in child protection and combines a role of supporter to her colleagues with that of education and development of their child protection knowledge and understanding. Margaret Reynolds is looking at child protection in a very different way by exploring the use of a developmental screening tool which, she argues, is most effectively used in targeted health visiting with children known to be at risk. Reynolds then goes on to discuss a tool which, is still at a pilot stage but which looks to have all the elements necessary for a very positive addition to evaluation methodology. Evaluation of parenting skills before and after interventions by the health visitor to improve parental knowledge and skills in child rearing, has shown that in the pilot stage at least, here is a potentially very exciting approach to measurement of health visitor effectiveness.

Health visiting and public health means that the discipline of health economics becomes a necessary addition to the supportive knowledge base from which the health visitor practises. Thus economic analysis is important to argue for, and work towards, in the quest for equity in resource allocation, equity in quality of life and equity in health status both from a lifestyle viewpoint and on a wider political and social basis. Jane Powell has examined health visiting from a cost-effective analysis and also has, in the same way as Robinson (1998), used randomised controlled trials to examine health visitor effectiveness in the reduction of health inequalities in Chapter 8. Powell has shown that health visitors can be instrumental in reducing inequalities in health if they address the structural determinants of health or include both information and support. The editors of this book are indebted to Powell's analysis of an economic appraisal of health visiting which will be so essential in developing health visiting within public health without losing any of the traditional ways in which health visitors have worked.

Clinical effectiveness belongs to the growing debate on the management of public health from a clinical governance approach incorporating clinical leadership and clinical supervision in risk management and health benefit. This must include a quality of practice, organisation and professional scrutiny which supports the government's drive to develop a system based on partnership within Health Action Zones in those areas with the greatest health and service challenges. Jane Harvey has been one of the lead health visitors in Birmingham in setting up programmes of clinical supervision in care and programme management and clinical effectiveness in risk assessment. Audit tools and outcome measures are essential to support economic appraisal of effectiveness in health visiting and there is a need to recognise that a positive attitude must be fostered among health visitors and their management to implement an essential part of the role of the profession in public health.

Health visitors from North Staffordshire

Combined Health Care Community Trust work in a uniquely interesting area from a geographical and demographic perspective. The traditions of the pottery industries and mining with the inevitable modern decline, the isolation of the area sandwiched as it is between Greater Manchester and the West Midlands but with surrounding rural areas of the Staffordshire Moorlands and the tail end of the Peak district, and until recent improvement in transport systems led to a population that rarely moved to other parts of the country, make this a fascinating place to work in. It could be imagined that health visiting only moved at the rate of the demographic changes but some areas of practice have been seen to be well in advance of health visiting elsewhere. This has given the editors an opportunity to bring together the work of five practitioners who have shown the research development of their work to improve the health status of their client groups.

Jean Glynn has shown how her interest in young people in relation to their sexual health is only effective when practised within the context of young people's perception of their health needs and varied life styles. Anne Plant argues for well developed child surveillance programmes which contribute to child health promotion and the equality of care within a changing population. Janice Frost has worked particularly in the area of child behaviour management and parenting skills and this focuses so well on the government's approach to supporting families and the development of Sure Start programmes. Randa Charles has published fairly widely on the need for accuracy, contemporaneity and relevance of records and record keeping. Readers will remember that not too long ago the Audit Commission, in the early 1990s expressed concern at nursing record keeping and were particularly concerned at some of the health visitor record keeping. This section of Chapter 10 is particularly pertinent in the light of the discussion in Chapter 3 over the use of information technology and in particular patient information systems.

Joan Leach, concerned about the number of child accidents occurring on her caseload, has developed an educational approach to raising awareness of, and lowering the incidence in childhood accidents in her GP practice. Individually you could argue that these health visitors are practising in a traditional manner, but viewed collectively they satisfy the public health perspective in working for both the community and the individual.

In the growing need to show economic use of resources there has been a push to move health visitors away from the home into working in clinics and health centres, thus fulfilling a need to show cost-effectiveness of human resources. However, domiciliary health visiting was where health visitors began and where they will always practice most effectively. That is not to say that there is not a place for working outside the home and the movement into community development demonstrates an equally effective use of health visitor education. Domiciliary health visiting nevertheless, as has been shown by studies (Clark 1973; Dobby 1986; Cowley 1991; Robinson 1998), will remain at the forefront of effective health visiting and Chapter 11 examines and discusses various methods of intervention that health visitors might use in the home. The case is made that health visitors, although not counsellors, nevertheless use counselling skills in their interventions and various appropriate approaches are explored. Some of the main situations that are best supported by domiciliary visiting are explored particularly using different intervention approaches and analysing the effectiveness of these.

Health visiting has always been aware of the ethical dilemmas that face the practitioner and Jan Rose with a health visiting and occupational health background is in an ideal position to explore these issues in relation to quality health care delivery. In an increasingly litigious society there is a need for health visitors to recognise that accountability is not just about ensuring correct qualifications and professional development for practice, but also about the need for an exploration of personal attitudes and values in effective healthcare delivery. Professional knowledge can be used in ways which can easily become unethical and health visitors are well aware of the need to understand and respond to ethical dilemmas that periodically arise with alternative approaches and advancing technology in relation to the delivery of health care. Health visiting can run closely alongside 'nannying', 'social policing' and 'coercion' to use some of the terms that are often thrown at central and local political strategies, and health visitors need to feel secure about their handling of some of the ethical dilemmas that they may meet in practice.

'Public Health and a Violent Society' is the title of one of the modules on the undergraduate public health degree programme at the University of Wolverhampton. Health visitors are among some of the more at-risk groups of professionals exposed to potential violence in their daily work. However, it is not about self-protection that this chapter focuses on but about the increasing violence within our society which is very much a public health issue. Ask the average person on any housing estate, public pavement or dimly lit alley what they most worry about and the answer will likely to be theft, burglary or violence to the person. These are examples of criminal violence but there is far more violence in the ways in which we behave to each other through verbal aggression, bullying, relationship breakdown and caring for the more vulnerable. Much of this seems to be a product of a less caring age but it is often within the family that the seeds are sown. Parenting has a major part to play – to the extent that the government are focusing on supporting families through Sure Start programmes and health visitors are recognised as being the professionals best able to support these initiatives. Health visiting education has probably only mentioned violence in passing but we would argue that more should be understood about violence between individuals, within families and in communities. To this end Chapter 13 examines the ways in which health visitors can influence by education, partnership and enablement, the parents, families and the community on how to understand each other and to work for the greater good rather than the individual.

This age is an age of knowledge and a seeking of answers to problems and particularly health problems. Since the Black Report (Black 1980) it has been apparent that a bigger and better health service is not going to solve the reasons for health inequalities, many of which stem from social inequality and marginalisation. In addition, allopathic medicine does not appear to have the answers to the health difficulties that individuals are experiencing, and so they are turning more frequently to alternative therapies which are used instead of or complementary to, the medicine practised in general practice. Pat Alexander is one of a growing number of health visitors who are also qualified in a branch of complementary medicine, and are able to practice alongside conventional medicine to provide a most comprehensive service to the patient or client. Alternative medicine has much to offer allopathic medicine, not least in the fact that it is far less likely to harm through extensive side-effects. If conventional medicine does not work there is a strong possibility that the patient may be left with unfortunate side-effects which may be very long lasting, but with alternative medicine the only side-effect is likely to be no effect. Allopathic medicine and alternative medicine can and should work alongside each other and Pat Alexander practises as a health visitor using complementary therapy skills, benefiting clients and giving her a satisfying and unique status of partnership within the practice.

Despite the discussion above concerning Chapter 14 and complementary therapies, health visitors are also gaining education to enable them to prescribe from the nursing formulary. Doctors and pharmacists expressed considerable concern about the prospect of nurse prescribing from education, practice and cost perspectives, and thus the availability of appropriate courses and the provision for nurse prescribing in general practice and in triage has developed slowly. The opportunity to include a chapter from a pharmacologist, Dr Iain Coleman, has added to the breadth and depth of this book. Dr Coleman has taught pharmacology to countless biomedical students and in recent years to practice nurses and nurse practitioners. To contain an entire course within one chapter has been a challenge, but the results are an opportunity to gain a greater understanding of pharmacokinetics and pharmacology and to recognise the part that health visitors might play in enabling their clients to understand therapeutic drug use. This chapter is also valuable from an education viewpoint because of the use of a problem-based learning method.

Practising health visiting in a multicultural society means that unless health visitors really understand the mores and practices of the culture in which they are working they are only partially effective. Trusts go to considerable lengths to employ health visitors who come from ethnic minority groups but there are insufficient numbers to successfully serve the population. In fact there is a major debate about whether like-cultural-group professionals should work with like-clients because this becomes divisive, racist and could lead to a more marginalised society. To overcome the arrogance of one culture, and the submersion of another culture, there is a requirement for each culture to develop an understanding and sensitivity to the needs of the others. The uniqueness of the domiciliary role of health visiting allows entry to all homes and the knowledge of health visitors about the culture of the home in which they are visiting will improve the partnership basis of their work with their clients. Shoba Gogna and Tejinder Hari both practise as Asian health visitors in a multicultural society and have come together in Chapter 16 to discuss customs, social mores and problems of south Asians and to show how a greater knowledge can aid health visitors from a different cultural background in their work with Asian clients. This chapter makes fascinating reading and the editors are indebted to these two health visitors for their time and energy in enabling the profession to explore the needs of south Asians.

It is likely that people from every country in the world are to be found somewhere in the UK and it would be a very ambitious book that attempted to explore the mores of each group. The three health visitors who have combined to produce Chapter 17 are exploring very different groups within our society. Joy Jeffrey has practised within the West Midlands for several

years and has a particular interest in the Afro-Caribbean culture with all its diversities. West Indians have been indigent in the UK population since the end of the Second World War and thus have become an established ethnic group in Britain, but they do have particular health problems and needs, not least because they are often to be found in some of the more deprived areas of this country. In discussing their problems Joy enables us to develop greater sensitivity within our practice. A totally different group who are even more marginalised are the travelling families within this country. Some people choose to drop out of society and have become the New Age travellers, others belong to an ancient nomadic tribe who attempt to live alongside other citizens in the UK. Joanne Davis and Helen Hoult have worked with travellers for several years and between them cover the bulk of the West Midlands area. The health needs of travellers are great but can only be responded to within the knowledge of their culture and a modification of the ways in which the NHS can respond to health problems in a nomadic people.

The final chapter of this book allows Karen Reeves Attwood to explore choice and opportunity in health visiting and she has thoroughly enjoyed being given free rein on what can and will be. It must be true to say that never has health visiting had greater opportunity, and a positive attitude to change, which is determined by health visitors and not imposed from above, will carry the profession forward. Karen has explored various ways in which health visiting can respond to internal changes within the profession and government initiatives which explicitly reuire the work of health visitors. Health visiting as a profession has in the past been criticised for its lack of initiative in taking up opportunities although there is plenty of evidence of the creativity of individual practitioners. This may be to do with education going too far down the community nurse route or because health visitors cannot let go of the traditional caseload to respond to the identified health needs of the profiled area.

Inevitably a text book, by the time it is published, comes onto a market that has moved on. However, the editors and authors have worked to ensure that the content of the chapters is as refreshingly up to date as is possible. It must be remembered that when one is in the middle of a busy active professional life, changes seem to occur with increasing rapidity. Nevertheless, in retrospect it is often possible to recognise the circular basis of some change and to realise that innovation also consolidates the recent past.

1

Health visiting – specialist and higher level practice

Anne Robotham and
Jane DeVille-Almond

INTRODUCTION

This chapter is about specialist and higher level practice and discusses whether there are indeed sufficient differences among the various ways in which health visiting is practised to be able to articulate a specialist and higher role. The term 'specialist practice' has been used in health visiting from the middle of the 1990s and came from the re-articulation of education; at the same time the term 'advanced practice' was mooted but without any clear idea of its definition or whether it is necessitated by formal education.

SPECIALIST PRACTICE

The United Kingdom Central Council for Nursing, Midwifery and Health Visiting (UKCC) proposed the Specialist Practitioner qualification for all post-registration professionals successfully completing a programme that was to be at least at university first-degree level. In effect, therefore, post-registered qualified practice leads to specialist practice. Specialist practice within the acute sector was based on the undertaking of a specialist practice course but there were no specific titles for specialist practice in secondary care. Within primary care eight discrete areas of specialist practice are identified. Inevitably, considerable concern was voiced within the general profession about the new specialist practitioners who, once newly qualified, immediately became 'specialists', and in particular, disquiet was expressed about health visitors who, newly qualified into specialist practice, were in effect totally inexperienced.

The debate, of course, centres on the meaning of the term 'specialist'. The comparable professionals within the NHS are medical or surgical consultants, often referred to as specialists, who acquire the title as a result of recognised seniority and experience. It is clear that the UKCC intended the terms 'specialism' and 'specialist practitioner' to distinguish between the area of practice and the higher level of practice but this was confused with the development of courses for practice in primary care. These implied that to become a specialist practitioner required the undertaking of a special course, which was probably not the original intention of the UKCC. Indeed there has always been a tension between specialist ability achieved through high level experienced practice but without educational underpinning, and an educational underpinning that can act as a springboard to higher level practice.

To return to the debate about the specific areas of specialist practice in primary care, these were coterminous with practitioner titles from previous courses, albeit modernised to fit a more flexible approach. Community Psychiatric Nursing became Community Mental Health Nursing; Community Mental Handicap Nursing remained the same but with the alternative, more politically correct title of Learning Disability Nursing. School Nurses and Practice Nurses became fully recognised as members of the community team rather than undertaking shorter courses as before, and a new specialism of Community Children's Nursing was introduced in recognition of the move towards nursing children with a variety of highly dependent conditions at home. The traditional community practitioners, health visitors and district nurses were assigned alternative titles of 'Community Nursing in the Home – District Nursing' and 'Public Health Nursing – Health Visiting'. Occupational health nursing fitted somewhat uneasily into community nursing and continues to argue its distinct identity.

It is probably fair to say that district nurses felt that they could live with their specialist title and, inevitably, it was shortened back into the comfortable and acceptably recognised traditional form. Health visitors, on the other hand, viewed their new specialist title with considerable scepticism and concern. 'Public health nursing' as a description was open to debate because there were implications for a hidden agenda. Health visitors had no problem with 'public health' – but 'nursing'? 'Nursing' had implications of reducing everything to illness and loss of a preventive approach to health care, implying the curative approach. As time has passed there has inevitably been a reconciliation between official descriptive titles and the more familiar terms, and the lack of enthusiasm for having Public Health Nursing as part of their title has allowed health visitors to retain the status quo. Suffice to add that the decision by the government in 1999 to continue to require health visitors to be registered separately will ensure a quality of practice and protection for the public in what is a very different area of community health care from nursing, requiring very different skills and knowledge.

Specialist practice in health visiting

The discussion above has traced the process by which health visitors become specialist practitioners as a result of Project 2000 initial nurse training and the subsequent Preparation for Specialist Practice. Before considering the appropriate content of courses for specialist practice in health visiting, the nature of the specialism should be reviewed.

In introducing a new standard for education and practice following registration, the UKCC coined the new term 'specialist practice'. They argued that preregistration programmes, while providing practitioners with the knowledge, skills and attitudes to provide safe and effective care, do not prepare them to meet additional specialist needs. Specialist practice, the UKCC stated, called for additional education for safe and effective practice and for the ability to exercise higher levels of judgement and discretion in clinical care. In proposing the use of the title 'specialist practice' the UKCC, while recognising the wide range of specialisms in general nursing, nevertheless only proposed named specific specialisms within the community. It is interesting that the proposed specialist practitioner programmes carried learning outcomes for standards for 27 common core outcomes, grouped under four headings of:

- Clinical nursing practice
- Care and programme management
- Clinical practice leadership
- Clinical practice development.

Further outcomes were identified for each named specialism in the areas of Clinical nursing practice and Care and programme management. For public health nursing/health visiting these are as follows.

A. Clinical nursing practice:

1. Assess, plan and evaluate specialist health care interventions to meet health and health-related needs of individuals, families, groups and communities
2. Undertake diagnostic, health screening, health surveillance and therapeutic techniques applied to individual, family and community health maintenance
3. Initiate action to identify and minimise risk and ensure child protection and safety, working in partnership with families

B. Care and programme management:

1. Build health alliances with other agencies for health gain
2. Influence policies affecting health
3. Search out health-related learning needs of individuals, families, groups and communities and stimulate an awareness of needs at local/national levels
4. Empower individuals, their carers, families and groups to influence and use available services, information and skills to the full and act as an advocate where appropriate
5. Identify appropriate resources to meet needs, plan and initiate measures to promote health and prevent disease
6. Support and empower individuals, families and communities to take appropriate action to influence health care and health

promotional activities by means of a community development approach

7. Initiate the management of cases involving potential or actual physical or psychological abuse and potentially violent situations and settings
8. Work with key personnel in health and other agencies to address and/or achieve agreed health goals and local policies
9. Collect and interpret health data and develop and initiate strategies to promote and improve individual and community health and evaluate the outcomes
10. Establish and evaluate caseload and workload profiles and devise programmes of care and monitor strategies of intervention.

This list comprehensively covers the whole range of work undertaken by health visitors. It is twice as long as all the other community specialisms except school nursing. On this basis alone the use of the term 'specialist practice', covering as it does all qualified health visitors, raises the question of the fundamental meaning of the word 'specialist' in such a wide-ranging field. Clearly the outcomes are specialist by the very nature of the breadth of knowledge and skills required to practise effectively in health visiting but, interestingly, they differ little from those identified for school nursing. The extra three outcomes for health visitors all belong to the area of community development and local policy issues.

Most health visitors agree that they incorporate all these tasks into their regular work patterns. In reality, there is a preference among health visitors to use the skills developed from these outcomes in the area of practice where they work most frequently, whether this is working with individuals and families or groups or communities. What is certain is that the outcomes identified are all regularly used whether the health visitor is working with an individual or on community development. Hyde (1995) argues that there are different levels of practice and uses Hamilton's (1988) analogy of community-as-background or community-as-foreground to distinguish between working with an individual in the community and working with a community of individuals. However, it could also be argued that the same specialist outcomes are used by all practitioners and thus there are no different levels, merely different spheres of work.

Scrutiny of the learning outcomes outlined above would suggest that the language and terminology used are appropriate to health visiting. However, when these outcomes are compared to those for other disciplines there are striking similarities, to the extent that the first Clinical nursing practice outcome for all disciplines apart from health visiting is:

1. Assess, plan, provide and evaluate specialist clinical nursing care to meet the needs of …

and for health visiting and school nursing is:

1. Assess, plan, provide and evaluate specialist health care interventions to meet …

In other words, the only difference between all nursing disciplines and health visiting is that the words 'clinical' and 'nursing' have been turned into 'health care'. It is thus very clear that care has been taken to ensure that the language used for descriptors for the learning outcomes for the programmes in PREP reflects a common framework, which could lead to a generic nurse.

On a similar scale of importance is the concern expressed by health visitor educationalists over course content. This was originally based on a CETHV syllabus reflecting the need for the disciplines of sociology, social policy and psychology as well as child nutrition and care and the principles and practice of health visiting. These subjects of study reflected the meagre coverage of these areas in initial nurse training and they were taught by lecturers who were specialists in those disciplines and without a nursing background. Students learned to apply the principles of these disciplines to health visiting rather than simply being taught 'applied sociology' or 'applied social policy'. Movement of colleges of nursing and midwifery into universities has now meant that in many cases lecturers in, for example, social policy, are nurses with a sociology/social policy degree teaching the applied subject as in a Project 2000 course. The problem with this is that it is not suitable for health visitors, who

need to be in a position to interpret the subject discipline for use in many different ways in their practice. Adapting an 'applied' discipline rather than the 'straight' discipline means a distorted knowledge base from which to draw principles.

The length of education and training courses gives rise to similar concerns among health visiting lecturers who were associated with previous courses. Prior to PREP the health visitor course was one calendar year in length, which included a minimum of 9 weeks' supervised practice. According to the UKCC standards (1994a), the new courses can be as short as 32 weeks, the unspoken reason for this being that the major acute post-registration courses are a maximum of 32 weeks in length and that there must be seen to be equity between acute and community education. Some recently validated courses have managed to retain supervised practice and the course is of comparable level to the pre-1995 courses, but other courses have been shortened, to the detriment of their content.

It is, however, becoming increasingly evident that the curriculum for health visitor education, if interpreted from a nursing approach, is too limiting for the breadth of work that health visitors wish to take on. Similarly, if a course equips health visitors with skills and opportunities that are subsequently stifled by organisational constraints practitioners feel equally frustrated, as can be seen in the following example.

Josie, a health visitor educated under the new degree programme at a university in the West Midlands, thoroughly enjoyed her course. She revelled in the opportunity that one of her assignments gave her: to go out into the community and find a group with which to work in order to raise the group's awareness of their health needs. She was talking to the head teacher of a local primary school and asked her whether her staff would like to have a discussion about their own health, rather than that of the children. This was duly fixed up for one late afternoon after the children had gone home. When Josie got there, not only did she find a capacity audience of the all-female teaching staff, but also the dinner ladies and the lollipop lady! A very full and wide-ranging discussion followed because it transpired that this group of women covered an age span of 30 years and they all had health needs, from stress to premenstrual syndrome, from asthma to raised blood pressure, from contraception concerns to worries about a husband's health. Six sessions followed and at the end a confident group of women thanked Josie for her tremendous support, knowledge and advice as a result

of their unspoken/unidentified health needs. Josie went on to qualify and practise in a multicultural area of the West Midlands but she became progressively disenchanted with health visiting as practised in her Trust because the health visitors were not encouraged to work outside the organisations for under-5s and their mothers. In the end, after practising as a health visitor for 4 years, Josie resigned her post to take up the post of community health development worker, at a lower salary but using all her skills and education. She remains very fulfilled in her work.

This vignette highlights the frustration felt by many health visitors emerging from progressive courses. In time, if they don't make a move then they make a conscious decision to comply with their organisation structure and lose the impetus to develop new ventures. However, this assumes that all newly qualified health visitors want to move into community development and this clearly is not so: the expertise of many is in working closely with families and the under-5s and their histories show their effectiveness (Chapter 11). The health visitor course needs be broad enough to ensure that all newly qualified health visitors can practise in any sphere – family, group or community – and with any age range.

In the light of clinical governance and primary care groups it is important that health visitor education takes on a far wider public health role and, additionally, that the organisation of health visitors is thoroughly reviewed within the primary care group, primary healthcare team and public health dimensions.

HEALTH VISITING IS HEALTH VISITING, BUT IS IT NURSING?

Chapter 5 discusses and analyses the skills of health visiting compared with the skills of nursing. The argument is that health visiting skills resulting from today's education and deployment systems build on and are constructed from a nursing basic education (Project 2000) and within Primary Healthcare Team organisation, including integrated nursing teams.

Prior to recent changes a far-reaching report, the *Community Nursing Review* (DHSS 1986), more universally known as the Cumberlege Report, was published. This was designed to look at human resource management within the

community and was based on the premise that there was considerable wastage of resources due to overlap between the different nursing and health visiting disciplines working in the community. Several years later a further paper, *New World, New Opportunities* (NHS Executive 1993), made similar statements about the need for teamwork in the primary healthcare team. Hyde (1995) explores the issues of tribalism within practitioners working in the community using such commentators as Goodwin (1983), Littlewood (1987), Butterworth (1988) and Cowley (1994a) to illustrate a lack of coherence within and between the various disciplines working within the community. The point is made by these writers that, despite every effort made to encourage them to work together, community nurses and health visitors continue to work in isolation. However, the last named, Cowley (1994a), recognised a softening of previously hardened attitudes and suggested that there was enhanced collaborative working between the different specialisms.

Health visitors have always been political animals and their education, in focusing on networking and alliance, has ensured that they have been closely involved in processes of decision-making at the optimum level. All has not been easy: criticisms have been levelled at the bulk of the profession for not taking up opportunities; the stability of community healthcare management has been questionable; a major debate has focused on the role of health visitors. In many ways it is easier to examine health visiting as a profession in relation to the political scene at government, Department of Health and local policy levels than it is to examine health visiting in relation to nursing and midwifery. Historically, a similar apparent conflict between the fields of social work and health visiting led to the work of the Jameson Committee (Ministry of Health 1956), which was established to advise the government of the day on the role, recruitment and training of health visitors. Robinson (1982) noted the 'difficulties in separating the respective roles of the health visitor and the social worker experienced by the two Councils for the Education and Training in Social Work and of Health

Visitors, established under the Health Visiting and Social Work (Training) Act 1962'.

Wilkie (1979) discussed the 1962 Act and commented on the change in entry requirements for the training of health visitors to include a State Registered Nursing Certificate and Obstetric Certificate. The 1962 Act was highly significant because it separated health visiting from social work (although in the immediate post-1962 years their training ran in parallel, with some shared content), and moved it into nursing. A changed conflict, with new opponents.

Subsequently, health visiting lost its most important asset – the Council for the Education and Training of Health Visitors (CETHV) – when the 1979 Nurses, Midwives and Health Visitors Act was passed and the responsibility for health visitor education was passed to the National Boards. At that time there was the proviso that no education and training changes could be made without the approval of the Health Visiting Joint Committee (HVJC), thus temporarily safeguarding the curriculum and content of health visitor education. With the passage of time the HVJC was lost to the UKCC's committees, and health visitor management and education became progressively squeezed by nursing into almost a generalist, marginalised and heavily criticised profession with, at the end of 1998, the very real prospect of losing its unique registration status.

Recent government papers and press releases have heavily underlined the need for health visiting, and the active intervention of Tessa Jowell as Minister for Public Health has ensured that registration will remain for health visitors in the light of the tasks outlined for them within the proposed radical alteration of NHS structures.

This section set out to respond to the heading: Health visiting is health visiting, but is it nursing? A brief discussion of the move of health visiting from public health in local authority control to the NHS as it was in the 1970s and 1980s has shown how health visitors, small in numbers in practice, were engulfed by the nursing profession, with a very large membership. The role of education has played an increasingly important part in shaping health visiting as more curative than preventive through an integrated education process wherein health visitors are educated through community healthcare courses. This next section explores the education process through role definitions.

A NEW HEALTH VISITOR EDUCATION

The development of a new education programme for health visitors does not require a dramatic modification of the PREP structure because the articulated outcomes, particularly in care and programme management (page 11), are both full enough and broad enough to sustain any revised course content.

It is in the actual course content itself that there needs to be far greater development of the public health role and this was proposed by Robotham (1998), in an attempt to raise awareness of the need for change. The rapid development of public health as the basis for *The New NHS – Modern, Dependable* (Department of Health 1997a) has further increased the need for a new approach to health visitor education. Direct entry to health visiting has long been advocated as a very positive way forward, provided that the health visitor course is of sufficient length to produce a well-educated practitioner, and it is clear that the emphasis for the way forward in the NHS – proactive healthcare – leaves the way open for alternative educational structures.

The increasing development of undergraduate programmes in public health developed on a social model of health responds to the very clear opportunities for tackling promotion and prevention outlined in *Our Healthier Nation* (Department of Health 1998a). Table 1.1 illustrates the design of the undergraduate degree at the University of Wolverhampton.

The seven subject areas are studied over 3 years full-time and, in addition, placements are arranged to support student learning in the various areas outlined. The placement opportunities are developed on a flexible basis so that part-time students can accommodate them within their work situation and, where it is possible for a student to undertake a sandwich year, then

Table 1.1 An undergraduate degree in public health (Robotham 1998)

Subject area	Types of module	Fieldwork experience
Science	Epidemiology; Immunology; Biology of Disease; Statistics; the Built Environment; Environmental Effects on Human Development; Nutritional Science	Practical experience within the Public Health Department; statistical experience; working in housing departments, traffic and transport departments; work in child development and surveillance; work with handicapping conditions – experience of listening and advising
Health	Health and Disease; Foundations in Health; Work and Health; Healthy Lifestyles; Sociology of Health and Disease; Perspectives in Health; Mental Health, Illness and Society; Transcultural Health; the Psychology of Health, Counselling and Intervention	Experience in work environments; general practice surgery; working in specialised clinics; working in homes for older people and sheltered environments – experience of listening and supporting
Economics	Business and the Economic Environment; the Economics of Public Policy; Economics of Health and Health Care	Experience in finance departments of the NHS or regional departments; experience of management in fundholding general practice – experience of listening and using business knowledge
Human Geography	Population Studies; Conflict and Change in the Countryside; Geographical Information Systems; Human Health and the Environment	Observation of geographical information systems within public health departments – experience of listening to the concerns of various public bodies
Politics	Social Policy and Public Health; Public Health Politics, Policy and Pollution	Experience of community health councils, local government departments, voluntary support agencies, charitable support organisations – experience of listening, supporting, handling of meetings, preparing reports, making representations
Law	Legal Promotion of Health and Safety at Work; Law of Environmental Pollution Control	Experience of environmental health departments, working with health and safety officers in a variety of settings – experience of listening and observing
Public Health	The Development and Scope of Public Health; Health Care Evaluation and Needs; Public Health and a Violent Society; Health Promotion: Foundations for Practice; Public Health Commissioning and Contracting; Perspectives in Public Health	Working in the community with identified groups – perinatal families, family groups, specific individuals, social work departments, police, Regional Health Authority commissioning, GP fundholder commissioning; the promotion and protection of child health – experience of listening, supporting, promoting health, educating, surveillance

longer periods of experience in public health departments and international organisations are advantageous. These provide not only work experience but also the necessary practical applications to underpin the theoretical concepts explored in the course. Students emerging at the end of this type of degree programme are very well equipped to work in public health departments, anywhere in the NHS that doesn't (for the moment) require a professional qualification, in voluntary and charitable organisations that fill the many supporting gaps the NHS does not cover, and in community development, housing departments and health promotion departments.

Criticism of this approach to education for a direct-entry candidate has focused on the current health visitor practitioner who has highly developed skills in support and intervention, e.g. with postnatally depressed women. It is felt that a practitioner from a public health degree would be unsuited to working closely on a one-to-one basis with clients who have, for example, mental health problems. This argument should be challenged on the basis that much of Project 2000 education takes a broader, more academic approach and no one questions the potential for supportive practice from Project 2000 diplomates once qualified. The fact that this academic undergraduate public health degree incorporates placements in a variety of areas within the whole spectrum of what constitutes a social model of public health makes it closer to the professional education course of PREP, and thus the graduates are in a better position to align their practice to professionals.

The undergraduate public health degree shown above would have the advantage of fulfilling the learning outcomes for specialist practice in health visiting and intending health visitors drawn from the ranks of nursing could enter halfway through the programme. As practitioners emerging from a Project 2000 course have the minimum of education in connection with child health and development it would be necessary to include a module or two specifically on this subject. Apart from that, there is little further requirement to differentiate the programme designed for professional background entrants from that for direct-entry students.

A DIVISION OF LABOUR IN SPECIALIST HEALTH VISITING

Health visitors currently in practice during this momentous change in primary care and public health are enthused by the prospect of greater opportunities which are opening up to them. The vision of a cradle-to-grave worker is coming ever closer but at the same time the cold reality is that there are not nearly enough health visitors to take up this work. Mention is made in Chapter 11 of the value of health visiting teams in domiciliary (specialist) health visiting, including a nursery nurse and a clerk. There is an equally compelling case for health visiting teams in the whole public health field.

If the concept of a universal service is to be truly taken up (see Chapter 5), then that service is most easily organised around three main thrusts, as in Figure 1.1.

Figure 1.1 can loosely be described as the universal range of health visiting in relation to its breadth, width and depth within the population in general. The skills within this are articulated in context throughout the chapters in this book but an outline of these is given in Box 1.1.

Clearly, the health visiting service is far more effective if a team approach allows development

---

> **Box 1.1** Universal health visiting skills
>
> - Health promotion
> - Health support, advice, guidance
> - Empowerment, partnership, enablement
> - Counselling, listening, hearing
> - Screening and surveillance
> - Community development
> - Networking, health alliances
> - Assessment, political strategies, policy influences

---

of practitioners from the traditional health visiting (specialist) qualification, public health workers with a public health degree (associate health visitors), staff nurse grade workers, other professionals (e.g. nursery nurses, as in Chapter 11), community link workers, interpreters, and social and healthcare assistants.

There may be many combinations of the above, but it is suggested that a universal team will consist of:

- For child and family health
  - Health visitor(s)
  - Nursery nurse(s)
  - Social and care assistants
  - Clerical support workers
  - Possibly interpreters
- For the population outside the family
  - Health visitor(s)
  - Staff nurse grades
  - Social and care assistants
  - Public health workers
  - Link workers or interpreters
  - Clerical support workers
- For the community
  - Community development health visitor(s)
  - Public health workers
  - Link workers or interpreters.

These teams should be linked to primary care groups (PCGs) and, depending on population size, there may be one or more such teams to a PCG. They are also part of the primary care health team (PCHT), and the most effective organisation would be for health visitors to liaise and work within the PCHT, each heading up their respective target groups, who function concomitantly with the integrated PCHT (Fig. 1.2).

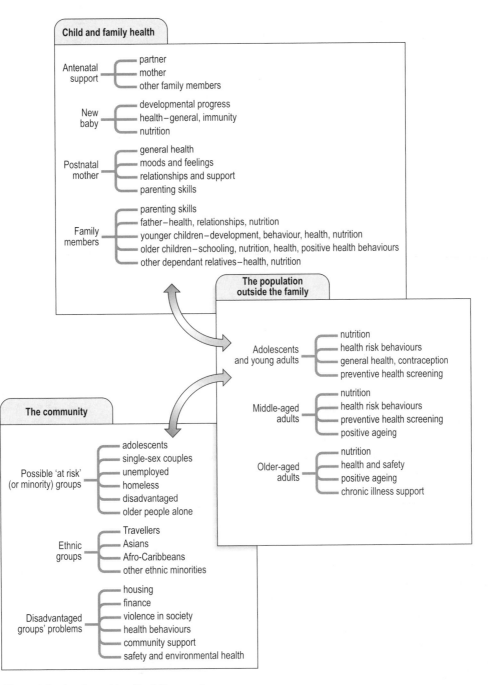

Figure 1.1   A universal health visiting service

A HIGHER LEVEL OF PRACTICE

The sections above have discussed the education and development of specialist health visiting, including an alternative organisational structure to enable health visiting to provide a universal service. In the introduction, mention was made of advanced health visiting and the development

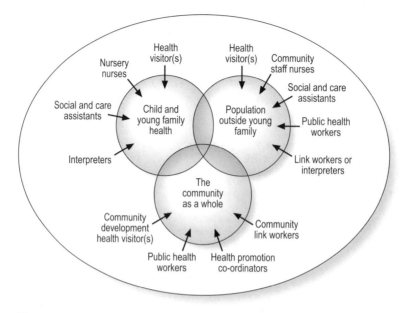

Figure 1.2   A primary care group health visiting team

of practitioners who might fulfil such a role forms an interesting analysis. It is pertinent at this stage to consider one or two other titles that have developed within community practice.

Nurse practitioner. This title has developed to respond mainly to the practice nurse area within primary care and specifically within general practice. There is no statutory or recordable title of nurse practitioner but there are now a number of educational courses designed for practitioners who wish to develop their roles. The average nurse practitioner course includes (at diploma or degree level) extra modules on subjects such as applied anatomy and physiology, pharmacology, health and clinical assessment techniques, conceptual frameworks for practice and reflective practice. This enables practitioners with this qualification to run their own clinics within general practice, to act as triage nurse in accident and emergency nursing and in general to work along a clinical medical model. Practitioners who also hold a health visiting qualification find that this type of post enables them to combine clinical skills with the promotion and prevention approach of health visiting.

Advanced practitioner. This title has fulfilled the growing need for some practitioners, parti-

cularly in health visiting, for recognition of the satisfactory completion of further education at master's level in clinical practice. In reality, the course content is little different from any similar course for nurse practitioners, albeit at a higher academic level. Clearly, both courses require a pharmacological baseline for nurse prescribing and health assessment (diagnostic) skills, as well as the ability to promote health and give nutritional advice. In addition, certain advanced practitioners have gained qualifications in complementary therapy areas – aromatherapy, reflexology, herbalism and other forms of alternative healing. This is discussed in Chapter 14. Pat Alexander practises in a GP surgery using health visiting and complementary therapy skills in an extremely effective and enlightened way.

The term 'practitioner' is common to both these titles above and the clinical skills acquired by reason of their education suggest that both types of practitioner practise along medical or alternative therapy lines. Discussions with both 'nurse' and 'advanced' practitioners reveal a professional who is practising in a fulfilled way using 'hands-on' clinical skills and judgement.

The main difference between advanced practice and an advanced practitioner is likely to hinge on the meaning of the terms 'practitioner' and 'practice', and comments and discussions in the health visiting and nursing press seem to confirm this. This has been confirmed by UKCC (1999): 'there needed to be a shift in thinking away from specialist roles, as represented by the community branches outlined in PREP, towards recognition of a level of practice, regardless of the environment or speciality in which the practitioner works' (CC/98/19 paragraph 9), and further: 'the term higher level practice (that is, significantly higher than initial registration) was adopted to denote the level of practice which the UKCC is seeking to clarify, as the term had no previous association with a particular role, organisation or group (UKCC, 1999).'

In a draft document, the UKCC (1999) have articulated a descriptor and standard for higher level practice that have been designed to: 'describe the practice characteristics of nurses, midwives and health visitors who are practising at a significantly higher level (the focus is on level of practice, not area of practice) and identify specific outcomes in the form of a professional standard that must be achieved for this attainment to be recognised by the UKCC and marked on the professional register'.

Descriptor of higher level practice

Health visitors working at a higher level of practice have developed their original skills and act as leaders of change with the public and individual clients, working directly with each group. Working from professional maturity and experience in the social, economic and political context calls for complex reasoning, critical thinking, reflection and analysis to inform health assessments, clinical judgements and decisions. Clients and fellow professionals will recognise their breadth of knowledge and expertise and their advanced communication skills and there will be wide networking abilities. Health visitors working at a higher level of practice have a track record of practice development and take a lead in implementing health and social care policy. They work across boundaries with a flexible innovative service, communicating extensively and effectively with clients, carers, the public in general, managers, other professionals and their own peer group to motivate and help develop practice and bring about change (UKCC 1999).

Standard of higher level practice

The standard for higher level practice suggests that there should be seven practice headings, which contain, in all, 45 criteria for higher level practice. The areas of practice identified are:

- Providing effective health care
- Improving quality and health outcomes
- Evaluation and research
- Leading and developing practice
- Innovation and changing practice
- Developing self and others
- Working across professional and organisational boundaries.

For recognition as practising at a higher level a health visitor would need to fulfil all the criteria under each of the seven practice headings, and it is made clear that, although an individual may meet some of the criteria, it is the integration of them all that signifies practice at a higher level.

Providing effective health care

Rita, aged 45 years, has left her husband and is homeless, and has come to lodge with her brother Fred. The council will not rehouse Rita because of a history of unpaid debts and antisocial behaviour. She has a daughter, Dawn, who is 15 years old, and two sons, 4-year-old Dominic and 18-month-old Damien. Dawn has started at the local school but does not like it. She does not attend and instead goes out with her 16-year-old unemployed friend, who gets drunk and takes drugs. Dawn has an 18-year-old boyfriend. She uses no contraception but Rita is sure she is sexually active and wants her to go on the 'pill'. Dawn also told Rita that she has a vaginal discharge and an itch but there is no way she is going to see the doctor. Dominic keeps scratching his head and Rita fears he may have nits, as he has had them in the past. He also has a skin rash, which is itchy. Rita says that she is very depressed because she is unemployed and Fred is hopeless and keeps getting drunk and they are all very overcrowded. She has come to the surgery to see the health visitor.

Marie, the health visitor, has completed a nurse practitioner course, has been health visiting for 5 years and is also family planning trained. She runs her own clinic in the surgery and patients/clients are given the choice of whether they wish to see Marie or the GP when they make an appointment.

As a higher level practitioner, Marie will use her skills to listen to Rita and hear all her problems. She clearly understands Rita's feelings of hopelessness and spends time initially hearing about her financial problems. It is likely that Rita is getting insufficient income supplement and Marie helps Rita to make an appointment to seek advice from an officer in the social security office. She also telephones the housing office on Rita's behalf to arrange an appointment for Rita to go to see the special needs officer and discuss methods of paying off her unpaid debts. At the time of this visit Marie arranges for a subsequent visit to undertake a health screening for Rita.

Marie encourages Rita to arrange for Dawn to come to the health visitor clinic, where Marie will take a vaginal swab and discuss contraception. She gets Rita's permission to discuss Dawn with the GP and explains the need for her clinic discussions with Dawn to remain confidential to herself and Dawn, although she will encourage Dawn to accept the GP's advice once the swab test results are known. Marie asks Rita whether she would be willing for the school nurse to work with Dawn at school. Marie arranges another appointment for the following day, so that Rita can bring Dominic and she can examine him for nits and see what treatment she can prescribe for his rash.

After the initial interview Marie sees Rita regularly, either at the surgery or at home. The school nurse has spoken to Dawn and found out that she dislikes school because she is ridiculed for her poor reading skills – the school has arranged supporting sessions to help develop her reading. Dawn has accepted the help of a particular teacher whom she thinks is wonderful because she listens to her. Gradually, the family's problems begin to resolve.

The health visitor in this vignette is able to work with this family to help them to resolve their problems and this has been expedited by the following facts.

- Marie's surgery appointments are for half an hour if necessary.
- She is able to take swabs for differential diagnosis and, in the case of Dominic, to prescribe therapeutic cream for his rash and teach Rita how to fine-comb his hair. The GP is happy for Marie to carry out all the consultation and examination for Dawn, and will prescribe oral contraception, with Rita's permission and with Marie keeping a regular check.
- Marie has good links with the housing department and the special needs officer is sympathetic to the situation.
- Marie's knowledge of the benefit system means that, when she advises Rita to go to the benefits office, she knows she is likely to get a positive response.
- Marie's good links with the school nursing

service mean that the school nurse is alerted to the situation and can liaise with the school pastoral service to help Dawn. The school nurse also spends some time talking with Dawn about handling her friend's alcohol behaviour and her own attitude towards alcohol.

- When the initial oral contraceptive does not suit Dawn, Marie discusses this with the GP, who changes the prescription, and Dawn is able to change her pills safely.

This is specialist health visiting practice, and also higher level practice because Marie receives direct referrals in the surgery and undertakes differential diagnosis using therapeutic communication and client-centred assessments that manage risk and are appropriate to the needs and culture of the individuals concerned. The health visitor manages their care and, in partnership with the clients and the GP, makes specific interventions informed by accepted best practice appropriate to their needs. Some aspects of the scenario are effectively delegated to other professionals. With appropriate advice, counselling and health promotion, the situation improves to the satisfaction of all concerned.

Improving quality and health outcomes

Jennifer, a health visitor, works closely with her practice nurse colleague, Lynette, in the Sneed & Partners practice. The practice meeting, which all GPs, health visitor, practice nurse and district nurses attend, is looking at the quality of healthcare interventions. Jennifer and Lynette have been discussing for some time the group of potentially at-risk menopausal women who currently attend the surgery and who are seeking support and information concerning HRT. The practice meeting encourages Jennifer to undertake an audit of all the women receiving HRT. Jennifer designs a questionnaire to circulate to all women registered with the practice who are over the age of 45. The practice team agrees that they should ascertain knowledge of and attitudes towards HRT in this target group and also what the women feel about their HRT treatment. The questionnaire has a high response rate, and indicates that the group contains several important categories of women:

- those who have tried HRT and are not happy with it
- those who have not yet reached the menopause but who wish to know more about HRT
- those who are in the menopause and are undecided about the use of HRT

- a small group of women who have had an artificial menopause treated with HRT.

After consideration with Lynette and the GPs, Jennifer sets up informal discussion groups with the women to respond to their wish for education. Jennifer and Lynette spend time in consultation with the groups and respond to their needs with advice, counselling and healthcare support. The GPs and Jennifer decide to explore the needs of those women who were unhappy with HRT and establish two or three different therapeutic regimens, which Jennifer carefully monitors with an audit tool. Gradually, the practice establishes an audit cycle – defining best practice, implementing it, measuring and taking action where necessary. Jennifer, Lynette and the GPs are pleased with the results of this initiative and Jennifer is thanked by her colleagues for leading them through the process.

The higher level practice demonstrated by the vignette shows the need for clinical leadership towards clinical effectiveness, and in the majority of situations it requires a team approach. The health visitor understood the audit process and her knowledge, in conjunction with the practice nurse, of the health needs of a target group within the practice population established a cycle of audit, risk management and clinical effectiveness. Challenging the original therapeutic regimens of the practice in relation to HRT was not without its difficulties, but good methodology in collecting information and establishing the situation soon convinced all the professionals concerned that this was an effective way forward.

Evaluation and research

Jane is part of the nursing forum that has been set up to support the nurse members of the local primary care group (PCG). Jane has an interest in research and is constantly encouraging her colleagues to collect data in relation to the healthcare needs of their client groups. Jane is particularly interested in hospital discharge care for older people and asks her colleagues to collect evidence of situations that they meet in their regular practice. Collection of this information over 6 months establishes several concerns, particularly about delays in the discharge information reaching appropriate professionals, but also about the number of times elderly clients complain that they have been visited by a series of professionals who do not seem to do anything and about whose function they know nothing. There also seems to be some doubt as to whether the link with the local social services for the elderly adviser is very clearly established. Jane hears of a good system that works in another part of the country and sets out to discover more about it. Her management realises the value of this work and arranges for her to visit the area concerned. Jane listens closely to all the information

she can obtain and makes copious notes to bring back to her colleagues. There is a wide-ranging discussion in the nursing forum and Jane's colleagues are impressed by what they have heard. A small pilot scheme is set up with one of the geriatric rehabilitation units that serves Jane's PCG area and the local social services adviser is invited to join in the scheme. At the end of 6 months the scheme is evaluated and patients and staff are pleased with the results. The nurse forum, through Jane, asks the nurse representatives on the PCG to discuss the results with the Board. This generates interest from the PCG, which establishes a larger pilot scheme to confirm the original results.

Higher level practice should continually evaluate and audit practice in relation to both self and others and Jane's ability to take the wider perspective was the trigger factor here. Using the nurse forum as a basis to sound out her ideas and recognising the need for improvement in this area meant that Jane could network outside her own immediate work group with the other organisations involved in elderly discharge planning and implementation. Always being alert to the need for research in areas where there is little evidence about practice and changes in health care delivery is a requirement for higher level practice.

Leading and developing practice

John is a health visitor who is also a team leader for the Westerby practice. This practice has bought in a community development that includes a self-managed primary healthcare team, including district nurses, health visitors, community staff nurses, care assistants and a nursery nurse. The GP practice nurse works closely with John and the team and they consider her to be a member although she is employed by the GPs. John acts as a leader rather than a manager and supports all the team members in their work and self-development. He holds a small budget and ensures that his colleagues can attend conferences or courses, provided they can justify how such attendance will enhance their practice. The budget also allows the employment of bank staff to underpin the study leave. John has worked closely with his colleagues, helping them to develop reflective practice skills, and they have regular sessions to maintain these skills. John is qualified in HIV and AIDS care and has a diploma in asthma care and in diabetic care. John acts as a resource to his colleagues and regularly holds small teaching sessions when they want new information that he can supply. He has actively encouraged his colleagues to produce information material for patients with varying chronic diseases and the team all take part in the approval process. Clinical supervision sessions, originally carried out on a one-to-one basis, have now changed to group sessions and John encourages a rotating clinical supervisor role among the more senior team members. A recent evaluation by the community trust has shown a positive response to this change by all the team members.

This is a clear leadership and development role undertaken by the health visitor. It embraces other disciplines and is facilitative rather than managerial, supportive rather than directive, and encouraging a positive ambience in which his colleagues can develop. Teaching and advice to colleagues in other disciplines and developing a climate conducive to learning and evidence-based practice is clearly working at a higher level, but John also thinks constantly about best practice to meet the needs of patients and clients. A patient/client consultative forum, set up by John, gives this group the opportunity to communicate the needs and aspirations of patients and their carers and the continual two-way communication between clients and professionals covering all manner of information helps to break down barriers and create effective partnerships in the practice.

Innovation and changing practice

Mary works as a health visitor for a community trust that believes in the 'grass roots' approach to introducing new practices. Mary has long wanted to introduce the use of the Edinburgh Postnatal Depression Scale (EPDS) on a regular basis to the health visiting team working in the trust. She discusses this with the development manager, who is very supportive of her ideas and suggests a pilot study. Mary and the two colleagues working in her clinic decide on a strategy.

- All three undertake a literature search about EPDS.
- Discussions are set up with the local midwives to tell them about the intended project and to seek their support and collaboration.
- They write a short paper on how they wish to set up the project and approach the GPs serving the area to seek their support. Two practices are very supportive; one only gives permission to use patients provided it does not interfere with the status quo.
- The manager, who is very supportive, finds some money to fund an evaluation study of the project, to be undertaken by the local University.
- Mary goes to see health visitors in another part of the country who have set up a project similar to the one she and her colleagues are planning.
- Mary and her colleagues contact Professor John Cox (Cox & Holden 1994) to seek any advice that he can give.
- A time scale is set up, materials are purchased and the project gets under way.

At the end of a year evaluation is undertaken and there are clear advantages to using the scale as a routine health visiting tool with postnatal women. Mary and her colleagues find that their practice with perinatal women has changed and that their clients have benefited greatly from the use of the tool. Mary and her colleagues are encouraged by their manager to disseminate their results to the rest of the health visitors in the trust. (See Chapter 11 for further information about EPDS.)

In wishing to change their practice as the result of research evidence, and in targeting a particular group with health needs, Mary and her colleagues are working towards higher level practice. They have used appropriate strategies to set up a project and have been proactive in managing the change required to alter practice. Not only is strategic planning required and much negotiating and networking, but also there are the 'invisible' changes that have to be planned for. These include aspects such as the changes that will have to be made to their weekly work data input to include a different approach to work, and ensuring that it is correctly coded for the information collection system.

Developing self and others

Jean works as a community staff nurse for the elderly, liaising with other professionals and assistants who care for and support older people in their homes. Jean was originally an enrolled nurse and converted to RGN 5 years ago. She enjoyed the conversion course and learned about reflection, which she uses in her practice. Jean selects a health visitor as her clinical supervisor and the sessions prove very fruitful to both herself and her supervisor. She gains so much from this that she undertakes the clinical supervisor's course run by her trust and then in her turn she acts as a supervisor to two colleagues caring for older people, both of whom are care assistants employed by the trust. Jean feels frustrated because she recognises that she needs further skills and education to work more effectively with her patients and clients. She applies for sponsorship for health visitor education and, at interview and subsequently, makes it quite clear that she wishes to continue to focus on older clients. Her enthusiasm and determination are recognised and she undertakes and successfully completes the health visitor course, eventually returning to work in her original post. Her confidence is high and she brings to her practice a wider dimension from her recent education. She undertakes some small-scale research with her client group and this is published in a peer-reviewed journal. Jean continues to clinically supervise care assistants and develops within them an enthusiasm for knowledge and self-development. They in turn take up opportunities for short education and development courses. In time, Jean and her colleagues, both in health and social care, set up a large support unit for carers and older people focused on the local community hospital. Jean reflects on her own development and that of her colleagues and recognises how much they have all progressed through sheer hard work, determination and desire for self-fulfilment.

This may sound almost trite in its positive outcome but it is based on a real situation. The health visitor in the vignette is not a high-flier and her practice is rooted in basic no-nonsense care, support and commitment. What characterises this scenario is determination. Jean did not have to undertake the health visitor course, indeed she was lucky that she got sponsorship because she might have been too focused in her approach to healthcare and illness prevention. The higher level aspects of this vignette are that Jean was self-aware and she was able to develop and use strategies to influence practice. The vignette says nothing about the high regard that patients and their carers have for Jean or how she fits into the wider health visiting team. Nevertheless, there is a great deal of higher level practice in this profile.

Working across professional and organisational boundaries

Sarah, a health visitor, works in a district chosen for a Sure Start trailblazer programme and has been chosen by her Trust to represent it at the local Sure Start planning meeting. The meeting identifies a housing estate that suffers from serious problems with services for children and young families. There is a well established voluntary organisation already running a good project in the area, with some informal drop-in parent groups. Sarah links with the voluntary organisation, the local authority, the residents' association and other service providers and together they set up a partnership to widen the scope of activities to include healthcare, family support and outreach and childminder networks. Sarah liaises and networks to gain information and evidence of interest from many groups, and actively encourages members of the partnership to adopt the same networking framework. They work with the advisers, provided free, to prepare an application and Sarah is identified as the person who will be trained to help as an adviser for another area who want to put an application in for the next wave. Sarah's group's application is successful and they begin actively developing their plan to transform existing services for the Sure Star programme.
Publicity is given to all parents and parents-to-be in the catchment area and introductory meetings are set up for parents to get access to services. Sarah is part of the organising group that sets up home visiting sessions for parents who wish to have this facility. She undertakes some visiting herself and draws from a group of nursery nurses,

linkworkers and some parents (who have had induction programmes in supporting) to undertake regular home visiting. Along with other planning group members Sarah sets up parent support groups, creche facilities, a housing advice centre and a special teenage support group.
The voluntary sector-run family centre offers open-access drop-in services and a play group, as well as a small kitchen and parents' room. With the extra funding received from Sure Start, Sarah is part of the group that plans and develops extra facilities within the extension that has been built, in which there are now meeting rooms, a playgroup and an outdoor play site. Nursery workers for the creche and day care are employed and further group activities for parents and children are developed.
As time goes on, midwives run regular preconceptual and antenatal clinics in the centre, the health visitors and the GP run regular drop-in health clinics such as well men's and well women's clinics, which are also attended by dietitians and health promotion staff. Cookery classes are set up and social services begin to develop a centre where children who are separated from one or other parent can meet and enjoy a social time together.

(This vignette is based on the examples from Sure Start – A Guide for Trailblazers (Department for Education and Employment 1999).)

Considerable debate has taken place both formally and informally on what should constitute higher level practice and it is clear that a master's degree does not guarantee higher level practice, neither does the holding of specific posts in areas such as education, management or research. Speciality-based knowledge and skill requirements for competence in particular areas of work will be articulated eventually by the UKCC but it is also likely certain administrative conditions will have to be met.

- Those practising at a higher level will have to periodically notify UKCC of their wish to continue to practise at this level.
- Those practising at a higher level may be able to add the suffix (H) following their initial registration.
- The assessment system for those practitioners wishing to be accredited as higher level practitioners should be founded on the attainment of clinical competence supported by postregistration.
- In order to enter the assessment process, practitioners must:
  - have a current first-level registration with the UKCC
  - spend the majority of their practice

planning and organising, carrying out work related to improving health and well-being
- hold a UK degree or equivalent in nursing, midwifery or health visiting or a health-related subject or hold a degree or equivalent in any other subject together with the successful completion of a postregistration education programme in their area of practice
- have practised for at least the equivalent of 3 years full-time in their chosen area of practice in order to collect the required evidence.
- Those wishing to be assessed for higher level practice may be asked to contribute towards the cost.

The assessment of practice for a higher level recognition is likely to include:

- presenting evidence of practice and knowledge against criteria specified for higher level practice, possibly in a portfolio
- the production of a written reflective account in a supervised setting
- final assessment at a panel interview.

Possible criteria against which higher practice may be judged

Chapter 9 discusses the process of audit based on the nursing process and it is possible to use the same process to prepare criteria against which to judge higher level practice, including the range and coverage of evidence and possible sources. Thus, for every aspect of practice that could be considered for higher level scrutiny there would be an assessment, planning, implementing and evaluating (APIE) approach, which may include:

Assessment
- Relationships and networks
- Purpose of the assessment
- Appropriate sources of knowledge and information
- The process of critically appraising and interpreting available information
- The selection of assessment methods to improve health and well-being

- Make assessments of risk that are valid and reliable
- Enable people involved in assessment to exercise, understand and manage the process
- Collate and structure the information obtained for later practice
- Synthesise the analysed information to develop and document a valid and reliable comprehensive assessment
- Negotiate and agree with relevant people the outcomes of assessment.

Planning
- Decide how to develop and sustain appropriate relationships and networks which have value for improving the health and well-being of individuals, families, groups and communities
- Develop appropriate strategies to influence others' practice and develop their potential
- Work out how to present information appropriately and clearly
- Enable relevant people to understand, manage and exercise judgement during the planning exercise
- Negotiate and agree with relevant people specific roles and competencies
- Improve the planning process by synthesising outcomes
- Develop plans consistent with theoretical frameworks
- Meeting needs and wishes.

Implementing
- Sustain appropriate relationships and networks to lead to improvement
- Contribute to the development of organisational climates conducive to learning and evidence-based practice
- Use appropriate strategies and opportunities to influence others' practice
- Offer information and advice – relevant, up-to-date, timely, consistent, user-friendly
- Monitor people's responses to information and advice and make appropriate modifications
- Make specific technical interventions to improve situations and that are appropriate
- Enable people who are involved in or affected by implementation

- Synthesise and apply outcomes of past evaluations and audits into practice to make improvements
- Actively monitor implementation and integrate it to achieve the interests of users and improve health and well-being, meet identified needs, reallocate resources available, meet priorities of service and manage risk.

Evaluating

- Select evaluation approaches and use evaluation methods that are consistent with the purpose and focus of evaluation, appropriate to assessed needs, consistent with theoretical frameworks, capable of reflecting the breadth and depth of perspectives
- Enable relevant people to contribute effectively to evaluations
- Alert appropriate people and organisations to questions and gaps in knowledge requiring resolution through research.

These are examples of the types of criterion that are likely to be piloted during the development of the process of setting standards for higher level practice. The opportunity to develop a mentoring process to support individuals working towards higher level practice will be an essential part of the exercise, as will the need to ensure that it is the development of practice that is the essential and not the development of the individual alone.

The following vignette is an extension of the previous one.

Sarah has been involved with this project from the outset and has decided that she wishes to collect evidence to apply for acknowledgement of higher level practice. She has a first degree from her Community Health Specialist Practice (Health Visiting) programme and undertook an MPhil 4 years ago, which she completed last year. She has been with the project for over 3 years and has amassed the following evidence:

- all reports and minutes of planning meetings for Sure Start application, showing her involvement
- extracts from her reflective practice journal
- records and care pathways for families involved in the programme
- records of all the negotiations in the development and organisation of the extension and its increased activities
- correspondence
- working notes and drafts for ideas and plans for activity developments
- clinical guidelines in relation to healthcare facilities

- audit records
- research papers she has written on some small-scale evaluative action research
- video recordings of new activities as they opened
- training materials she prepared for induction programmes for home visitors
- written and audiotaped comments from participants in the various programme activities.

Sarah also prepares papers and reports to respond to the criteria discussed above. With the advice and guidance of her mentor she selects those areas that demonstrate more clearly the development of the project and its successful practice rather than simply showing how she has developed. She applies to have the evidence scrutinised and a date is sent to her for attendance for a viva at the higher level practice assessment centre. In due course, Sarah hears that her application for higher level practice status has been granted and she is formally recommended to apply the suffix (H) to her RGN qualification.

This vignette is hypothetical at this stage of the development of higher level practice criteria and procedures. However, it is likely that the procedure will be along somewhat similar lines and it is hoped that the intensity, breadth and depth of the process are evident. It is likely that health visitors will be in a position to apply for higher level practice because of the skills that their professional practice allows them to develop. Clearly, good practice is not higher level practice and there will be many very good practitioners who will not be in a position to apply for higher level practice, nor will they wish to do so, because the process is rightly extensive and prolonged.

As health visitors grow and develop within the wider opportunities that have been created through health improvement programmes, healthy living centres and Sure Start, there will be a number of ventures with which they will wish to be involved and become confident. The following three aspects are totally dissimilar and at the same time can be closely related:

- becoming a Primary Care Group Board member
- working on committees and learning how committees work
- project development and management.

These aspects are discussed in some detail, although the reader is advised to seek information from several sources to gain alternative perspectives.

HIGHER LEVEL HEALTH VISITING PRACTICE – PRIMARY CARE GROUP BOARD MEMBER

The New NHS – Modern, Dependable (Department of Health 1997a) heralded one of the most dramatic changes in the NHS since its inception, with the introduction of PCGs. The PCG Resource Unit, part of the Public Health Resource Unit in Oxford and dedicated to supporting the development of PCGs, set out to develop a consultation exercise for deciding the education and training needs of PCGs.

A two-part Delphi survey was undertaken in April and May 1998, followed by a conference in June 1998 in order to provide information about education and training priorities that need to be addressed by PCGs. Round 1 of the survey concentrated on identifying the main skills and areas of knowledge felt necessary for each PCG and round 2 identified three categories of PCG participant and looked at the skills and knowledge felt necessary for each.

Three categories of PCG participant were identified:

• Board Member (or Director), who oversees the PCG but may not have responsibility for day-to-day running
• Doer, who will run the PCG day to day – this includes the executive/management and those involved in working groups, or those co-opted to perform tasks for the PCG
• Stakeholders – all those within the PCG who contribute to patient care or are patients themselves (e.g. GPs, nurses, local authorities) not included as Directors or Doers.

It is necessary here to include information that will be reiterated in Chapter 2, concerning levels of operation of PCGs. These are:

• *Level 1*, an advisory body to the Health Authority with no budget
• *Level 2*, as level 1 but with a nominal budget
• *Level 3*, holding a budget for almost all health care services except some specialist services
• *Level 4*, as for level 3 but becoming a trust responsible for community and primary care delivery.

Table 1.2   Skills required by primary care group members

Skill	PCG level
Communication	All levels
Critical appraisal	All levels
Strategic planning	All levels
Financial planning	Levels 2, 3, 4
Information analysis	All levels
Team working	Level 1

The Delphi exercise showed that the top five skills required for each PCG level were as listed in Table 1.2.

At a NHS Executive workshop (NHS Executive 1998a) on nurse involvement in primary care groups there was debate about the skills and attributes that nurses have to bring to PCGs. In particular it was felt that nurses:

• had a whole-system approach
• were good at working in partnership and collaboration
• understood quality and quality systems.

The key areas that were considered a priority for development were to do with strategy and management and included: strategic thinking skills; new styles for managing complex change; understanding clinical governance; understanding general management services structures and processes; process of commissioning and decision-making skills; personal development; recognising transferability and value of current skills, confidence building and assertiveness skills. Although the conference was concerned with nurse involvement there was a strong feeling that such competencies were equally relevant to all members of the PCGs, not just nurse members. In particular, it was felt that nurses had a particular contribution to make to the education and training and workforce planning agendas of PCGs, and that these could be areas that they were mandated to lead.

Concerns were raised at the conference regarding the future roles of nurses working in health authorities, who will have a much reduced role from hitherto. Again, the need to promote the principle of multiprofessional structures, processes and learning opportunities concerned participants in the conference. It was felt particularly that there was a need for resources to support the organisational development of PCGs and the personal and professional development of those working in them – this may well be enhanced by a good relationship between the education and training consortia and PCGs. Other concerns raised related to: the fact that PCGs start with a financial deficit; how nurses will be released from clinical work to participate in PCGs; how to secure inclusion of nurses and other healthcare workers in the development of PCGs.

A large health authority in the West Midlands secured funding from the local education and training consortia to underpin an education programme for the newly elected nurse members of several PCGs. A 2-day conference was held to pool knowledge about PCGs, for the newly elected members to meet each other, and to begin to develop ideas for the way forward. A local university was contracted to support the venture and to deliver appropriate education. The competencies that the PCG members felt they would need included:

- Good communication skills
- Team working
- Budgeting/financial skill
- Strategic planning/thinking
- Negotiating
- Willingness to learn/ability to say you do not understand
- Flexibility
- Managing information
- Corporate governance
- Networking
- Respect for other opinions and disciplines
- Assertiveness
- Good time management/diplomacy
- Photographic memory/good recall
- IT skills
- Leadership skills
- Management of change
- Ability to get on with others
- Commissioning.

Further questioning elicited from the members that they would particularly like education support in these areas identified. It was decided by the university that a monthly study day would commence over a period of a year and that during that time three modules covering those areas would be studied at level 3 to enable some of the members to complete a first degree. Roughly half the group were health visitors and the remainder spanned district nursing, practice nursing, mental health nursing, midwifery and learning disabilities nursing.

The training programme began and attendance was good. Members were positive, enthusiastic and highly motivated. Early facilitation focused on electronic information sources to ensure that health service information could be rapidly accessed. Initially, members were unsure of what was required of them and daunted by the apparently massive task ahead. Handling committee work was also covered at an early session and it soon became clear that they were settling down and beginning to find their feet in the PCG process. The university facilitators noticed rapid development of confidence in the group and recognised early on that they needed plenty of time to chat to each other to acquire knowledge of how colleagues on PCGs throughout the city were faring. There was considerable sharing of information and experiences and it was clear that some PCGs were functioning better than others, mainly through better relationships between more forward looking GPs and the nurse member. Alliances were quickly being built between the non-GP PCG board members and there was a healthy sharing of support for the lay members.

At this stage of the development of PCGs the learning curves of all those involved are very steep and there are still a huge number of untapped areas to cover. Health visitors who become involved with PCGs will find as time goes on that their background and experience stand them in good stead in some of the work covered, particularly in communicating, networking, health needs assessment and many management functions. One of the healthiest aspects of the situation outlined above is the very close collaboration that is developing between individual members of the PCG boards. There is an immediate recognition that the tribalism of professional disciplines is no longer necessary in the broader approach to the massive problem of effective healthcare provision.

HIGHER LEVEL HEALTH VISITING PRACTICE – WORKING ON COMMITTEES AND HOW COMMITTEES WORK

It is very likely that health visitors practising at a higher level will be involved in committee work. Indeed, specialist practitioners are already in this position, although they are less likely to be chairing committees. It is important that it is recognised that committee work is an effective method of communication and networking and that to be an effective committee member/chair is a means of positive promotion of health care, whatever the function of the committee.

Committee functions

The functions of a committee are set out in the constitution or in a resolution passed by a meeting or higher level committee. For PCG boards the constitution is likely to be set out on the basis of the Health Authority constitution, and subcommittees set up by the PCG board are likely to adopt the constitution principles of the PCG board, but this needs to be checked with the PCG board chair.

Subcommittees can be:

- *advisory*: a group of people who are specialists in particular areas and simply act in an advisory capacity – the main committee may take their recommendations on board or reject them
- *standing committees*, which are often set up for a specific purpose, e.g. finance committee, education committee
- *ad hoc committees*, which prepare a report on a specific aspect/topic and are then disbanded.

Procedure

The rules of the committee are contained in the constitution of the health authority and its standing orders. These include guidance on items such as:

- Admission of the public and the press – when they may be excluded, how much the public or the press may record
- Calling meetings – regulations concerning when the chair can call a meeting or whether members can do so
- Notice of meetings – the regulations are likely to be that the agenda and documentation must be delivered or be sent by post at least three clear days before the meeting
- Setting the agenda – certain items may be decided to appear on every agenda. If a member wishes to put an item on the agenda there is a minimum time limit within which to put the request to the chair
- Chairing the meeting – guidelines on who chairs in the absence of the designated chair or vice-chair
- Notices of motion – motions and amendments:
  - *Motions*. In rigorous, formal procedures for meetings no business can be done unless a

motion has been proposed and seconded. In less formal committees the chair allows discussion of the topic before the wording of a motion summarising the proposals is worked out. Only then does the committee switch to the formal procedure for motions and amendments.
  - *An amendment* is a mini-debate inserted in the main debate. An amendment is always taken after the motion. Amendments cannot simply reverse the motion.
  - *A procedural motion* can suggest that the meeting proceeds to the next business, i.e. it can cut the proceedings short, and the chair, generally speaking, has to give it precedence over the debate.
- Voting – there are several ways of voting:
  - *A clear agreement*. The chair may realise that everyone more or less agrees and can say: 'Is it agreed that the motion is carried/ defeated?' There is a pause for breath and unless there is any protest the motion is carried/defeated.
  - *Out loud*. Some meetings ask for members to say aloud 'Aye' or 'No' and there is a judgement on which vote has the most support.
  - *By show of hands*. The commonest method of voting is for members to raise their hands and be counted. In a small meeting the chair counts the votes for and against, including those abstaining.
  - *Card vote*. When members cast a vote on behalf of those they represent, a show of hands may not represent the actual number of votes recorded when representation is accounted for.
  - *Secret ballot*. Members mark a piece of paper that cannot be identified as theirs – this is unlikely on formal committees.
  - *Co-opted members* do not have a vote unless the rules say they do.
  - *Proxy*. A person who cannot attend the meeting may ask someone else to vote on their behalf, but only if the rules provide for it.
  - *Chair's vote*. In a formal meeting the chair does not have a vote unless there are equal

votes cast for and against the motion, in which case the chair has a casting vote. In committees of, for example, local authorities, the chair usually has two votes, one cast with everyone else and another casting vote should the number of votes be equal – but the two votes are not cast together.

- Recording of votes – if they disagree with the motion, members may request that this should be officially recorded in the minutes
- Minutes – regulations about the drawing up, signing and discussion concerning the minutes
- Suspension of orders – unless in contravention of any statutory provision or direction by the Secretary of State, any of the standing orders may be suspended provided at least two-thirds of the membership are present, including one executive and one non-executive member, and the majority are in favour
- Record of attendance – the names of all present must be recorded in the minutes
- Quorum – this is the number of members that must be present for the decisions of the meeting to be valid and is usually one-third of the total number of the chair and officers appointed, including at least one non-officer member and one officer member
- Legally, there is some doubt as to whether the courts would support a challenge to any possible breach of the constitution but there is a political and moral issue for committees that are part of public control – if they break their own rules and take a decision that is against the constitution the courts could allow an injunction against the illegally taken decision.

Officers

The Chair

The chair is responsible for running the meeting:

- opening the meeting
- getting through the agenda (in good time)
- giving people a chance to put their views
- seeing decisions are taken and agreed
- conducting votes on resolutions
- upholding the rules or constitution of the organisation

- being neutral
- being in charge.

But there are limits: the meeting can

- challenge a ruling of the chair
- approve a resolution calling for a speaker whom the chair has ignored
- vote for a procedural motion, e.g. that an item or motion should not be considered
- in some cases, continue a meeting if the chair has adjourned it unreasonably.

In a formal meeting, the chair says very little and is charged with the responsibility for the procedures and progress of the meeting. The job is to check that the meeting has been properly convened, follow the agenda, introduce items (not with a speech), select speakers, conduct votes, rule on points of order and ensure that the debate is conducted according to the rules. The chair should say nothing except about procedure and uses some judicial umpiring when contentious motions are being proposed and opposed by warring factions – one thing at a time – one speaker at a time – one vote at a time – everything in its proper order and no-one speaks while the chair is speaking! The more conflict and disruption, the more formal and neutral the chair.

In smaller, friendlier, more business-like meetings the chair is more likely to leave the heights and join in the discussion. However the role remains essentially that of a clarifier and conciliator rather than a protagonist of one point of view. In a committee that is of one mind, a subcommittee or a working party the chair may get involved in proposing a particular course of action, even winning over some members.

Responsibilities of the chair. Several responsibilities are commonly expected of the chair:

- acting on behalf of the committee between meetings
- reporting the committee's decisions and work to higher level committees and meetings
- carrying forward the organisation – pursuing decisions made in meetings
- resolving conflicts or clarifying issues to prepare for meetings

- representing the organisation to the public or other bodies, and campaigning.

Chair's action. In some formalised structures the occasions and limits of the chair's action may be written down in the rules. Some circumstances require urgent action by the committee before the next meeting. Chairs of local authority groups, for example, may be delegated to agree contracts following a set of procedures without having to submit prior details to the committee, and sometimes the committee authorises the chair to negotiate and come to an agreement on its behalf. Other factors may be:

- how much the chair is trusted
- the size of the decision – it might be that a holding action is taken rather than doing something irrevocable.

Chair's action is a powerful device – it would take a brave committee to subsequently overturn a decision.

The Secretary

The secretary is responsible for the smooth process of meetings. Some health authorities appoint the secretary to the PCG and they may work closely together so that the health authority knows what is happening in the PCG. The secretary is responsible for accurate minute-taking, including the times members arrived and left, ensuring that the committee is quorate before any formal business is recorded. The secretary must be conversant with the rules and procedures of the committee and be prepared to handle voting procedures. The secretary does not usually have any voting powers within the committee unless s/he also holds another office. The secretary is also responsible for ensuring that:

- the agendas and minutes are sent out on time
- any requests for motions, amendments and agenda items are handled correctly prior to the meeting, particularly ensuring that these are put before the chair
- the minutes are accurate, are distributed appropriately prior to the meeting and, having been approved and signed, are sent to any approved recipients (other committees, the senior committee, the public or press).

The ordinary member

Ordinary committee members must be aware of what is happening. The way in which information is structured and presented tends to fix the terms of the debate. Once people have heard a case presented in one way, they find it harder to hear another point of view. To be alert to these ploys is important if one is to have any impact. Some suggestions about getting your own point across are:

- Speak firmly, early in the debate, preferably just after the main speaker, or
- Speak quietly, right at the end, appearing not to expect to influence the outcome but nevertheless leaving the impression with people of reasonable dissent – they may remember you another time and look to you to participate
- Speak disarmingly to defuse any hostility or resentment, unthreateningly: 'Can I just throw out for discussion some of my instant reactions to what's been said...?', or 'I've got to say I am a little worried about the way the debate has been going. Look at it my way...'
- Plant an idea nervously, casually 'What about ... setting up a project?', then step out of the discussion to see if the idea flowers. Some time later, one of the more powerful people says, as though they have thought of it themselves, 'What about ... a project?'
- Even if nothing happens, you have edged in and it is easier to pick up the idea later: 'What I was thinking about in suggesting a project, was ...'.

Prepare for the discussion, even write out your speech so that you feel secure in your knowledge and in command of the issues. Prepare for the meeting by reading the agenda and the papers.

Know the rules that are used at the meeting. Play them at face value. Even if the regular members have got into the habit of shouting over each other when they want to speak, we should raise our hands and try to catch the chair's eye.

Be brave: stop the meeting to get your bit in. Seize the chance of a relevant specific point to make a general statement like 'This raises basic problems about ...'.

Conventional behaviour of members is based on the House of Commons – a principal feature is that all remarks should be addressed to the chair. Members who wish to speak should indicate to the chair by raising their hand.

Declaration of interest

We need to know as members of a committee if other people are or might be influenced in a discussion by an outside interest. The convention is that as the item is raised a member should say, 'Can I declare an interest?' and would then only take part in the discussion if asked or in a circumspect manner. The member would not vote.

Point of order

A point of order is an objection made by a member about the conduct or procedure of the meeting. A speaker may deviate from the subject, use unpleasant language or break a rule of the meeting. The chair may miss an agenda item or run an election incorrectly. The member must put up a hand immediately and say clearly: 'Point of order, Chair.' The chair must halt the proceedings, stop the speaker and ask the member to say what the point of order is. The chair will then rule on the point but can be challenged by the meeting.

Apologies for absence

Members who are unable to attend the meeting should write a brief note of apology to the secretary. The names of the members who have apologised are read out at the beginning of the meeting.

The differences between a meeting and a committee

At a meeting:

- the chair is, or claims to be, entirely nonpartisan and does not participate in the discussion, making only procedural statements
- no business is conducted except on the basis of a motion
- a motion must be proposed and seconded
- there is a strict order of debate, with speeches for and against the motion
- speakers stand.

On a committee:

- the chair may join in the discussion
- business can be discussed as a topic and, if an agreement is going to be formalised into a motion, then it can be worked out during the discussion (rather than being presented at the beginning)
- motions only need to be proposed
- speakers remain sitting down.

The above are some of the conventions and rules of meetings and committees but the main rule is the constitution that guides the conduct of meetings and committees. Subcommittees will follow the same constitution and may be conducted in much the same way.

Health visitor's checklists for chairing

Health visitors working at higher levels of practice may well be involved in the work of committees/meetings and it is worth considering the value of an effective chair in moving work forward and developing ideas. The purposes of meetings that health visitors may be chairing are likely to be included in this list, itemised by Kieffer (1988):

- to consult
- to create or develop ideas
- to decide on aims
- to delegate work or authority
- to establish or maintain relations
- to give or exchange information
- to inspire
- to persuade or involve
- to share work or responsibility
- to socialise and have fun.

Most health visitors will have been present at meetings with very different chairing styles, and it is often very evident which meetings are more productive and how much this depends on the chair. There are a number of issues that the reflective chair should constantly bear in mind.

It is important that meetings start and finish on time – people with busy timetables will be more positive towards your meeting if they know that it is punctual. It is important that the chair has a clear idea of the purposes and outcomes of the meeting and that these are also stated clearly to members. Chairs often need to keep discussions relevant to the topic and restrain the more vociferous or dominant members without alienating them. It is also important that more reserved members are encouraged to participate and that all members feel that they have the chair's support and that their contribution is valued. A good chair will try to promote discussion between members rather than just with the chair and it is important to be even-handed over giving members the opportunity to speak. Sometimes the chair may need to resolve or defuse conflicts, disputes or tensions and, if the discussion gets bogged down, a good chair should be able to move it on. If there are difficult points, a chair should clarify these and summarise the discussion periodically so that all members are aware of the stage that the debate has reached. Finally, having successfully managed the time, the chair should succinctly review the meeting and, if relevant, confirm arrangements for the next meeting.

HIGHER LEVEL PRACTICE – PROJECT DEVELOPMENT AND MANAGEMENT

In considering the priorities for change, the Department of Health (1998b) makes the following statement: 'It will be important not to let change overwhelm us. The philosophy will be to take it one step at a time: plan the pace of change and prioritise and understand that the aim is evolution not revolution.'

Implicit within this statement is the impetus for a considerable amount of project work within the healthcare sector, for therein lies the opportunity for improving cost-effectiveness and maximising health gain. As will be discussed in Chapter 3, expertise in project management in the health service is often focused on areas such as information technology. However, there is now a pressing need for project work in relation to, for example, service delivery, human resource management, setting quality standards for practice, implementing research studies and setting up training and staff development programmes, to name but a few. It may well be that an experienced health visitor will be in a position to head up a project.

The six stages of setting up a project are somewhat similar to writing a research proposal.

- Stage 1 – developing a project idea (clarifying the problem to be resolved or developing a new way of working)
- Stage 2 – bringing together an appropriate team to implement the project
- Stage 3 – planning the project
- Stage 4 – implementing the project (the better the planning the easier the implementation)
- Stage 5 – completing the project
- Stage 6 – evaluating the project

Stage 1: Developing the project

Most projects will be based on some evidence of need or as the result of a feasibility study or strategic planning meeting. It is important that as much data or literature evidence is gathered as is possible and that this is closely examined to judge its reliability and validity. As in research proposals the clarity of the research question is all important, so in project development the clarity of the aims is critical. In the early stages the project team will be small but as the project develops it may be necessary to bring in particular expertise.

The position of stakeholders is clearly important at this early stage. If they are providing funding, then key stages and the resources required will be a dominant factor. If the stakeholders are, for example, clients or the local community, they will need to be in at the development stage. Similarly, if the project involves work pattern changes then the staff, who are stakeholders, will need to be involved. Not to involve stakeholders in a project early on means almost certain failure.

Stage 2: Bringing together the team

The project leader (or manager) must have credibility through adequate seniority within the organisation, and have the support of management.

The sponsor(s) who is funding the project, may, for example, have put the project out to tender, or the project team may have applied for funding from local authority or health authority sources.

The stakeholders may be users of the service (staff or patients/clients) or suppliers of materials or technology. They could possibly also be the sponsors.

Partners, e.g. the local authority or a charitable organisation, might be contributing funding, expertise or resources.

The project team are those people who are undertaking the work of the project. Team members are usually selected for their skills, enthusiasm, motivation and drive, and possibly their technical expertise. The team should have very clear roles and responsibilities and there should be good communication channels. The project team may have a *steering committee* that is able to approve decisions and progress the work of the team.

Stage 3: Planning the project

In-depth brainstorming may be facilitated by an 'away-day' to allow concentration on the task in hand. This also allows team members to get to know each other better if they do not work regularly together. The project aims and objectives are determined early on and these lead to outcomes that may be linked to the time scale set. Tasks may be identified in the early planning stages and these may be linked with staffing needs and possible training requirements.

Costs and resources needed will be included at this stage, as will the need to ensure quality of the project design and its strategy for evaluation. It is essential that all stages of the planning and implementation of the project are clearly documented and that team members and key personnel have access to records and reports. Feedback from team members is an essential element in the whole process and this must be well documented and scrutinised for appropriateness in relation to the original aims and objectives.

Another important aspect to consider at the planning stage is dissemination of the results of the project. This may occur at regular intervals, by means of a newsletter for example, or at a more formal event such as a conference or workshop. The idea is to share good practice and prevent duplication of work and consequent waste of resources.

Stage 4: Implementing the project

As was said above, the better the planning the easier the implementation. It is important that the leader/manager has good control of the whole process. There will be a need to be able to see the whole picture and compare this with the original plan, decide if the project is moving away from the original plan, decide what action needs to be taken and then take that action.

Control of a project must involve time management, resource and cost management and quality management. Human resources management, through good communication, interaction and good working relationships, and then feedback and corrective action, are essential to good control.

Contingency planning is also important to good control – what to do if something goes wrong, e.g. if materials requested don't arrive on time or if someone pulls out of the project team.

A good project leader recognises that there will be rises and falls in the speed of implementation of the project. Communication skills are essential to keep the team involved, motivated and supported. The project leader is mindful of the stress that change can bring and needs to monitor team members. In addition, project leaders need to have a highly developed sense of self-awareness, recognising their own personal traits and the effect that these may have on other people. People management may also mean conflict management, and this is essential to good project leadership. Above all, the ability to listen to people involved in the project, be they stakeholders or team members, and hold an unconditional positive regard for each individual will help to carry the work forward.

Stage 5: Completing the project

This involves pulling together all the information, ensuring that the aims and objectives have been met and that all changes/products have been delivered on time. All documentation must be up to date so that an evaluation can be made and also that standards and quality can be shown to have been met. The process of dissemination may have been staged; if not, preparations should be underway to set up the formal event.

Stage 6: Evaluating the project

Many projects have evaluation built into the implementation process, e.g. data on clients who have attended a clinic each week, or interim report forms from staff who are changing their work practices. These can then be drawn together to form a summary report. The team may wish to put together an evaluation report on the process of the project and their roles within it. Stakeholders may be canvassed for opinions, using questionnaires or interview schedules.

Many health visitors have been involved in projects and have discovered the process to be similar to a research proposal for an undergraduate honours degree programme. Certainly, the writing of a project proposal follows similar guidelines to the average research proposal. It is important that such proposals are characterised by succinct and clear writing to give the sponsors, stakeholders and team members a clear picture of what is to be achieved. Roberts & Ludvigsen (1998) have put together a useful and simple text containing tools and case study examples for carrying out project management in health care, and this is recommended to readers.

CONCLUSION

The discussion in this chapter has ranged widely over specialist and higher level health visiting practice. As stated earlier, many health visitors will be practising at a higher level in one aspect of their practice and may not wish to diverge into other areas in order to become a higher level practitioner. As this book unfolds further, it will become apparent that the skills of health visiting are higher level in themselves, but the range of practice may prove too wide for effective health visiting, except in certain circumstances. There are enormous opportunities for health visitors and from this chapter through to Chapter 18 it is hoped that the reader will find material and ideas that will encourage and inform specialist and higher level practice.

USEFUL DATABASES

Use these to locate articles, studies and research on clinical, medical and nursing practice, to inform arguments and to back up your research contribution. All offer full references and abstracts and a few give the full text of articles.

Medline

Nine versions of the international database Medline are collected together at:

www.omni.ac.uk.

Pubmed is the most popular as it includes current material and up-to-date Clinical Alerts:

www.ncbi.nlm.nih.gov/Pub

There are several other databases at this site, including CancerLit, Toxline, Aidsline, Bioethicsline and Healthstar (for health planning). Set up your search terms and then indicate which database you wish to search – but note that all are American in origin.

ENB Healthcare Database

Search for different types of resource, as well as journal articles. Up-to-date and with short abstracts, this database concentrates on UK material and is a useful base for articles on the National Health Service:

www.enb.org.uk/cgi-bin/hcdsearch

Health Promis

The national health promotion database for the UK. There are also databases of material on health-related resources for Black and ethnic minority groups, learning disabilities and older and younger people, which can be accessed separately.

Government sites

A rapidly expanding area of current, relevant information, documents and statistics. Use these sites to keep abreast of the latest legislation, circulars and press releases.

COIN – Circulars on the Net

This site includes health circulars on the Internet since 1997 and, recently added, pre-1995 local authority circulars. Search by title (alphabetical), by series or by full text (keyword) search:

www.doh.gov.uk/coinh.htm

Department of Health

The essential site for locating White and Green Papers, Health of the Nation information, circulars, press releases and information phone lines. Click on Public Health, Health Care or Social Care for the opening menu to explore subject collections, or on Search to search across the Department of Health site by keyword:

www.open.gov.uk/doh/dhhome.htm

Department of Health Press Release Menu. Press releases for the last three months:

www.coi.gov.uk/coi/depts/GDH/GDH98Q4 .html

Department of Health Statistics. Explore the latest NHS performance tables, health and personal social service statistics and community care statistics, among others:

www.doh.gov.uk/public/stats3.htm

Official documents

Access to material published by HMSO and other authoritative bodies. Click on UK on the main menu and choose whether to search by date, title, department or category. Category searching can be by Acts and Bills of Parliament, Command Papers, Consultative Documents, Public Information, Statutory Instruments and Green or White Papers:

www.official-documents.co.uk/

Evidence-based sites

This site, developed in Sheffield, is absolutely essential for finding material on this complex area of growing importance. It will help to develop skills to find, critically appraise and, ultimately, change practice in line with effectiveness. It is arranged alphabetically with over 100 links to the main sites of evidence-based health care:

www.shef.ac.uk/~scharr/ir/netting.html

2

The development of public health in health visiting

Anne Robotham and Jane DeVille-Almond

THE DEVELOPMENT OF PUBLIC HEALTH IN ENGLAND

This chapter is about health visiting and public health and could easily simply trace the history of health visiting from the appointment of respectable women by the Ladies Sanitary Reform Association in 1867 to the present day. However, the public health role of health visiting is not all that simple, because it has been influenced and even distorted by: the changing role of doctors; the tensions between public health doctors and general practitioners; the introduction of the NHS in 1948; the reorganisation of the NHS in 1974; the Acheson report of 1988; and the 'new NHS' of 1998. A brief glance at the changes in title given to doctors working in public health during the last 250 years gives an idea of the changes in focus.

- The 'Heroic Age' – the later part of the 18th century and the early part of the 19th century – showed that public health was basically about healthy conditions in relation to the basic necessities of life. There were three phases in the developing knowledge of public health doctors:
  - the age of environmental sanitation, 1840–1890
  - the age of developments in bacteriology (isolation, disinfection) 1890–1910
  - the age of education and personal hygiene, 1910 onwards
- During the Second World War public health became 'social medicine'

- In the 1970s public health became 'community medicine'
- After the Acheson report of 1988 public health became 'public health medicine'.

Community medicine 1960–1988

The government's Green Paper on the NHS (1968) and the Seebohm Report on the Social Services (1968) provided the push from declining social medicine into community medicine. J. N. Morris first defined the role of the community physician as being 'responsible for community diagnosis and thus the intelligence for effective administration of health services'. The new community physician was the key to effective integration of the health services, linking lay administrators to clinicians and co-ordinating the work of the NHS with that of local authorities. The community physician was recognised as a specialist adviser with special skills in epidemiology.

The 1974 reorganisation of the NHS

This brought all local authority health services into the NHS, i.e. district nurses, community dentistry, chiropody, physiotherapy, health visitors. Environmental health officers came into existence in local authorities (instead of public health inspectors); these took over all aspects of food hygiene, pollution, noise radiation, water and sewer inspections, infestation nuisances, and some health and safety work in small and Crown premises.

Medical Officers of Health became District or Area Medical Officers and were sucked into NHS medical administration. (Many resigned.) The new 'community physicians' were supposed to use their knowledge of epidemiology to tackle the epidemic diseases of the late 20th century:

- heart disease
- strokes
- cancers
- smoking related respiratory and circulatory diseases
- accidents
- chronic disability and handicap.

Infection was thought to be a thing of the past. The Medical Officer of Environmental Health was the health authority community physician who had the statutory responsibility as 'proper officer' to the local authority for the control of notifiable infectious diseases and food poisoning.

The Alma-Ata declaration from the World Health Organization (WHO) declared the goal of 'Health for All 2000'. This included designating the 1980s as the decade of safe water, the expanded programme of immunisation (against diphtheria, tetanus, polio, whooping cough, tuberculosis and measles) and the Control of Diarrhoeal Disease programme to increase knowledge of the use of oral rehydration programmes in childhood diarrhoeal illness.

'Health for All' was not confined to developing countries, however: in 1985 the European Office of the WHO produced 38 Targets for Health for All in the European Region – from environment (water, housing) through to healthcare and health research.

The Acheson Report (1988) was the first official enquiry into public health in Britain since the 1871 Report of the Royal Sanitary Commission. In his report, Acheson used the WHO categories (1951) to define public health as: 'the science and art of preventing disease, prolonging life and promoting health through organised efforts of society'. This definition, in conjunction with one put forward by Brotherston (1988): 'the organised application of resources to achieve the greatest health for the greatest number', gives a fairly comprehensive definition of the philosophical, economic and organisational basis of modern-day public health. The Standing Nursing and Midwifery Advisory Committee report *Making it Happen* (Department of Health 1995a) goes to some length to show that Public Health is a worldwide concept and that the Maastricht Treaty (Article 129) provides for European Community action in the field of public health. This action is limited to the principles of taking action if it is more effectively achieved by the Community rather than the member states, or taking action over issues relating to public health but not to delivery of health services. The bovine spongiform encephalopathy (BSE) crisis regulations of the early to middle 1990s, involving mainly the agricultural industry, were nevertheless imposed under principles of public health.

Public health is concerned with the protection and improvement of the health of populations and communities and is based on the collection of health and social information in order to draw up accurate profiles on the health needs of the population.

THE AVAILABILITY OF HEALTH INFORMATION

To profile the health needs of a community we need at least three types of information:

- information to describe the basic characteristics of the community (number of individuals, age, sex, etc.)
- information to describe and monitor the health status of the community
- information on the determinants of health in the community.

Basic characteristics

These can include a wide range of data that are all relevant when viewed holistically but whose constituent parts are often overlooked because the relevance is not recognised. Personal data are the most easily accessed by health visitors because of the types of record available in NHS databases: these include age, sex and occupation. However, economic data about the individual that include employment require more intensive enquiry to tease out and raise to the surface the hidden problems of deprivation and poverty. It is often difficult to ascertain the numbers of families and individuals who receive income support and yet this may be fundamental to their health status. Similarly, leisure data and support networks such as religious activities and other community activities, which play an indirect and important part in health status, are less easy to find except on individual enquiry and are often considered difficult to access and therefore unimportant. Data on housing occupancy and condition can be collected fairly easily and the

importance is evident, but environmental issues such as noise and pollution can be viewed from different contexts and these are less easy to pursue. For example, noise from traffic or industry is constant, although it may affect sleep and personal thinking space, but noise from neighbour behaviour is variable and possibly more threatening, creating an environment that may ultimately become more prejudicial to health.

Health status

Certain aspects of health status are easier for health visitors to find out, such as mortality and its causes and therefore, by implication, morbidity. However, most health workers argue that morbidity cannot ever be completely ascertained and that there are individual personality and coping factors to be considered. Quality of life and well-being assessment is possible both on an individual basis and from a family or community viewpoint but the tools available vary in reliability and are time-consuming to administer. Bowling (1991) argues that recent indices of health status have focused on ill-health and were based on negative concepts of health – for example, mortality and morbidity rates, the self-reporting of symptoms, illness and functional ability. Healthcare professionals and social scientists are now looking more closely at the measurement of health status through the development of tools for positive measures of health. These include concepts of 'social health', 'social well-being' and 'quality of life', which influence the individual as well as the family and community.

Determinants of health

It is probably helpful to consider these under:

1. influences on the individual
2. influences to do with the local social, economic and physical environment
3. influences to do with the wider social, economic and physical environment.

1. Influences on the individual are mainly concerned with lifestyle and will include important factors such as normal diet and exercise taken, and whether the person smokes or abuses alcohol or drugs. Knowledge of and attitudes towards health issues, and the actual clinical health of the individual, are also important health determinants and can be linked with personality and response to stressful situations. Finally, employment and the educational background of the individual are inseparably linked to lifestyle.

2. **Influences of the local social, economic and physical environment** are of varying relevance as health determinants depending on individual and community response. Factors such as crime and vandalism, quality of housing, levels of traffic and accidents, and levels of pollution all have a very clear impact on health and have been the focus of a number of research reports that have contributed to the Green Paper *Our Healthier Nation* (Department of Health 1998a). Other important local factors are access to good food, health care and leisure facilities, and the employment and educational opportunities in the area.

3. **Influences of the wider social, economic and physical environment** all have importance and yet are less likely to be taken into consideration when determining health. Seemingly less immediate factors such as the advertising and pricing policy on tobacco and alcohol, road safety legislation, legislation on contraception and abortion may all be important to the individual, depending on their circumstances. Political issues such as national economic and employment policies and environmental issues such as the effects of greenhouse gases and global warming are some of the wider issues that are relevant for current and future health status.

Health visitors who are working to raise awareness of health issues will be very aware of these influences and, although many feel overwhelmed by their inability to influence policy, nevertheless there are good examples of health visitors who have worked with communities to effectively change policy.

Community profiling

The methods by which health visitors have collected information about the area in which they work have changed little over the past 20 years and reflect earlier epidemiological enquiries, which commenced during the Victorian public health era. Health visitor profiles have been described by several commentators as the most comprehensive source of information available about communities, particularly during the period covered by the Acheson Report (1988).

However, despite a heightened knowledge of their working area, health visitor practice has not responded to identified needs, primarily for two main reasons. Firstly, the organisational management of health visitors has meant that their work has been directed in the main by local policies and management structures. Health visitors who in the early 1990s were managed by the Child Health Directorate of their Trust were required to reflect the work of that directorate, i.e. to work primarily with under-5s and their mothers. This may well have been in direct conflict with the revelations of their area profile, which might have indicated a persistent health need among, for example, the 40–55-year-old members of the population. Health visitors who were determined to overcome this became creative in the way in which they recorded the statistics of their work in an attempt to respond to the originally identified health needs of their particular profiles. In a study on Marketing in Health Visiting, de la Cuesta (1994, p. 352) calls this a 'tailoring strategy... developed to meet the deficiencies in the health care and social systems, and to make the service relevant to the client's perceived needs'.

Secondly, social data have become increasingly available as a result of many audits and surveys carried out by both statutory and voluntary organisations. These are often based on an assessment of need but in addition they cover a wide range of aspects of social life. Social audits have as their basic premise the requirement to balance resources against need in many areas such as housing, employment, the natural and social environment and so forth. It is this difficulty in balancing the ways in which these valuable data can be used by health visitors who are basically working in health promotion and illness prevention that leads to the lack of response from many health visitors in practice.

Health needs assessment has formerly been the basis of the health visitors' community health profile and useful data have been collected for many years, much of it remaining shelved because health visiting has never taken the initiative in determining its practice on the basis of identified need – rather on the traditional need, based around the mother and baby unit. In addition to this there has always been the tendency to collect information on a yearly basis and only rarely to link this in with any assessment of the effectiveness of health visiting interventions.

Health visiting in both specialist and higher level practice will be most effective if it collects data that straddle the social and health needs of the public. Hawtin et al (1994) consistently argue that community profiling requires actively involving the community, as well as using data already in existence such as home ownership and employment rates. The following definition of a community profile best fits this: 'A comprehensive description of the needs of a population that is defined, or defines itself, as a community, and the resources that exist within that community, carried out with active involvement of the community itself, for the purpose of developing an action plan or other means of improving the quality of life in the community'.

Epidemiological data in health visiting profiles

Despite the fact that information collection and audit has become increasingly comprehensive it must be remembered that epidemiological data should always be viewed critically in terms of:

- *Accuracy*: for example, hospital records of admissions will log readmission of the same person as a separate admission. Another example is that death certificates are required by law to state the immediate cause of death followed by the underlying cause of death, but in Western countries few deaths are recorded as due to 'mental illness' or 'degenerative joint disease'.
- *Completeness*: for example, only those road traffic accidents reported are counted. Another

example is that, although doctors are required by law to notify the Public Health Department of infectious diseases and are paid a small fee for doing so, underreporting is common.

- *Timeliness*: how up to date is the information? It frequently takes the National Office of Statistics some time to collect all information, and it is often 2 or 3 years behind with some types of information.
- *Validity*: for example, lung cancer morbidity can be based on mortality statistics because most people affected die within a short space of time. For diabetes, a chronic disease, morbidity statistics cannot be based on mortality data.

Concern has been expressed by health visitors working in specialist areas related to public health departments that many of them collect data about the frequency of health problems but this has in the past been glanced at superficially where interventions have not been measured. The public health audit tools of the 21st century will require accurate interpretation to enable effective intervention analysis. We need, therefore, to be quite clear about the meanings of epidemiological descriptors and measures.

Measuring the frequency of health problems

Rates

Over the course of 2 years 123 children were seen in a hospital fracture clinic with broken arms following a bicycle accident. Details of the main types of accident were as follows:

- Accident with a car – 25 cases
- Accident with an immovable obstruction – 23 cases
- Accident with a person or animal – 15 cases
- Accident on a slippery surface – 10 cases
- Accident due to bicycle fault – 20 cases.

Does this mean that children are more likely to be injured while riding on roads alongside motor vehicles?
Answer: It is not possible to make a judgement until further information is available:

- How many bicycle riding children are there in the area surrounding the particular clinic?
- How many children ride safe or faulty bicycles among cars, people, animals or on slippery surfaces?

To make a valid comparison we need to relate

the number of children who ride bicycles, faulty or otherwise, to the number of bicycle riding children in the area, or to the number of children who ride their bicycles in each set of circumstances. In other words we need to use *rates*.

A rate is a measure of how frequently an event occurs. All rates are ratios, which means they consist of one number divided by another number:

$$\text{rate} = \frac{\text{number of accidents over a specified time period (numerator)}}{\text{average population of bicycle-riding children during the time period (denominator)}}.$$

The figure is usually multiplied by, for example, 1000 to convert it from a fraction to a whole number.

Incidence and prevalence

A secondary school has 100 children in the third year. On the first day of November, 10 children were away with a cold. Over the month of November, another 18 children developed colds and were away from school.

Assuming that the number of children in the year did not change during November, answer the following questions:

- What proportion of children had a cold on the first day of November? (point prevalence)
- What proportion of children had a cold some time during the month of November? (prevalence)
- What proportion of children who didn't have a cold at the start of November developed a cold during the month of November? (incidence).

Point prevalence refers to the proportion of people in a population with a disease or condition at one point in time – 10% (10/100).

$$\text{prevalence} = \frac{\text{total number of cases in a specified time period}}{\text{total population in the time period}}$$
$$= 28\% \ (28/100).$$

$$\text{incidence} = \frac{\text{number of new cases in a specified time period}}{\text{population at risk in this time period}}$$
$$= 20\% \ (18/90).$$

Population at risk is important – it refers to

all people who could become new cases – 90% (10 children already had a cold on 1 November therefore 90 children were at risk). The population at risk can require some careful selection to ascertain true (rather than assumed) numbers.

You are interested in the incidence of testicular cancer in your area. You find out the number of new cases over the past year from the cancer registry. This gives the numerator for calculating the incidence. The denominator is the population 'at risk'. Imagine that you start with the total population of your area for the past year. Make a list of everyone who should be excluded from this to leave you with the true population 'at risk'.

Your list should include women, men who have had testes removed and men who already have diagnosed testicular cancer.

As can be imagined, it is difficult to calculate the size of the population at risk; however if health visitors aim to work with this population then they must be sure of the validity of their data and the means by which they seek to achieve their ends. The same initial questions are posed for any medical epidemiological problem:

- Consider your 'at risk' population
- Consider the source of the data and their collection methods
- Consider the accuracy and validity of the source data
- Make comparisons with other similar populations
- Consider relevant social data.

It is reasonable to seek out health problems using medical epidemiology based on available morbidity and mortality statistics and not to consult the community *per se*. However, most empirical evidence suggests that members of the community are less aware of medical problems and far more concerned about social issues.

Profiling with the community

It is unlikely that a community has only one need that is common to all its members and thus various groups will identify different needs depending on factors such as age, socioeconomic status, political persuasion and available resources.

Profiling with the community will require constant dialogue with representatives of the many groups and subgroups that contribute to the diversity and richness of community life. Hawtin et al (1994) suggest that to profile with the community it may be necessary to enable the community to:

- become motivated to come together
- understand the nature of its oppression
- identify its requirements
- plan its action
- take part in developing services and resources for the community.

DeVille-Almond discusses later one way of getting a community to come together by increasing communication through the production of a newspaper, and this can be effective in small homogenous communities. For larger and more heterogeneous communities, however, one of the striking features can be conflict, possibly stemming from a variety of divisions such as race, age or class. Hawtin et al quote Haggstrom's (1970) concept of the two appearances of community – community as object and acting community. The first is the network of interest groups, political parties, bureaucratic organisations and so forth that is acted upon. The second identifies its own needs and problems, participating in the decision-making and engaging in collective action.

An example of community as object (acted-upon community) was seen when, on behalf of a charitable organisation, a researcher was profiling child care needs in a community in a deprived area. From going round and speaking to all the leaders and organisers it became clear that they were very enthusiastic about their own particular project. Potentially, there was enormous energy and some excellent work was being done in many aspects of community support, from children's holiday play schemes, through groups for young mothers run by an elder citizen to discuss problems of parenting, to classes in the local community school for the unemployed to learn computer skills. However, each of these groups was beavering away independently of the others. When one worker was asked why he thought this was, his response was: 'You are all doing to us.' Reflection on this helped the researcher to understand that this community area, although deprived, had had quite a lot of money invested in it for a number of projects, all of which had been quite successful. However, what this worker was saying was: 'We cannot work together because we are not encouraged to take responsibility for the distribution and effective use of the money invested in us – give us

the money to use and we will make it effective.' He was clearly right and thus the recommendation to the organisation who wished to donate money to set up a scheme was: 'Just give them the money and they will use it effectively – don't put in any other project organisers.' Sadly, the donating organisation felt unable to let their money go without retaining control themselves and so a further small project started up, running alongside and overlapping with others, and the community came no closer together.

Profiling for primary care groups within public health

If primary care groups are to function effectively, there must be far closer dialogue with the community, and clearly health visitors have the skills to be proactive in this area. This will require a profile elicited by the traditional health-visiting approach, based on data collection from existing healthcare sources, health visitor and other community professional caseload profiles, epidemiological, social, housing and environmental, education, employment and other sources. These are the passive data essential to underpin the next stage of active community participation in profiling. As has been suggested above, communication is the most important part of the process and there are two stages at which the community can be consulted. Firstly, publicising in all public places and in local newspapers that profiling is to be undertaken and requesting the assistance of all interested parties; or secondly, publicising the current health visitor type profile results and requesting active comments and criticisms from the local community.

The former method is to be recommended so that an active community approach is encouraged. Publicising the intention to survey will draw in a core of interested professional, social, political and volunteer group leaders. They will all have something to offer in relation to their focal interests. It must be made clear at this stage that the purpose of profiling is to ascertain health needs and to improve resource allocation, and that the results will be made available at each stage to check for accuracy and the range of need dimension.

If possible, the community should be surveyed directly by questionnaire. The costs of this need not be too great and the local newspaper may be prepared to print the questionnaire for little or no charge. The cut out/tear-off section can then be collected from posting boxes at central points such as the post office, library, community hall, leisure centre and so forth. Again, a clear explanation must be attached to the questionnaire of the reasons for the survey, and it must be made clear that there is no way in which respondents can be identified. The final profiling method would be for members of professional healthcare services to undertake face-to-face surveys of opinion from all the main groups and organisations active within the community.

This 'acting community' approach may be undertaken on a regular basis: probably biennially would justify the effort. The principal reason for profiling in this way for primary care groups is that the profile will inevitably show far more interest in social concerns than health issues. For example, if questions are posed about what members fear most in their street the response may well be burglary or car break-ins. Health visitors and others who work in the community are well aware of the distress that theft and burglary causes and the relationship between this and despair in deprived areas. Health visitors who are members of, or keep closely in touch with colleagues on these primary care groups, will continually lobby to raise awareness of these issues and encourage active networking with local authorities as part of primary care within the social model of public health.

This approach reflects the report of the Working Group on Public Health and Primary Care (Department of Health 1997b), who have recognised the valuable strategy adopted by some Trusts (see below) for structuring the public health time of health visitors. Health visitors can be appointed as part time neighbourhood health strategy co-ordinators and, once established in that role, they have a wide range of opportunities for development. The co-ordinator can act as advocate for the local population and has delegated authority from the health authority to make representations on behalf of the neighbourhood residents in, for example, objecting against a local planning application.

Health needs

Bradshaw (1972) first classified social need into the four areas of: *normative need*, which is defined by experts/policy makers and is often a desirable standard laid down and compared with the standard that actually exists; *felt need* is want, desire or subjective views of need that may or may not become expressed need; *expressed need* is demand or felt need turned into action; and *comparative need* has to do with equity. Student health visitors have become familiar with these definitions but recently Bradshaw (1994) modified his original comments to suggest that real need would exist when all the four elements were present at the same time. Despite health visitors' familiarity with Bradshaw's defined elements there are problems in imposing this structured approach. For instance, normative need can be very urgent and yet may not be felt or expressed. Similarly, comparative need can exist in one area or group and at the same time not be felt, expressed or recognised as normative.

To illustrate the above situations, a health visitor may visit a mother who has recently had a baby and lives in a fairly affluent area. However, she is in a detached house, has no access to a car, her family live far away, her husband works long hours and she has a highish score on the Moods and Feelings questionnaire. This woman satisfies all the elements for need and yet none may be expressed or recognised until searched for.

MODELS OF HEALTH AND HEALTH VISITING IN PUBLIC HEALTH

Models of health

There are broadly two models of health that health visitors are interested in and on which they spend a disproportionate amount of time. Both models belong to the sphere of public health and are closely interrelated, but they are structurally far apart. The *medical model of health* emphasises cure rather than prevention and its effective response is measured by the absence of disease through cure rather than prevention, or the reduction in hospital waiting lists by treatment rather than health promotion. Historically health visiting began with the *social model of health* based on prevention and health promotion but, as Western medical science has grown in the latter half of the century, so the organisation of health visiting, particularly since the transfer of health visitors into the NHS in 1974, has become more closely allied to the medical model.

Health visitors are often sharply divided in their views about working in a medical model of health. Many value the work they undertake with the individual, and the organisation of their work, bringing them closer to general practice, lends itself to this work with individuals. Although many health visitors would challenge the idea that work in postnatal depression, for instance, is using the medical model, yet working with the individual on a curative basis is fundamentally a medical approach. Similarly, working with individual older people to ensure compliance with packages of care that include medication is also using a medical model approach. However, there are few health visitors who subscribe to the social model of health who would not argue that the medical model also has a place within the wider social model.

The social model of health embraces the curative model but also emphasises the place of prevention and promotion of health within the social and environmental context. Immediately the social and environmental context is raised, the importance of equity and equality becomes fundamental. To examine health needs out of context is meaningless because it is the structures within which people live that determine their health needs, and it is these structures that include all the material resources that must be included in an analysis of the meaning of a social model of health.

Organisation of health visitors into primary care teams runs the risk that the social model of health will not be sufficiently well embraced if the leadership of primary care teams remains with general practitioners. However, it is clearly possible to practise within the social model of health if the basis of solution of problems lies in influencing and negotiating within the social networks of professionals working in the community.

Empirical evidence emerging as the result of health visitors discussing alternative approaches to problems in 1998 seems to indicate that many general practitioners are far keener on social solutions to medical problems than they used to be. In the past, the curative approach was the only option open to GPs who were not intimately familiar with the community of their caseload, and despite knowing that allopathic medicine was not an effective solution to many problems, they had little alternative but to prescribe expensive drugs. Indeed, they were often forced into this solution by their patients, whose expectation of a satisfactory consultation was that they should emerge with the familiar prescription form. Epidemiological evidence has shown the ineffectiveness of this type of approach in dealing with common medical problems, e.g. bronchitis or anxiety. The value of the health visitor and primary care team attempting a social solution by approaching housing departments to improve living conditions, using support and counselling mechanisms or even referring clients to local health and recreation clubs, is that the patient has the opportunity to be 'cured' by a social model of healthcare.

Pietroni (1996) discusses the vision offered to general practice by Vickers (1984), who 'emphasised the need for the concepts of personal doctoring (general practice) and social medicine (public health) to come together to enable the new field of community care to flourish'. In many ways this vision was precipitated by two earlier pilot projects of general practice – the Peckham experiment and the Glyncorrwg Community Practice. The Peckham experiment operated as a form of club at which individuals could participate in healthy activities. The activities included being given information on how to improve health and the quality of life and health examinations were periodically made. Out of this, the pioneer health centre was built in 1935. The Glyncorrwg Practice grew as the result of 48% of the male population being out of work in 1986 following local pit closures, and emphasised the importance of the family group and community in sustaining health around a purpose-built swimming pool in an architecturally pleasing environment.

Pietroni's (1996) own vision carried the former experiments further when the Marylebone Health Centre was developed in 1987 to include not only an orthodox medical practice but also other forms of community care including complementary therapies, a counselling and psychotherapy unit, a social care unit, a health promotion and health education unit and a patient-run and -staffed patient participation programme. Pietroni comments that it is most probable that the enduring element will be the social unit, which is co-ordinated by outreach workers and includes:

- transport service for patients and relatives
- decorating and minor repair service
- befriending and sitting service
- once a month telephone contact for over 75s
- single parent club
- newsletter, three times a year
- language interpreter centre
- homeless accommodation service
- crisis listening or drop-in service
- swimming club
- movement to music
- choir
- elderly–toddler sessions
- yoga classes
- reminiscence group
- help in the practice, volunteer groups

and other activities. A number of GP practices around the country are adopting this approach and involvement of practice population volunteers has led to the development of many of the innovations outlined above. A greater sense of community around the practice develops and, with the enthusiasm that accompanies these initiatives, considerable sums of money are raised to buy extra equipment.

In many ways the approaches outlined above epitomise the approach that health visitors have traditionally always been educated for and yet have been unable to easily slip into, that of involving people in social ways to the benefit of their health. Clubs to bring young people together with elders are recognised as beneficial to psychosocial health because of the natural affinity of the young with the old. Tedesco (1997) showed how, in a rural community, the bringing

together of older people into an exercise club satisfied both health and social needs.

Interest is seen in the 'new public health' that grew out of the Lalonde report of the 1970s (Lalonde 1974), followed by the work of Ashton & Seymour (1988) in the UK. A growing awareness of the new diseases menacing society today, such as AIDS, *Salmonella*, Legionnaires' disease and new variant Creutzfeldt–Jakob disease, led to the Acheson report into communicable disease and the public health function of 1987. All this has produced a new interest in public health and communicable diseases and the re-emergence of tuberculosis in the UK has reminded us that health visiting was established to deal with such concerns. Unfortunately, during the second half of the 20th century health visitors were unable to make the impact that their education suggested they should, and the opportunity to try again in the 21st century, and succeed, cannot be allowed to disappear.

Models of health visiting

In Chapter 4, Carnwell shows how health visiting practice should use models that can truly respond to a far wider approach to health promotion and illness prevention. She particularly discusses the advantages of the model of Chalmers & Kristajanson (1989), Beattie's (1996) accounting for health using the biopathological model, the ecological model, the biographical model and the communitarian model, and the adaptation of these by Twinn (1991). Importantly, Carnwell points out that models designed for public health are inappropriate for use with individuals, and if health visiting maintains its practice with individuals and communities then it will be important for practitioners to have practical knowledge and understanding of models suitable for both approaches.

There has been wide discussion prior to and following the report of the Standing Nursing and Midwifery Advisory Committee (SNMAC 1995) about suitable models for the public health role of health visitors, nurses and midwives and the conclusion drawn by the SNMAC is no standard model is advised. Opinions vary among health visitors themselves over whether health visiting should be practised solely in any one domain (see Chapter 12). The profession recognises that, clearly, traditional work with mothers and children should carry on, especially through home visiting. A systematic review of the literature related to domiciliary health visiting carried out by Robinson (1998) shows a wide range of effectiveness outcomes. Robinson comments that health visitors are most successful when functioning in a non-directive, supportive way that tends to be regarded by their employers as non-work. Increasingly, health visitors are being directed by their managements to work through groups invited into health centres and GP surgeries although there is limited evidence to suggest that this is effective except in a very general way. Groups that tend to be more effective are those established by health visitors that bring together same-problem-focused clients – who in time, and with health visitor empowerment, are able to take over the control and running of these groups. They exist, however, as the result of established effective domiciliary visiting.

Other models of health visiting that involve work outside the home cover a wide range of initiatives, which all contribute to public health and yet appear idiosyncratic to the context in which they arise. Group initiatives are more likely to be found in the health promotion approach and can serve the needs of like-minded/problem-solving approaches. There is a definite limit to the number of group initiatives that can be run in the community: most of these centre on the general practice and thus have a medical/illness-based reason for their existence.

A COMMUNITY DEVELOPMENT PROJECT

Jane DeVille-Almond

I was employed by Walsall Community Health Trust in September 1995 as a part-time Public Health Nurse in Moxley in the West Midlands. Moxley is a poor socioeconomic area with a high incidence of many common health problems.

My task was to help improve the health status of the Moxley residents by setting up appropriate health clinics and assessing local health needs. Unlike previous attempts at public health, which seemed to use statistics as a passive tool, I felt it was important to integrate health professionals working in the area with the community and other local agencies so as to truly assess Moxley's needs – as an active tool.

When a neighbourhood needs assessment is undertaken, it is of vital importance that the appropriate structures and mechanisms are in place and that these are ready to respond to issues that might be discovered. Collecting 'local knowledge' is not just a matter of data collection; it also involves political and policy commitments.

On reflection, this was easier said than done. To truly get the feel of a community I felt it was important to integrate with and more importantly to be accepted by the community. However, before being able to do this I had to ask the question: 'What is a community, and should we expect everyone to take us on board?' Communities are very hard to define – just because there is a natural boundary in terms of either houses or area the people inside those boundaries do not automatically see themselves as part of the community. I found there to be a very definite divide between the elderly and the young, the youth and the 'grown ups' and the men and women. However, if the elderly had grandchildren and great-grandchildren in the community it gave them a link with the young. There was also a 'class structure' within the community, which at times became quite complex. This appeared to be defined by several factors, including:

- which road you lived in
- how long you had lived in the area
- whether you were married or were single with a child
- whether your family was a long established name that had dominated the community for many years or whether you were new to the area
- whether you or your partner was presently in work.

There were several other factors that defined a community, but trying to work within these complex rules often caused friction between others and myself.

An example of this became apparent when I first set up a keep-fit class: many of the younger mothers came, which put some of the older residents off attending. There were also a few local notorious members of the community who had dominated other sections of it for many years. Once these people became involved in any new initiative it put many others off. It became quite a task to decide whether to exclude the dominant people, thus making room for many others, or to try to integrate them with the other members of the community without frightening the others off. After working within the community for a while it became apparent that it would have to be a mixture of both. There were also barriers created by working from a church-owned building. Some people felt that the fact that events were run in the Community Centre, which was owned by the church, would put a large number of local residents off attending. I had to try and make sure this did not happen.

When I began in Moxley over 60% of the residents lived in local authority housing and the unemployment rate was around 26%. The GP's facilities were very poor, with only one consulting room, no hot running water and a very small waiting room. Residents were often kept waiting for up to 2 hours before seeing a GP and services such as cervical smears were only offered on Thursday mornings between 11 and 12 – it was little wonder that the uptake was poor. The area had already been highlighted as having high incidences of all major illnesses but the nearest health centre was almost 2 miles away. As 53% of families did not own a car, access to this health centre was often difficult.

I was asked by the Trust to address women's and children's needs, in accordance with the *Health of the Nation* (Department of Health 1992) targets, and to progress from there.

My main aim was to ensure that I worked collaboratively with all the people in the area: this included social services, the local council, local churches, local schools, the local commu-

nity association, local health professionals, local voluntary bodies and, most importantly, local residents. I soon discovered that there was an immediate need for many health provisions and as a starter I decided to address two that I could rectify almost immediately. The women who lived locally expressed concern over there being no adequate baby clinic in the area and also they felt that some sort of keep-fit class would be good. There had been a Weight Watchers group in the area for a while and, although there was a great need for such a service, it had closed down as many found it far too expensive.

I needed to find a suitable building to run the clinics in and I was unable to use the GP's surgery. However, the local health authority had given some funding towards the building of a community centre owned by the church. These funds were given on the understanding that the local authority could have free room space for 10 years for all health activities. The community centre was in the heart of Moxley and made an excellent venue. My only concern was that the fact that it was a Church building might be a bit of a stumbling block with some of the local residents.

I asked local schoolchildren to help design posters to promote the forthcoming clinics and asked local businesses to donate prizes for these. I awarded eight prizes for the best posters and well over 100 local people attended the awards ceremony. I announced to all when the two new clinics would be starting. This all happened within 6 weeks of taking up my job.

One of the first comments I had from local residents was that people often spoke about what was needed but then nothing ever got done! They also expressed concern that no one ever consulted them on issues such as what day and time would be best for the clinics. I therefore had a panel of local residents to help me with these issues. I felt that it was important for people to see that things were being done. Within weeks both these clinics got off the ground.

We started a baby clinic in the Community Centre, which we ran on a much more informal basis than is commonly done. We provided a creche facility for older children, had complimentary light refreshments, and encouraged mothers to discuss issues not only with health visitors in group sessions but also between themselves. Many of the mothers now help with the running of this clinic. The demand has been so great that we now have a Child Medical Officer on a monthly basis and a second clinic has been started for new babies only. Here two of the local health visitors encourage the mothers to set up support groups and run discussions on the specific health needs of newborns and their mothers.

On Tuesdays we have a 'weigh-in' clinic, two keep-fit sessions (the local community association pays for the instructor), a blood pressure clinic, a reflexology clinic and invite speakers on a whole range of topics, talks for which we provide creche facilities. I also run 6-week cooking courses where cheap, low calorie meals are prepared within half an hour and everyone gets a taste. At the end of the 6 weeks each person is issued with the recipes and a breakdown of cost and calorie content. Women in the audience help me to buy and prepare the food and also supply me with recipes. We make a small charge for the keep-fit classes and 'weigh-in' clinic and this money goes towards monthly prizes for achievement by participants, food for the cooking courses and the complimentary refreshments. Every 6 months, for extra-special effort, I offer the opportunity for two women to attend a health farm for the day. At least six of the local women have lost 35 kg or more in weight.

Many of the women said that they would like to attempt other sports but felt they were not the type to join a tennis club or go to the gym. The keep-fit instructor and I decided to work together with the local sports and leisure services and get tennis coaching, swimming lessons and other activities organised at a knock-down price. Many of the women took advantage of this and I also used some of the award money to fund these events. Over 40 women completed tennis courses that were offered and some have continued playing. We will hopefully run similar events this year.

I was given an initial £500 by the Trust and opened an account in the name of Moxley Community Clinics. Any money raised from the charges for the 'weigh-in' clinic and keep-fit classes and any other funds I receive are paid into this account. This then enables us to run these clinics at a relatively low cost to the Trust. Much of my equipment is provided by sponsorship from outside the NHS, by fundraising by the local community or by applying for research based money.

I have instigated the setting up of a chiropody clinic in the Community Centre on the same day as around 55 pensioners meet for bingo, making the clinic more accessible for the users. This was started at the request of the local pensioners and the Trust provided a session every 2 weeks. It soon became apparent that the need was for more than this and the service is now provided on a weekly basis. Very few appointments are missed as many of the attenders are on site on this day anyway.

I have also worked with a community arts team to get local young people involved in a theatre workshop looking at health issues.

Men's health

After working in the area for a while locals soon started to approach me about other health issues. Many of the women were concerned about their menfolk not being included in the health initiatives, so I decided to address some of the men's health issues and looked at setting up a clinic for men.

I worked with other nursing colleagues to improve men's health awareness and uptake of services. I did this by taking services out into the community and held men's health clinics in pubs, betting shops, local shops, the library and other venues.

The clinics that were available to men were often in medical settings such as GP surgeries or hospitals and men often defaulted on their appointments. It seemed when I questioned them about these clinics that many of them felt that they were wasting the doctors' and nurses' time by going to see them if there was nothing wrong. Even when things start going wrong, men are four times less likely than women to see their doctor about health problems.

The main aim of this project was to try and inform as many men as possible of the importance of early detection of health problems and to encourage men to become more health-aware. I also attempted to compare uptake between a clinic in a community setting and one in a surgery. I particularly aimed our health programme at men from the lower socioeconomic groups, whom I felt would not go and seek such advice in traditional settings.

Apart from the weight, exercise, drinking and smoking problems I also focused on testicular awareness in the younger men and prostate awareness in the older men. Prostate cancer has doubled in incidence in the last 30 years and accounts for four times as many deaths as cervical cancer. Testicular cancer is also on the increase and is the commonest cancer in men aged 20–44 years. I decided to run two pilot projects and see how effective each might be.

Surgery screening. In the surgery I targeted men between the ages of 40 and 50. I sent out a questionnaire randomly to around 25% of the men in this age range to see what time would be most appropriate, in particular for those in work. I then sent birthday cards out on the patient's birthday asking him to make an appointment with the practice nurse at his convenience. The response was poor: only 18% returned the questionnaire and of those who attended the clinics only 4% had one or more health risk problem. It seemed that the men with the real problems stayed away.

Community screening. For the community screening I decided to take the screening to the men rather than expect the men come to the screening – and where better than a public house, a traditional male domain. The first pub in which I carried out the health checks, the Moxley Arms, is in a very deprived area and has a regular local clientele. This 3-day event was so successful that I and my colleagues held a further five events at pubs, betting shops and public places in the area. I also got the bar staff to wear T-shirts printed with health messages relating to testicular cancer. This proved to be very effective in promoting open discussion.

Findings

In total we saw over 200 men and many were found to have health risk problems. At the first event 68% of the first 50 men screened were found to have one or more health risk problems: many of these related to excessive smoking, drinking, obesity and high blood pressure.

In the second pub, 72% were found to have one or more health risk factor. We also picked up a diabetic, who is now on insulin, and two men reporting lumps in their testes, which were subsequently investigated by their GPs.

We did a follow-up 8 months later of the first 50 men that we had seen and recorded any changes in lifestyle. The follow-up clinic had an attendance rate of 48% and of these 6% had made substantial changes to their lifestyle, with a subsequent improvement in health, and a further 12% had made small changes such as reducing alcohol intake, cutting down on smoking and taking a little more exercise.

I feel that services such as these could easily be taken in to other areas with limited costs. More importantly, I feel that by going out into the community and attempting to screen the most vulnerable men in their normal settings we will achieve much more in our quest to inform those most at risk from ill health. Many of the men we screened, although reluctant at first, showed a great deal of interest in their health once problems were discovered. Many confessed to feeling silly when visiting their general practitioner with headaches, despite some of them having systolic blood pressure readings of over 200 and diastolic readings of over 120.

Local committees

I became very closely involved with all local committees and represent health-related issues at Agenda 21 and Single Regeneration Budget (SRB) meetings. I attempted to get local industry interested in funding certain aspects of community life that I felt would benefit the health of the local population. I also successfully campaigned to have adequate street crossings put on a busy main road where a child was killed and others injured and, through SRB, became involved in a programme that looked at the installation of central heating and double glazing in all council houses in Moxley, the provision of better street lighting, environmental improvements and working with the local police and residents to address local crime problems. I feel that all these issues play a big part in the health and happiness of a community and should not be underestimated by nurses in a public health role. I also worked persistently alongside the SRB committee to ensure that something was done about the GP's surgery. In October 1998 we were still awaiting the date on which the first brick of our new Health Centre was to be laid.

After attending an Agenda 21 meeting it became apparent that there was a problem with local news reports. Moxley is on the borders of Walsall and Wolverhampton: the local shops sold the Wolverhampton edition of the local newspaper but Moxley was reported under Walsall. This meant that many residents could not read about local stories. To address this situation we decided to run our own newspaper. Local residents, council representatives and I now run a newspaper called *Moxley Big Gob* ('gob' being local slang for 'mouth'), which is issued to every household in Moxley. I write regular articles and features to do with health, including what clinics are running, with times. I also put in regular photos of local residents taking part in the clinics. Walsall council has promised to fund this for the foreseeable future.

The future

Local officials, businesses and voluntary groups were useful sources of information but the most valuable source was discovering the knowledgeable members of the community and working closely with them. Once people started to approach me with health issues within my area and put forward agendas of their own I realised that I was on my way to a successful partnership.

We had over 380 kg shed at our 'weigh-in' clinic during 1997–98 and we now have well over 100 men, women and children of all ages using the various clinics weekly. There are always new issues to be addressed and new people to empower, and part of my role as a public health nurse should be to ensure the sustainability of services on offer and where possible to pass them over to the people to run themselves.

It would be arrogant of me to suggest that there have not been problems in working with the local community and other agencies, and there have of course been failures as well as successes. Some of the failures were brought about by lack of communication between myself and other community members and some by personality clashes. However when working in the public heath arena one has to remember that upsetting one person can often have a knock-on effect to 50 others, especially where the community contains very close knit groups. I had a great deal of difficulty in delegating work. This was mainly because there was no one to delegate it to. However, once I became involved with the community, many people were willing to commit themselves to helping in the setting up and running of projects. I also had a great deal of difficulty persuading other professionals within the Trust about the value and priority of the role. I feel, however, that for the project to work successfully it is important to learn from the failures and build on the successes. This type of work takes lots of commitment and a 9-to-5 approach would be out of the question. I have often worked evenings and weekends to truly involve myself with the community and feel that now, more than 3 years into the project, this hard work has started to pay off.

Walsall Community Health Trust has been very supportive of me and has allowed me to develop the services even when my approach has challenged existing systems and policies.

It became apparent that I had truly started to empower the local residents when I mentioned recently that I would have to close down some of the classes for a week because the nursery nurses and myself would not be there.

'You can't do that,' was the reply 'We don't need you lot here. We can run this on our own.'

It is often difficult as a health professional to let go and it was at this point of the project that

I realised that I had stopped being the instigator of better health in this community and the community had started to take over. I was simply a player in the team. Changing attitudes is possibly the most difficult task one has to encounter in the public health field and it takes more than a few years. However once the seed has been set it will soon start to spread and hopefully in years to come it will be possible for this community to truly reap the benefits of better health for all.

Community development models as exemplified by DeVille-Almond are becoming increasingly popular but rely heavily on a project approach with a limited lifespan and defined objectives to be realised within a relatively short time scale. While the reasons behind these time scales and limited objectives are recognised and understood they are self-limiting and degenerate into a fund-seeking exercise in order to prolong their lives. They serve a purpose but this tends to be lost with the passage of time after the completion of the project. However, with the changes envisaged in healthcare organisation and delivery in the White Paper *The New NHS* (Department of Health 1997a) it is hoped there will be a totally different approach to the delivery and organisation of health care through Health Improvement Programmes and Primary Care Groups.

HEALTH ACTION ZONES AND THE INFLUENCE ON HEALTH VISITING

One of the major concerns that health visitors have constantly identified both in their profiling work and their interventions with individuals is the ever-widening gap in health equality. The distance between the haves and the have-nots is at an all-time high and, more than ever before, requires two distinct methods of health visiting intervention – the high-profile type of work with the knowledgeable, access-to-all-relevant-materialistic-opportunities client suffering from competition, isolation and stress; and the make-do, find-an-alternative, lowest-cost client who has health needs and no means of responding to them. To fight these articulated inequalities the

government set up, in 1998, 10 first-wave 'health action zones' to bring together a partnership of health organisations, including primary care, with local authorities, community groups, the voluntary sector and local businesses. As a direct reversal of the competitiveness of the NHS internal market, these health action zones are to encourage partnerships and alliances across local organisations and groups to target specific health issues and introduce innovation.

Health action zones are designed to be more long-term than many recent changes – between 5 and 7 years. This will allow the setting of agreed milestones between the national and local partners, the establishment of better economic strategies across the period, and evaluation methods to ensure specific outcomes at regular intervals during the lifetimes of the zones.

Healthy living centres

'Healthy living centres' are being set up using lottery money, and the local voluntary, public and private sectors will be drawn together to design, set up and quality-assure the effectiveness of these centres. It is specifically envisaged that there will be opportunities for health and fitness facilities for all, as well as meeting rooms for opportunities for raising awareness of good health behaviours. These are the opportunities that health visitors should not let slip and if they are at the forefront of advising, guiding and delivering the health promotion and education sessions they will be in a position, through their active profiling, to advise on the health problems evident in the area. Within the health action zones are the three main settings that the government has identified as focal points for health inequalities – healthy schools, healthy workplaces and healthy neighbourhoods.

Healthy schools

'Healthy schools' is a an initiative particularly designed to take the opportunity to encourage healthier lifestyles in children. Health psychology has shown that lifestyle habits taken up during younger and middle childhood will become lifelong habits and thus, if there is a clear focus on health, particularly in relation to healthier eating, regular exercise and a warm and happy environment, children will respond positively. There are a number of initiatives in different schools around the country, which have established enterprising approaches to projects such as a breakfast club, healthy tuck shops, homework clubs, latch-key support clubs. All these and other initiatives have been set up as the result of an alliance involving the school, local supermarkets, local business organisations and the children and their parents. School nurses and health visitors have been involved and there are opportunities for health visitors to support the development of further initiatives. Health visitors in particular have knowledge of lonely or isolated people who are free during the day and would be willing to give up some of their time to support these ventures. The upshot of these activities is that, with a continual focus on health, there should be some reversal of the increased development of poorer health behaviours resulting from the modern technological, health-awareness-lacking age. It is important also for health visitors to recognise that inequalities in health will become less obvious among children where healthy eating support ventures ensure that costs are kept to a minimum and that the numbers of children who qualify for free school meals are not reduced by such ventures.

Healthy workplaces

Health visitors are in a strong position to raise awareness of the problems of employees who work in smaller organisations and businesses where there is no occupational health department. In particular, women often discuss with health visitors visiting their homes their employment concerns about their partners. These women are concerned about raising awareness of the need to adhere to health and safety regulations, particularly where there are work risk factors that could influence the health of the family. For example, men who work in small units such as car repair garages should be aware of the need to ensure that heavy oils do not seep through their clothing, especially in the groin area, which would put them at risk of testicular cancer. It is useful to work through women to raise awareness of the risk factors that men face, but also for health visitors who are working in the community to make direct approaches to small businesses, offering regular health discussion sessions to minimise risk-taking and build in better health practices. Empirical evidence from health visitors working in areas with small pockets of industrial units has shown that employers welcome help and support through health teaching programmes and well-person advice sessions.

In working in partnership with women in the home, health visitors are often in the position to discuss women's concerns about the health of their men.

Transport initiatives

The government White Paper *A New Deal for Transport: Better for Everyone* (Department of Environment, Transport and the Regions 1998) particularly stresses a new integrated strategy for transport in general, but there are local measures aimed specifically at improving health that health visitors can bring to the attention of the women they are working with. It is not suggested that health visitors should take an active role in transport initiatives on a national level, but at a local level they may well be involved in traffic-calming measures, setting up school crossing patrols or safety initiatives to reduce the incidence of accidents outside the home. Raising awareness in families of ways in which health could be improved might include:

- encouraging more people to walk to work or use cycles
- encouraging safer routes for children to walk or cycle to school
- encouraging mothers to try to keep children in pushchairs away from vehicle exhausts
- encouraging fathers to press employers to introduce green transport plans to help them use alternatives to driving to work alone
- encouraging women to influence the family

decision on car purchase towards the use of lead-free petrol.

Health initiatives in the office

Employers in some areas have allowed small labour forces to have an hour out of the office/shop periodically for discussion of health topics that the employees had themselves requested. Unlike large industrial organisations, in businesses where employees number fewer than 100 there is no requirement for an occupational health service, yet they may face similar health risks with only health and safety inspections to ensure compliance with regulations and no occupational health promotion or education. Health visitors in some areas of the West Midlands have responded to that need.

Health visitors also should take up opportunities to link with other offices and businesses who have little or no access to health advice and information. In particular, guidance on handling stress, bullying in the workplace, repetitive strain injury and other problems associated with continued computer use could all be introduced, taught and supported by health visitors. These programmes could be set up as part of the health action zone initiatives and, if necessary, could draw on the lottery funding available.

These healthy workplace initiatives require the skills of professionals such as health visitors who are trained and able to approach a wide network of businesses and organisations, possibly initially through Rotary, Inner Wheel, the Townswomen's Guild or other business people's organisations. They have access to funds, some charitable, to underpin small health promotion/well-people initiatives but, more importantly, raising awareness of health issues leading to a healthier workforce and workplace would greatly improve the public health.

Healthy neighbourhoods

A number of initiatives have been developed over the last few years to help to improve environments, particularly in inner city and urban areas. Monies under the Healthy Cities (Davies & Kelly 1993) and Single Regeneration Budgets programmes have meant that many new pockets of housing development and improvement have been set up in run-down and derelict former industrial areas. Health improvement programmes have been identified and money sought from central funding to enable local authorities to tackle regeneration of cities and large towns to bring people and life back into the centre from the suburban fringes whither they had moved. Development strategies for cities and large towns now mean that these are safer areas for people to come into, especially at night. Policing and improved lighting, closed-circuit cameras and pedestrian-only zones have meant that personal safety after dark has also been improved. The Healthy Cities initiative had its first success within 4 years of commencement but the uptake across the UK has been patchy, with an uneven variety of grassroots work and high-level publicity. The initiative was based on the sharing of information about health, including data analysis and strategic planning, across the community and including the public. Many commentators note the value of this approach and effectiveness evaluations have shown some health gain, albeit on a limited basis.

In large, former local-authority housing estates and other smaller private estates local people have come together to introduce Neighbourhood Watch schemes, traffic-calming initiatives and more school crossing patrols to raise levels of safety and reduce fear among residents, especially older people. Surveys among older people have shown that fear of burglary and theft is their greatest anxiety and keeps them trapped in their homes after dark. Health visitors have been instrumental in helping some neighbourhoods to set up such schemes as Neighbourhood Watch, and the networking necessary with local leaders, councillors and organisations does mean that these skills should continue to be taught to and used by health visitors.

An initiative announced by central government under the Social Exclusion Unit's report *Bringing Britain Together: a national strategy for neighbourhood renewal* (1998), is a new fund, worth £800m over 3 years, which is intended to help the poorest neighbourhoods. These are neighbourhoods that have severe multiple problems, which usually include:

- poor job prospects
- high levels of crime
- a run-down environment
- no one in charge of managing the neighbourhood and co-ordinating public services that affect it.

The programme started in 1999 with 17 pilot areas, selected because their problems are particularly severe. However, health visitors are in a position, because of their overview of the neighbourhood area, to be able to lobby for changes to be made even if their area is not selected for this developmental money.

HEALTH VISITORS AND HEALTH TARGETS

The Health of the Nation (Department of Health 1992) and *Our Healthier Nation* (Department of Health 1998a), White and Green Papers, have set targets for improvements in illness rates initially in five key areas (*The Health of the Nation*) and later in four key areas (*Our Healthier Nation*). The main difference in the focus of the two papers was that the first focused on epidemiology and the second on the socioeconomic–environmental causes of ill health. It has become abundantly clear since the publication and shelving of the Black Report (Black 1980) that, whatever initiatives were set in place involving NHS organisation and ill-health targeting, there would be limited improvement unless there was full cognisance of social factors.

Health visitors are in a good strategic position to respond to target-setting in major areas of ill health. Previously they have promoted health and illness prevention as a major part of their work, but response has tended to be on the individual level as a result of promoting healthy living in homes, schools and community groups. Health visitors, however, have been acutely aware that women do know the best foods for their families but that to feed a growing family on a limited income means that, with all the best health advice in the world, good-quality fruit, vegetables and a balanced diet are beyond the pockets of many of their clients.

Health visitors are aware that there are high rates of heart disease and stroke in ethnic minority groups as well as in indigent caucasians and for some time have been seeking ways to retain cultural influences while at the same time encouraging healthy eating to lower blood pressures and reduce weight gain. An example is the high rate of diabetes among older Afro-Caribbean people. Discussion with their children, the next generation, shows that they are quite clear that the cause has been their parents' eating habits. These have partly been due to the fact that the traditional West Indian diet is based on many fruits and vegetables that have only been available in this country in the last decade. Discussing such epidemiological facts encourages the younger generation to improve their eating and also to raise awareness among their parents. In south Asians, as is discussed in Chapter 17, communicating the dangers of using quantities of ghee in cooking is difficult because of the high regard in which this food product is held and its place in the social mores of this culture. To introduce the concern raised by the medical evidence about high levels of saturated fats in the diet often means that health visitors need to work through the leaders of Asian groups, the spiritual temple leaders, in order to raise awareness and highlight the dangers. To change something so seemingly innocuous and yet fundamental to a culture calls for good levels of cultural knowledge, skilful use of link workers where there are language problems, and clearly articulated concerns that do not mock cultural beliefs and yet allow for the adoption of healthier approaches. Empirical evidence shows that health advice is often delivered through younger family members and that health visitors have a big part to play in illness prevention by disseminating all relevant knowledge and information.

The unique position of health visitors in relation to health promotion across all cultures and groups means that they approach target-setting with a certain diffidence. If, for instance, health breakdown in the four *Our Healthier Nation* target areas is improved by better screening and swifter and more effective treatment, this is measurable. The problem for health visitors tackling reduction in illness targets is that, to be effective, their work must be long-term. Thus, recipients who benefit would not be among the identified victims of the targeted disease area. This has always been a problem for health visitors and there is now an even greater need to find ways of recording and measuring the effectiveness of health advice and healthy lifestyle support.

HEALTH VISITORS AND HEALTH IMPROVEMENT PROGRAMMES

Health improvement programmes (HImPs) were announced under the White Paper *The New NHS – Modern, Dependable* (Department of Health 1997a) and are a local initiative for improving health and healthcare to be based on the annual report of the Director of Public Health. Health improvement programmes will involve the health authority drawing up the strategy in consultation with local trusts, primary care groups and other primary care specialists working in the community (such as pharmacists, dentists and opticians), and will also include the public and other organisations in partnership. Health improvement programmes commenced in 1999 and, although partially reviewed each year, will cover 3-year periods. This will mean that strategy can be planned for longer periods than the 1 year that was the rule during the early 1990s. Health visitors should ensure they are involved in the planning of these strategies because they require a programme from a health and social focus that will meet the most important health needs of the population. For local planning it is the people working on the ground with the population who should be able to bring forward, or encourage local people to bring forward, their health concerns.

The actual implementation of health improvement programmes will fall into the hands of the management structure of either primary care groups or health trusts, but it is the health authority who will monitor the running and effectiveness of the programmes. The actual responsibility for commissioning more joint health and social care services to satisfy local health need will belong to primary care groups, and these will be built into their service agreements with NHS trusts. This means that health visitors need to know who their local nurse representatives are on the primary care groups and keep in close contact with them to ensure that their voices are heard on behalf of, and with, their clients. It may well be that the nurse members of the local primary care group will look to health visitors to provide them with information about the health needs of the local population.

PRIMARY CARE GROUPS

Primary care groups have grown out of the various commissioning models developed in recent years. Some GP fundholding initiatives have proved very successful, others less so, and it is envisaged that primary care groups will represent GPs who were both within and outside the original commissioning groups. These primary care groups are strongly supported by their health authority, which has a nonexecutive director on the primary care group board. Boards will be composed of GP representatives, nurse members, a member from the local social services, a lay member, the chief officer and the aforementioned health authority member. Other representation from professions allied to medicine will be co-opted when necessary to provide knowledge and expertise. Once members are elected to the board their tenure of office will be 3 years.

Primary care groups became operational in April 1999 after an initial shadowing period alongside the commissioning groups. Their starting points varied around the country depending on the security of establishment of commissioning or fundholding groups. There are four options for the form that any primary care group may adopt:

- supporting the health authority in commissioning care for its population, acting in an advisory capacity

- formally taking devolved responsibility for managing the budget for health care in their area, as part of the health authority
- becoming established as free-standing bodies accountable to the health authority for commissioning care
- becoming established as free-standing bodies accountable to the health authority for commissioning care and with added responsibility for the provision of community health services for their population.

It is possible that in time a primary care group may become a trust – a primary care trust (following the appropriate government legislation) – and it could be that this occurs in partnership with the current community health NHS trust in order to better integrate services and management support.

The functions of primary care groups are to:

- contribute to the health authority's health improvement programme
- promote the health of the local population, working in partnership with other agencies
- commission services for their local populations from the relevant NHS trusts within the framework of the health improvement programme
- monitor performance against service agreements with NHS trusts
- develop primary care by joint working across practices: sharing skills; providing a forum for professional development, audit and peer review; assuring quality; and developing the new approach to clinical governance
- better integrate primary and community health services and work more closely with social services on both planning and delivery.

The relationship between primary care groups and public health

The term 'primary care' immediately summons up concepts of the medical model of health care, which is individual and tends to focus on the practice as community. In addition the concept of the primary health care team appears to be coterminous with the concept of primary care

and, although the team members focus on the practice as community, in many cases they do not really feel a team – rather individual professionals focusing on one working area. Although the concept of primary care is embedded in the care packages delivered by social services to help maintain and support people in their own homes, nevertheless there has been a distinction made between the primary care of the GP practice team (primary medical care) and the primary care of social support. This does not appear to have the same kudos as medical care and yet has the same, if not greater impact on the ability of the client/patient to retain their independence as part of the community.

Within general practice the primary health care team has developed a number of public health skills to support the traditional role of the primary care practitioner:

- health promotion programmes
- community development projects
- child health surveillance and immunisation
- screening for undetected disease
- drawing up of protocols and guidelines
- deciding what health care need is needed by the practice population
- involvement in the commissioning of services
- designing formularies
- data collection and patient registers

and, traditionally, much of this was based on short-term, immediate treatment responses to individuals, whereas public health tends to take longer-term, strategic views of the health needs of populations and communities, working across agencies. With the new primary care group focus there will have to be a balance between these perspectives. Primary care and public health also share common themes, such as a generalist and multidisciplinary approach, a holistic view of health, a concern for clinical standards and quality, and working across the health and social care interface.

Primary care and public health are interdependent. There are many examples around the country of individuals in public health departments in health authorities and in primary care already taking a combined approach. Some primary care practitioners, such as health visitors, health promotion specialists, community workers and others, are involved in health needs assessment, interagency work on wider public health issues, health promotion, screening and health protection programmes and community development work. In order to tackle inequalities and address *Our Healthier Nation* priorities, this work will need supporting and strengthening (NHS Development Unit, 1998).

The report of the Working Group on Public Health and Primary Care (Department of Health 1997b) was issued prior to *The New NHS* and *Our Healthier Nation* and was designed to prepare for the debate of exactly how public health and primary care are interrelated. The working group recognised local difficulties, such as the lack of coterminosity between practice population and geographical patch, and the wider difficulty created by the fact that their remit was to focus only on health authorities, general practitioners and nurses in primary care, thereby excluding other models of public health practice. It also recognised the wide variation in public health initiatives across the country, often dependent on a handful of enthusiasts, and the tension between public health and primary care, which the group considered stemmed from a lack of understanding of each other's ways of working and priorities. It used Tables 2.1 and 2.2 to identify the differing perspectives.

The common themes that run between public health and primary care are equally important when exploring the health visiting response and are probably similar to Table 2.3.

The Working Group on Public Health and Primary Care (Department of Health 1997b), in identifying the tensions between public health and primary care were mindful of the impending changes of *The New NHS – Modern, Dependable* (Department of Health 1997a) and *Our Healthier Nation* (Department of Health 1998a) as well as the introduction of many of the initiatives mentioned in *The New NHS* such as health improvement programmes, health action zones, the chief medical officer's project to strengthen the public health function, primary care groups, Supporting Families. It is likely that these initia-

Table 2.1   A summary of the different perspectives of public health and primary care

Public health	Primary care
Longer term, strategic view	Short term, operational view
Population focus	Individual patient focus
Larger populations (geographical)	Practice population
Prevention orientated	Treatment orientated
Needs assessment of groups and populations	Needs assessment of individuals
Work through others (manage change)	Direct work with patients

Common themes:
Multidisciplinary and generalist approach
Holistic and concerned with health
Consider people not just as 'patients'
Clinical standards and quality
Longer term relationships and concerns
Whole spectrum of health and disease issues
Concerned with health/social care interface
Achieving value for money

tives look overwhelmingly public health policy and yet they are to be run in collaboration with primary care. The problem is that the medical model underpins current definitions of primary care and public health and inhibits the development of community perspectives on health.

Numerous studies have confirmed that there are inequalities in health status between deprived and affluent communities, both in mortality and morbidity. It is premised that geographical and social factors as well as individual characteristics, perhaps to do with education and self-esteem, may be the causal elements. The effect on health status is thus dependent on the relative strength of these circumstances. The approach of previous governments has been to attempt to strengthen the individual against circumstances, with little noticeable effect. The attempt to strengthen the medical model through a contract culture for the individual resulted in deterioration of professional relationships at GP/administrator level and further imbalance in the equity of services offered.

Attempts to involve the community have also met with mixed reactions. Highly motivated community volunteers can only function with the support of their fellow lay members, and this

Table 2.2   Health visiting in the differing perspectives of public health and primary care

Public health perspective	Health visiting response
Longer term, strategic view	As a result of assessment and working through others, help communities to influence local policies – especially improvement in housing, reduction in noise and pollution, improvement in amenities, improvement in safety and accident prevention
Population focus	Work within the population; understand the socioeconomic status and perspective; know many individual family networks; work closely with playgroups, nurseries and schools; understand demographic characteristics; local employment opportunities; local homes for older people; numbers who are cared for at home; cultural and ethnic dimensions; Sure Start initiatives
Larger populations (geographical)	Understand population projections and movements; large and small area profiles; very aware of birth rates; collation of records to produce health status and trends (e.g. breast feeding rates); have knowledge of housing, transport, employment, pollution, crime, clubs and groups; trailblazer action for health action zones
Prevention orientated	Use data on smoking, screening uptakes, maternal mood status, family eating patterns, local shopping habits, local health awareness, available morbidity and mortality data – all to focus health promotion and health education; health improvement programmes; helping to set up food co-operatives
Needs assessment of groups and populations	Use national morbidity and mortality data, health visitor community profiles, local health visitor and other community workers' caseload profiles, GP caseload profiles, population rapid appraisal methodologies and community links – all to plan for strategic focus and campaign for change.
Work through others (manage change)	Work with families to develop parenting skills, improve nutrition, reduce negative health behaviour; work with groups to increase health knowledge and health awareness; work in community development to improve facilities, bring communities closer together, foster caring, reduce violence and crime
Short term, operational view	Formulate annual targets based on caseload and practice caseload health and illness data; plan health education and health promotion in response to identified health and illness requirements; monitor and evaluate outcomes
Individual patient focus	Work with individual mothers and babies to maintain optimum growth and development; maintain growth and development surveillance and screening; work with individual older people to maintain health status and reduce potential ill-health; work with individual families to reduce accidents, improve dynamics, develop healthy lifestyles; work with individuals with health needs
Practice population	Help to develop care pathways following hospital discharges; plan and work in practice clinics to improve health knowledge and surveillance; help to develop health and fitness ventures both within and outside practice premises
Treatment orientated	Set up and develop clinics to support long-term chronic disease (e.g. asthma, incontinence, family planning and HRT clinics); set up and develop clinics to support post coronary heart disease and stroke; evaluate effectiveness
Needs assessment of individuals	Family history, pregnancy and birth history of new babies to establish genetic risk factors; social, economic and living style knowledge to bring accumulative potential risk knowledge; close working with parents to establish potential behavioural and lifestyle risk factors in young children
Direct work with patients	Supporting and listening work with mood-affected mothers; parenting management work with mothers and fathers; supportive work with child or adult following acute illness; work with special needs child; supportive work with chronically ill child or adult

support often diminishes through apathy or as a result of the time it takes to be effectively involved in community issues.

THE PUBLIC HEALTH ALLIANCE

The Public Health Alliance was set up in 1987 as an independent group to lobby for public health improvements. One of its research projects was to examine the potential for the reality of working public health and primary care together and as a result, *A Public Health Model of Primary Care – From Concept to Reality* (Taylor et al 1998) was published. This proposed a public health model of primary care with three components – public health, which has a key role in promoting equity; primary care, which has a key role in promoting and developing collaboration; and the

Table 2.3 The common themes between public health and primary care

Common theme	Health visiting response
Multidisciplinary and generalist approach	Health visiting teams of nursery nurses and link workers can link with other agencies to support families (e.g. where there are child-handling problems); health visiting can link with social service providers to respond to the health and care pathway needs of older clients; health visiting remains a universal service with a targeted focus as a result of a generalist approach
Holistic and concerned with health	Health visiting particularly works within the bio-psycho-social model of health; the bio-psycho-social response is applied both to individuals and communities; health visiting rejects the victim-blaming approach of some health promotion initiatives, choosing instead to focus on the stresses impacting on people's lives
Consider people not just as 'patients'	Health visiting sees a person as part of the family or community group; health status is against family context; any disease focus is contextualised against socioeconomic situation
Clinical standards and quality	Health visiting is concerned with measuring the effectiveness of prevention, which is a long-term issue; health visiting recognises the needs of the individual within screening and immunisation programmes by providing research-based knowledge on which to make decisions
Longer term relationships and concerns	Health visiting is concerned with networking both within the NHS and with non-NHS organisations; working in health alliances with, for example, the voluntary sector; developing communication networks (e.g. through a community newsletter)
Whole spectrum of health and disease issues	Health visiting particularly works with homeless people to reduce risk of diseases of deprivation and social epidemics (e.g. drugs); health visiting uses a socioeconomic basis on which to promote and educate good nutrition practices
Concerned with health/social care interface	Health visiting works closely with social workers in child health, safety and protection concerns; health visiting should work closely with care organisations in determining care pathways for older people
Achieving value for money	Health visiting is concerned with long-term effectiveness issues; health visiting should use accurate annual profiles against which improvements in health can be measured; health visiting could aggregate the goals they have negotiated with clients to provide information about the health needs of communities and hence the effectiveness of the service in meeting the community's needs

community, which has a key role in promoting participation (Fig. 2.1).

The Public Health Alliance group has gone further in helping to establish frameworks whereby active development of the individual circles of Figure 2.1 can be broken down into 'quality indicators', as it has called them. These are reproduced in full with permission of the Alliance and are an invaluable way in which health visiting can see itself working across sectors and with groups to achieve a harmonious marriage of the two systems of healthcare (Fig. 2.2).

Examples:

1. Primary healthcare worker helping an individual patient cope with the limitations of their chronic illness, such as asthma or diabetes
2. Healthcare professional or professions providing advice or treatment to patients to prevent the progression of ill health or shorten episodes of treatment (e.g. dietary advice and education about medication)
3. Primary healthcare team working to prevent the worsening condition of particular groups of patients within the practice through recall systems, co-ordinated activity and special clinics
4. Multisectoral, community-based health promotion to prevent the onset of ill health (e.g. establishing a food co-operative and addressing local environmental health issues)
5. Establishing a help and advice service (including health assessment and treatment) for, for example, homeless people (Taylor et al 1998).

It is likely that health visiting is to be found to a certain extent in zone 2 of the framework and very definitely in zones 4 and 5.

The next 'quality indicator' identified by the

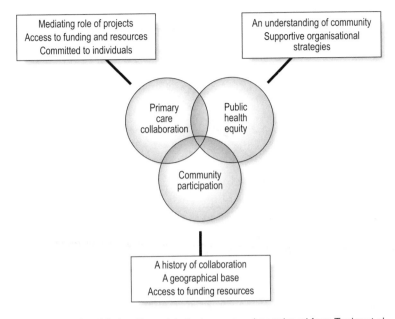

Figure 2.1 A public health model of primary care (reproduced from Taylor et al 1998 with kind permission from Public Health Alliance)

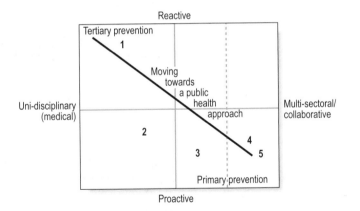

Figure 2.2 Primary care and public health (reproduced from Taylor et al 1998 with kind permission from Public Health Alliance)

group is truly focusing on the public health aspect of the model and uses all those initiatives and fundamentals that are the basis of health visiting (Fig. 2.3).

Examples of the various stages within the framework:

1. Evidence-based medicine
2. Infection control
3. Secondary and tertiary health promotion
4. Planned approach to community health – collaborative health needs assessment
5. Healthy schools programme
6. Community-based public health action, e.g. food co-operative (Taylor et al 1998).

The final breakdown of the model produces a framework that assumes community participa-

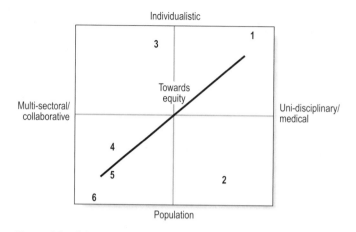

Figure 2.3   A framework for public health (reproduced from Taylor et al 1998 with kind permission from Public Health Alliance)

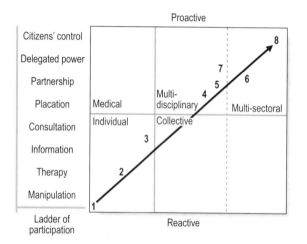

Figure 2.4   Community participation and primary healthcare (reproduced from Taylor et al 1998 with kind permission from Public Health Alliance)

tion within primary care and demonstrates the absorption of public health and primary care into a new public health model of primary care (Fig. 2.4).

Examples of the various stages within the framework:

1. Patients receive treatment
2. Practice newsletter – health education sessions
3. Patient participation group/practice volunteer schemes
4. Self-help groups
5. Health forum
6. Collaborative community profiling exercise
7. Community development project with resources to set up community activities
8. Joint campaign to win regeneration funding for an estate (Taylor et al 1998).

FITTING A PUBLIC HEALTH MODEL OF PRIMARY CARE INTO THE NEW NHS

A number of sociopolitical considerations must be recognised when the new approach to health care delivery is challenged. From the two recent papers *The New NHS – Modern, Dependable* (Department of Health 1997a) and *Our Healthier Nation* (Department of Health 1998a) it is apparent that the government has bowed to the power of the general practitioners and assured them of their contractual status within the organisation. One chink in the armour can be seen in the discussion about salaried GPs that emerged in the earlier paper *Choice and Opportunity – Primary Care: The Future* (Department of Health 1996a), when new possibilities were raised for GPs to become salaried, either within partnerships or with other bodies such as NHS trusts. Some general practitioners will wish to take up the option but the dominance of general practitioners on primary care group boards will mean that the medical model of public health will also be dominant. A second concern is that, although the government has approached proposed healthcare as set out in the Green Paper *Our Healthier Nation* (Department of Health 1998a) – on three fronts from macro, meso and micro levels – there is little firm evidence that there will be a power base from which to achieve this.

In *Our Healthier Nation* the government chose four priority areas that it considered were significant causes of premature death and poor health. Significantly, they chose to drop sexual health as a priority area, although it had been one in the earlier White Paper *Our Healthy Nation* and despite concern over the world HIV and AIDS epidemic. Sexually transmitted diseases are also of public health concern because of their link with lowered fertility, particularly the so-called 'silent' sexual disease of *Chlamydia trachomatis* infection, sufferers from which are frequently unaware that they have contracted it until chronic responses become apparent. It was felt that the health contracts to deal with the targets identified in the later Green Paper reflected the full range of social, economic and environmental factors that impact on the four disease areas:

- heart disease and stroke
- accidents
- cancer
- mental health.

The contract for health in relation to the four above target areas covers a three-pronged attack through a four element approach, as set out in Figure 2.5.

This approach marks a change in government thinking by acknowledging that the first element, social and economic issues, should be tackled on three levels – the national, the local and the individual. If all three put equal energy into finding solutions, it will be hailed as one of the greatest responses to public health since comparable efforts in the heroic age against equally daunting barriers. Similarly, suggesting that government also has a part to play in the other categories is certainly a positive move. Structures being set up within NHS organisation through collaborative ventures, such as primary care boards with their lay and wider professional influence on commissioning services, must be applauded. The only problem that is immediately obvious is that there still is an over-representation of the medical profession, with its inevitable medical model approach.

Contract target area:	Government and national players can:	Local players and communities can:	People can:
Social and economic			
Environmental			
Lifestyle			
Services			

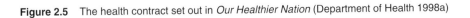

Figure 2.5   The health contract set out in *Our Healthier Nation* (Department of Health 1998a)

CONCLUSION

As a result of these recent government papers on new approaches to healthcare the opportunities for health visitors within this framework are greater than ever, and with doubts about registration removed health visitors must be prepared to be among and behind players in all three approaches to the four areas. From the outset, health visitors should have close links with the nurse members of their primary care group boards, if they are not the members themselves. This will allow feedback to health authorities and the government about issues that must be addressed, particularly in relation to the disadvantaged and socially excluded. Health visitors' knowledge of local issues is critical to effective primary care group functioning and the need for contemporary profiles based on active rather than passive data is of great importance.

At the middle level of local players and community, health visitors, with their public health knowledge and skills, can raise awareness of issues and encourage and support the community in making relevant demands to satisfy need on all counts, but especially in social need. To become active in community development calls for health visitors to exhibit a certain degree of confidence and this must result from good initial professional education as well as from taking every opportunity for continued professional development.

It is in working with individuals that health visitors have been most effective so far (Robinson 1998), and continued work with mothers and young families through Sure Start initiatives is essential. The opportunities to respond to local need through the emergence of flexible initiatives for people in similar circumstances can offer cost-effective and cost-benefit approaches responding to fluctuating circumstantial changes to help and support all young families in an equitable and participatory way.

3

The use of health informatics in health visiting

Ruth Wain and Judith Shuttleworth

INTRODUCTION

In this chapter, the current and potential use of health informatics in health visiting will be reviewed. Firstly, it is important to define the concept of health informatics and to consider the background to the development of health informatics in the NHS as a whole and in the community setting in particular. The reasons why development in this area has been slower than elsewhere are discussed, and then the potential uses of information and the vision for health visiting are outlined and put into the wider context of the NHS as a whole. Finally, two examples of implementation of this vision are outlined.

The main theme of this chapter is to determine how information can best be used to improve patient care, both at the individual and population level. The White Paper, *The New NHS – Modern, Dependable* (Department of Health 1997a) states that 'better care for patients, and improved health for everyone depends on the availability of good information, accessible, when and where it is needed'.

Central to this development is the new NHS strategy, *Information for Health* (NHS Executive 1998b), which outlines the development path for information for the period 1998–2005. Frank Dobson, in the foreword to this document, describes the strategy as 'a radical programme to provide NHS staff with the most modern tools to improve the treatment and care of patients and to be able to narrow inequalities in health by identifying individuals, groups and neighbourhoods whose health care needs particular attention'. These business objectives are not only relevant to the NHS as a whole, but to health visitors in particular as they are in the unique position of carrying out all of these functions at a local level.

DEFINITIONS

What is health informatics? It can be described as 'the defining, storage, processing, analysing and retrieval of information, either in the form of data or knowledge' and encompasses the different aspects of people, skills, processes, systems and technology required to carry out these functions. Wyatt (1996) defines it as 'the term used to describe the science of information management in health care and its applications to support clinical research, decision-making and practice', and the Enabling People Programme (1997) as 'making effective use of information and technology for communication, decision-making and learning in health delivery and management'.

The kinds of activity encompassed by this view of health informatics include:

- audit
- management of resources
- self-management and professional development
- research
- communication among healthcare professionals/organisations
- using information for managing services
- using information for patient management
- decision support
- evidence-based clinical practice
- activity analysis
- monitoring quality of care
- epidemiology
- tracking patients
- development of clinical services.

The term 'health informatics' is synonymous with 'information management and technology' (IM&T) and the more recently used term 'information communication technology' (ICT). However, because of the way that IM&T has developed, in

that it has concentrated on the development of information systems and technology and has failed to address the issue of information management, it has not been seen as part of the domain of those primarily involved in the delivery and management of healthcare. As a result of this, health informatics tends to be a term with which clinicians can more readily identify, as it may be seen to be approaching the subject from the information management perspective, although in reality the content is the same.

However, IM&T should not be seen as an entity in itself but as an integral part of the delivery of healthcare services. According to the study of the Massachusetts Institute of Technology, *Management in the 90s*, in rapidly changing organisations it is essential that there is effective planning and integration of the strategies for business activity, human resources, and for information management, systems and supporting technology (Adams et al 1992). This concept is illustrated in Figure 3.1, and maintains that if any of the circles representing the three strategies shift in relation to the others there will be a consequent effect on the ability of the organisation to streamline, innovate or respond to change.

The process of strategic alignment is related to a conceptual framework. On the one side of the framework is the organisation's business domain

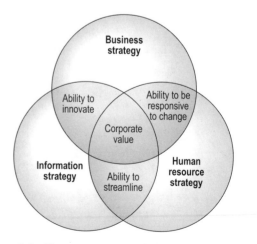

Figure 3.1 The strategic alignment model (redrawn with kind permission from Adams et al 1992)

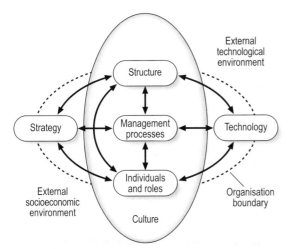

Figure 3.2 The Management in the 90s framework (redrawn with kind permission from Adams et al 1992)

and on the other side are the information systems, their management framework, IM&T specialist staff and supporting technology. In the middle of the framework sits the human resources domain reflecting the culture of the organisation (Fig. 3.2).

It is within this framework that the role of IM&T in healthcare, with particular reference to health visiting, will be considered.

BACKGROUND

The computing revolution which engulfed the health service during the early 1990s has had little impact on community services in general and health visiting in particular. The majority of the investment in IM&T has been in the acute sector – this may be partly due to the fact that community services are still seen as the 'Cinderella services', and therefore have not been able to accrue the enormous financial investment in IT that has happened in the acute sector, but also to the fact that it is much easier to implement IT systems in a single-site hospital than in community services. These are not only multi-site but also consist of large numbers of domiciliary workers such as health visitors and district nurses. An additional factor is undoubtedly the dearth of information systems available to support community services. However, this is

a cyclical argument, as with no commitment to investment in IM&T in this area there is little incentive for systems suppliers to develop these systems nor is there any clear national picture as to the sorts of system that are required. However, the fact that patient care in the community can be greatly improved by better information is well recognised: the Audit Commission (1997) estimated that improving information could save community trusts in England and Wales up to £30m annually through reduction in administrative support. A further £180m of clinical time could be released to invest in patient care. This represented an average avoidable cost of £200 000, plus £1.2m in clinical time that could be released in each trust annually.

The key principles that information should be person-based, shared, derived from operational systems and secure, together with the philosophy of the new strategy *Information for Health* (NHS Executive 1998b) of providing access to clinical information to support patient care and the development of the electronic patient record (EPR), are fundamental to all parts of the NHS and have real potential benefits for health visiting should they be embraced by the profession. In addition, the infrastructure that was developed and implemented as part of the first national IM&T strategy (Adams et al 1992) – the new NHS number, the use of national definitions such as read-coded clinical terms, and electronic communications via the NHS Net – provide the central building blocks on which to base any future developments.

However, the reluctance of community health professionals to accept this new technology is to some extent understandable, as it is obvious that their previous experience of computer technology has not enthused them. They have become fatigued by what is commonly termed 'feeding the beast', the process by which they have been required to complete diary sheets for input to the legacy systems for monitoring purposes and from which they have not received any feedback of useful information in return. This has made them feel that it has been a futile exercise and one that has used valuable time better spent on patient care. There are two issues identified here:

first, it is only by 'closing the loop', i.e. feeding back information to those who provide it, that the quality of the information improves; and second, the information itself needs to be of use to the health professional in supporting the delivery of clinical care. Such clinical information is currently mainly kept on the parent-held record rather than by the health visitors themselves. A further problem is the nature of the health visitor's record, which is fundamentally different from other health records that focus much more on illness and disease. The type of information kept about children under 5 is more about objectives for child stimulation and development, along with psychosocial and physical dimensions. Records also contain information about immunisation status, level of growth and development attainments and other factors relating to parenting skills.

THE NEW NATIONAL IM&T STRATEGY

As part of its modernisation plans, the government set out its information strategy for the modern NHS in the document *Information for Health: An Information Strategy for the Modern NHS 1998–2005* (NHS Executive 1998b). The purpose of the new strategy is to ensure that information is used to help patients receive the best possible care by enabling NHS professionals to have the information they need both to provide that care and to play their part in improving the public's health.

In order to do this, the strategy commits to:

- lifelong electronic health records for every person in the country
- round-the-clock on-line access to patient records and information about best clinical practice for all NHS clinicians
- genuine seamless care for patients through GPs, hospitals and community services sharing information across the NHS information highway
- the effective use of NHS resources by providing healthcare planners and managers with the information they need.

The key issues which the strategy supports are:

- tackling inequalities in health as outlined in the Green Paper *Our Healthier Nation* (Department of Health 1998a)
- a primary-care-led NHS
- collaboration between the NHS, local authorities and others in order to improve health
- preparation and evaluation of health improvement programmes
- development of primary care groups
- improving the quality of care and supporting clinical governance arrangements.

The information principles on which the strategy is based are:

- information will be person-based
- systems will be integrated
- management information will be derived from operational systems
- information will be shared across the NHS
- information will be secure and confidential.

These support the concept of 'integrated care' and are based on the fundamental premise that good clinical practice and service performance management will only flow if the strategy is focused on delivering the information required to support day-to-day clinical practice.

The strategy states that healthcare professionals need:

- fast, reliable and accurate information about the individual patients in their care
- fast, easy access to local and national knowledge bases that support the direct care of patients and clinical management decision-making
- access to information to support them in the evaluation of the care they give, underpinning clinical governance, planning and research, and helping with their continuing professional development

and that policy-makers and managers need to have good quality information to help them better target and use the resources deployed in the NHS and to improve the quality of life of patients and local communities.

Electronic records

Central to the strategy is a move towards electronic records, as they are likely to be more legible, accurate, safe, secure, available when required, and can be more readily and rapidly retrieved and communicated. Also, they can be integrated with other records and made available for audit, research and quality assurance purposes. The strategy clearly defines the terms electronic patient record (EPR) and electronic health record (EHR) – phrases often used to define similar concepts. The EPR describes the record of the periodic care provided mainly by one institution, whereas the EHR is used to describe the concept of a longitudinal record of a patient's health and healthcare – from cradle to grave. It is defined as a combination of information about patient contacts with primary healthcare and subsets of information associated with the outcomes of periodic care held in the EPRs, as illustrated in Figure 3.3.

This model can be seen to be flawed, however, as it represents the primary care record as an EHR when in fact it is an EPR in its own right. An alternative model is shown in Figure 3.4, in which the EHR is seen to be made up of all of the constituent parts and data can flow in both directions so that all NHS providers can both provide data for and view the EHR.

Whether the EHR is real (i.e. is held centrally in a data warehouse) or virtual, in that the various components are kept by the supplying organisa-

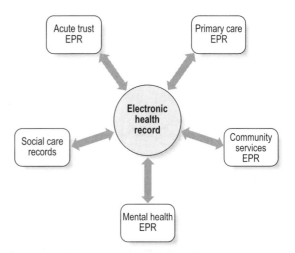

Figure 3.4 Electronic health record: an alternative view

tions but can be viewed by means of an interface, is still under debate. Regardless of how the data are to be held, it is essential that healthcare professions agree the nature and content of the component data sets so that a consistent model of EHRs can be constructed. The unique NHS number will play a crucial role in facilitating linkage and in improving confidentiality in data transfers and the use of data for audit and research purposes.

The main use of the electronic health record is for providing routine patient care, and one of its main benefits is seen as improving the integration of care across organisational boundaries. In addition, aggregated anonymised subsets of the EHRs can be used for other purposes, as shown in Figure 3.5.

For EHRs to benefit patient care it is essential to create and maintain accurate, complete, relevant, up-to-date accessible datasets. However, currently there is no agreement on either the content, structure or potential use of individual patient summary records.

From its inception the NHS has pursued the goal of seamless care. In most aspects it has been hampered by the sheer volume of communications about patients, coupled with the number of organisations and professional boundaries involved.

Where co-ordination and communication between different parts fall down, the consequence

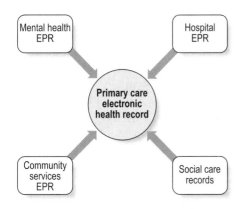

Figure 3.3 *Information for Health*: electronic health record (redrawn with kind permission from NHS Executive 1998b)

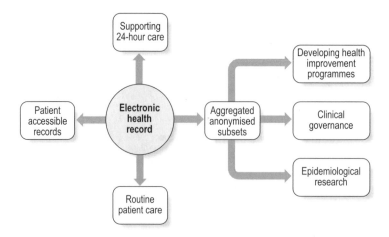

Figure 3.5   Use of the electronic health record (redrawn with kind permission from NHS Executive 1998b)

is inevitably poorer care. Considerable time costs are involved in chasing up information and resolving problems caused by incomplete information. Developing EHRs will facilitate the shift from profession-specific and institutional records to integrated lifelong person-based records. As a minimum, co-ordination of care should improve across the following organisational boundaries:

- within the full primary care team
- between hospitals and general practice
- between health and social care.

Accessing primary care data

Developing these new sources of data will take some time and an urgent issue for health authorities and primary care groups is the relative lack of access they normally have to information about primary and community care. At present much of the Korner data is of little value – knowing how many patients actually received a particular service is not the same as knowing that patients who need the service actually received it.

'The case to abandon the development of a single episodic MDS [minimum data set] for community health services is strong' (NHS Executive 1998b). An equally urgent concern of community-based clinicians is the substantial amount of time taken up by recording data for central statistical returns that does not flow

naturally from the care process and is of little or no value to their treatment of individuals or for retrospective evaluation. There is little evidence that the collection of Korner data in community services offers managers anything useful for gauging either value for money or effectiveness in community services.

The successful development of the EPR and EHR requires a common coded clinical vocabulary to facilitate reliable and accurate electronic communication of clinical information and enable consistent activity analysis. The NHS has made considerable investment in the Read Codes and the subsequent Clinical Terms project to produce version 3, which extends the vocabulary from a medical to a clinical thesaurus. This development of the Read Codes as the NHS standard terminology is supported by the clinical professional bodies, including the Royal College of Nursing, the Royal College of Midwives, the Community Practitioners and Health Visitors Association (through the Strategic Advisory Group for Nursing Information Systems – SAGNIS). The group, which was set up to develop the coding for nursing, midwifery and health visiting, produced their final report in August 1995, although, like the development of all of the Read Codes, development will be ongoing. The report nevertheless provides the basis for the development of an EPR for health visiting.

Defined aggregations of clinical terms, agreed at national and local levels as appropriate, are also required to ensure the development of good quality data for statistical use. Healthcare resource groups (HRGs) and health benefit groups (HBGs) are useful tools, but to date they have been developed mainly in the acute inpatient care setting. Healthcare resource groups are used to group together similar conditions that have similar resource implications. Community HRGs are defined as 'descriptions of care given by community professionals' and 'activity is described in groupings which are comparable in terms of costs and resources used' (NHS Executive 1997). However, this may need revisiting, as their groupings are at a very high level (e.g. individual case management). Within this there is likely to be wide variation in the amount of resources required, depending on the circumstances.

As NHS clinicians address the obligation continually to review and improve personal effectiveness through evidence-based practice and clinical audit, they face several problems:

- the variable quality and reliability of information
- a dearth of local clinical informatics expertise
- a lack of personal keyboard skills
- pressure on their time.

The vision

The vision that is proposed is not new. The Chief Nursing Officer and Director of Nursing at the Department of Health, in her address to the British Computer Society Nursing Specialist Group, spoke of the importance for strategy, organisational structure and information technology to be managed together (Moores 1991) and at the same conference the following year stated that 'the integration of compatible and accessible data is essential for the future' and that 'a workforce capable of using information to manage both clinical care and the nursing resource is essential' (Moores 1992).

These three ideals – the full integration of information alongside strategic and organisational development, the accessibility and compatibility of data regardless of source and the ability to use information effectively to improve patient care and service delivery – still form the basis for the vision, with the addition of the use of the NHS Net, the 'information superhighway', to provide a private network with speed, reliability and security for the transfer of clinical information, links to other NHS sites and organisations from the desktop, and access to the Internet and sites containing rich sources of health information (including the National Electronic Library for Health, which is currently being set up).

In the not too distant future, all health visitors should have access to a computer at their main place of work, which will allow:

- use of e-mail as a quick and efficient means of communication to liaise with other professionals, e.g. to inform a GP of concerns about a particular client
- use of an electronic appointment system to make appointments for the client with self and other health professionals across organisation boundaries
- easy and rapid access to current and standardised guidelines
- access to evidence-based data
- continual update of knowledge by access to electronic textbooks and journals
- input of clinical information to support client care at point of delivery
- the use of this clinical database in different views to produce information for other purposes such as management information, rather than collecting it separately
- use of an up-to-date multidisciplinary information base to inform programmes of care
- continual monitoring of processes and outcomes at the individual and caseload level
- automatic aggregation of clinical information across the service for audit purposes.

Once the information needed is available and the benefits can be demonstrated, this will provide the basis for a business case to support the investment required to allow health visitors to be provided with the equipment to enable them to access this type of information in their clients' homes.

USES OF INFORMATION IN HEALTH VISITING

Managing clients

Most client-related activity is recorded on the health visitor's diary sheet, but these sheets are often handed in at the end of the week and used for monitoring purposes rather than directly to support the provision of support and care. Health visitors often keep their own records of visits, but these are not generally shared nor in a format in which they could be used for other purposes such as monitoring activity against the agreed care plan or monitoring the outcome of interventions.

Measuring effectiveness

One of the main challenges for health visitors is to demonstrate that their work is effective. It is widely acknowledged that there is a lack of information about outcome and therefore about the effectiveness of interventions and different forms of service provision. Demonstrating the effectiveness of health visitors is not easy as many of their interventions are nonclinical; the whole range of input from health education to general advice and support to mothers cannot easily be measured by tangible indicators but some of it can and it is these areas that can form a starting point to collect evidence on effectiveness. The use of quantitative measures such as the Edinburgh Postnatal Depression Scale (EPDS), sleep diaries, centile charts, and measurements such as attitude Likert scales and environmental/ social vulnerability scales are not only useful assessment tools in their own right but also provide good measures of the effectiveness of interventions at both individual and group level to demonstrate the overall effectiveness of the role of the health visitor.

Managing caseload

As part of the Putting the NHS Number to Work programme, Walsall used the new NHS number to identify the active patient caseload in one GP practice that had a high turnover of patients. It was found that, while patients were removed from the GP's list when they changed to a new GP, there was no mechanism in place for notifying the health visitors so that the patients could be removed from their list. This meant that health visitors wasted time visiting clients who were no longer at that address, but perhaps more importantly were not able to hand over to the new health visitor. There was also the problem of health visitors' lists containing both active and nonactive clients. If at the individual patient level the care plans could be stored, and activity monitored against these plans, then at the end of one intervention a further intervention could be instigated if necessary. This would provide one way of distinguishing between active and nonactive clients.

Supporting clinical governance

A First Class Service (Department of Health 1998b) highlighted the fundamental importance of improving the quality of care throughout all areas of the NHS. This is because performance management processes designed simply to target outliers will eventually eliminate the extremes of poor performance but may not improve mediocre or average performance, and will therefore fail to benefit the vast majority of patients. There is another aspect of this: simple identification of outliers is a very simplistic assessment of quality – once identified, a 'drill down' procedure into the underlying data is required to explore possible reasons for being in that position, particular aspects of the community to which the data are referring, interventions that may themselves be more time-consuming or expensive but that may in fact relieve the burden from another area of the service. A more comprehensive database would allow these other possibilities to be explored.

Continual improvement of clinical service quality across the NHS must be supported by information on current comparative effectiveness and outcomes. It also requires a culture among clinical staff where the obligation on individuals to assess personal performance continually is

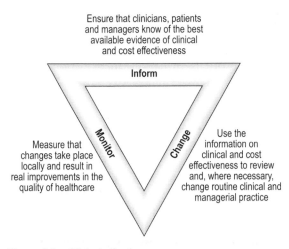

Ensure that clinicians, patients and managers know of the best available evidence of clinical and cost effectiveness

Inform

Monitor

Change

Measure that changes take place locally and result in real improvements in the quality of healthcare

Use the information on clinical and cost effectiveness to review and, where necessary, change routine clinical and managerial practice

Figure 3.6 Clinical effectiveness

accepted as a natural and important element of being a professional. This is an area with which health visitors can be seen to be already conversant in terms of their reflective practice; however, what they have not developed is a culture of developing the information flows to support it in a coherent way.

Implementing a framework for clinical governance requires a comprehensive programme of quality improvement such as clinical audit, evidence-based practice and processes for monitoring clinical care using effectiveness information and clinical records systems (Fig. 3.6).

To achieve this, information must be drawn from:

- local clinical audit data
- national comparative data
- local care pathways and clinical protocols
- national best practice guidelines
- National Institute for Clinical Excellence evidence
- international research evidence.

This requires statistical data to be linked to textual reference material.

Reference material

The rapid expansion of the use of electronic media has revolutionised the storage and ex-change of information, and access to the World Wide Web provides vast amounts of material available directly on to the desktop. In relation to the professional knowledge base, it is growing ever faster, and clinicians and managers find it impossible to keep abreast of the vast amounts of information available.

There is a need to critically appraise the growing body of medical literature and evidence to ensure that clinicians receive fast and convenient access to appropriate knowledge bases to provide real-time support to their care of individual patients.

There is now an opportunity to begin to develop from scratch an NHS-accredited National Electronic Library for Health (NELH). Once placed here, the material may be regarded as 'official'. The National Institute for Clinical Excellence (NICE), established by *The New NHS* (Department of Health 1997a), has a remit to 'produce and disseminate clinical guidelines based on relevant evidence'. NICE will therefore be one of the major sources of accredited material placed in the NELH.

Senior managers in the NHS must lead their organisations into the information age 'from the front' (NHS Executive 1998b). They too have a need for access to up-to-date accredited information and so an 'NHS Information Zone' containing on-line reference material for the NHS management community is also planned.

Information for Health (NHS Executive 1998b) states that 'the NHS must have accurate and reliable data to support:

- local clinical governance
- National Service Frameworks, local care pathways and clinical protocols
- Health Improvement Programmes
- the national 'Framework for Assessing Performance'.

Risk management

Risk analysis can be defined from a number of perspectives. The strategic guidance on effective use of information to support the management and delivery of nursing and midwifery care (NHS Executive 1995a) states that the management of risk can be broken down into four stages; identification, analysis, control and cost.

- *Identification*: What can go wrong?
- *Analysis*:
  - How will it go wrong?
  - How severely?
  - How frequently?
  - How likely?
- *Control*:
  - What changes can be made to prevent it?
  - What will reduce the effect?
- *Cost*: How will any loss be paid for?

Information is required to manage risk effectively, but collecting too many data, or the wrong data, or not using them, wastes resources and time.

Supporting national service frameworks

Gathering the best evidence of clinical and cost-effectiveness and relating that to the views of service users to determine the best ways of configuring the provision of particular services is an important new approach that relies on information.

While technology is not a solution in itself, in some circumstances it will enable change, e.g. through the introduction of systems to collect and audit data along a care pathway and share information between organisations.

Developing local care pathways and clinical protocols

There is a need for those involved in planning and managing services to have ready access to a wide range of other information to support the best use of the national evidence base. Locally, there needs to be agreed guidance on service delivery in the form of local care pathways and protocols that can be accessed on an internal 'Intranet'.

Health improvement programmes

The three major functions of health improvement programmes are health needs assessment for a population, planning interventions to address those needs and monitoring their outcome. These are distinctly similar to those outlined by the Public Health Information Specification Project (PHIS), which was commissioned by the National Health Service Management Executive to develop the public health aspect of the common basic specification (CBS) data model. This project produced a model comprising three views. In the functional view, health needs assessment, intervention planning to address identified health needs, and outcome monitoring are disaggregated into their elementary processes (Fig. 3.7).

The other two views are the entity model, which shows the data used and produced by the processes and the relationship between the data, and the behavioural view, the sequence in which processes may be carried out. There is an infinite variety of behavioural views since processes may be continuously reiterated, in any order. The whole model can be seen as a planning cycle in which activities can be continuously influenced by feedback of information and, as such, its use enhances the effectiveness and efficiency with which resources are used.

The New NHS and *Our Healthier Nation* (and other recent initiatives) have created a substantial information agenda for the collation and inter-

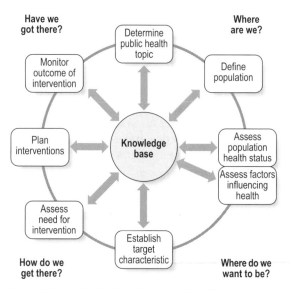

Figure 3.7 Public Health Information Specification model (redrawn from Wain & Holton 1993)

pretation of information to support the local HImP and the commissioning priorities of primary care groups in identifying the needs and measuring the health of different local communities to support the provision of more effective healthcare. All of which are an important part of the public health function, so it is not surprising that this model remains relevant.

Health needs assessment

The public health function is also central to the role of the health visitor. Health needs assessment has been part of their role since the new syllabus for health visitors was introduced in 1965 and they have become increasingly proficient in the development of community and caseload profiles that include 'bottom-up' approaches to the epidemiological assessment of need. 'Through their contribution to the delivery of local health care and by the application of epidemiological, psychosocial and social science principles and knowledge, they act both as community participants and local researchers' (Robinson & Elkan 1996). Their broad knowledge base and their intimate knowledge of the local community makes their contribution invaluable and complementary to the 'top-down' approach to health needs assessment carried out at district health authority level. Of particular value is the fact that health visitors are in a position not only to identify needs from a professional viewpoint but also to engage their clients in the process of negotiating care packages to meet their individual needs and to amass collective views on clients' perceptions of their health needs. 'The communication skills which many nurses, midwives and health visitors acquire during their professional education can equip them to participate in consultation with groups and individuals about their health needs' (NHS Executive 1993).

The national framework for assessing performance

Accurate and timely data are essential for management purposes, if actions are to be appropriate and evidence-based. The reasons for poor data quality are:

- a backlash against the collection of information that supports only management needs
- a failure to feed back useful analyses to those from whom the information is collected
- no incentives to collect good quality data and in some cases perverse incentives to provide inaccurate and untimely data to avoid censure for poor performance.

The introduction of the national framework for assessing performance focusing on service quality and effectiveness offers the opportunity to create a new attitude in the NHS to information quality, especially if:

- a responsive and credible benchmarking service can be delivered locally, to support clinical governance and health planning, that is respected and valued by the clinical community
- there are inclusive processes for local staff, especially clinicians, to own the information and make active use of it to promote local clinical improvements.

The knowledge base

All the above functions require a vast knowledge base to support them. The new IM&T strategy states the government's commitment to providing information at a national level but there is a pressing need for information to be collected locally. There is much information already available that has been collected by individual health visitors, but a local strategy needs to be developed for making it available to all.

The knowledge base will be used to inform decisions made in the various ongoing developments, and these will feed back into the knowledge base, making it continually richer. Figure 3.8 shows the flow of information.

The community information agenda

There is no doubt that the new information strategy is ambitious for all parts of the NHS, but nowhere more so than for community and primary care. The inadequacies of health systems to support community health staff have been apparent

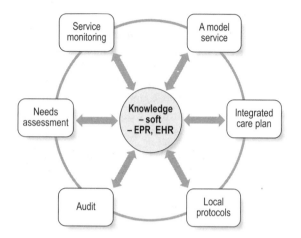

Figure 3.8   The knowledge wheel

for many years and, as stated in *Information for Health* (NHS Executive 1998b), 'Even without the organisational changes signalled in the new NHS, the development of integrated primary community care systems would have been sensible. The new NHS proposals make this inevitable.'

The agenda therefore is to:

• develop a knowledge base to support all aspects of care provision
• modernise primary care information systems
• integrate primary and community care information systems
• use information captured in operational clinical systems to provide secondary data flow
• develop primary and community care effectiveness indicators for local and national performance management
• develop the means to extract the information needed automatically from primary and community care information systems to meet the needs of the national framework for assessing performance.

MAKING INFORMATION WORK – IMPLEMENTATION ISSUES FOR HEALTH VISITING

Information framework

The first building block in providing appropriate

information and information systems for health visiting is to agree a robust information framework that adequately describes the range and complexity of services provided and supports the development of a health visiting patient record, which will form an integral part of a multiagency child health record and support a cradle-to-grave electronic health record. The framework will need to contain elements that can be recorded consistently by different professionals so that information will be valid and comparable irrespective of where or by whom it was recorded. *Information for Health* and the discussion paper on casemix groupings for community services both view information collection as focused upon that needed to support a full clinical record supporting clinical service delivery and used by clinicians as the prime information source. Specific extracts and aggregation of information from these records will be used for costing, planning and commissioning (Fig. 3.9).

The Community Health Care Resource Group's consultation document (April 1997) used the four principles of health visiting underpinning all health visitor activity – the search for health needs, the stimulation of the awareness of health, the influence of policies affecting health and the

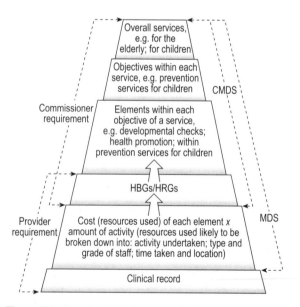

Figure 3.9   Levels of detail for commissioners and providers

facilitation of health enhancing activities – and from these identified the following groupings and elements:

Groupings:
A. Individual case management
B. Assessment
C. Health education/health promotion
D. A programme of monitoring individual health and development with associated health promotion
E. Parenting/caring skills
F. Child protection – on the register
G. Protection of individuals or families at risk
H. Counselling/psychological support including bereavement
I. Management of diagnosed condition/problem
J. Nutritional guidance
K. Public health function

Core elements of health visiting that underpin their activities:

- Advocacy/empowerment
- Caseload management
- Clinical supervision
- Formal communication
- Interagency working
- Liaison
- Management
- Prioritisation of work and workloads
- Professional development
- Record keeping
- Referrals
- Reflective practice
- Research and Development
- Systems management and management
- Teaching of other grades and professions.

The exercise was focused specifically on uni-disciplinary care, although it was acknowledged that it could be applied to multi-disciplinary care. It aimed to include all activities, including those that were not necessarily patient related. It was acknowledged that there was a need to identify the key activity where several activities occurred as part of a single contact. This issue, however, is not new to health visiting and, although the need to identify the key activity or service recipient is similarly essential to ensuring comparable

and consistent data collection, it has not been an area that has been successfully addressed. The model described in the Community Health Care Resource Group's consultation document was very complex. Each of the 11 groupings identified was defined and a range of activities included in the grouping was identified or details of the tools used were given. Items identified as a grouping can also occur at a lower level as an activity under another grouping heading. For example, 'assessment' is identified as a grouping in itself but also as an activity in six other groupings. Although the model reflects the range of health visiting services, it is perhaps too complex to be achieved in one move from existing information recording. It relies heavily on concepts that were proposed within the Community Minimum Data Set. This has not been implemented, possibly because of issues of user acceptability and ability of existing systems to collect the information. In addition this model has not resolved many of the issues regarding clear identification of the key activity and key recipient of the service that currently cause difficulties in collecting high-quality information.

The model for deriving information indicated by *Information for Health* proposes that the core building block would be the EHR. By means of common record structures and headings and use of standard clinical terms, information could be derived that was standardised and comparable. However the current situation for health visiting seems to be a long way from achieving this, even in a paper-based system.

To make progress it may be advantageous to begin by defining a simpler model than that identified in the Community Health Care Resource Group proposals and Community Minimum Data Set, while incorporating some of the features of these proposals that clinicians find easy to apply with some consistency and set about implementing them. This will ensure that health visitors will have more confidence in discussing and owning informatics issues and the quality of existing data will begin to improve. This must form a safer platform from which to embark on more ambitious information developments in the future.

What information to collect

The complexity of the health visitor's workload results in lack of consistency when trying to describe the services they deliver. A distinction can be made between the generic basic package of care, comprising advice, surveillance and immunisation, that is delivered to every child and the additional services that may also be required relating to special needs, behaviour management, child protection, etc. However in practice elements of two or more different care packages may be delivered as part of an integrated care plan during a single contact. There are differences in how this information is currently recorded on diary sheets, which can result in double counting in terms of contacts. This complexity is also mirrored in attributing the recipient of the contact. Although a specific child may be the reason for a visit, advice may still be given even if the child is not present, e.g. if a child is exhibiting a specific behaviour problem that the health visitor feels is related to parental management or behaviour. There is often difference of opinion among health visitors as to whether the contact is attributed to the adult, the child or both. Although data definitions allow recording of a proxy contact this often does little to illumine the decision regarding recording of contacts. Advice may also be given regarding another child or to an adult relative or even a visiting friend. These opportunistic contacts are not always recorded in the same way by different health visitors, even those working within the same trust. Even where definitive written guidance is provided to ensure consistency of data collection this is often not felt by professionals to be helpful as it does not accord with how they view their service provision.

The introduction of the parent-held record, often known as 'the Red Book' meant that the records became the joint responsibility of the parent and the professional. Parents were encouraged to make entries in the book and it was envisaged that it would be taken along to GP visits and that the GP would make relevant entries, although there has been a reluctance among some GPs to participate in this joint record-keeping. Most of the information held here, except for the child health surveillance record, is not replicated elsewhere. The health visitor only keeps additional information where there are specific concerns about child protection issues or where it is necessary to retain information about other family members. The only other record kept by the health visitor is what is known as the 'tracer card', which contains minimal details of care pathway contacts. This lack of uniformity and consistency in the manual records supporting health visitors is another factor contributing to the difficulty in providing good information to support service delivery.

This confusion is frequently mirrored in the provision of computerised information systems for health visitors. Typically the generic surveillance and immunisation elements are supported by a version of the national Child Health System. These were often the earliest systems implemented and therefore the information collected on them was often extended as far as possible to capture other elements of the service. In many trusts a community information system was introduced at a later date in addition to the Child Health System. This type of system would be structured in line with data manual guidance to provide information to support Korner returns. This entails a distinction between advice and support contacts, which are related to individuals, and health education and surveillance contacts, which are related to specific groups and tend not to be related to individuals. However the fact that both types of contact are frequently fused within a single time-slot has led to considerable disparity in the information provided on these returns and recorded on the systems. The advent of GP fundholding caused a further twist when it became apparent that health education and surveillance contacts for a specific practice not delivered at the practice premises were not identifiable unless assigned to an individual client, i.e. as part of the advice and support recording mechanism.

Methods of data collection

Another problem is the fact that health visiting

services are typically delivered in the client's home, a busy baby clinic or GP surgery. Although some community trusts have gone some way to provide appropriate technology, such as palm top computers, to allow use of information in the workplace, frequently this level of investment has not been possible. Most trusts have provided clinic-based computer access, with information input by clerical or clinical staff. Both approaches have their defenders. Clerical input is seen to be more cost-effective, can ensure that information is recorded in a fairly consistent way and can be more timely and accurate than input by less computer-literate clinicians. However, as the need to record more clinical information to develop a full health record including assessments and care plans develops, the use of clerical staff becomes less appropriate. Clinical input can improve ownership, data quality (and quantity) and the use of information. However this may not be an automatic result of installing computers for use by clinicians, as without significant staff support and organisational development programmes clinicians may revert back to using manual information sources. Birth books, clinic books and address books are often retained in tandem with computerised systems and are often maintained and consulted as the prime information source, to the detriment of computerised data quality.

Information systems

There are major decisions to be made by community trusts as to the development of information systems to support the collection of clinical information. The future of legacy systems such as the Child Health System will be decided nationally but in the interim the solution may be to create a data warehouse linked to existing systems. This would allow incremental development of front-end interfaces and tools for data manipulation.

The need to integrate community and primary care systems has already been recognised as part of the new structure of the NHS, but there are many GP systems on the market as well as many different configurations of service delivery. Although some GP system suppliers have developed community service modules, this may not in reality be the best way forward. It may be more beneficial for systems to be developed to meet the needs of the specific professional groups, with interfaces being created that will enable them to be seamlessly linked. This would have several advantages. It would allow information to be more readily available to all the relevant teams, some of which are not primary-care-based. For example, although it is clearly beneficial to have the information within the primary care record for services that are part of primary healthcare, there is a risk that for other services provided by community trusts, such as supporting children with special educational needs or district specialist services, linking this information directly to GP systems would mean that it was not available to those needing it. It would also allow the system to capture information for the total population served by the community trust rather than only for the practice population and would also allow the records to move with patients if they changed GP.

The most important criterion for the development of this new generation of systems is that they should enable multi-disciplinary clinical information to be available to the health professional at the point of contact with the client. The only way forward is for clinicians and IM&T specialists to work together in their development to ensure that everyone's needs are met. Health visitors need to be very actively involved in this process.

CASE STUDIES

The following two case studies demonstrate two different approaches that community trusts have taken incorporating IM&T into health visiting practice.

Case Study 1 – Southmead Health Services NHS Trust

This case study is reported in *Case Studies of the Successful Use of Clinical Information by Practising Clinicians*, produced by the Enabling People Programme. The objective of the study was to manage clinical information to support clinical practice. Their starting point was similar to that found in most community health trusts – practitioners inputting information willingly 'but irritated and exasperated with the resulting reports'. The approach taken was to use a model to link technology to the management of clinical information. In setting up the project, they posed the following questions:

- How can the management of clinical information be more effectively linked to technology?
- How can a coherent approach be developed to give consistency to the service?
- How can strategic objectives be realised at field level, maximising the use of technology?

Their starting point was also similar to that of many other community trusts, in that computer codes were numerous and ambiguous and levels of intervention and outcomes of care were not recorded on the system. As a result any useful analysis of the retrieved data was impossible.

The project determined the following requirements:

- a theoretical framework to give structure
- a model to identify levels of interventions (primary, secondary and tertiary), to establish trends and match them to resource availability
- technology to track and record clinical input and outcomes of care
- in the longer term, that the system be used for, for example, 'cost of quality' exercises and audits of protocols used
- 'cost of care' could be developed from the system.

They reviewed the systems that were being used internationally and chose Neuman's systems model. This, it was felt, created a common language between clinicians and technology experts, allowing both perspectives to develop at the same time while staying in touch with the demands and limitations of the other's remit and resources.

Data was collected from two perspectives: first, the assessed need, carried out on an annual basis, and second, the day-to-day recording of client activity. As a result of this, they were able to monitor:

- day-on-day clinical input and levels of intervention required based on assessment of need
- subject matter covered
- length of contact
- grade of staff.

The project, however, was only funded as a pilot for 1 year, and has now been completed. Further funding has to be found for the work to continue.

Case Study 2 – Walsall Community Trust

Walsall has taken a very different approach, in that the information project has been integrated into the Trust's overall development plans. In 1998, a small project group involving health visiting managers and health visitors was set up to improve the quality of information available for health visiting staff and managers. It specifically addressed the following issues:

- development of an information framework to reflect caseload, complexity and casemix
- a systems analysis
- changing the culture
- developing the infrastructure.

Information framework

The first step was to review the information requirements; clinicians identified that their key requirements were to record information that was simple to use, consistent across practitioners and measured workload effectively. The model proposed was a simplified version of proposals within the Community Minimum Data Set and Community Health Care Resource Group models. Separate episodes of care would be set up for the same individual relating to the different care programmes they were receiving. Each of these programmes could then be assigned a weighting based on the typical care package associated with it. Separate programmes would only be set up when a clinical care protocol had been defined by the health visiting service to support it. This would ensure that care programmes were clearly distinguishable by clinical staff and thus the sophistication of the information recorded would develop as their ability to identify boundaries between types of care developed. This should address the current difficulties encountered in ensuring a common and consistent recording system.

The programmes would distinguish between standard care programmes for the client groups – children, mothers, adult and elderly. In addition, there would be additional care programmes for areas such as the child protection register, behaviour/parenting, specific problem/special need, and so on (Fig. 3.10).

Programmes of care can be ordered concurrently, as with Client A, or successively, as with Clients B and C. The model also attempts to identify workload measures across the full caseload by means of the weightings for each care pro-

gramme. Historically, dependency measures and the information frameworks for health visiting have focused on child and maternal health and have not provided adequate mechanisms to measure the increasing workload, particularly with the elderly.

This framework, therefore, is a local attempt to identify an information model that reflects current clinical practice and protocols, is achievable within the short term and will form a bridge to more sophisticated information models. The model is capable of identifying care packages delivered by a single discipline but can also be developed so that these form an integral part of multi-disciplinary programmes.

Systems analysis

Having formalised an information framework it is then possible to undertake a systems analysis to identify how this can be implemented. Often, changes can be made to existing systems that will allow some piloting of the framework and enable users to identify gaps and pitfalls that will be invaluable in specifying a replacement system. In Walsall the group has reviewed and rationalised the existing coding structures to reflect the information framework as far as possible. The number of codes has been reduced in an effort to get consistent recording and improve data quality. A decision was taken by the clinicians that every intervention should be recorded on the community system so that the client summary represents a complete electronic patient record. A specific code was used to indicate that full details of the intervention could be accessed through the Child Health System module. In addition, a means of recording the programme of care information has also been identified.

The review of the computerised information formed part of a wider review of information sources and information flows. As a result of this, duplications were identified and awareness and training sessions have been undertaken to ensure that uniform working practices are agreed and duplicate systems such as birth books and address books are removed.

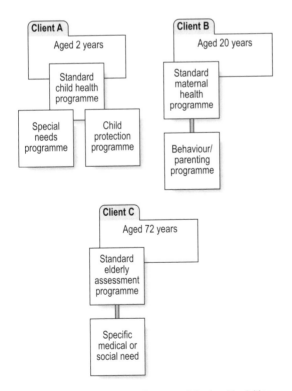

Figure 3.10 An information framework for health visiting

Changing the culture

To achieve the changes outlined, various aspects of the organisational culture will need to change. The most significant changes include:

- developing competence and confidence in contributing to information issues
- developing understanding and ownership of the information framework and information systems (computer and manual)
- developing familiarity with and confidence in computers as a prime source of information
- developing willingness to change and ownership of the change process.

Walsall has undertaken a project, 'Making Information Work for You', to address these cultural issues. This project is led by the chief executive and specific resources were identified that enabled five clinicians to be seconded for 1 day per week to undertake specific information projects in their clinical areas. Two of the project co-ordinators are from a health visiting background. There has also been an Information Week at five sites across the Trust where staff could view poster displays, attend presentations and discussion groups on key information issues and every person attending was able to fill in a User Needs Questionnaire and a Training Needs Questionnaire. In addition, they received a copy of the locally produced booklet *Working with Computers – What You Need to Know*, which included guidance on confidentiality and security issues. Clinical staff were also able to identify areas of interest for them. As a result, clinicians are now much more proactive in identifying information requirements and the support they require from information services and a large number of projects have been initiated by clinical staff. The cultural change has required additional resources but once begun seems to develop its own momentum.

Infrastructure – making life easy

To achieve the vision of information being generated from an EPR and sustaining a culture where clinicians use computers as part of their clinical toolkit requires considerable investment

from a community trust. However, progress can be achieved by adopting a project-based, incremental approach. Walsall Community Trust has started on a small scale by providing more PCs at clinic bases so that clinical staff can use them to support their basic caseload management and have information accessible for office-based queries, checking addresses, etc. The trust has also worked with other members of the natural community, including the health authority and the hospitals trust to provide access to community and hospital information systems from several GP practices so that information relating to health visiting is available to practice staff who have system security clearance and to the health visitor. Health visitors who wish to develop their use of computers have been trained in data input and report generation and are also being developed as local information champions. This approach has developed the use of computerised information within the workplace and is an essential precursor to establishing effective use of portable information systems.

To ease the burden on clinical and clerical staff and to shift the emphasis to use of information rather than 'feeding the beast', a successful pilot of bar-code input of clinical activity has been completed. Scanning of manual diary sheets is being piloted and this will free clerical time to provide better information feedback to clinical staff. Obviously, these are only interim steps along the way and will not provide clinical staff with clinical information, including assessment and care plans in the client's home. However, they will help develop a better understanding of the benefits of using information and the necessary confidence and commitment to make use of portable technology likely to be much more effective. This will be the next step. In addition, this type of approach will enable the Trust to develop a system specification for use within the next 12–18 months that is owned by clinical staff who feel they have been fully involved in the process.

CONCLUSIONS

It can be seen that the new national IM&T

strategy is an ambitious one, particularly for community trusts, which for many reasons have lagged behind other areas of the organisation. However, in some ways this can be seen as a challenge, as they are able to start with a clean sheet of paper. This has to be an advantage for health visitors, as more recently there has been a definite move to involve clinicians from the outset and this gives a wonderful opportunity for them to set the agenda and make sure that the systems work for them, that data collection is manageable and that access to the information they need is available where and when they need it, whether in the client's home or in remote clinics. By making this information readily available to them, data quality will improve and so will patient care.

ACKNOWLEDGEMENTS

We would like to thank Maureen Chaudhry and Juli Wilson, health visitors at Walsall Community Health Trust, and Judith LeMaistre, IM&T Programme Director at Gloucestershire Health Authority, for their comments on previous drafts of this chapter.

4

Models of specialist and higher level health visiting

Ros Carnwell

INTRODUCTION

The use of models has followed a different course in health visiting from in nursing. Nursing theorists provided the impetus for nursing to define itself more clearly in conceptual and academic terms. Despite difficulties in the application of models to nursing practice (Kenny 1993), the use of models has provided the nursing profession with a wealth of opportunity to debate its professional development. Most nursing models do not 'fit' health visiting practice, because of such fundamental concepts as self-care deficit (Orem 1985) or disequilibrium (Roy & Andrews 1991). Such concepts arguably imply a state of ill-health rather than health, which is irreconcilable with the health emphasis of health visiting. One of the few nursing models that fits well with health visiting (Peplau 1952) provides an ideal framework for understanding the transition of the health visitor–client relationship, but is limited to individual work with families, rather than communities.

The search for suitable models for both nursing and health visiting has not been helped by ambiguity in language. Robinson (1992), for example, argues vehemently that nursing uses such terms as 'model' and 'paradigm' inappropriately. McFarlane (1986) too, comments on the inconsistent terminology and convoluted language used in discussions of nursing models.

Health visiting, then, has probably been wise to reject the drive to use nursing models, most of which would require to be adapted for health visiting. The use of a single model might also reduce complex human characteristics and situations into something that can be conceived within the components of a model. Health visiting does, however, need to consider ways of demonstrating and evaluating its activities. The models discussed in this chapter focus on two important components of health visiting – health promotion and public health. Community work, rather than work with individuals is, therefore, the predominant focus of this chapter. Prior to discussing health promotion and public health models in relation to health visiting, it is necessary first to distinguish between concepts, theories and models.

CONCEPTS, THEORIES AND MODELS – DEFINITIONS AND DEVELOPMENT

Concepts can be simply described as labels ascribed to images and objects. Britt (1997) likens concepts to blocks in a Lego set but argues that, unlike the tangible building blocks, concepts are elusive, changeable and tentative. Labelling such elusive concepts fulfils the purpose of categorising them in order to make sense of experience (Carnwell 1998). Concepts are categorised by grouping things together that have properties in common and separating things that have different properties in common (Britt 1997). The concept of culture, for example, can be derived by grouping together such properties as beliefs, attitudes, norms, religious practices and mores. Properties such as skin colour, stature and other biological characteristics would be separated out, as these are properties associated with race rather than culture. Properties associated with culture and properties associated with race could then be linked to each other to allow deep understanding of complex issues. This linking together of concepts is fundamental to the development of models.

Models can be defined as: 'organizing devices for a continuing, explicit dialogue between multiple sources of data and assumptions … models summarize what we have learned about the dynamics of phenomena in patterns woven from

different contexts, in different historical periods and with different individuals and social groups' (Britt 1997, p. 2).

Britt (1997) also distinguishes between four different types of model: descriptive, interpretative, explanatory and predictive. These categories are cognisant with Akinsanya et al's (1994) view that models describe, explain and predict practice. The capacity of models to fulfil these functions is derived from their development. Most models emerge either from empirical research findings or from the literature. The different types of model could emerge from either qualitative or quantitative findings, or indeed a combination of the two (Britt 1997). A rich description of a culture could, for example, form the basis of a descriptive model. An interpretative model might attempt to make sense of some of the relationships between concepts in more detail. An explanatory model would look for causes of phenomena, such as why certain concepts, rather than others, emerged as important and whether there were causal links between concepts. A predictive model would attempt to anticipate whether the same phenomena would emerge in the same way in the future or in different circumstances.

Although models tend to be theoretical and research-based, they also have utility value. Models help practitioners to organise their thoughts and justify how and what they do (McClymont et al 1991). Moreover, according to Fawcett (1992), there is a reciprocal relationship between conceptual models and practice. Models guide practice, for example, while practice provides evidence for the credibility of the model.

Developing models also guides theory development. Britt (1997) views models as more explicit than theories as they 'tentatively specify what variables we believe are important, our current thinking about what their natures are, and how we believe they are related to other variables in context' (p. 16). The subsequent testing of these relationships is the beginning of theory development. A model, for example, might make propositional statements about relationships between perceptions of health, subsequent health behaviour and health status. These relationships could then be tested empirically in order to develop a theory around health behaviour and outcomes. The emerging theory might then be used to guide future practice, such as how to deliver health education messages or how to promote health at an organisational level.

It cannot be assumed, however, that because a model has been derived from theory or empirical evidence it has sufficient credibility to benefit practice. For this reason, various authors (Fawcett 1985, Britt 1997) have developed criteria for the evaluation of models.

Evaluating models

On the basis of the work of Fawcett (1985) and Britt (1997), 10 criteria for evaluation are proposed (Box 4.1).

The criteria are divided into three categories of questions for evaluation: questions concerning the clarity of concepts within the model; questions concerning the accuracy of concepts within the model; and questions concerning application

---

Box 4.1   Questions for evaluation

Conceptual clarity
1. Do the concepts within the model appear factually accurate within their context?
2. Do the concepts within the model hang together in a logically congruent way?
3. Is the definition and description of concepts sufficiently detailed to give confidence in the ability of the model to reflect reality?

Conceptual accuracy
4. Do the concepts within the model reflect the reality of the situation and people to whom they apply?
5. Does the model include all expected concepts and are irrelevant concepts avoided?
6. Are the concepts within the model grounded in theory and empirical evidence?

Application to practice
7. Do predicted relationships between concepts accurately depict real life events both in the future and in different contexts?
8. Is there potential contradiction between theories emerging from the model and the reality of practice?
9. Can theories emerging from the model be tested in practice?
10. Does the model have practical significance and offer guidance for future practice?

---

of the model to practice. Unlike Fawcett's criteria, which are nursing-orientated, these criteria are appropriate to models in a wider sphere of professional practice. The criteria will be used, as appropriate, to evaluate the models in this chapter.

HEALTH PROMOTION MODELS APPLIED TO HEALTH VISITING

Several concepts characterise models designed to promote health. These include concepts relating to changing behaviour, maintaining behavioural change, understanding individual perceptions and cognitions concerning health, and explaining health behaviour in terms of sociostructural variables. The simplest of these approaches, such as Procaska & DiClemente's (1984) model of change, focuses exclusively on changing and maintaining changes in behaviour. Slightly more complex models (e.g. those of Becker et al 1974, and Pender 1987) locate behavioural change within a societal context. More complex still is an attempt to consider the nature and impact of structural variables on different phases of diagnosis, such as that used in the model of Green et al (1980). Each of these models will be discussed and evaluated in relation to health visiting and public health.

The transtheoretical model of change

Procaska & DiClemente (1984) developed a transtheoretical model based around the process of change. They developed their model specifically for the treatment of addictive behaviours. Their intention was to develop a comprehensive model of change that was applicable to the broad range of ways in which people change the variety of different behaviours that people wish to change; the various types of treatment available (e.g. therapy programmes, self-help); and the course that people follow when bringing about change.

Procaska & DiClemente's model uses the revolving door model of change (Fig. 4.1) developed by McConnaughy et al (1983).

According to Procaska & DiClemente's (1984)

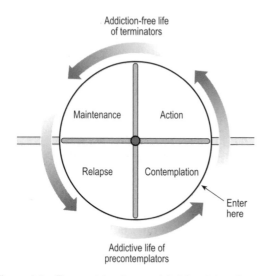

Figure 4.1 The revolving door model of the states of change (redrawn with kind permission from Procaska & DiClemente 1988)

model, people at different stages of the change process exhibit different psychosocial character-istics. Thus, as each individual progresses around the cycle his/her own psychosocial characteristics will change. People at the precontemplation stage, for example, are likely to see few benefits and many problems related to changing their behaviour and are therefore low in self-efficacy in comparison to people who have progressed through to the maintenance stage.

The precontemplation stage is quite crucial, as the efforts of either themselves or other people to persuade them to change their behaviour often fail. This might explain why many attempts made by health visitors to persuade people to change their health behaviour fail. Traditionally, health visitors would have offered advice to people without necessarily taking into account their personal circumstances or motivation, as will be seen below in the discussion of Beattie's health accounts. Once on the cycle, however, people become motivated by the potential benefits and a successful outcome becomes possible. People may then reach the active or maintenance stage, often regressing to the stage before rather than giving up completely. Thus, once on the cycle of change, such people are receptive to health visiting advice so that health visiting

intervention can be construed as successful. It is arguable, however, that such people might have changed their own behaviour without health visiting intervention provided that they had access to the appropriate information.

In addition to the revolving door model of change, Procaska & DiClemente identified 10 change processes of the transtheoretical approach. Furthermore, they argued that seven of these processes could be exploited during the four different stages of the change cycle (Fig. 4.2).

Consciousness-raising, for example, tends to occur when people are contemplating change. During this time they become open to inter-ventions likely to confront the target behaviours. A well-timed visit from the health visitor could enable people to re-evaluate their health behaviour and assess which values they want to work towards (Procaska & DiClemente 1988). During the action phase, a process of self-liberation occurs. This process enables people to relinquish dependence on the therapist and become self-efficacious in bringing about change. The helping relationship is crucial during the action stage in providing the support needed to overcome nega-tive feelings associated with change. During this stage, for example, the health visitor might discuss with the client the negative feelings asso-ciated with the change, what situations trigger such feelings and how they could possibly be resolved. As individuals move towards main-taining change, their management of the changes in their behaviour will need to be reinforced by the health visitor so that they do not relapse to the contemplation stage. Maintaining changes in behaviour also requires counterconditioning and stimulus control. This would involve the health visitor in discussing the client's circumstances so that the client gains a thorough understanding of the conditions under which they are likely to relapse and the ways of controlling such conditions.

The left-hand side of Figure 4.2 presents five different levels of psychological problem requir-ing intervention. Procaska & DiClemente (1988) argue that the symptom/situational level repre-sents the primary reason for people entering therapy. They further argue that the lower down

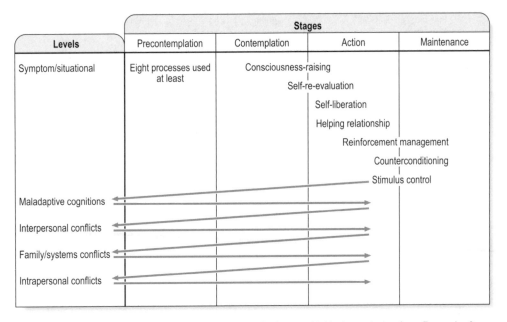

Figure 4.2   Levels, stages and processes of change (redrawn with kind permission from Procaska & DiClemente 1988)

the hierarchy, the less aware the person is likely to be of the determinants of the problem and therefore the more resistant to change. Intrapersonal conflicts, for example, could represent unresolved childhood conflicts of which the person may not be fully aware. Such conflicts could include patterns of health behaviour rooted in childhood, which could be resolved through health visiting guidance. Some conflicts, however, might require sensitive counselling and may be beyond the scope of the health visitor. The health visitor in this situation would probably recommend professional counselling prior to working with the client towards changing health behaviours.

Procaska & DiClemente's model is relatively simple. It is designed to respond to complex personal problems requiring therapy. Fundamental to this model is the belief that therapists should be as complex as their clients. This should enable the health visitor to shift the nature of their intervention, focusing on different change processes and levels of intervention during different stages of the change cycle. Although this model does cater for the complex nature of

human behaviour, it does so at an individual behavioural level. It does not therefore fully acknowledge societal influences on health behaviour. A model that moves some way to achieving this is the health belief model.

The health belief model

A slightly more complex explanation for health behaviour than that offered by Procaska & DiClemente is the health belief model (Becker et al 1974). It is a development of social psychological theories postulated by Lewin (1935). Following Lewin (1935) Rosenstock (1974) developed a theory in which people make decisions about health on the basis of two factors: how severe they perceive an illness to be and what they consider to be the benefits of preventive action. The theory holds that cues to action might bring about changes in these perceptions (Fig. 4.3).

Becker et al (1974) criticised the original model for its emphasis on negative aspects of health such as the threat of disease. They argued instead that positive health motivations exist and account

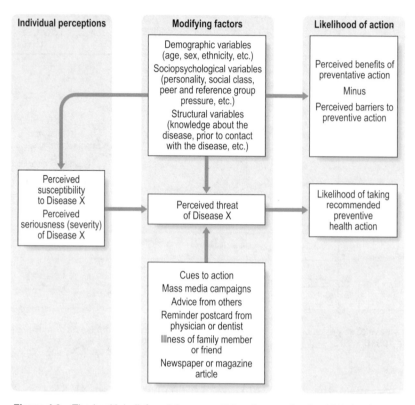

Figure 4.3   The health belief model as a predictor of preventive health behaviour (redrawn with kind permission from Becker et al 1974 A new approach to explaining sick role behaviour in low income populations. Am J Pub Health 64: 205–216, copyright ©1974 American Public Health Association)

for some portion of health-related behaviour. They also proposed that there is an 'incentive' value of compliance in which the threat of a present illness provides an incentive to reduce the threat. In relating this to the readiness of mothers to take recommended action when their child is ill, Becker et al suggested that mothers make an estimate of the likelihood of the physician's instructions reducing the threat. In making this estimate mothers take into account their perception of: the accuracy of the diagnosis; the usefulness of medication prescribed in the past; and the usefulness of modern medical practices.

Becker et al's (1974) health belief model has been used in various health education contexts, such as family-based health visiting (Diment 1991) and school health teaching in primary schools (While 1991). For the purpose of this

chapter, the model will be considered in relation to the community context of public health. The value of this model to public health lies in an analysis of modifying factors, which are evident in the central column of the model. The model has been criticised 'for not explaining the nature of the influence of modifying variables upon the individual's perceptions and beliefs and how these are expressed in resultant behaviour' (While 1991, p. 102). This criticism implies that the impact of sociostructural considerations of society on individual perceptions of health and disease is unclear and therefore contentious. Crossing the boundaries between individual perceptions and sociostructural variables is a particular expertise developed in health visiting.

Knowledge of demographic, sociopsychological and structural variables relies on a public health focus. Health visitors using this model use data from community profiling to identify risk variables in a particular community. A high proportion of ethnic minority groups combined with lower social classes in a given population might be indicative of certain conditions such as poor nutrition or substandard housing. These factors, together with poor education, might suggest that a given population would have a lack of perception of susceptibility to, or the severity of, a particular disease. It is at the public health level, therefore, that health visitors would attempt to modify these factors by mass media campaigns.

While (1991) also argues that the model assumes that the individual person is the ultimate unit of analysis. The importance of modifying factors to the model, however, does counteract this argument. Modifying factors exist outside the individual and impact upon and interact with the individual. Thus the ultimate unit of analysis is arguably the individual within a social context. Individual perceptions, together with the likelihood of action, might also suggest a predominantly individual focus. The model could, however, be applied at a community level. A reminder postcard sent to remind parents about their children's immunisation, for example, has the advantage of increasing the herd immunity of a whole population as well as protecting the individual child. Equally, a 'traffic-calming' campaign in a particular neighbourhood might alert both the public and politicians to the susceptibility of the local population to traffic accidents. It is possible, therefore, for susceptibility to be perceived and acted upon at a wider level than the individual. Nevertheless, whether susceptibility is an individual or collective perception, the ensuing action will ultimately become collective, if only due to the accumulative action of individual changes in behaviour. It is this collective action that is fundamental to public health initiatives and hence the success of Becker et al's health belief model.

The health promotion model

A model which has some similarities with Becker et al's health belief model is the health promotion model (HPM; Pender 1987). The HPM (Fig. 4.4) uses social learning theory as its basis, which, like Becker et al's model, is drawn from social psychology.

Pender's modifying factors resemble those proposed by Becker et al, while both models focus on cues to action and the likelihood of changing behaviour. Pender (1996), however, argues that, unlike the health belief model, the HPM does not include 'fear' or 'threat' as motivating forces for health behaviour. Pender further argues that avoidance-orientated models are of limited use in motivating healthy lifestyles in some groups.

Two versions of the HPM will be explored in this chapter. The first version (Pender 1987) was developed following the initial formulation in 1982. The second version discussed here (Pender 1996) is the latest version, which was developed on the basis of considerable research and testing of the earlier version.

Pender's 1987 version has its theoretical foundations in expectancy-value theory (Feather 1982) and social cognitive theory (Bandura 1986). Expectancy-value theory holds that individuals are rational and will persist with a given behaviour as long as it produces positive personal value and is likely to produce the desired outcome. Social cognitive theory relies on interaction between the environment, the person and the behaviour, each being capable of modifying the others. Fundamental to the HPM is the belief that individuals play an active role in shaping and maintaining health behaviours and in modifying the environmental context for health behaviour.

The revised HPM (Pender 1996) included three new variables: activity-related effect; commitment to a plan of action; and immediate competing demands and preferences. The headings at the top of the model (Fig. 4.5) also differ from the original version. Pender divides the model into three discrete sections: individual characteristics and experiences; behaviour-specific cognitions and effect; and behavioural outcome.

Individual characteristics and experiences include prior-related behaviour and personal

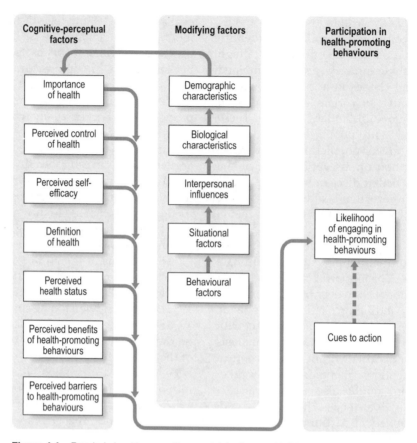

Figure 4.4 Pender's health promotion model (redrawn with kind permission from Pender 1996)

factors. Drawing on empirical studies, Pender concluded that the best predictor of behaviour is the frequency of the same or similar behaviour in the past. In other words, people who have a habit of engaging in unhealthy behaviours are likely to continue to do so. For Pender, existing bad habits also influence personal perceptions of self-efficacy, as well as perceptions of the benefits of healthy behaviour and barriers to achieving it. Barriers to healthy behaviour experienced in the past are therefore seen as hurdles to overcome. Personal factors include: biological (e.g. age, sex), psychological (e.g. self-esteem, definition of health) and sociocultural (e.g. race, education, socioeconomic status) characteristics. According to Pender (1996), these directly influence both behaviour-specific cognitions, as well as health-promoting behaviour.

Behaviour-specific cognitions and effect are important to Pender's model as they can be modified by healthcare intervention. These cognitions include certain perceptions that people hold. The benefits of engaging in healthy behaviour, for example, might be sufficient to motivate some people towards healthy behaviour. However, barriers to action, such as unavailability and expense, might decrease the likelihood of engaging in healthy behaviour. Pender concludes that when readiness to act is low and barriers are high, action is unlikely to occur. Thus, health visitors attempting to change behaviour through advice-giving are often unsuccessful because there are too many barriers to action, such as the high cost of nutritious food. Such barriers might maintain a state of low readiness. When readiness to act is high and barriers are low, how-

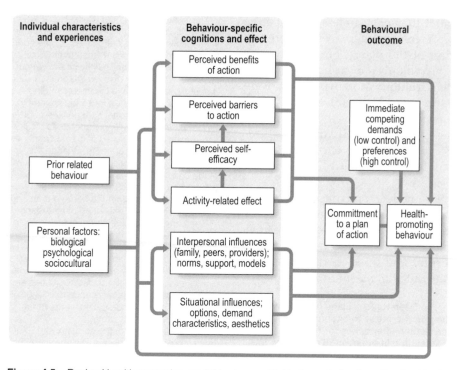

Figure 4.5   Revised health promotion model (redrawn with kind permission from Pender 1996)

ever, the probability of action is much greater. A person's perception of their own self-efficacy (Bandura 1986) is also important in influencing behaviour. Not only is a feeling of being efficacious likely to encourage future engagement in the target behaviour, it also lowers the perception of barriers to the target behaviour so that it seems more achievable. Thus, health visitors would be wise to function at a public health level by reducing barriers to action through public health campaigns and collaborative action. This, in turn, would enable people to feel more efficacious in overcoming barriers to healthy behaviour.

Self-efficacy is also influenced by the activity-related affect. This means that the emotion resulting from the health activity, whether it be positive or negative, will influence whether the activity is repeated in future. This, in turn, will influence the person's perception of self-efficacy. A person who experiences pleasure from a health activity, for example, is likely to feel efficacious in relation to that activity and is therefore likely to repeat it. The different individual perceptions

discussed above, together with the activity-related effect, will impact on people's decisions to commit themselves to a plan of action.

Other factors likely to influence commitment to a plan of action are interpersonal and situational influences. According to Pender (1996) 'individuals are more likely to undertake behaviours for which they will be admired and socially reinforced' (p. 71). People vary, however, in the extent to which they are susceptible to the influence of others. Situational influences on health behaviour include perceptions of the aesthetic features of the environment in which the health behaviour will take place (Pender 1996). Pender views situational factors as having both direct and indirect influences on health behaviour. A feeling of reassurance and compatibility with an environment, for example, will indirectly influence health behaviour. More direct influences will occur in situations where health behaviours are enforced by rules such as no smoking.

The final component of Pender's (1996) model, behavioural outcome, is predicated upon by the commitment to a plan, unless a competing demand or preference intervenes to prevent implementation of the plan. Commitment to a plan needs to be reinforced by a strategy in order for it to reach fruition. Moreover, even well-thought-out strategies for health improvement can be influenced negatively by unexpected demands over which the individual has little control; or by competing preferences over which the individual has more control but that are difficult to resist.

Like the two models previously discussed, Pender's health promotion model focuses on individual behaviour. It does, however, give fuller consideration to the social context in which health behaviour occurs. The three models presented thus far are illustrated in the following vignette.

The health visitor in Deep Hayes village has been working with the practice nurse to encourage breast awareness. In particular, attendance for routine mammography screening in the over-50 age group has been poor and they are concerned to improve the uptake. They begin by interviewing women opportunistically to ascertain their stage in Procaska & DiClemente's transtheoretical model. They discover that some women are at the precontemplation stage, do not see breast screening as a priority and do not believe that it has any benefits. Other women have moved to the contemplation stage, but have been deterred from taking action because, having weighed up the pros and cons of mammography and talked to women who have attended for the procedure, they have decided that the procedure is likely to be too uncomfortable and to have limited benefits. A few women have progressed as far as attending for mammography, but have only attended for one screening. These women are in their mid-fifties and have not been screened for 4 years. They have therefore failed to maintain the screening programme and have relapsed to their preprogramme behaviour. The health visitor and practice nurse want to achieve two outcomes: to increase the attendance for all women and to increase the annual attendance of the same women in order to increase the detection rate of early breast changes. Procaska & DiClemente's transtheoretical model is useful in enabling them to assess the women's stage in the change cycle, but has limited use in promoting attendance. Indeed, the therapeutic nature of the model makes it more valuable in changing addictive behaviours than in promoting healthy activities. It is unlikely, therefore, that the health visitor and practice nurse would move to a deeper level of therapeutic intervention than focusing on the situational context. Furthermore, the change processes might well be limited to consciousness raising, thus moving the women from precontemplation to contemplation, but no further. The health belief model, however, proves useful in promoting screening.

The health belief model (Becker et al 1974) enables the health visitor and practice nurse to identify perceived susceptibility and the seriousness of the condition. As a cue to action, they target all women over 50 with a breast awareness campaign. They invite the women to group sessions where they discuss the predisposing factors to breast cancer, so that all women can diagnose their own susceptibility. They then invite the women to share with the group their own personal experiences of breast cancer. A former patient also willingly attends to discuss her personal experience of being cured of breast cancer as a result of the breast screening programme. Sharing this knowledge also acts as a modifying factor by increasing women's knowledge of the condition. It is anticipated that, following the campaign, the women will weigh up the benefits of attending for screening, together with the barriers to attendance, and that this will increase the likelihood of attendance.

The campaign proves largely successful in enabling the women to progress through the cycle of change, although there are a number of women who remain resistant to change. Not wishing to give up on these women, the health visitor uses Pender's health promotion model as an aid to analyse the behaviour-specific cognitions and effects that might account for this resistance to change. The health visitor and practice nurse discover a variety of perceptions that explain their behaviour.

For several women, the complex nature of their lives makes breast awareness a low priority. Although they can see the benefits of screening, these are outweighed by the barriers, such as time to attend and lack of transport. A minority of women do not have financial problems but have such a low perception of their own self-efficacy and so little control over their lives that the future and their health status do not matter to them. Two women have other health problems: one suffers from multiple sclerosis and one has a severe heart condition. What all of these women share in common is a sense of health as 'destiny' that is beyond their control. External attempts to control health on their behalf are not considered significant. Furthermore, previous attendance for screening programmes, such as cervical screening, have not been a pleasurable experience either in terms of the effort required to attend or the procedure itself. This activity-related effect, therefore, only served to reinforce their perceived self-efficacy. Interpersonal and situational influences served to reinforce this further. Experiences of screening programmes shared with family and friends concurred with this view of a negative experience, often requiring long waits in crowded, impersonal waiting rooms.

Pender's (1996) HPM revealed some critical factors in explaining health behaviour. The health visitor had a difficult decision to make. She had to balance attempting to raise the self-esteem of some women against interfering with their right to make their own decisions. Moreover, some of their decisions seem quite reasonable, given the circumstances.

Although both Becker et al's and Pender's model do take into account structural variables, structural factors are not considered from the point of view of their specific impact on health behaviour. This factor could be crucial in developing public health initiatives and is fundamental to Green et al's PRECEDE model, which will be discussed next.

The PRECEDE model

The PRECEDE model (Green et al 1980) centres on the need to initiate change in behaviour by analysing its preceding causes. Seven phases represent the process through which behavioural change takes place. In phases 1 and 2, to the right of Figure 4.6, an epidemiological and social diagnosis is made.

In particular, phase 1 focuses on quality of life indicators such as the individual's or community's own subjective definition of their quality of life. Of particular interest to the health visitor at this stage would be population factors such as age distribution, the percentage of different

ethnic minority groups, the unemployment rate and housing facilities, as well as numerous other social factors. Edet (1991), for example, used phase 1 of Green's model to identify risks associated with adolescent pregnancy. Quality of life is preceded, and therefore predicated upon, by nonhealth-related factors and health problems (phase 2). Health visitors would therefore be particularly aware of the different dimensions (incidence, prevalence, etc.) of different diseases and conditions, and how they impact on and interact with subjectively defined quality-of-life perceptions as well as objective quality-of-life indicators. During phase 2 the health visitor would isolate the specific indicators and dimensions that were thought to impact on the subjectively defined quality of life. In an area with an aging population, for example, the effects of disabling conditions on the quality of life might be identified as important. In Edet's study of adolescent pregnancy phase 2 involved

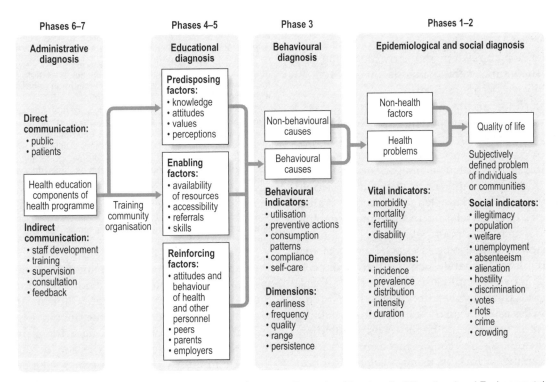

Figure 4.6 Green's PRECEDE model (redrawn from *Health Promotion Planning: An Educational and Environmental Approach, Third Edition* by Lawrence W Green and Marshall W Kreuter. Copyright ©1999 by Mayfield Publishing Company. Reprinted by permission of the publisher)

using available data to identify specific health problems that contribute to adolescent pregnancy, such as high infant and maternal mortality rates associated with adolescent pregnancy.

Phase 3 refers to the behavioural diagnosis needed to identify different causes, both behavioural and nonbehavioural, that impact on health problems. Early, frequent and persistent consumption of cigarettes, for example, would represent a behavioural cause of health problems. Non-behavioural causes of health problems could relate to the local environment. Traffic congestion, for example, might increase the incidence of road traffic accidents, or industrial pollution might be responsible for chest diseases. The health visiting response to these two categories of cause would differ considerably. The non-behavioural causes would be addressed through community action and participation, the health visitor engaging in political action by association with relevant local groups. By contrast, Green et al's model would adopt a health education response to the behavioural causes. Phase 3 of Edet's study involved the identification of both behavioural causes such as early exposure to sex, greater sexual freedom and early menarche, and nonbehavioural causes such as unemployment and low socioeconomic status.

According to the model (Fig. 4.6), phase 3 is preceded by, and therefore affected by, predisposing, enabling and reinforcing factors represented in phases 4 and 5. Returning to the example of early, frequent and persistent smoking, the educational diagnosis used at phase 4 would identify existing knowledge, attitudes, values and perceptions relating to smoking. Enabling factors, such as support systems to discourage the habit, would also be assessed. Finally, factors that reinforce the habit, such as attitudes of peers and employers, would also be considered. Phase 5 would then involve deciding which of the three classes of factor – predisposing, enabling or reinforcing – should be the focus of attention. The health visitor could, for example, focus on enabling factors by using available support systems to attempt to counteract the effects of predisposing and reinforcing factors.

The final two phases of the model, phases

6 and 7, involve the factors that precede the educational diagnosis. Edet's use of the sixth and seventh phases, for example, involved the implementation and evaluation of the health education programme of sex education. At this stage, then, it is assumed that for an educational diagnosis to take place an administrative diagnosis must first occur and an evaluation strategy be negotiated. This includes communication with the public, training of both the community and the organisation staff, staff development, consultation and feedback. Health visitors are particularly effective at this stage, as they are able to work at the interface between healthcare organisations and the public. Their role therefore includes both direct and indirect communication, as well as consultation and feedback.

A health visitor in Old Town has recently moved to a new post in which most of her work involves working with travelling families on an newly established caravan site. This is a newly formed post and she is responsible for developing an outreach service to these families.
On examining quality-of-life nonhealth factors she discovers that the travelling families are alienated from the local community, which is hostile towards them. There is a high incidence of absence from school because the children are ostracised by their peers. The caravans, and indeed the site, are overcrowded. Vital indicators of potential health problems include the fact that most families have more than four children and prefer not to use contraception because of their religious conviction. Behavioural causes of this overcrowding, therefore, relate to nonuse of birth control. The health visitor appreciates that the predisposing factors leading to this include religious values and beliefs and respects this. The desire for large families could, however, be reinforced by familial norms passed down generations. It is probably at the enabling level that the health visitor has the greatest impact. Using skills of communication she works with the site as a 'community' to discuss the value and norms associated with having children. Through discussion she encourages the families to see the benefits of limiting family size. She also discusses natural family planning methods and the benefits of this.

In evaluating her performance, the health visitor communicates with both the families themselves and her employer. Clinical supervision is needed to enable her to make good judgements. She could be in danger, for example, of working so closely with the site occupants that she ignores wider health issues such as the alienation and discrimination occurring from the local communities.

The four health promotion models discussed

thus far have been successfully applied to health visiting practice in the public health domain. The four models will be evaluated next, before discussing public health models.

EVALUATION OF HEALTH PROMOTION MODELS IN RELATION TO HEALTH VISITING

Using the evaluation criteria listed in Box 4.1, it is evident that all four models discussed thus far have considerable credibility. The three main elements of evaluation – conceptual clarity, conceptual accuracy and application to practice – will be considered separately.

Conceptual clarity

All four models appear to be logical in that clear lines of association exist between concepts. The concepts embraced within Procaska & DiClemente's model and Green's PRECEDE model, however, seem to be less clearly explicated than other models. The transtheoretical model (Procaska & DiClemente 1988) focuses more on processes and theories than on description of concepts. Likewise, Green's PRECEDE model describes different stages without explaining concepts underpinning the derivation of the model. Descriptions of concepts are evident from the original development of the health belief model (Becker et al 1974), the detailed components of which were reviewed by Rosenstock (1966), thus demonstrating the grounding of the concepts in theory. Supporting empirical evidence for the health belief model can be found in Mitchell's (1969) review of research into Rosenstock's original variables. This revealed that the health belief model provided satisfactory explanation for most research findings relating to preventive health behaviour. Pender's health promotion model also demonstrates conceptual clarity through the explication of each of the concepts within the revised model.

Conceptual accuracy

The accuracy of the models is depicted in the vignettes, which illustrate the relevance of the models to the people to whom they apply. Pender's and Green et al's models did, however, appear to more accurately reflect complex health behaviours, while Procaska & DiClemente's model of change, and to a lesser extent the health belief model, were limited in this respect. These latter two models, therefore, could arguably be lacking in expected concepts related to causal influences of health behaviour. Green et al's (1980) main value seems to be in its recognition of the impact of causes and factors on health problems and how these can ultimately affect quality of life. The nature of factors preceding other factors is unique to this model and demonstrates the need to always consider what lies behind the evidence presented. The limitation of the model lies in its tendency to focus exclusively on a defined problem to the detriment of other possible problems and solutions. The health visitor in the vignette, for example, chose to focus on family planning rather than alienation or absenteeism. This potentially reductionist approach could result in a narrow focus on identifying problems and the necessary changes in behaviour required to resolve them. The model could therefore be in danger of subordinating autonomy and self-empowerment to its main aim of initiating behaviour change (Naidoo & Wills 1994). Empowering both the local community and the travelling families to meet and discuss their similarities and differences in culture and lifestyle might have relieved alienation and absenteeism at the same time. Following this, a change in behaviour relating to family planning might be easier to achieve.

Theoretical or empirical grounding of concepts is clearly evident in the health belief model, the health promotion model and the transtheoretical model. The health belief model is grounded in theory of individual perceptions as well as research into how changes in perception can be brought about (Rosenstock 1974). The health promotion model is grounded in theory (social learning theory) as well as in research and testing of the original model. Most of these studies attempted to predict health behaviour from the variables within Pender's original model, such as value of benefits, perceived self-efficacy, perceived barriers and demographic characteristics (Frank-Stromborg et al 1990; Pender et al 1990; Lusk et al 1994; Garcia et al 1995). Pender (1996) concluded from an analysis of these studies that the variables that were most successful in predicting health behaviour were perceived self-efficacy, benefits and barriers. These findings then formed the basis of the revised model. Procaska & DiClemente's model is based on change theory (McConnaughy et al 1983) and, like the other models discussed, is also based in self-efficacy theory (Bandura 1977a).

Application to practice

The predictive ability of the models is dependent on the intended purpose of the model. Green's model is interpretative, rather than predictive while Procaska & DiClemente's is explanatory. It is therefore not possible to evaluate the predictive ability of these models in relation to time and place. Some support for the predictive value of the health belief model, however, has been found in relation to breast self-examination (Fung 1998) and alcohol consumption (Minugh et al 1998). Certain variables within Pender's health promotion model, too, have proved useful in predicting health behaviour, as indicated above.

The only potential contradiction between theories emerging from the models and the reality of practice occur with Procaska & DiClemente's change cycle and the health belief model, for they arguably provide a limited theory of health behaviour in so far as they omit the entire life context. Nevertheless, the transtheoretical model has proved successful in examining the processes of change in a behaviourally oriented weight-loss programme (Suris et al 1998), smoking cessation in pregnancy (Stotts et al 1996) and specific opiate-dependent patients (Tejero et al 1997). The value of this model seems to be, therefore, in planning interventions that target specific stage-dependent causal mechanisms (Pollak et al 1998).

In all cases the models can be tested in practice, as is demonstrated through the two vignettes, as well as the extensive research evidence discussed above. The practical significance of these models can be translated into guidance for health visiting practice. What seems to be evident, however, is that health promotion models are insufficiently complex to take into account the sociocultural constraints that influence people's lives. The use of public health and health visiting models might, therefore, prove more worthwhile in guiding health visiting activities.

HEALTH VISITING AND PUBLIC HEALTH FRAMEWORKS AND THEIR APPLICATION TO HEALTH VISITING

The dynamic and unique nature of health visiting, combined with uncertainty about defining and measuring its outcomes, have led to attempts to conceptualise and hence describe and explain health visiting at different stages of its development. Health visitors need to rely on a variety of concepts and models if they are to explain the complexity of their professional activities. The remainder of this chapter will consider a variety of frameworks for health visiting and public health. Beattie's health accounts will provide the predominant framework for this discussion. Other models discussed are Chalmers & Kristajanson's (1989) models of community nursing and Neuman's (1989) systems model. In addition, certain theories and paradigms will be considered, namely: Twinn's (1991) paradigms of health visiting and Chalmers's (1992) theory of giving and receiving in health visiting.

Beattie (1993) makes an important contribution to debates about the future of health visiting. He argues that health researchers have made a paradigm shift towards focusing on explanations of health emanating from negotiated meanings through conversational exchanges. This, he argues, is only one way of explaining health and fails to explain what influences people to select particular accounts. This resonates with While's (1991) criticism of the health belief model. Both criticisms seek further explanations than simple structural explanations appear to offer. It was suggested above (see discussion of the health belief model) that applying individual explanations at the community level can integrate individual perceptions with sociocultural considerations of society. Beattie's health accounts develop this argument further by identifying links between what people believe and the social worlds they inhabit.

According to Beattie (1996), what people believe can be defined in terms of two dimensions: modes of thought and focus of attention (Fig. 4.7).

Each dimension can be viewed as bipolar. The modes of thought dimension comprises hard (mechanistic) and soft (humanistic) poles. This reflects the seriousness that the professions and society ascribe to different approaches to analysis. Hard approaches, according to Beattie, dominate, as they are in keeping with the natural science tradition. Soft approaches, by contrast, are equated with lay as opposed to expert views and are therefore seen as 'trivial'.

The focus of attention dimension comprises the polar opposites of individuals or collectivities. Work in the individual pole focuses on individualist philosophies of health behaviour. Solutions to problems arising from the health behaviour of individuals, therefore, lie either in understanding individual personal biographies in order to explain behaviour or in attempting to correct behaviour. By contrast, work in the collective pole looks for collective causes and solutions relating to health behaviour.

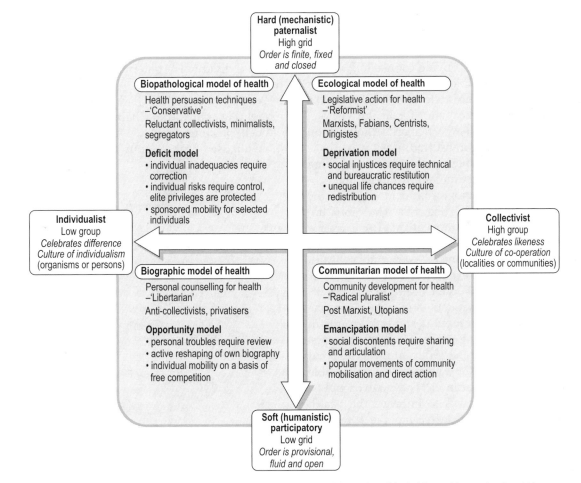

Figure 4.7   Beattie's accounts of health in relation to ways of knowing, sociopolitical philosophies and cultural bias (adapted with kind permission from Beattie 1996)

The two dimensions of hard versus soft approaches, and of individual versus collective approaches, reflect the dilemmas of health visiting. Health visitors ascribe to both the soft (humanistic) approach to healthcare and the hard (mechanistic) approach, depending on the changing and dynamic demands of their work, and their particular orientation. Recent debates concerning the health visitor's public health function represent a return to the hard mechanistic approach to public health and hence a return to the roots of health visiting. However, when this hard mechanistic view is combined with current trends in health visiting towards work with collectivities rather than individuals, then health visiting is firmly located within the reformist rather than the conservative tradition. The soft approach to health visiting remains an important facet of practice, both at the individual and the collective level. At the individual level, health visitors provide counselling within the libertarian tradition. The use of the soft approach within the collective level perhaps marks the most radical shift for health visitors, in which community participation and action occurs within the pluralist tradition.

Beattie also identifies four ways of accounting for health – the biopathological model, the ecological model, the biographical model and the communitarian model (Fig. 4.7). The biopathological model, in the top left quadrant, uses a mechanistic mode of thought, focusing on the individual as an organism. At a public health level, the model is exemplified in Chalmers & Kristajanson's (1989) public health model.

According to Chalmers & Kristajanson the public health model identifies at-risk groups in the community, using epidemiological concepts. It was developed in the 19th century to respond to threats to healthcare such as communicable diseases and malnutrition. The goal of public health at that time was to improve the health of the population by decreasing the spread of disease. According to Chalmers & Kristajanson (1989) the public health model assumes that disease is determined by exposure of a susceptible host (the individual) to the agent (the disease). This interaction between the individual and the environment is known as the host–agent environment interaction. The public health nurse intervenes in this relationship using primary prevention, such as promotion of good nutrition, and secondary prevention, such as screening the population for disease and case-finding. In this way the health of the entire population is protected by reducing the spread of disease. During this early stage, the emphasis of health visiting was on defining health problems and providing therapeutic interventions rather than addressing the underlying causes of disease. The agenda, therefore, would have been determined by the 'expert' (Beattie 1979). The focus would also have been on using persuasion techniques, thereby correcting and repairing the defective individual (Beattie 1984). The deficit model would have been prevalent, requiring expert-directed intervention in which the social distance was high (Beattie 1984).

The individualist, paternalistic and conservative characteristics of the top left quadrant can be seen in Twinn's (1991) adaptation of Beattie's model (Fig. 4.8) and in Chalmers's (1992) theory of health visiting.

Twinn used Beattie's four quadrants and some

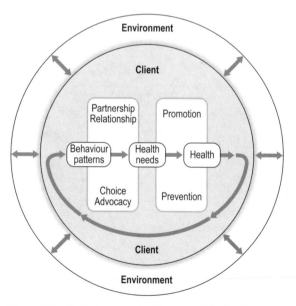

Figure 4.8 Twinn's conceptual framework for health visiting (redrawn with kind permission from Twinn 1991)

of his dimensions (directive versus nondirective, and collective versus individual) as well as the general principles of the model as the basis for a conceptual framework. For Twinn, intuition and professional artistry, together with professional reflection, are central concepts. Twinn's framework is based on a belief in the client as the central focus in the health visiting strategy. Although this might be seen as endorsing the traditional individualised practice of health visiting, Twinn argues that the client is seen in the context of the community and that 'this does not restrict the framework to an individual or collective paradigm, but is central to the formation of strategies in either setting' (Twinn 1991, p. 971). She further argues that a relationship of partnership must exist between health visitor and client in order to determine strategies that are appropriate to the client's perception of their own health needs. Furthermore, she identifies choice and advocacy as fundamental to both facilitating partnership and responding to the political dimension involved in promoting health and preventing ill health.

Twinn describes health visiting activity in Beattie's top-left quadrant as the 'individual advice-giving' paradigm. She argues that individual advice-giving is the traditional approach to health visiting practice, involving the provision of advice and health teaching to mothers about the care of infants and young children. This individualist, paternalistic approach to health visiting is also reflected in Chalmers's (1992) theory of giving and receiving in health visiting. Chalmers identified three phases of the health visitor/client relationship:

- the entry phase
- the health promotion phase
- the termination phase.

During the entry phase the health visitor gains access to the client within either an 'open context' (in response to an identified problem or need) or a 'closed context' ('routine' initiation by health visitor). Depending on the context, the health visitor will either make a routine offer of information or will focus on needs identified by the client. In either case the client's perception of the value of the offer will determine whether it is received positively enough to progress to the health promotion phase. Advice and help is offered during this phase to promote health, its success again being determined by its value to the client. Help viewed positively will enable the client to share a range of health issues, which can be addressed throughout the relationship. Alternatively, the client may 'block' any offers not perceived as of value. The interaction between the health visitor and client is therefore regulated by the type of offer made by the health visitor and the perception of its value by the client. The termination phase is characterised by either negotiated or non-negotiated termination. Negotiated termination is characterised by preparation of the client for the termination of visiting. In contrast, visits are terminated without any input from the client in non-negotiated termination.

The top right quadrant of Beattie's model (1993) can also be seen in Twinn's (1991) analysis. Twinn (1991) argues that this public health focus represents the 'environmental control' paradigm of health visiting which she equates with Beattie's ecological model of health. This model represents the hard, mechanistic side of health visiting, concerned with communities rather than individuals. The epidemiological expertise of health visitors is used to analyse the interaction between individuals and the environment so that risks to health can be identified. Twinn (1991) argues, further, that this reflects one of the principles of health visiting, 'the search for health needs' (CETHV 1977). For Twinn, the public health (ecological) model involves health visitors in establishing the health needs of a particular population from a health profile of the community. The findings from the profile would then be used to target priorities and practice. The professionalist use of health persuasion techniques, evident in early public health initiatives (top left quadrant), gives way to a managerialist philosophy that relies on legislative action for health. The agenda, therefore, is determined by bureaucratic rules rather than by the expert (Beattie 1979).

The ecological approach is also similar to Chalmers & Kristajanson's (1989) community participation model. This model differs from the public health model in that it involves the community in planning and delivery of health services. This radical shift in emphasis changes the power base from health professionals to the community. In assisting the community to identify its own solutions prior to seeking outside assistance, health visitors encourage communities to identify the causes of health problems as well as solutions. According to Beattie (1984), health professionals working in this quadrant direct their expert power towards custodianship of health, guarding and protecting communities against environmental risks. The community participation model reflects much of health visiting practice, as well as that of other health professionals, during the 1980s and 1990s.

The community participation model is also at the heart of public health initiatives that rely on models of prevention (Caplan 1966). Neuman's (1989) model is particularly suited to the public health role of health visiting as it relies not only on theories of prevention but also on systems theory. The value of systems theory to health visiting and public health lies in its assumption that a system can only be understood in relation to its totality (Haggart 1993). Health visitors attempt to understand individual clients in relation to their wider environment but also attempt to understand the community within its wider social and political context.

Central to Neuman's theory is a belief that individuals have a defence system, represented as a series of circles referred to as lines of resistance with a normal line of defence and an outer flexible line of defence. According to Neuman (1989), stressors break through this normal line of defence when the outer flexible line of defence fails to protect the individual from stressors. When this occurs the internal lines of resistance attempt to restabilise the individual. The concept of lines of resistance can also be applied at the community level. Communities could be viewed as having an outer flexible line of a defence, which gives the community its geographical or social structure. Stresses can come from both within the community and outside it to threaten the lines of resistance. The community exists within and interacts with the wider system. Neuman identifies intrapersonal, interpersonal and extrapersonal stressors to explicate this interrelationship. From the community perspective, intracommunity stressors would be those stressors arising from within the community, such as crimes against property committed by local youth. Indeed, Haggart (1993) raises the point that some communities 'have lines of resistance and normal lines of defence which may include behaviours or strategies considered by the nurse to be damaging to health' (p. 1919).

Intercommunity stressors arise from interactions between communities. This might occur if a major link road was planned to benefit one community and in doing so disadvantaged another. Extracommunity stressors would occur when stress stems from right outside the community. The development of a new factory would be an example of this.

Neuman's model is also based on assumptions concerning primary, secondary and tertiary prevention (Caplan 1966) and their capacity to prevent stress. This, of course, makes the model particularly pertinent to public health and health visiting. Interventions by the health visitor would therefore take place at three different levels of prevention: primary, secondary and tertiary. At the primary prevention level the health visitor works in partnership with community groups. Through participation with voluntary and statutory organisations the facilities within the community can be continually enhanced in response to the expressed needs of the local population. At the secondary prevention level health visitors work with communities to identify potential problems before they arise. Knowledge of epidemiology enables them to recognise morbidity and mortality trends within the population and to work with communities to identify potential local causes and solutions. The tertiary level of prevention involves working with populations to contain situations to ensure that they do not become worse than they already are, to provide support and monitor the situation. An example of this could be traffic-calming measures, which, although they would not reduce the problems caused by traffic, would provide supportive and controlling measures to prevent the worst elements of traffic congestion. Application of Neuman's model to health visiting is illustrated in the following vignette.

High Town is a small community on the outskirts of a large urban city. The town is characterised by a north/south divide. The south side of the town consists predominantly of socioeconomic groups I and II. The north side houses mainly people in socioeconomic groups IV and V and unemployment is very high. The town is approximately 1 mile from the main city centre. A large ring road has recently been completed, which creates a geographical divide between the north and south sides of the town. This also makes access to the main city more difficult for people on the north side.

One of the health visitors has been working in High Town for some 5 years. He has noticed increasing discontentment and isolation of the population on the north side. In collaboration with a community group he decides to use Neuman's model to assess the stresses within the community, the consequences of these stresses and the preventive action that can be taken to alleviate the problems. Table 4.1 outlines the types of stressor identified within the categories intracommunity, intercommunity and extracommunity.

Having identified the stressors and possible consequences it was possible to consider how the consequences could be limited within the different levels of prevention. Examples of preventive measures are listed in Table 4.2.

The use of Neuman's model in public health provides an useful framework within the bottom right-hand quadrant of Beattie's health accounts. However, health visitors might also adopt both the biographical and communitarian models at different times. Both these models, being at the bottom of Figure 4.7, use soft humanistic approaches, but the biographical model (in the left-hand quadrant) focuses on personal and private troubles, using counselling to facilitate coping. Beattie (1984) describes work within this quadrant as being client-centred with low social distance, involving counselling and empowering individuals. Twinn (1991) refers to this as the 'psychological development' paradigm in which health visitors provide personal support. She distinguishes this from the more directive 'advice-giving' paradigm by focusing on partnership in which clients participate in decision-making. This partnership approach reflects Beattie's (1979) 'consumerist' approach, in which the agenda is determined by the customer. This individualist approach is also evidenced in Chalmers' (1992) theory of giving and receiving. Moreover, it is probable that Chalmers' theory illustrates how health visitors vacillate between Beattie's two left-hand quadrants on the paternalistic (hard) and participatory (soft) approaches to their individual work with clients.

The focus of the communitarian model is on groups and how individuals interact within groups. Health visitors would act as advocates in this context, working with other community workers and campaigns to improve health. Beattie

Table 4.1   Examples of types of stressor and their consequences

Type of stressor	Example	Possible consequences
Intracommunity stressors	High rate of unemployment Local authority housing in poor state of repair Lower than average car ownership Lack of state nursery provision No local facilities for youth	Reduced standards of living Deprivation and poor health Poor access to facilities in city Isolation of women Increased vandalism and crimes by local youth
Intercommunity stressors	Division of single community into two separate communities by ring-road Alienation of population on north side from rest of population and from main city	Crime against south side by youth from north side Increased fear of crime
Extracommunity stressors	Shortage of local authority housing Major developments to main city increase traffic flow on ring road and local residential network The Accident and Emergency department and many wards at local City hospital are to be closed	High incidence of homelessness Increased accident rate Poor access to health care

Table 4.2   The use of different levels of prevention to alleviate stressors

Level of prevention	Action
Primary prevention	Liaise with local councils to establish job opportunities arising from local city developments
	Work with local organisations (e.g. schools and voluntary groups) to provide sports facilities and clubs for youth
	Liaise with local communities to develop Neighbourhood Watch schemes
	Lobby local council to improve street lighting to reduce fear of crime
	Lobby local government to improve public transport to main city
	Lobby local government to improve walking access between the two sides of the ring road and walking access to main city
	Employ a multiagency approach to health needs, health education and health promotion
Secondary prevention	Lobby local authority to repair local authority houses and to provide additional housing stock
	Liaise with local schools to improve nursery school provision
	Liaise with local authority to increase traffic-calming measures in residential areas
Tertiary prevention	Work with local organisations to develop skills training for unemployed and youth
	Liaise with local groups to monitor provision of services

(1979) describes this as a syndicalist approach in which the agenda is determined by collective negotiation between allies. Moreover, as Twinn (1991) points out: 'where health visitors have been successful, they have shared their knowledge and expertise openly, and worked in partnership with community members, making decisions jointly' (p. 968).

This communitarian approach also bears some similarity to Chalmers & Kristajanson's (1989, p. 572) community change model. This model is characterised by an examination of underlying social, political, and economic factors affecting health as well as making systemic efforts to alter destructive structures. Thus, all sectors of the community are involved in creating systems that work towards improving health. The emphasis here is not only on community participation, but also on collaboration of different professional and voluntary groups towards a common goal – health improvement. This communitarian model is given legitimacy by the present Labour government in its White Paper *The New NHS – Modern, Dependable* (Department of Health 1997a). The emphasis on primary care groups within the White Paper, together with health action zones and health improvement programmes, encourages collaboration between professionals and lay people towards health improvement. Such

an approach fosters community change through community participation and action.

Central to this belief in community change is the change from health education, which would have involved advice-giving in the early public health model, to health promotion. Health promotion is a much wider concept than health education, involving health visitors in advocacy, mediation and community empowerment. Health promotion thus involves health visitors in political activities in challenging the distribution of power and resource allocation and therefore influencing policies affecting health (CETHV 1977).

Sociopolitical philosophies also are of concern to Beattie (1993) and these too reflect the tensions in health visiting. The dimension of paternalist and participatory (Fig. 4.7) is indicative of the top-down and bottom-up approaches to policy-making in healthcare. One of the principles of health visiting is 'the influence of policies affecting health' (CETHV 1977). This involves health visitors in participatory action. Using the communitarian model enables them to mobilise communities to direct action and is therefore typical of Beattie's radical pluralist philosophy, in which individual problems gain recognition in the public domain.

The final component of Beattie's (1993) analysis

to be discussed here is four types of cultural bias (Fig. 4.7). 'Grid' refers to rules and constraints that a culture imposes on its people (Beattie 1996). 'High grid', which is associated with paternalism, refers to a precise definition of roles and statuses and separation of roles. This typifies the public health model described by Chalmers & Kristajanson (1989), in which the power base lies firmly with health professionals. 'Low grid', associated with participation, is characterised by negotiation within a society in which nothing is fixed. The responsiveness of health visitors to the needs and preferences of the client and the client's capacity to choose whether to accept or reject offers of help (Chalmers 1992) are typical of a low-grid culture.

'Group' refers to the boundedness of a group. 'High group' is characterised by a strong sense of belonging to a well-defined social group, to the extent that the interests of the group are more important than individual interests. This, combined with the 'low grid', would characterise the communitarian view of health visiting. In contrast, working with 'low group' characteristics is less typical of contemporary health visiting, although some work with individuals' interests is still carried out.

In tracing the changing nature of health visiting, it is possible to locate the profession within different quadrants of Beattie's accounts at different points in time. The early public health model adopted by health visitors (Chalmers & Kristajanson 1989) seemed to adopt a biopathological model of health, in that advice was given to individuals to enable them to improve their own health and consequently the health of the whole community. This top-down, biopathological approach can also be seen in contemporary health education campaigns aimed at persuading individuals to change their behaviour. Indeed the health belief model (Becker et al 1974), and the transtheoretical model of change (Procaska & DiClemente 1984) are based on this belief. It seems, therefore, that a paternalistic approach has dominated health visiting to some extent throughout its history.

More recently, health visiting has moved towards the collectivist (high group) rather than individualist (low group) pole of Beattie's accounts. The profession continues to struggle with the dilemmas created by working in both ecological and communitarian models. The ecological model is paternalistic and involves health visitors in striving for more formal recognition of their public health role in legislation. This represents a shift from the communitarian model with which they have had some involvement for the past two decades. Beattie's accounts are illustrated in the following vignette.

The health visitor in Low Town has become aware of the high incidence of smoking during pregnancy. She wants to work with the midwife to set up a Quit Smoking group to help pregnant women to stop. The biopathological model of health can be applied here, in which health behaviour is seen as a deficit in the individual. The conservative philosophy holds that individuals are responsible for their own health and, therefore, that they should be responsible for changing their own behaviour. Using this model it is assumed that, once given the correct information, the women will change their behaviour. This proves difficult, however, as the context of women's lives in Low Town is such that the deprivation and lack of facilities they experience causes undue pressure. The way in which they alleviate their sense of hopelessness is by smoking.

In working with these women the health visitor has to take cognisance of the ecological model of health, which embraces a social reformist rather than a conservative philosophy. This approach therefore assumes that social reform is needed to alleviate deprivation by redistributing life chances and addressing social injustice. It is at this level that health visitors draw on one of the principles of health visiting: 'the influence of policies affecting health' (CETHV 1977). Although they can do this at both macro (societal) and micro (individual/family) level, the collectivist, 'high group' approach within this quadrant would imply that the health visitor would adopt a political stance, working with local communities to improve their facilities.

Working with local communities and instigating political action to shape change also requires the health visitor to adopt the radical pluralist philosophy of the communitarian model. Working closely with the local community enables the health visitor to emancipate the women so that they can help to change the negative forces affecting their own lives. It is only when this process is complete that the health visitor can move to the individualist approach, perhaps addressing personal biographies and how they shape smoking behaviour.

The above vignette has illustrated how health behaviour, and health visiting responses to it, do not happen in a vacuum. Indeed, Beattie's four accounts could be seen as a dynamic cycle, in which health visitors move around and between the four quadrants according to the needs of the individuals and groups with whom they work. It is this dynamic nature of contemporary health visiting that separates it from the different disciplines within nursing and also from specialist branches of medicine and public health.

A review of public health and health visiting models reveals the extent to which health models support and to some extent are built upon Beattie's health accounts. The models discussed above will now be evaluated.

EVALUATION OF HEALTH VISITING AND PUBLIC HEALTH MODELS

The evaluation of health visiting and public health models is complex as most are defined differently than the health promotion models discussed above. With the exception of Neuman's systems model, none of the 'models' discussed above is defined as such by the authors. Chalmers's theory of giving and receiving, for example, is defined as a theory rather than a model. Twinn (1991) describes her analysis of Beattie's work as four conflicting 'paradigms'. Beattie (1993) describes his work as four health accounts. The following evaluation will therefore take into account these differences in definition. The evaluation, as before, will address issues of conceptual clarity, conceptual accuracy and application to practice.

Chalmers's (1992) theory of giving and receiving was probably described as a theory as it emerged from empirical research using a grounded theory methodology. Hence, the theory is high on conceptual clarity since it emerged from empirical interview data from 45 experi-

enced health visitors from 13 different health authorities. Grounding of the theory within the data would ensure that concepts were factually accurate within their context. Chalmers argues that health visitor interactions with clients are influenced by the meaning that events have for them within the context of past experience. This view seems logically congruent both with the theory of giving and receiving and with the reality of health visiting practice. The central concepts within the theory, giving and receiving, reflect the pattern of interaction between health visitors and their clients, and how each controls this interaction. The explanatory nature of the concepts adds conceptual clarity to the theory as the concepts appear factually faithful to the reality of health visiting at the individual level. The concepts are also linked to phases of health visiting and the type of work carried out at each phase. This adds to the congruence and descriptive detail of the theory. It may be concluded, then, that Chalmers's theory of giving and receiving is high on conceptual clarity.

Conceptual accuracy is reflected in the use of grounded theory in Chalmers's research. Use of grounded theory makes it likely that the concepts within the theory reflect the reality of the health visitors studied. Besides being empirically based, the model also has a firm theoretical foundation in concepts from symbolic interactionism (Mead 1934, Blumer 1969). Exchange theory (Homans 1961, Blau 1964) is also used by Chalmers, who suggests that health visitor–client interactions that are not providing any benefits or are creating feelings of lack of self-worth, rejection or powerlessness will be avoided. The use of grounded theory would ensure saturation of the data to the extent that all expected concepts were reflected in the theory. Nevertheless, there can be no guarantee that all possible concepts in client–health visitor interactions were represented within the interviews, or throughout the interpretation of transcripts. Health visiting exchanges within this theory, for example, are located in only two of Beattie's health accounts. The theory, therefore, does not include all necessary concepts reflecting the public health collective dimension.

Chalmers' theory seems successful in its demonstration of application to practice. A potential contradiction might emerge if health visiting developed its focus on public health to the exclusion of individual work with families. This contradiction also reflects the theory–practice gap, in that some of the work identified by Chalmers is routine and child-focused, which is more in keeping with traditional health visiting practice. Chalmers' research was, however, published in 1992, the data possibly being collected in the late 1980s. The theory can be tested in practice and the phases of the health visitor–client relationship are, to some extent, supported by the phases evident in Peplau's (1952) model, which focused on the development of the relationship between mental health nurses and their clients. As a theory grounded in empirical practice, Chalmers' theory provides a good explanatory framework for the reality of practice and thus might offer guidance for future direction.

The three models discussed by Chalmers & Kristajanson (1989), by contrast, are less easy to evaluate. Chalmers & Kristjanson appear to use the term 'model' rather loosely in describing the historical and political changes in public health. The absence of clearly specified concepts results in a lack of conceptual clarity and accuracy. Nevertheless, the changes they identify, although perhaps not overtly testable in practice, do reflect the contemporary dilemmas of health visiting. This grounding of the models (though not concepts) in empirical as well as theoretical evidence, therefore, does ensure that the models have practical significance and therefore contribute to current debates about health visiting practice. The three models are based on existing theories. Biological theories of the host–agent environment and susceptibility, for example, underpin the public health model. Moreover, theories about professional power, co-operation and political activity underpin both community participation and community change models. Furthermore, the three models lend theoretical support to Beattie's (1996) four health accounts as well as Twinn's (1991) four conflicting paradigms in health visiting.

Unlike Chalmers & Kristajanson, Beattie (1996) does not proclaim that the four health accounts are a model. It would therefore be unwise to treat them as such. Beattie does, however, draw on four models of health (deficit, deprivation, opportunity and emancipation), which he subsumes within four broader models of health (biopathological, ecological, biographical and communitarian). These models are derived from Beattie (1991). A variety of philosophies are explicated within the four health accounts, while conceptual clarity is produced through the use of bipolar dimensions. The four quadrants derived from these two different dimensions produce logical congruence, and concepts such as 'high group' versus 'low group' and paternalist versus participatory are sufficiently described to reflect reality. The complex nature of the four quadrants could result in some conceptual inaccuracy, although this needs to be balanced by the danger of omitting concepts that are important to a complex social scene. Like Chalmers & Kristajanson's three models, Beattie's health accounts offer thought for the future of health visiting. It is thus in their practical application that Beattie's health accounts have their greatest power. Beattie's health accounts also proved valuable in forming the basis of Twinn's (1991) conflicting paradigms.

Twinn's four conflicting paradigms of health visiting were used as the basis for a conceptual framework for health visiting. Concepts used included partnership, promotion, choice, advocacy, prevention and health. Despite the obvious use of these concepts, the framework lacks conceptual clarity. The flow of influence between the arrows within the model (Britt 1997), for example, would suggest that health influences health behaviour, which in turn influences health needs, and that the influence of health needs completes the cyclical influence of these concepts upon each other. Twinn does not, however, define health in relation to her framework, nor does she clarify the links between health, health promotion and behaviour patterns or how they relate to partnership, advocacy, promotion and prevention. Instead, she links these concepts to professional artistry and reflection. For these reasons also, the concepts lack logical congruence and there is insufficient description of the concepts to provide confidence in their ability to reflect reality.

Because of the logical incongruence of Twinn's (1991) conceptual framework it is difficult to estimate conceptual accuracy. Some concepts, for example, might be irrelevant. The lack of conceptual clarity and accuracy within the framework also makes it difficult to develop theories from the model that can be subsequently tested. This conceptual framework is an example of the difficulty experienced in applying models to practice when the defining concepts lack clarity and coherence.

The final model, Neuman's systems model, is typical of many models used in healthcare. It relies on concepts derived from existing theory, i.e. Seyle's concept of stress (Seyle 1956), which it contextualises within different levels of personal interaction. This gives conceptual clarity to the model. The categorising of stressors, for example, enables community groups to enumerate stressors from the perspective of the different stakeholders, and therefore to prioritise the different preventive actions.

Logical congruence is enhanced in Neuman's model by the application of Caplan's (1966) model of prevention. This also provides sufficient confidence in the model's ability to reflect reality. The model was grounded in both theory and empirical evidence and has since been tested in a variety of contexts, including public health nursing (Benedict & Behringer Sproles 1982),

mental health, and community nursing (Beitler et al 1980). This lends accuracy to the model.

The evaluation of health visiting and public health models, theories and paradigms suggests that most are valuable tools to analyse contemporary health visiting practice. Although theories and paradigms are defined differently from models they make valuable suggestions for the future of health visiting in public health.

SUMMARY

The models, theories and paradigms discussed in this chapter reveal not only the complex nature of health visiting but also the complexity of defining, evaluating and applying models to health visiting practice. Simple health promotion models have proved useful in explaining health behaviour and possibilities for behavioural change. More complex health promotion models were more successful in explaining behaviour within a cultural milieu. Thus, such models have more value for public health initiatives. Public health models, however, seem to offer a more critical framework for considering future directions in health visiting. Such frameworks offer alternative paradigms for health visiting that may co-exist.

The different types of model and framework discussed in this chapter present a challenge for evaluation. Nevertheless, the evaluation criteria developed in this chapter were used successfully in evaluating a range of models, theories and paradigms.

5

Skills in health visiting

Doreen Sheldrake and Anne Robotham

INTRODUCTION

This chapter is designed to discuss the fundamental skills of health visiting. At present there is no direct entry to health visiting, so health visitor education follows on from nurse education. Nurses and health visitors work closely together in many spheres and may be said to be using the same skills. However, we contend that health visitors interpret these skills and use them for a different body of knowledge. This may be because the skills are used for different theoretical perspectives or in a proactive rather than reactive forum. This chapter will therefore begin by comparing the skills learned in nurse education and the modification and extension of these for health visitor education.

NURSING KNOWLEDGE

General nursing practice requires that practitioners be alert and sensitive to the needs of their patients but in many situations patients are unable to function without the care of nurses. In a sense, nursing care begins with the nurse 'doing' for the patient, anticipating the patient's needs, enabling patients, for example, to articulate their pain level and generally taking over from them, albeit temporarily. The management of the patient's treatment is determined in discussion with the patient and a care plan is formed. In the ideal world a patient undergoing treatment that requires the care of nurses is gradually led towards self-efficacy as they move through their illness to a state of wellness. In addition, patient health education is also running alongside the care tasks performed by nurses.

Thus within this process of illness treatment within the health service, the patient experiences a number of clearly defined skills from nurses:

- care through practical nursing tasks
- assessment of illness care needs
- care programme management determined by the demands of the illness
- anticipation of physical and psychological needs
- health education around the illness focus
- preparation and planning for care on discharge.

In addition, patients have understanding and expectations of:

- nurses' roles
- the meaning of nursing care and medical treatment.

Clearly outlined above is a general analysis of the range of areas that nurses cover and in many cases this includes considerable competency in areas of technical/clinical expertise and

management – all requiring high levels of communication ability.

The interesting factor in this brief analysis of nursing skills is that they are so focused on an approach that may be recognised as reductionism. Thus the person from the community becomes a patient with a condition – an individual who has needs that are pertinent to them and possibly to their immediate family. This reflects the reductionist approach of medical treatment within individual illness and this is both important and acceptable within illness and healthcare.

Figure 5.1 was first introduced in a document dated June 1983 as the result of a statement on the development of interprofessional education and training for members of primary care teams by the then Council for Education and Training of Health Visitors (CETHV), the Panel of Assessors for District Nurse Training (DNTRB), the Royal College of General Practitioners (RCGP) and the Central Council for Education and Training in Social Work (CCETSW).

Although the intention here is not to discuss education methods, the diagram clearly illustrates situations where the skills of the different practitioners involved are determined by the

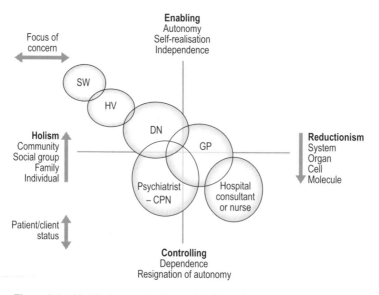

Figure 5.1   Modified example of a model of care (redrawn from Baraclough et al 1983)

Table 5.1   Comparison of the skills of nursing and health visiting

	Nursing skills	Comparable health visiting skills
1	Care through practical research-based nursing tasks	Care through practical research-based advice
2	Assessment of illness	Assessment of health needs and behaviours
3	Care plan management determined by the demands of the illness	Management of care pathways as identified by the client
4	Anticipation of physical and psychological needs	Anticipation of physical, social and psychological needs
5	Health education around the illness focus	Health promotion on a holistic health basis
6	Preparation and planning for care on discharge	Planned activity management
	In addition, patients have an understanding and expectations of:	*Clients without contact rarely have an understanding and expectations of:*
7	Nurses' roles	Health visitors' roles
8	The meaning of nursing care and medical treatment	The meaning of disease prevention and health promotion

status and focus of concern. Despite this caveat, however, it is clear that the thinking of 15 years ago is still highly relevant for today's practice.

The reductionist approach is not pejorative in the sense that nurses' skills are reduced by the focus of their work; rather they are centred on the nature of the closeness of the interaction between nurse and patient within an illness paradigm. Developing this theme in relation to the foci of concern highlighted in the diagram may enable health visitors to recognise what it is that is different about their education in terms of the skills required in health visiting.

Re-examination of the list of nursing skills above in comparison with health visiting skills shows a change (Table 5.1).

At this stage it is worth detailing the identified health visiting skills, which become apparent as the discussion ensues.

1. Care through practical advice

One of the charges formerly levelled at health visitors is that they never ceased to give advice and that on many occasions it was unsolicited. The development of the public health role of the original sanitary nurses from which health visiting grew was to advise and teach in homes on health and hygiene relating to babies and young children. The point of this is to emphasise the word 'advise' and to examine it in the context of modern health visiting within the arena of a far-better educated public. Originally, the advice given by health visitors was paternalistic,

assuming complete ignorance of the basic tenets of child health and hygiene, and in the majority of situations the health visitor was working only with working-class people. Today's health visitor is working in a knowledgeable society, which central government considers to be classless and whose hopes and aspirations are based on material acquisitions. Both these statements could be criticised for their generality but are included to show the changes apparent in the society in which the health visitor of today is working. Clearly, the skills of the earlier health visitors were based on a didactic approach, albeit with kindly intentions. Those skills would be challenged today and found to be unacceptable by their recipients.

A young family has a 4-year-old daughter with a carcinoma of the kidney with bone secondaries. She was treated by surgery and chemotherapy but sadly a recurrence of the bone metastases took place several months later. The family 'surfed the Internet' and discovered a drug used in America for this particular recurrence. They informed the paediatric consultant and requested this treatment.

The vignette is included to illustrate the depth and breadth of information available to clients, which clearly means that health visiting has to approach from a totally different stance than in the early part of the 20th century.

The practical advice that may be sought from health visitors falls into three main areas:

- social and environmental problems
- problems of child rearing
- family health problems.

Social and environmental problems

Care must be taken when discussing such problems not to assume that the health visitor is working in a socially deprived area. Social problems in families living in more affluent circumstances can be as severe and different as those of families living in material poverty.

The practical advice offered depends, of course, on how important the problem is to the client. Clients living in damp and run-down property need urgent advice on how best to solve this problem, and this is one of the most frustrating areas of the health visitor's work. It is easy to empathise with families in these situations and it is also not difficult to recognise the problems of housing departments with dwindling stock and rising lists of needy clients – coupled with a greater tendency on the part of clients to seek litigation against local authority housing departments.

Health visitors may attempt to help clients by writing to housing departments on their behalf or encouraging them to enlist the help of local councillors in their fights for rehousing. Many families are in despair over their situation and one of the skills of the health visitor is to encourage clients to take positive action to enhance their demands by, for example:

- documenting the instances of nuisance
- taking photographs of damp or other unhealthy situations
- drawing other tenants together in an effort to collectively influence the housing department
- documenting health problems experienced by children which may lead to school non-attendance.

The type of advice discussed above is designed to develop people's confidence and motivation to do something themselves to alter and improve their situations, and requires the health visitor to have a wide knowledge of the whole system of housing in both the public and private sector. Often, this gives the health visitor a better chance of developing good links with clients and the 'giving and receiving' concept proposed by Chalmers (1992) is a clear result of advice over the initial problem. In this concept, Chalmers argues that each party 'gives' and 'receives' in order to mange health visitor–client encounters. The health visitor gives the focus of 'routine' (thus not making it intrusive) and 'client centred' in the entry phase. This is followed by information, teaching and support in a health-promotion phase and finally a negotiated or non-negotiated termination phase. The client 'gives back' information and interest and 'gives' positive reception that the help has been well received. It is important that the entry work is successfully established before attempting to move into subsequent phases.

Isolation is a problem in urban areas with large detached houses. Some professional women with small babies have high expectations of their own mothering abilities and cannot run next door to seek help without appearing to concede personal failure. The health visitor making a planned visit may be consulted on a presenting problem, e.g. infant colic, which may have little to do with the real problem of isolation. The perceptive health visitor can see the real problem but has to allow the client to take agenda leadership over the secondary problem, working to find an appropriate management strategy for the colic until the real problem becomes apparent to the client. Again, Chalmers's work on giving and receiving becomes the underlying theoretical perspective within care and advice in health visiting. Provided the health visitor and client have satisfactorily achieved a solution to the colic then it may be possible to open up the debate on isolation. However, if the colic is not satisfactorily resolved, will the client allow the health visitor to challenge the situation by suggesting that isolation may be the principal problem?

The skill of perception in health visiting is essential to satisfactorily identify the root cause of problems. Clients are very close to their own difficulties and ascribe reasons for problems from a narrow selection of choices. Health visitors coming with wider perspectives can work with the client in partnership (analysed more fully in Chapter 11) by offering alternative coping strategies.

Problems of child rearing

The care and advice given in this area is endless and is the recognised focus of health visiting work. Advice can be as detailed as guidance relating to feeding or dealing with infant constipation, or fundamentally broad-ranging in relation to child development and behavioural management. Child protection also draws on every aspect of the health visitor's knowledge in relation to the law, research on at-risk situations, material evidence of abuse or neglect, and family dyadic relationships.

The skills of care and advice in health visiting duplicate those of nursing in response to practical guidance, e.g. on infant feeding practices or home safety. Health visiting skills used must be in partnership with clients because authoritarian approaches compromise future working relationships. The approach 'Have you tried...?' is often more acceptable than 'You must ...'.

Where there are issues of possible risk to or neglect of children, approaches determined by Trust guidelines must be employed. Here health visitors must be vigilant about potential risk factors, honest with clients if there is a doubt over an explanation given about, for example, an injury, and confident enough to record openly in the client-held records the concerns identified. Advice given must be immediate and the situation must be observed regularly and frequently. Clearly, formal policies must be adhered to by health visitors but the fundamental work in the initial stages has translated 'advice' into 'instruction'.

The trap that health visitors can fall into is that they are so concerned about maintaining working relationships with carers that they may minimise the potential risk to the child.

Family health problems

Health visitors are often drawn into family discussions on the best way of solving health problems. This is often a fruitful partnership approach in which the client can discuss their own health solutions and the options open to them until they reach an appropriate and satisfactory outcome. In this scenario the family tests its own

knowledge against that of the health visitor to see whether compromises or alternative strategies are needed. Other situations that can develop are when a client is unaware that there is a problem, e.g. in an area of child development where the client sees no problem but the health visitor recognises abnormality or delay. An example here might be a speech delay identified by the health visitor that has been accepted as normal by the parent.

However, it is also important to recognise that health visitors who adhere too strictly to developmental tools and do not take into account family and cultural factors are guilty of raising anxiety levels unnecessarily if they make an issue of the situation.

Advice on family health must be tailored to family circumstances and this may mean the health visitor compromising and negotiating acceptable advice. The beginning of the process is about determining the problem in relation to the family knowledge level and then building upon this knowledge level. This may mean that the same problem from one family to another elicits an entirely different response from the health visitor – depending on family circumstances.

2. Assessment of health needs and behaviours

The wider debate over health needs assessment has been covered in Chapter 2. In this chapter we are more concerned with basic health visiting skills in relation to families and individuals, and, to continue the comparable analysis with nursing skills, health visitors need to be skilled in health needs analysis in relation to both the current and long-term situation.

A number of tools are available to health visitors to structure their assessment of health needs. Traditionally, health visitors have annually analysed their caseloads and the information that this revealed was enormously important, giving a clear view of how their work was progressing. Unfortunately, the evidence produced from these caseload analyses was, as mentioned previously, never acted upon. The ways in which they viewed their work were restricted by the overwhelming need to ensure that the 'box of records', for which they felt acutely responsible, was worked. Interestingly, if challenged on the number of families they were really working with, most health visitors would identify some 30–50, and the remainder were visited regularly because it was 'routine', whether the client wished it or not.

Despite the criticisms above, the annual caseload evaluation does allow health visitors two essential pieces of information and we would argue it is important to continue this practice. Firstly, the results can reveal a true evaluation of the health visiting practised on that caseload, e.g. details of infant feeding patterns, child behaviour problems, maternal depression, family disorganisation problems, and many other factors. All of these should be used as a basis to examine how health visiting input has influenced any recorded changes. Perhaps an emphasis on antenatal classes in relation to infant feeding can be measured against an emphasis in the following year on individual discussions with pregnant women in their own homes. This would allow a clear analysis on which has been more effective – group work or individual work. Balanced against this must be cost-effectiveness, in terms of time and effort, in achieving improvements in infant health. Previously, health visitors have ignored this opportunity to undertake true evaluation, for the reasons outlined above.

Secondly, caseload evaluation should be used in conjunction with regular community profiling to determine the focus of health visiting practice. This may lead to a shift from the prime focus on mothers and under-5s to another age group in need – for example, a rise in breast cancer rates in the area for women aged 44–60. It could be argued that working with the under-5s allows the health visitor to undertake an assessment of the health needs of all the family. However, a criticism of this argument is that often the assessment of health needs of all the family is not undertaken in relation to the wider perspective, of the epidemiological and social factors of the area. Good caseload evaluation should be undertaken annually to allow for the use of these two important results.

As a result of the evaluation of health visiting

interventions outlined above it is possible to recognise that outcomes of health visiting practice are essential to satisfy the health needs of the individual, the community and the purchasers. Health visitors must recognise that successful health visiting interventions may be perceived by both client and purchaser to be the result of their own work, not that of the health visitor. It is therefore important that health visitors clearly identify what they have done and measure this against clearly defined outcomes related to accurate evaluations of health needs. It must be borne in mind that identified health needs are peculiar to each individual client or family. It is they who identify their own needs in conjunction with the health visitor, and it is important for health visitors to document where they have raised awareness of health needs towards which they and the family are working, as well as working with the client's own agenda. Good examples of this are seen in relation to smoking and similar health behaviours.

Many community trusts have developed tools for use by health visitors on initial contact health-needs assessment. These are based on a scoring system for risk factors in a similar way to the public health scoring systems such as the Jarman index (Jarman 1983), although on a more personal basis. Some health visitors find these useful for giving a baseline of family need and they are known to have been used by purchasers to establish resource allocation. Many other health visitors challenge the whole basis of risk scores on the premise that these can change so rapidly that they become meaningless as a tool to influence intervention and are out of date the minute they have been completed (Lightfoot 1994, Hudson 1997). There is also the criticism that families are being labelled by their score and indeed, who is making the assessment – the health visitor or the family? These tools do, however, have a value in providing a checklist so that in moments of concern about overriding problems a brief response can be inserted for use at a more convenient time.

The skills of dialogue between client and health visitor to establish health needs are essential and in many ways will override any tool designed for the purpose.

During an antenatal visit, a health visitor discusses with the client general family support systems and the influence of meaningful family members in her life. All the time the health visitor is alert to other health needs. The physical needs are very evident and have been dealt with by the midwife. However, discussion on the wider family brings to the fore a realisation that the client hasn't thought through sibling rivalry and has not yet prepared the toddler for her loss of unique child position. There will be a host of other factors but this one identified item is used to illustrate preparation for the psychological health needs of the toddler.

3. Management of care pathways as identified by the client

There are no clearly defined management programmes for this area of health visiting skills. Few nursing models are appropriate in these situations and it far more likely that health visitors will borrow health psychology models based on Bandura's self-efficacy model (1977a) or Becker et al's health belief model (1977b). In most situations these necessarily require adaptation to the client's needs but the value of flexible models is shown in Chapter 4. Here, the skills of health visiting are twofold: first, being able to identify and use the most appropriate model and second, enabling the client to solve the problem using the health visitor in client-listening sessions. In this second aspect the health visitor is probably using a variant of Rogers's (1967) person-centred approach, discussed in Chapter 11.

Many client problems are long-term and health visiting skills are mobilised towards helping the client to set short-term goals that are achievable. Positive reinforcement of what clients have already achieved is essential in raising self-esteem and this is done without any aspect of paternalism on the part of the health visitor. It means that the health visitor takes time to listen to the client story, to help them unpick the complexities of the situation, and for the client to recognise their own strengths in the process.

The health visitor can help the client to record what they are doing, to keep a diary of the problem, e.g. where there are toddler sleeping problems and it is necessary to see how repetitive the problem really is. Other ways in which clients may be encouraged to keep a record may be: a food diary (see Chapter 10), a diary of moods

and feelings in relation to postnatal depression, management of infant crying or temper tantrums and so forth. The management skills of the health visitor are to enable discussion and analysis of diary contents, recognise the severity or otherwise of the problem, pick out themes and patterns and negotiate a planned programme of change suitable for the client's agenda.

Present-day life circumstances (stress, pace, pressure, change) require health visitors to enable individuals to find a way around the difficulties they face, and this means a focus on changing the circumstances or situations in which people live rather than concentrating solely on individual behaviour and knowledge. Helping clients to change their focus calls for health visitors' ability to promote discussion, challenge their belief system where appropriate and offer alternative frames of reference. For example, modern family behaviour has, in many cases, lost the rhythm of regular mealtimes. Young children do not respond to erratic patterns in their lives and thus do not settle into established eating behaviours. Helping mothers to recognise the benefit of their own childhood patterns and rhythms in establishing beneficial eating behaviours may mean establishing better rhythms within the family, encouraging family conversation and relaxing harmony. The circadian rhythms identified in relation to sleep (Kerr et al 1997) apply equally well to eating behaviours in young children. If mothers have not experienced regular patterns and rhythms in their own young lives then health visiting skills of suggestion and education are prominent here.

4. Anticipation of physical, social and psychological needs

Anticipation in the nursing care field is designed to prevent the occurrence of further physical problems in relation to the immediate illness, and to prepare patients for interventions to minimise adverse psychological responses. In a sense the anticipation is clearly relevant and immediate.

Anticipation in health visiting enables clients to identify the possible impact of wider issues. This includes both short-term and long-term responses to client situations. For example, health visitors working with mothers of growing infants draw on and extend the mother's knowledge of infant development, encouraging aspects of safety such as ensuring that the rolling infant is not placed on an unsecured surface above floor level. In addition, situations that may not yet have occurred are identified and discussed by health visitors. Examples include dangers in relation to equipment that has become apparently necessary for infant growth, such as baby walkers, but in reality has no part to play in child development. Health visitors help mothers to challenge some of the traditional practices of child-rearing that have been found by research to be unsafe, e.g. placing a young baby to sleep in the prone position.

Anticipation of social needs is more difficult to conceptualise and yet there are many ways in which health visitors can enhance mothers' social situations. Examples here include introducing new mothers to other mothers in similar circumstances to establish peer-group support networks. Helping women to understand their social circumstances is also included in the anticipatory work of health visitors, particularly women who are trapped in unhappy marriages and who need to realise that there are ways out. This theme is further explored in Chapter 13 on violence and health.

One factor that has often concerned health visitors relates to very young girls who become pregnant and whose own mothers are very critical of the situation, to the extent that the self-esteem of the young mother is lowered. The provision of an intermediary who allows both sides to express their anger and concerns and then encourages the positive aspects of the situation to create harmony and self-efficacy is beneficial to all concerned, and health visitors are often in the position of being this intermediary.

Social needs of older people are anticipated by health visitors and frequently these involve networking and liaison with other agencies to access group activities or social support visits. Often, health visitors listen to the reminiscences of older people and are criticised for apparently social visits. However, current work on reminis-

cence therapy (Chapter 2) has shown that these are vital for social health and as such are important aspects of health visitor anticipation.

Research (Browne et al 1988, Cox & Holden 1994) has shown that health visitors are well equipped to anticipate psychological needs and health breakdown. Listening to women and allowing them to express their concerns is one well-used method, as is knowing the vulnerability of women with particular personal histories. Examples include the knowledge that women who lost their own mothers before the age of 11 are more at risk of postnatal depression, or that parents who had harsh childhoods themselves are more likely to deal harshly with their own children. These exemplify the very real need for health visitors to listen to families and seek for possible at-risk factors during the early getting-to-know-the-family period. It is critical that health visitors do not gain information through question-and-answer sessions; rather, they use skills to draw parents out and discuss with them the relevance of information about past situations to current or future situations. This is discussed further in Chapter 11.

When it comes to working with other age-groups, some health visitors are in a position to target adolescents and have set up clinics particularly to provide support, again in the form of listening sessions to enable adolescents to work through problems in emotional development. Often these are in relation to family-planning advice and counselling and the adolescent is encouraged to anticipate their needs and health behaviour.

5. Health promotion on a holistic health basis

Bunton & Macdonald (1992) suggest that health promotion is the disciplines of psychology, education, epidemiology and sociology; it also embraces other disciplines such as social policy, communications theory, marketing, economics and philosophy. Health education is a means whereby recipients have health promotion communicated to them. In a sense it is the didactic sharing of health promotion, and is less frequently seen as part of health visiting because it cannot be presented in partnership with the client.

Health visiting skills in health promotion range from working with individuals through working with groups to working with communities. In Chapter 2 DeVille-Almond relates how she has worked with a community to promote health and raise their awareness of health issues. In many ways, promoting health in communities is about bringing people together and encouraging them to work for the health and safety of the community. Examples of this include the student health visitor who worked with a group of mothers in North Staffs. They were particularly concerned that their children had to cross a busy main road to reach school. By bringing the mothers together and helping them to realise that they shared the same concerns, the student encouraged them to make representations to the local council and police department – the upshot of which was that a pelican controlled crossing was installed. This might be criticised as not being health promotion because there is a pre-conceived idea that health promotion is targeted at the individual, albeit possibly using group methodology. However, the skill in health visiting is about being able to mobilise communities to promote the health of their more vulnerable members (see Chapter 2).

Neighbourhood Watch schemes have often been set up as a result of health visitors raising awareness of the anxieties of local people about burglary and theft. The pulling together of the community has not only reduced the threat to its more vulnerable members but has also enabled other members to become actively involved in its organisation, giving them a clear application for their skills and the satisfaction of having a worthwhile part to play.

Health visitors promoting health to families often build on concerns expressed by women discussing their families. A classic example of this is the mother of a family of growing children who is concerned about their predilection for junk food. With the support and encouragement of the health visitor she is able to confidently make changes to the meals that are offered and discuss with her family the reasons why such changes have been made. Work by Mayall & Foster (1989) has shown that mothers often have a wide knowledge of what their families ought to eat but financial constraints force them to forego more expensive nutritious foods in favour of more filling ones. Health promotion in these circumstances means that health visitors encourage and support women in their concerns and discuss with them ways of making cheaper food equally as nutritious as more expensive items.

Promoting individual health sees health visitors taking a different approach from nurses, who promote individual health as a result of illness or health-damaging behaviour. In many ways, health visitors promote health to apparently healthy individuals as well as to those who are exhibiting health-damaging behaviours. For instance, promoting dental health in a young school-child means that clear explanations are required at a level that is meaningful for the child. Anticipation, therefore, is not the basis on which the health promotion is made, rather the opportunity to help the child to see that dental caries can be prevented by their own actions with toothpaste and brush, and moreover that this goes hand in hand with the responsibility of growing up.

6. Planned activity management

This skill of health visiting differs from the nursing skill of preparation and planning for care on discharge in that it is client-driven in health visiting rather than being carried out in consultation with the patient and other care organisations, as in nursing.

Activity management can cover topics such as working with families with disabled children, working with children with behaviour problems, working with families with chronic illness in one of the parents, and working with families with dependent elderly relatives.

Mr and Mrs B are both teachers with seven children ranging from 17 down to 6 years, and at her last and eighth pregnancy Mrs B gave birth to a baby with Down's syndrome. There was good support from the outset, with neonatal nurses, midwives, paediatrician and GP all combining to help in the care. The health visitor was also involved from the beginning but recognised that in this case the greatest need was support of the family rather

than the new infant, who was supported by other professionals.

This brief vignette shows the need for perception in the health visitor to recognise where within the family is the greatest need for support. The initial focus of activity in the beginning meant that all concerned were caught up in planning and work with the new baby. Often, having made the initial introduction to the family (and, of course, knowing them from past contact), the health visitor steps back and appears to have a limited input into what is going on. However, the health visitor and the mother have agreed a home visiting programme, which is revised regularly. It is critically important to recognise that the health visitor skills here are to maintain contact with the other professionals in order to keep abreast of the situation, and possibly to remain in the background until the situation is normalised. The health visitor realises that the family supports each other but visits or makes periodic contact to monitor family dynamics and minimise any breakdown. What is vital about this type of scenario is that the health visitor is more effective when observing from the outside than when working from within. There are other professionals dealing with the day-to-day matters, but knowledge of family dynamics means that the health visitor is working to identify any changes that may lead to long-term difficulties. A common situation is that when the health visitor is discussing the needs of the family the mother remembers that, when she picked the second-youngest child up from school earlier in the week, the teacher had mentioned that he was becoming more disruptive in class. Because the mother's attention is focused on the needs of the baby she has not recognised the needs of this other child. The opportunity to look at the whole family that has arisen from the health visitor's visit means that together the health visitor and the mother can discuss the situation and plan how she can perhaps focus more attention on that child, whose behaviour is possibly demonstrating lack of his mother's attention.

Dependent elderly relatives can influence family dynamics by disrupting normal family home life, if brought into the family home, or by creating pressures and drawing a parent from the family home in order to attend to their needs. The skills of the health visitor centre on dialogue with both the elderly relative and the family to ascertain the needs of each, linking in with other agencies to provide alternative support. The health visitor plans with the family and the relative a programme of activity that meets the needs of each, reduces the elderly relative's feeling of dependency and helps the family to function with less guilt and pressure.

THE PRINCIPLES OF HEALTH VISITING

The section above has been designed to show how health visitors use skills originally identified at the beginning of the chapter as those of nursing.

Health visitor skills are founded on four principles of practice that have stood the test of time since their definition by the CETHV in 1974. They were adopted by the UKCC for postregistration education and were quoted in *Making it Happen* (SNMAC 1995) in relation to child health promotion, good parenting and family health visiting. The SNMAC believes that the skills that health visitors apply to their practice equips them to assess the health needs of communities. The principles of health visiting, which were re-examined in 1977 and 1992, have remained unchanged and are:

- the search for health needs
- stimulation of an awareness of health needs
- influencing policies affecting health
- facilitation of health-enhancing activities.

The search for health needs

In a re-examination of the principles of health visiting (Twinn & Cowley 1992) there is a discussion of the interpretation of the words 'search' and 'needs'. At that time it was felt that the words should be left unchanged but many health visitors have expressed concern that 'search' implies that this is not the basis for their work in health needs. Search can be based only on what is overt; however health visitors use all their senses to assist them to identify and explore what is actually worrying the client. Thus, where the needs are not obvious to either client or health visitor, the process of discussion and enabling the client to draw out their beliefs and values creates a partnership in which client and professional both search for covert health needs. If covert health needs are uncovered the client may be enabled to understand their significance on both an individual and a family basis.

Health visitors use advanced skills of listening and empathy to practise in partnership with individual clients and community groups during this searching process. A model may be the tool outlined by Carnwell in Chapter 4, identifying stressors using Neuman's (1989) systems model.

It is important in the planning of health visiting practice to consider whether health visiting focuses on targeted intervention or maintains a generalist approach. If the organisation of health visiting is based on targeted intervention where there are known areas of vulnerability, then the importance of this principle is lost. In other words, generalist health visiting practice allows for every opportunity to search for health needs, whereas targeted practice is based on overt health needs.

Health visitors use both qualitative and quantitative research methods to collect epidemiological data to establish community health needs, as discussed in Chapter 2, but the uniqueness of the work that health visitors undertake with individuals realises the richness of the methodology in establishing health needs.

Continued health visiting practice in relation to the principle of searching for health needs means that health visitors should take every opportunity to keep primary care groups informed of health needs that are uncovered.

Stimulation of an awareness of health needs

Past NHS planning did not allow for those health needs associated with demographic changes, specific lifestyles (such as poverty, homelessness and unemployment) and ethnicity to be readily identified and included in the business plans and subsequent service provision. This emphasises the importance of alerting people to health needs and any potential help that may be available. The stimulation of awareness of health needs by health visitors encompasses three different levels of action – clients (individuals and communities), health service managers (commissioning authorities and provider units) and politicians and policy-makers at a national level (Twinn & Cowley 1992).

From a superficial point of view there would seem to be little difference between *searching* for health needs and *stimulating awareness* of health needs and yet health visiting has always differentiated between these two terminologies. Stimulation of awareness of health needs is at the heart of why in many ways, the medical model/approach to healthcare is only semi-successful. This is because it fails to do more than acknowledge health needs resulting from social inequalities, need and deprivation. The only way in which the medical model approach will ever be entirely successful is if social needs are not only acknowledged but acted upon. The Labour government, in its two documents *A New NHS* (Department of Health 1997a) and *Our Healthier Nation* (Department of Health 1998a), has grasped the nettle in accepting that for healthcare to succeed there are social factors that must be dealt with. This is where health visiting has always striven to play a part – in raising awareness of inequality, badgering agencies on behalf of the disadvantaged, encouraging and empowering individuals and communities to demand equal opportunities for healthcare. It is to be hoped that the new primary care groups will be more focused on redressing social inequality issues, and, with their fundamental skills, health visitors will continue to stimulate the awareness of primary care groups of such inequalities.

Influencing policies affecting health

In *Making it Happen* the SNMAC committee (1995) made the following statement: 'SNMAC believes that the skills that health visitors apply to their practice equips them to assess the health needs of communities, and that this should be built upon for locality-based health need assessment and primary care purchasing' (p. 16). Since the adoption of the 'New NHS' this has become an even more important statement in relation to influencing policies affecting health. As discussed in Chapter 2, health needs assessment is an integral part of public health delivery and the current movement towards primary care groups as the hub of public health means that health visitors, through their membership of them, are in an even stronger position to influence policies affecting health.

Health visitors have consistently and persistently used their professional bodies to lobby members of parliament, local government officials and indirectly, from time to time, the public through press releases and other statements. An example of a press release has been criticism by health visitors of prominent advertising of artificial infant formula milks, to the detriment of breast feeding. A further example is the strong support voiced by health visitors of stop-smacking campaigns – End Physical Punishment of Children (EPOCH – Cook et al 1991).

Health visitors are natural cross-boundary workers with experience in networking across healthcare and other statutory and voluntary sectors, thus enabling them to influence other agencies and professional groups in relation to healthcare needs and provisions. Health visiting provides a voice for women and their concerns and, as a predominantly women-based profession, is instrumental in highlighting the real concerns of women's issues.

Health visitors practise in managed primary healthcare teams and are responsible for developing teamwork and responding to the policies of the health authority/NHS trust. They are thus in a position to promote innovative practice development in response to general practice and primary healthcare needs. The marketing process (de la Cuesta 1994) can be used to develop a relationship with the purchaser/GP in order to agree a service package. This should be based on outcome measures specific to the requirements of the Children Act 1989, Caring for People (Department of Health 1989a), The Patient's Charter (Department of Health 1991) and Our Healthier Nation (Department of Health 1998a).

The facilitation of health-enhancing activities

More than ever before, this health visiting principle is central to the concept of public health.

Personal confidence and self-esteem are crucial to individual client development and in many instances are developed through group settings. Health visitor stimulation of lay and community groups can improve health facilities in an area and also lead to safety and environmental campaigns.

The promotion of health is central and pivotal to all the principles of health visiting practice, particularly when it is associated with primary prevention and with creating structural or community change.

The specialist health promotion roles of health visitors in general practice may involve health-enhancing activities for individuals or in response to a specific need, such as stress or anxiety management. It might mean targeting wider groups across GP practice boundaries, e.g. a mobile clinic site for travellers or a monthly health market stall (Twinn & Cowley 1992). It could also mean campaigning for resources to help people to live more healthily – safer roads, better housing, more realistic levels of income support.

Our Healthier Nation (Department of Health 1998a) makes the point that previous health strategy – The Health of the Nation (Department of Health 1992) – was limited because of its reluctance to acknowledge the social, economic and environmental causes of ill-health. The redefined targets in relation to heart disease and stroke, accidents, cancer and mental health each have an attached national contract. Within these there is very clear scope for health visitors to introduce health-enhancing activities and empower the public to take these up or introduce new ones themselves.

SKILLS AND ART OF HEALTH VISITING PRACTICE IN DIFFERENT SETTINGS

Health visitors currently practise within primary healthcare teams and the skills they use are often related to the setting in which they practise. The more regular settings for practice include:

- the home
- the health centre/GP surgery
- community-based centres
- homeless accommodation or women's refuge hostels.

Health visiting in the home

The earliest fact impressed upon any student health visitor is that health visitors do indeed enter the home as a visitor and are there with the permission of the individual or family. There is no statutory right of entry in relation to visiting a new baby – the requirement is that health visitors *make contact* 11 days after the baby's birth.

Different skills are involved in the initial entry into the home from those employed when the health visitor makes regular visits. In the comparison of nursing skills with health visiting skills earlier in the chapter, it was mentioned that it is very likely that the client has little idea of what health visiting is or why the health visitor is there, particularly on first contact.

Until the middle of the 1980s most health visitors visited unannounced, at their own convenience, and it has only become apparent in the last 8–10 years that this was one of the most common reasons for the suspicion of social policing being attached to them. In the late 1980s the changing relationship between patients and healthcare professionals led to the White Paper *Working for Patients* (Department of Health 1989b). Health visitors' response to this was a recognition that home visiting was more effective when clients were prepared for and had agreed to the visit rather than when they were caught unawares and unprepared.

In the light of the above, the client now receives a letter requesting a date and time for a visit. The reason for the visit may or may not be stated at this point. Assuming that this is a first contact, clear identification of the health visitor's role in general and the relevant background of the individual practitioner, coupled with an open-mannered approach, form the baseline for

productive work. Evidence shows that good first impressions carry the greatest weight. The client is given an opportunity to question the process so far and the conversation progresses to the initial health visiting agenda. The health visitor uses all the senses to detect untoward tensions and inconveniences that may inhibit this. The art of health visiting then lies in the practitioner's ability to enable the client to pick up this agenda and follow it for their own ends. It is possible that the client may unwittingly be following dangerous procedures and it is important that the health visitor attends to these without prejudicing further work.

The health visitor is visiting a client for the first time. She is invited into the home and sees the mother holding the baby and a toddler of 2 running around in front of an unguarded fire. When asked to sit down she kneels on the carpet in front of the fire, commenting that maybe it would be useful if she could be there to protect the toddler from the fire. The conversation proceeds following the initial agenda and it is only later in the visit that the health visitor feels it is appropriate to raise the issue of safety and discuss the particular health needs relating to this dangerous situation.

Clearly, immediate adverse comment on this unsafe practice at the outset of the visit might alienate the client and yet it must be addressed before the visit is terminated.

This home safety issue would be documented in the personal child health record book, and indeed the whole area of child safety might be opened up at this time and the mother encouraged to look at other potential dangers in the home, which would be listed in the record book. Charles suggests in Chapter 10 that few clients lose the record book; if this has been the case, however, it is important that a supplementary record sheet should be used and left with the client. A copy of the sheet can be retained by the health visitor.

Health visiting skills encourage the client to pursue their own agenda once the purpose of the visit is understood. If clients raise a number of issues then the client and health visitor list and prioritise these. This means that less important issues are not overlooked and the health visitor may add one or two of her own that she has noted and that the client is happy to include.

Together the client and health visitor negotiate a series of tasks to satisfy some of the more important issues, each recognising the need for the client to feel in control of the process. Client and health visitor determine the length of time that this will take and agree a timetable for the next visit or contact.

The effectiveness of health visiting is dependent on the art and skills of meaningful dialogue and negotiating techniques and is essentially the entire basis of the giving and taking identified by Chalmers (1992). However, good documentation, well-planned follow-up programmes and clarity in the relationship between health visitor and client will enable measurement of effective health visiting in the home.

In relation to the vignette above, Robinson (1998), in a search of the literature, has shown that domiciliary visiting is effective particularly in relation to reduced unintentional injury and, to a lesser extent, the prevalence of home hazards.

Other home visits

Visiting older people in their homes can be instigated in the following ways:

- a referral from the GP
- a referral by another agency
- a referral from a colleague from another discipline
- referral by relatives or neighbours
- a self-referral as the result of an initial visit.

The skills are very similar to the visit outlined above, again requiring the health visitor to arrange the visit by letter or telephone. Either way, this is a planned visit and again requires skills of entry and agenda setting, as outlined above. Skills of health visiting require listening closely to the presenting problem, bearing in mind the possibility that it may not be the real issue. The nursing models of Roy (1975) and Orem (1991)are very useful when working with this age group because it is the activities of daily living that the client and the health visitor are negotiating.

If there is a carer in the home, the health visitor has another agenda with the carer alongside and yet separate from that of the older person. In these situations the alert health visitor often seeks to avoid any secret agendas and ensure that all concerns are fully explored. Chapter 13 discusses elder abuse, and sensitivity to this possible situation must be maintained.

Robinson's (1998) work on effectiveness of health visiting in the homes of older people found that it reduced carers' coping stress, enhanced their quality of life, reduced mortality among older people and reduced hospital admissions. In addition, work on the effectiveness of reminiscence therapy is also relevant – the very dialogue that health visitors have with older clients is likely to include reminiscence.

Other home visits are likely to be planned, perhaps in relation to child or family needs. In the majority of instances the health visitor and client will already have established a relationship and thus the skills of initial entry are minimal. The skills and art of meaningful dialogue, however, remain of paramount importance, as does the need to work in partnership with clients. Criticism of the reality of true partnership diminishes the better the working relationship between health visitors and their clients. Once they can work and negotiate in trust established by frank dialogue, there is a wider field in which they can work, covering many more topics and aspects. Chalmers (1992) suggests that good early entry work forms the basis for effective further work and calls the second phase 'the health promotion phase'. Where work in the entry phase has been poor, Chalmers suggests that clients are less likely to accept health teaching, will possibly refuse the health visitor further entry to the home and may well default on clinic appointments.

Health visiting in the health centre/GP surgery (Box 5.1)

The health visitor working in the health centre, and to a lesser extent the GP surgery, is very much part of a team. However, in larger health centres health visitors may be a team in themselves working within the wider team of paramedical staff. This approach is not the intention of the philosophy of integrated teams because

Box 5.1   Types of session that may be undertaken by health visitors within the health centre/GP surgery

Clinics (in the medical model sense)

- Well baby/child health (perhaps with the nursery nurse)
- Child health promotion/surveillance/screening
- Immunisation (often with the practice nurse)
- Well-woman (possibly with the practice nurse)
- Family planning (possibly with the practice nurse or in practices where the health visitor is the only professional with a family planning qualification)
- Asthma (where the health visitor has the additional qualification)

and others

Groups (in the health education sense)

- Parentcraft (often with midwives)
- Postnatal (usually a structured 8-week course)
- Mother and toddler (often with the nursery nurse and for children of different ages)
- Postnatal support (for mothers with personal and postnatal problems)
- Twins support (often with the nursery nurse)
- Weight control education (often with other team members)
- Exercise (often with other team members)
- Smoking cessation (often with other team members)

and others

None of the groups is a fixed entity: they depend on the expressed needs of the attending community

---

among the professionals there is in effect still only the concept of 'working alongside' rather than working in a truly integrated manner. Integrated team work is slowly being introduced into GP/community care but the models used differ widely across health authorities and trusts. It is assumed that when primary care groups really get under way not all will subscribe to the same model of integration, because of the diverse nature of the communities they serve and the human and material resources available.

Various examples of integrated teams have been publicised.

Lawton (1996) was an early commentator on an integrated team approach introduced into a Welsh general practice. In this model the main focus was on the inclusion of all practice professionals in a team with regular meetings and joint discussion on responsibilities; for example, each discipline was responsible for running

certain clinics within the practice. The team was managed by a member of one of the professional disciplines (at the time of writing, the health visitor). Future objectives were to use audit and undertake PREP requirements, staff appraisal and practice profiling. In addition, the team was looking at: shared records, practice guidelines and treatment protocols; monitoring continuity of care; developing health promotion initiatives, and setting up library facilities within the practice.

The CPHVA (1997) issued a professional briefing paper that included full references and bibliography on various models available. They included a useful definition of integration: 'A team of community based nurses from different disciplines, working together within a primary care setting, pooling their skills, knowledge and abilities in order to provide the most effective care for the practice population and community it covers' (p. 229).

The CPHVA particularly commented on the often-raised concern that the concept of integrated teams would lead to a generic community nurse and recommended that it was important that professional disciplines worked together not to compete but to recognise each other's philosophies, values, roles and responsibilities and to promote both differences and areas of commonality to GPs. There was also the concern that within integrated teams the public health remit might be lost in overriding concern for 'care' of the individual rather than the needs of the wider community. 'The wider community' may also come to mean the GP practice catchment area only, and thus practice concerns may override the social concerns of the community.

It is most likely that this competitive element will disappear with the loss of general practice fundholding and its divisive effects, and the growth of primary care groups. The very composition of the new primary care groups should ensure an equal balance between social and healthcare needs. The most appropriate model of integration should ensure, among other things, that the whole primary healthcare team produces an annual plan of action, building on the community nursing profile and identifying specific public health issues.

In many ways the organisation of health visiting within general practice is secondary to the different skills necessary to practice in centres and surgeries, and within or outside teams. The siting of health centres in the heart of the community acts as a central focus for clients seeking the health visitor, and the knowledge that the health visitor is to be found in the health centre means that clients have easy access without the need for appointments. In some areas health visiting teams who work closely together have organised themselves to allow for someone always to be available in the centre during opening hours. Criticism of the cost-effectiveness of this system was avoided by the fact that the health visitor is thus readily available and may well be running clinics or groups during this time, or catching up on the volume of paperwork that seems necessary to today's practice. A survey undertaken in one centre in the West Midlands (Windsor 1990) to evaluate the number of callers for the health visitor during a week showed that the number of client contacts easily surpassed those made by all health visitors away from the centre except at the beginning and end of the day. Clearly, this method is only effective where there is a health visiting team working together. It does not replace planned home visits but it does give clients the possibility of immediate access.

Where there is one health visitor in a GP surgery, or smaller teams in health centres, a combination of fixed health-centre times and home visiting remains the more cost-effective method. Cost-effectiveness in this sense is not about contact numbers but about the immediacy of access to a health visitor that some clients in deprived areas have found so useful. This system can also operate in rural areas provided that there is a sufficiently large team of health visitors to be able to organise it. Marley (1995) describes the need that was identified for a 'duty drop-in rota' of health visitors within the Strelley nursing development unit project. Because of resource issues in the GP practice it proved impossible to continue this. Analysis of 1 week's client-initiated contacts showed 62 as against 46 planned contacts and clearly demonstrated need

that in this instance it was, unfortunately, not possible to meet.

There is a major difference between the client visiting the health visitor in the health centre, on independent territory, and visiting at home on the client's territory. Thus the environment of the health centre has to be welcoming and give the client what they want. If the client is coming to attend a group then the organisation of that group should be such that clients have control over what they want from it. They may organise the group themselves or want to be sure that it is not too large or too small, with the attendant difficulties of being overwhelmed or exposed. Clients come to health centres, whether for individual discussion or group activities, with their own agendas. Thus it is easier for the health visitor to concentrate on their needs and what is being said. Despite this, alert health visitors will be aware that occasionally the problem is secondary to another unspoken difficulty. What is necessary here is for health visitors to have the astuteness to identify those healthcare concerns that can be safely tackled within a group setting and those that merit one-to-one conversation.

Another factor that must be considered by health visitors is time management, which may particularly be addressed by attendance at clinics or group sessions (Box 5.1).

Too much time spent with one client means someone else waiting and it may be necessary to suggest a home visit, after ensuring that the urgency of the problem is not affected by delay. The important skill in working with clients in clinics is the ability to recognise immediacy and to help clients themselves to prioritise health visiting time.

Skills in a group setting rely on the education of health visitors to work with groups, understanding their dynamics and characteristics. Tuckman's (1965) model of group behaviour is a useful knowledge base for group interaction, as is Belbin's (1993) model of team roles at work. The two models mentioned are most useful because they clearly aid the organisation of groups in the initial stages by health visitors, and then later give health visitors an understanding of how to withdraw successfully, enabling the group to continue functioning productively. In addition, health visitors' group skills and knowledge encourage group attendance and participation by shy attenders, allowing them to feel secure and comfortable in the group situation. Similarly, the same skills enable more controlling members of the group to use their skills without detriment to the shy ones. It is a skilled health visitor who enables the first-time mother to feel confident enough to sit alongside the experienced mothers, who also do not feel held back by the novices.

Health visiting in community-based centres

This area of practice has usually only been open to those health visitors who have the opportunity to undertake project work in communities. It must also be made clear that there is a difference between this and health visitors who have used community centres as a base to work from in the absence of physical space in a GP surgery or health authority clinic. These latter situations call for skills similar to those identified in the previous section. It calls for vision on the part of a trust or health authority to recognise that health visitors have the special skills to enable them to undertake community work, and it also calls for a special type of health visitor to carry it out.

In modern health visiting, one of the earliest workers in the community was Drennan (personal communication, 1984), who set up and developed health-promotion initiatives in Paddington and Kensington Health District communities. She worked against considerable difficulties in finding centres to use for group discussions and activities, ascertaining residents' health needs and requirements and encouraging and motivating colleagues to help. It is largely as a result of the knowledge and experience that she gained from this work that other centres have been set up as a result.

The inclusion of DeVille-Almond's contribution as part of Chapter 2 allows us to examine the skills necessary for this work. Clearly, one of the major skills is networking – with other professionals, non-health agencies, community leaders and vocational and charitable organisation workers. This particularly calls for patience, ignoring frustrations resulting from other workers' differing agendas and recognising that it is often difficult to create interest in the community for the enthusiasms of the few who are motivated. DeVille-Almond particularly highlights the difficulties of communicating with communities and, increasingly, community development workers attached to social services find that an early task is to motivate a small group of community leaders to take responsibility for the organisation of a newsletter. This may call for a round of discussions with local businesses and organisations to seek support to cover production costs – possibly by charging for the opportunity for local advertising.

Both DeVille-Almond and Gilbert (Gilbert & Banks 1997) have shown the need for health visitors to develop community projects to provide information to funding bodies about:

- the aims, objectives and achievements of the project to date(s)
- the work that needs to be achieved at periodic reviews
- the work at risk of not being achieved
- options on the possible way forward, with returns on investment.

The objectives of Gilbert's work are included here to show the potential value of health visiting in the community in developing the public health role for the benefit of the population of a particular area:

- to work with mainstream services to develop a health-related focus in the community
- to work with children and their families to:
  - increase their level of social and financial support
  - increase the developmental opportunities for young children
- to create structures for health action by tenants and services
- to improve the resettlement of new tenants by the provision of new information about a wide range of services

- to develop a model by which health gain can be achieved at the level of the GP practice population.

Possibly one of the most important skills attached to working in the community, with the community, is enthusiasm. Closely following this is an ability to be creative, to be able to work in any ambience (see DeVille-Almond about working in the local pub) and an infectious, challenging manner. It also calls for a resilience that outweighs despondency when one of the best ideas 'bites the dust' because of lack of resources.

Health visiting in homeless accommodation or women's refuge hostels

Health visitors work in hostels or homes on two organisational bases – either because they are working as specialist visitors or because the home or hostel is part of the general practice caseload.

Health visitors working as specialist practitioners often cover the whole catchment area of the health authority and thus become the specialist expert for their colleagues, receiving referrals and linking with colleagues when clients are moved on. The skills of health visiting in the specialist approach are a knowledge of all aspects of homeless law, knowledge of alternative options to bed and breakfast accommodation, and skills of negotiation for and on behalf of the client. The work of the specialist health visitor service for homeless families has been well discussed by Hutchinson & Gutteridge (1995), who detail ways in which the health of homeless families has been improved by the introduction of this specialism.

In many cases the plight of homeless families in bed and breakfast accommodation includes the problem of temporary registration with local GPs, and there are particular problems in the London area, where a few GPs are unwilling to accept homeless families on to their caseloads.

Some bed and breakfast accommodation facilities are so poor that health visitors working with families living there are in constant distress

about what they see. There have been a number of research projects detailing the health problems of families in bed and breakfast accommodation – foremost among these was the SHAC/Shelter report of 1988, which has been followed by others (Amina Mama 1996, Barrie-Foy 1997). The skills of health visitors here are to work as positively as possible, endeavouring to arrange for children to be admitted to play groups and nurseries as a matter of urgency and helping mothers to reduce the accident potential of totally unsuitable accommodation. It is also important that as far as possible the health visitor arranges for domiciliary services, e.g. family planning, immunisation and child surveillance. Helping parents to find somewhere to go during the day is also a priority in this type of health visiting as is ensuring that they have every benefit they are entitled to by encouraging them to apply to local family benefit centres.

Health visiting in single-parent hostels calls for yet another group of skills from the health visitor. Personal selling is particularly relevant to this aspect of promoting the service (de la Cuesta 1994). Adjusting the approach through physical appearance and language to appear trendily acceptable is a means of gaining a client's confidence. Many young mothers in single-parent hostels are deeply suspicious of possible paternalism and resent any suggestion of criticism of their child-rearing practices. Often they have been in the care of the social services themselves during part of their lives, lack experiences of positive parenting and are fearful that their children may be taken away because of their present circumstances.

The skills of the health visitor in these circumstances lie in breaking down barriers, trying to create trust and confidence in the young mothers and at the same time promoting parenting and teaching child care and maternal health. Group work is often a way forward, particularly if a young member of the team takes this on, but the contents of sessions for discussion have to be determined by the group and the skill here is in introducing areas of health or child care that have not initially been seen by the group as relevant. Often, young women are under considerable pressures from their families, the baby's father and other friends, and in many cases resent the herding together of people all with the same difficulties into one hostel, added to which they may be separated from their extended family because of lack of space in the family home, the breakdown of relationships or merely the absence of accommodation nearby.

A major concern of young single mothers invited to group sessions is that they will be subjected to a school approach; in many cases they have not completed their schooling or failed to gain any qualifications and thus have a negative concept of education. This work will be further discussed in Chapter 12.

PSYCHOLOGICAL SKILLS OF HEALTH VISITING

The Hyland–Donaldson Psychological Skills Scale for Health Visitors (Hyland & Donaldson 1987) was a tool developed for teaching and assessment of students. It consists of a scale of eight sections each dealing with a different psychological skill:

- Basic nonverbal communication skills
- Basic verbal communication skills
- Advanced communication skills
- Assessment skills
- Adult management skills
- Child interaction skills
- Family management skills
- Professional relationship skills.

It is not the intention to analyse each individual skill here or to assume poor knowledge of them, but without these skills the entry phase of Chalmers (1992) discussed above cannot succeed. There is further discussion of communication approaches in Chapter 12. One of the criticisms occasionally levelled at health visitors is apparent lack of empathy, i.e. failing to understand the problem from the client's perspective. Health visitors can be deflected from the client by a need to reassure because of a desire to put things right – to be seen as helpful.

Thus, active listening requires the identification of emotions portrayed through verbal and nonverbal communication, and reflection back to the client to find out whether your interpretation of what has been said is correct, including an assessment of the nonverbal messages that have been received.

Assessment skills – accurately summarising the content of discussion at the end of the intervention – encourage the client to feel that active listening has taken place and that there has been no misunderstanding on the part of the health visitor. This gives the client hope that action will take place and that her dignity and self-confidence have been preserved.

Adult management skills include the need to be very aware of your own and the client's attitudes to health values and behaviours. Avoidance of stereotyping, not judging by first impressions and recognising that the client's behaviour is caused by the situation rather than a personality problem, are clearly part of empathy and comprehension in the effective health visitor.

Health visiting is often important in maintaining family harmony. It is not suggested that the health visitor should acts as an arbitrator in family disputes but the skills to support both partners, or the absent partner, and to defuse emotions are sometimes necessary.

Finally, in professional relationships it is clearly important that health visitors recognise the difference between assertion and aggression. Of all the community professionals, health visitors are at greatest risk of being interpreted as aggressive. This because they often need to deal firmly with other professionals or agencies to communicate their concerns about the intolerable circumstances in which clients are living or their anxiety about potential child neglect or abuse. At best, this is interpreted by community nurses as 'bossy', at worst as aggressive.

CONCLUSION

This chapter has discussed how the education of health visitors builds on the skills of nurses and modifies these in different contexts to create alternative perspectives. In the process these initial skills are modified from a reductionist approach to a holistic approach. Students newly into health visiting education complain that they feel they are being deskilled, but what is actually happening is this modification from reductionism to holism. Baraclough's figure (Fig. 5.1) is a very good way of viewing the major conceptual shifts that newly qualified health visitors must make.

The principles of health visiting have been explored as a process rather than as an outcome, because each of the four principles demands a very different research and communication ability in the practitioner. This approach has been maintained when discussing the main venues that health visitors work in: homes, clinics, community and other centres.

The psychology of communication has always been important in health visiting and the work of Hyland & Donaldson (1987) in clustering these into aspects of health visiting communication has proved invaluable in determining the similarities and differences in approach to individual clients and families. Health visiting is moving forward into the public health model of primary care, and the skills learned in practice remain a formidable basis on which to continue development. The only skill that possibly requires strengthening is that health visitors should be prepared to recognise that the traditional approach of working in the home with families must be better balanced by more work with communities. This demands developed networking abilities, the motivation to seek out and the skills to empower people acting on behalf of the community to which they belong.

6

Reflective practice in health visiting

Anne Robotham and Doreen Sheldrake

INTRODUCTION

Health visitor education has for many years taught its new practitioners to evaluate their work during debriefing sessions. At different stages of the educational process, students are encouraged by the practice teacher to describe what they have done with the client and relate it to their current knowledge. The debriefing sessions allow the community practice teacher to explore with the student the content of their intervention work with the client, the relationship between the work done and their present state of knowledge, and finally their own feelings about the experience. These feelings include an assessment of the purpose and outcomes of the intervention, all aspects of communication with the client and an analysis of the student's values and behaviour in relation to the client contact. These debriefing sessions between community practice teacher and student begin as regular, frequent meetings (even twice a day, initially), but as time goes on their structure changes from description to critical analysis and evaluation.

This chapter is designed to follow the process of education of a student health visitor, including theory of practice, reflective practice, knowledge, critical analysis, conceptual frameworks and mapping, and finally creative thinking.

To begin any process of evaluation or reflection one must initially consider what health visiting is and what its practice consists of.

HEALTH VISITING PRACTICE

It is appropriate here to give the full definition of health visiting practice as formally defined in 1977 (CETHV 1977), which has remained germane to health visiting practice in the new millennium:

The professional practice of health visiting consists of planned activities aimed at the promotion of health and prevention of ill-health. It thereby contributes substantially to individual and social well-being by focusing attention at various times on either an individual, a social group or a community. It has three unique functions:

(i) identifying and fulfilling self-declared and recognised, as well as unacknowledged and unrecognised, health needs of individuals and social groups

(ii) providing a generalist service in an era of increasing specialisation in the health care available to individuals and communities

(iii) monitoring simultaneously the health needs and demands of individuals and communities, contributing to the fulfilment of these needs, facilitating appropriate care and service by other professional health care groups.

Robinson (1982), in a masterly work on the evaluation of health visiting, struggled with the idea that health visiting contains a body of knowledge upon which practice is built, and over the past 18 years there have been many attempts to evaluate health visiting practice (Luker 1982, Robinson 1982, Dobby 1986, Twinn 1989, Cowley 1991, Chalmers 1992). Despite these and other careful analyses, there has been no clear articulation of the body of knowledge unique to health visiting. Robinson (1982) and Twinn (1991) consider that health visiting practice is both a science and an art. Goodwin (1988) suggests that health visiting, as a science alone without the art, becomes mechanistic, routine and even mindless, with the measurable product being a numerical list of contacts. It could be argued that skills and knowledge are fundamentally entwined in the philosophy of health visiting and that to disentangle these within the individuality of practice will reveal both the science and artistry that Robinson (1982) and Twinn (1989) discuss.

The opening statement in this chapter recognises the community practice teacher as pivotal in teaching health visiting practice. In the very title 'Community Practice Teacher' lies an assumption that there is a definable type of work in professional life that is called practice and means just that – practice of an art or science. Jarvis (1992) suggests a theory of practice, and that to understand professional practice it is necessary to understand health visiting action with which to underpin the theory. He draws on the work of Schutz (1972) to posit an idea of meaningful social action that he argues is an adequate description of professional practice. However, many professional practitioners would challenge the notion that practice is all action, and Jarvis accepts this point and suggests that within professional practice there is also nonaction.

On the basis of this it might now be appropriate to identify categories of action as part of practice (Table 6.1).

Table 6.1   A theoretical analysis of conscious action (Jarvis 1992)

Category of action	Level of consciousness		
	Planning	Monitoring	Retrospecting
Nonaction			
Anomic	None	None	High
Prohibited	Low–High	None	None–High
Nonresponse	None–High	None	None–High
Action			
Experimental	High	High	High
Repetitive	High–None	High–Low	High–None
Presumptive	None–Low	None–Low	None
Ritualistic	None	None–Low	None–High
Alienating	None	None–Low	None–High

ACTION IN PRACTICE

In identifying categories of non-action it is important to recognise their value in eliciting what has occurred (or not) in practice – i.e. what was considered by the practitioner but rejected because intuitively it was felt that alternative actions would be more appropriate in the circumstances. It is recognised that all activities ought to be client-led. However, there are many situations where the health visitor suggests a variety of options, one of which the client selects. Within these options are categories of action and, if considered, they reach the level of conscious planning by both client and health visitor. It still means that there may be unexpressed options that fall into the anomic category with its attendant consciousness level.

For example, in a moment of desperation the client may fleetingly consider suicide. It is neither expressed to the health visitor nor, indeed, seriously planned by the client. It thus becomes an anomic action because the health visitor, reflecting on the situation, has the sensitivity and perception to recognise that it could have been an option. In other words, at the time the health visitor and client did not plan or monitor the option but retrospection suggested the possibility. Each health visiting situation is unique, with attendant unique categories of nonaction.

It is necessary to consider levels of consciousness because it is only on the basis of their recognition that reflection can take place. Thus reflection must encompass the ability to articulate consciousness levels – was something planned, was it monitored by the practitioner (or client), was retrospective thought given to the process within the situation?

The premise that there is an art and a science to health visiting was mentioned earlier. Using analysis of categories of action enables the reflective practitioner to recognise that one can only measure action, not nonaction. Thus nonaction, which is an essential part of health visiting practice through its consideration and rejection by practitioner and client, becomes part of the art of health visiting because the nature of science is that it is measurable. Continuing with this theme, the measurement of the scientific aspect is in effect the measurement of tasks undertaken because the categories of action are all based on visible planning with clearly identified outcomes.

The two other categories of nonaction identified in Table 6.1 can be treated similarly. For example, a health visitor who is a community practice teacher is running late for a planned appointment with a client. She drives over the speed limit and arrives at the venue reasonably promptly. A later debriefing session with her student focuses on time management. The health visitor uses as an analogy the difficulty of keeping to planned visits and realises that in reaching her earlier appointment on time she has used a prohibited category of action. To help the student to understand the process they consider together whether consciousness levels are part of this category of action. Together they consider whether driving within the law is part of health visiting practice. They also consider whether breaking the law was conscious or unconscious – simply being so focused on the management of her work that an unconscious action occurred. In the normal course of events the community practice teacher would not have given this another thought but in searching for an example to illustrate levels of consciousness to the student she has selected this example and thus there was a retrospecting level of consciousness.

Non-response is, for example, when people involved in situations do know how to respond but choose not to at that time. A health visitor is passing through the GP surgery waiting room when she sees a client at reception whom she knows is coming to her with a difficult problem. She decides not to approach the client in anticipation and to wait until the receptionist rings through to say that the client is waiting to see her. She selects this non-action in the knowledge (high-planning level) that she can check her records in order to prepare herself for the intervention.

Turning to categories of action, it is useful to be able to discuss them all, finding examples in practice to enable the student to recognise that level of consciousness is essential to the reflective process.

Experimental action is seen as being creative, new actions being worked out in the process of health visiting practice. This typifies health visiting because each intervention is practised within a new contextual situation and, for practice to be relevant, previously tried methods will have to be modified (experimented with) to satisfy the new situation. For this process to be effective a high level of consciousness is required at all stages. This could be interpreted as the artistry within experimental action.

Repetitive action can be either highly conscious, as in Table 6.1, or involve limited levels of consciousness. Highly conscious repetitive actions in health visiting include the constant repetition of feeding or weaning advice, e.g. in the well baby clinic, articulated to suit each individual client. Poor practice would be to repeat the same advice irrespective of client individuality; good practice means that the entire communication is consciously underpinned by being tailored to the client.

Presumptive action has little place in sensitive and perceptive health visiting. There are few, if any, instances when a health visitor would programme an action with the client without a detailed communication process to ascertain its appropriateness to their needs. All communicative action is therefore assumed to have a higher level of consciousness than that identified with presumptive action.

Ritualistic action has been seen as the bedrock of past traditional health visiting practice – 'we do it this way because we have always done it this way'. The importance of research-based practice carried out in a challenging and questioning atmosphere is to eradicate all ritualistic practice. Again, the low levels of consciousness required are inappropriate except in retrospection, which is the hub of reflection. *Reflection therefore, is the safeguard against ritualistic practice.*

Finally, **alienating action** mitigates against any meaningful further work with the client. As discussed in Chapter 5, effective initial entry work by health visitors will ensure the continuation of planned programmes of activity.

It is also useful here to discuss the dangers to practice of:

- experiment without safeguards or experience

- repetition without consciousness
- presumption without communication and checking-out
- ritual without conscious thought – habitual practice may be dangerous practice
- alienating, which will prevent client participation and empowerment.

Discussion of action moves the process of reflection through learning from action.

LEARNING FROM ACTION

Retrospection (Table 6.1) can be seen as the precursor to reflection, which is most likely to occur when retrospection indicates that the action has not produced the expected outcome, e.g. when the probability factor has been greater than was anticipated. Learning occurs during the process of translating retrospection to reflection. Dictionary definitions (*Penguin English Dictionary*) identify the process:

- Retrospect: to look back
- Retrospection: act of looking back on past experience
- Reflection: act of reflecting, thoughtful consideration, meditation.

Thus, moving from retrospection to reflection must include learning from the experience, and to learn from experience there must be an analysis of that experience from which to learn.

Learning from practice is experience and therefore becomes experiential learning.

Argyris & Schön (1974) conducted a number of studies across a variety of professional groups to develop a theory of competent interpersonal practice and explain how individuals learn in practice situations. They concluded that there are theories of action, including values, strategies and underlying assumptions, that form individuals' patterns of personal behaviour in professional practice. Argyris & Schön identified two levels of theories in action – *espoused theory* and *theory-in-use.*

They suggested that espoused theory is what an individual, when questioned, says (s)he would do, and theory-in-use is what the individual, when observed in practice, actually does. Argyris (1982) later challenged this by showing the incongruence between espoused theory and theory-in-use and suggested that espoused theories may be seen as a representation of the accepted norms of a profession and theories-in-use the practitioner's intuitive response to the particulars of a given situation, which are difficult to describe but can be observed in the practitioner's behaviour.

Twinn (1991) uses Schön's (1983) work to argue that intuition and artistry are complex aspects of professional practice but are nevertheless fundamental to the process of professional judgement, which is essential to effective action in professional practice and can only be learned from experience.

Jarvis's earlier work (Jarvis 1987) demonstrated how reflective skills and reflective knowledge stem from disjuncture, i.e. questioning why the outcome has occurred, particularly if something has gone wrong. From this premise he formed a typology of learning (Table 6.2).

Each of the reflective forms of learning can have two possible outcomes – conformity or change. Scrutiny of Table 6.2 in relation to health visiting suggests that there is a similar process in nonlearning to the nonaction in Table 6.1 and that therefore the same analysis is appropriate.

Nonreflective learning belongs to the early days of student health visiting practice where the knowledge level is insufficient to work without preconscious skills of briefing, prior to an intervention, as the result of the preparation between community practice teacher and student. This is part of the early shadowing process essential to build experiential knowledge. Thus,

during debriefing sessions in these early days, the community practice teacher and student identify the action/nonaction processes and thus the learning/nonlearning processes will follow. Moving through the nonreflective learning aspect of Table 6.2 enables student reflective learning and making sense of situations as they evolve.

Boyd & Fales (1983), considering the link between knowledge and learning, examined learning from experience and argue that research on learning from experience tended to focus on the *outcomes* of such learning rather than the *process*. They contended that experiential learning must be conceptualised as a process and that most of this type of learning goes on without the benefit of a structured learning environment, much of it is unintentional and some of it is even unconscious. The main advantage of the teacher/ practitioner–student relationship is that the environment is structured to a greater or lesser extent, and for this reason the student may learn more quickly from experiential learning – particularly when there is active reflection through the debriefing process. This process requires the use of a reflective journal (to be discussed further).

TEACHING LEARNING BY INTERPRETING REFLECTION

To facilitate the preceding discussion, it is recommended that the student uses the model illustrated in Figure 6.1 during shadowing, for reflecting with the community practice teacher.

With the client's permission the student records the visit in the journal, including as many aspects of the cycle as possible. The journal entry for this visit is discussed using Socratic dialogue. The community practice teacher adds further comment, using his/her professional knowledge and judgement, to explore all aspects of the visit from the perspective of all the participants concerned, using the Gibbs categories outlined in the cycle. This process is time-consuming but the community practice teacher who makes time in the early days finds that this is compensated for by the speed with which the student absorbs experiential learning. Empirical evidence (Sheldrake et al 1998) shows that students move

Table 6.2 A typology of learning (Jarvis 1992)

Category of learning	Type of learning
Nonlearning	Presumption
	Nonconsideration
	Rejection
Nonreflective learning	Preconscious skills
	Memorisation
Reflective learning	Contemplation
	Reflective skills
	Experimental knowledge

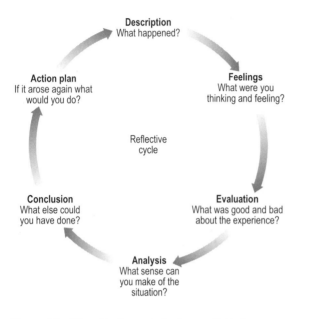

Figure 6.1   The reflective cycle (redrawn with kind permission from Gibbs 1988)

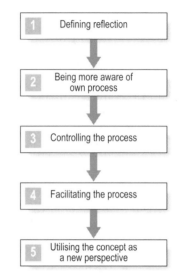

Figure 6.2   Towards a progression of reflection (redrawn with kind permission from Boyd & Fales 1983)

far more quickly through the stages of novice to advanced beginner and hence to competence, as suggested by Benner (1984).

Reflective learning is the *process* of learning and makes the difference between whether a person repeats the same experience several times, becoming highly proficient at one behaviour, or learns from experience in such a way that he or she is cognitively or affectively changed. To explore the process of learning how to reflect Boyd & Fales (1983) used qualified counsellors who were accepted by their peers as 'reflective persons'. In repeated interviews with nine counsellors Boyd & Fales showed a progression of focus shifts within the activity of reflecting on the process of reflection and these are represented in Figure 6.2.

To examine this figure briefly:

Stage 1. Defining reflection means initially exploring its parameters. The greatest difficulty is pinning down what we mean by reflection – what is it? what is it not?

Stage 2 proceeds in the light of 1: one is now more conscious of reflecting even if not sure what it is. A suggestion is that it is self-revealing,

i.e. that really it is all about ourselves and our response to a situation.

Stage 3. Boyd & Fales's group found that with this emphasis on reflection they were actively able to control decision-making – the reflective process enabled them to speed up active thinking. They did, however, feel the need to control the process and, if they were stuck, to stop going round in circles. Interestingly, the counsellors felt that at times the focus was unwelcome and they had to learn how to turn it off – to distract themselves.

Stage 4 created some excitement in the counsellors as they allowed the client/student to become more aware of what s/he does and let them come to their own conclusions.

Stage 5 The study group found they had used reflecting as a concept to enhance existing knowledge and understanding.

As a result of this initial study with their group Boyd & Fales were able to construct a set of components of the process of reflection based on an analysis of self (Table 6.3).

Clearly, this is based on a counselling process, and the teaching of health visiting practice is similar because the demands of counselling

Table 6.3   The process of reflection based on the analysis of self (Boyd & Fales 1983)

Stage of reflection	Process descriptors
1. A sense of inner discomfort	Awareness that something doesn't 'fit'. A feeling as though we have 'forgotten' something
2. Identification or clarification of the concern	A key characteristic appears to be that, unlike thinking or problem solving, the reflective process is conceptualised in relation to self
3. Openness to new information from internal and external sources, with ability to observe and take in from a variety of perspectives	Openness taking the form of reviewing past experience, foregoing the need for immediate closure on the issue (i.e. forming a conclusion), intentionally structured lateral thinking, intentionally setting aside the problem. For the community practice teacher/counsellor this is a useful intervention stage by enabling the collecting of this information but without forcing it into a pattern
4. Resolution, expressed as 'integration', 'coming together', 'acceptance of self-reality' and 'creative synthesis'	This is the 'eureka' stage of reflection, when insight is gained and at which point people experience themselves as changed, having learned or having come to a satisfactory point of closure in relation to the issue (i.e. reached a satisfactory endpoint or conclusion)
5. Establishing continuity of self with past, present and future	There is a recognition in terms of similar solutions from past experience, reviewing past values in relation to the changed perspective, evaluating the change as better for self, applying the new perspective to a variety of additional issues in the present self-structure, planning for future behaviour consistent with the changed perspective, or examining the implications of the change for future behaviour
6. Deciding whether to act on the outcome of the reflective process	The change or resolution is evaluated in terms of the individual's own subjective criteria, the intensity of the subjective sense of the rightness of the resolution, its consistency with the individual's existing or aspired value structure, and with other desired goals of the self. The need to test one's self-changes against the mirror of others is an essential component of all growth

mirror the demands of the unique health visiting context. In teaching the practice of health visiting it is impossible to divorce the influence of self (i.e. the practitioner) from the structured enablement of client power.

To extend the above discussion, Saylor (1990) described research analysis of student nurses' ability to evaluate self in terms of a job well done. Students from early seniority levels were most likely to base their evaluations on positive re-actions from the client, contrasting with experienced seniors, who were most likely to base their evaluations on objective data. For example, they often described thinking back on the day and reviewing vital signs, pain and level of anxiety, understanding the rationale for procedures and medication as a measure of competency. On the basis of this work, Saylor suggested that reflective self-evaluation using appropriate indicators is essential for professional education. In addition to being a means of appropriate self-evaluation, reflection is also necessary for experiential learning.

Thought processes in learning

In developing a theory of reflection and teacher education Goodman (1984) was concerned that the meaning of the term 'reflection' should be clarified and his argument focused on the need to recognise that reflection is not just quiet rumination. If reflection is to be a worthwhile goal within teacher education (and thus health visitor education), our notion of it must be comprehensive.

Firstly, reflection suggests a need to focus on substantive rather than utilitarian concerns, i.e. the categories of action/non-action. Secondly, a theory of reflection must be legitimate and integrate both intuitive and rational thinking, i.e. the categories of conscious thinking. Finally, certain underlying attitudes are necessary in order to be truly reflective, i.e. the process descriptors of Boyd & Fales's (1983) stages of reflection.

Dewey (1933) referred to *routine thought*, which is a process of thinking and may lead to problem-solving but is in direct opposition to that of reflection. Routine thought is about how we confront, manage and deal with immediate situations, but it does not allow time to reflect because it lacks the patience necessary to work through one's doubts and perplexity. Goodman (1984) identifies *rational thought*, which is clearly distinguishable from routine thought and which some observers equate to reflection. However, Goodman argues that rational thought does not encompass *intuitive thought*, which is associated with the spark of creative ideas, insight and empathy. He thus posits reflective thinking as occurring with the integration of rational and intuitive thought processes. It is possible that this is the art and science of thinking in health visiting practice.

Up to this point the emphasis has been on the student, but it is important that the ability of the community practice teacher is not forgotten: drawing again on Dewey (1933), Goodman identifies three attitudes as prerequisites for reflective teaching:

- *open-mindedness*: an active desire to listen to more sides than one
- *responsibility*: there must be a desire to synthesise ideas, to make sense out of nonsense and to apply information in an aspired direction. This attitude fosters consideration of the consequences and implications beyond questions of immediate utility
- *wholeheartenedness*: the internal strength necessary for genuine reflection and the ability to work through fears and insecurities.

It is suggested that both teacher and student work within these parameters. Goodwin identified three levels of reflection. In the light of the analysis of thought processes, these could be assigned similar levels (Table 6.4).

At the third level, if practitioners relied on reflective criteria only then there might be a constraint in the development of practice. Heath (1998) uses Porter & Ryan (1996) to postulate that reflection is not necessarily the dominant factor in higher level practice and that it is the combination with a comparable level of thought that spearheads expert practice. If reflection only is used then practitioners may conclude that practice cannot be developed because of the constraints of organisation or policy and go no further. Thus creative thinking (level 3 thought) must be seen to precede level 3 reflection in order that practice can move forward, albeit on the basis of reflection. This suggests that levels of thought might be one step ahead of levels of reflection. However, creative thought requires high levels of reflection. To explore this further other models of reflectivity should be examined.

Levels of reflectivity

In writing on a critical theory of adult education and learning Mezirow (1981) proposed levels of reflectivity within the learning process (Box 6.1).

Mezirow (1981) proposes that the first four levels are of a lower order, likening these to consciousness. The remaining three are thus at a higher level, likened to critical consciousness. The link between Mezirow's proposition and reflection via consciousness is illuminated by the statement made in the first section of the chapter – here repeated – 'It is necessary to consider [the] levels of consciousness because it is only on the

Table 6.4 Comparative examination of levels of reflection and thought

Level	Levels of reflection (Goodman 1984)	Levels of thought (Dewey/Goodman)
1	*Reflection to reach given objectives*: Criteria for reflection are limited to technocratic issues of efficiency, effectiveness and accountability	*Thinking encompasses formulations of ideas (routine thought)*: Criteria for thinking include situational observation, previous and current knowledge
2	*Reflection on the relationship between principles and practice*: There is an assessment of the implications and consequences of actions and beliefs as well as the underlying rationale for practice	*Thinking is about processing the information (rational thought)*: Criteria for thinking include the absorption and assimilation of all evidence (including policies) to formulate a recognisable structure for strategic action
3	*Reflection which, besides the above, incorporates ethical and political concerns*: Issues of justice and emancipation enter deliberations over the value of professional goals and practice and the practitioner makes links between the setting of everyday practice and broader social structure and forces	*Thinking is about creating and using information for new ideas (intuitive thought)*: Criteria for thinking include assimilated evidence within research-based knowledge: it relies on the ability to rise above policy and organisational constraints to allow far-sighted flexible practice

> **Box 6.1** Levels of reflectivity (Mezirow 1981)
>
> - **Reflectivity** – awareness of specific perception, meaning or behaviour of our own or of habits we have of seeing, thinking or acting
> - **Affective reflectivity** – becoming aware of how we feel about the way we are perceiving, thinking or acting or about our habits of doing so
> - **Discriminant reflectivity** – we assess the efficacy of our perceptions, thoughts, actions and habits of doing things; identify immediate causes; recognise reality contexts in which we are functioning (play, dream, religious, musical or drug experience) and identify our relationships in the situation
> - **Judgmental reflectivity** – involves making and becoming aware of our value judgements about our perceptions, thoughts, actions and habits in terms of their being liked or disliked, beautiful or ugly, positive or negative
> - **Conceptual reflectivity** – becoming aware of our awareness and critiquing it, i.e. critical awareness or critical consciousness
> - **Psychic reflectivity** – this leads one to recognise in oneself the habit of making precipitate judgements about people on the basis of limited information about them
> - **Theoretical reflectivity** – differs from the previous two in that it encompasses them both in a process central to perspective transformation. Theoretical reflectivity represents a uniquely adult capacity and, as such, becomes realised through perspective transformation

basis of their recognition that reflection can take place. Thus reflection must encompass the ability to articulate consciousness levels – was something planned, was it monitored by the practitioner (or client), was retrospective thought given to the process within the situation.'

It is assumed, therefore, that using the technique above to compare Goodman's three levels of reflectivity with the levels of thought process, it should be possible to identify seven levels of thought process. However, the exercise is not conducive to the momentum of the chapter and it will therefore be left to the reader to attempt this task.

A more recent hierarchy of levels of reflection has been identified in Table 6.5, which is a model proposed by Kitchener & King (1990) to facilitate learners to become critically reflective.

The reflective judgement model describes changes in assumptions about sources and certainty of knowledge and how decisions are justified in the light of these assumptions. That is, the model focuses on describing the development of epistemological (theory and nature of knowledge) assumptions and how these act as meaning perspectives that radically affect the way individuals understand and subsequently solve problems. The model has seven stages, and each stage includes assumptions about what can be known and how certain one can be about knowing it; it also includes assumptions about the role of evidence, authority and interpretation in the formation of solutions to problems. This model goes beyond the first tentative stages for student learning, but can certainly be used by the time they are halfway through their practicum.

Clearly, Table 6.5 has led us into an extension of the reflecting and thinking processes into an analysis of knowledge, whether there is a body of knowledge called health visiting and whether it is possible to reflect on knowledge identified as belonging to one professional discipline alone.

Knowledge

Schön (1983) proposes that the professions are bound by a form of professional knowledge that fails to take into account the indeterminacy of practice. Schön argues that the dominant epistemology (a branch of science that deals with the nature and validity of knowledge) of practice is *technical rationality*, which relies on the assumption that empirical science – based on positive facts and observable phenomena – is the only source of objective knowledge about the world. Schön suggests that there is an area in professional practice where practitioners can make use of research-based theory and technique, but equally there are other areas where there are uncertainties and value conflicts that are incapable of technical solution. Benner (1984) also makes the point that not all knowledge embedded in expertise can be captured in theoretical propositions or in analytical strategies that depend on identifying all the elements that go into a clinical decision.

Eraut (1985) argues that there are different kinds of professional knowledge. He suggests that there is knowledge of the kind that does not

Table 6.5 The reflective judgement model (Kitchener & King 1990)

Stage of reflective judgement	Characteristics (modified to suit health visiting)
Stage 1	Knowing is characterised by a concrete, single-belief system: what the person knows to be true is true. Knowledge is both absolute and concrete: beliefs do not need to be justified. This is unlikely to be seen in student health visitors as it probably only belongs to young children.
Stage 2	Knowing takes on more complexity since individuals assume that, while truth is ultimately accessible, it may not be directly and immediately known to everyone – some people hold 'right' beliefs while others hold 'wrong' ones. There is an assumption that the source of a knowledgeable answer will be an authority, e.g. teacher, doctor. This might be apparent in initial nurse training. It can concern the student health visitor because they may have to revisit this level having come into training as an experienced practitioner. The client might expect knowledgeable answers from them in this new professional approach.
Stage 3	There is a belief that authorities/professionals hold the truth although it may be at times inaccessible. However, they believe that absolute truth will be manifest in concrete data sometime in the future and argue that, since evidence is currently incomplete, no one can claim any authority beyond his or her own impressions or feelings. Individuals at this stage do not understand or acknowledge any basis for evaluation beyond these feelings. This may well be seen during the first semester in average and above students and for weaker students may last considerably longer.
Stage 4	The uncertainty of knowing is initially acknowledged at this stage and usually attributed to the limitations of the knower. Without certainty, individuals argue that knowledge cannot be validated externally; thus, they argue, it is idiosyncratic. The fact that uncertainty is clearly accepted at this stage as an intrinsic characteristic of knowing is, however, an important development. It allows individuals to distinguish between well- and ill-structured problems (Churchman 1971, Kitchener 1983, Wood 1983). Well-structured problems, e.g. an arithmetic problem, can be described completely and solved with certainty. Ill-structured, real-world problems, e.g. how to reduce pollution, are such because all the parameters are seldom clear or available and it is difficult to determine when and whether an adequate solution has been identified. When students in stages 1, 2 and 3 cannot acknowledge that some problems do not have an absolutely correct solution, they cannot acknowledge the existence of real, ill-structured problems. This stage may be seen in the student health visitor prior to health visiting practice.
Stage 5	Individuals believe that knowledge must be placed within a context, an assumption deriving from the understanding that interpretation plays a role in what a person perceives. This is beyond the idiosyncratic justifications of stage 4: it is only at stage 5 that they are able to compare and evaluate the relative merits of two alternative interpretations of the same issue. This should be typical of all students about to complete the health visitor course.
Stage 6	Knowing is uncertain and knowledge must be understood in relation to the context from which it was derived. Knowing involves evaluation and some perspectives, arguments or points of view may be evaluated as better than others. These evaluations involve comparing evidence and opinion across contexts, which allows an initial basis for forming judgements about ill-structured problems.
Stage 7	Individuals still believe that knowing is uncertain and subject to interpretation, but they can argue that epistemically justifiable claims can be made about the better or best solution to the problem under consideration. As with Dewey's (1933) description of reflective thinking, individuals claim that knowledge can be constructed via critical inquiry and through the synthesis of existing evidence and opinion into claims that can be evaluated as having greater 'truth value' or being more 'warranted' than others.

normally get included in syllabi. This knowledge may be as significant as the quality of 'getting on with people', which may simply be assumed as part of the job, although it could be academicised as 'interpersonal skills' or 'psychology' and is the basis of Chapter 6. Another form of knowledge,

Eraut claims, is professional codified knowledge derived from an analysis of such activities as problem-solving, decision-making and communication, and is clearly different in kind from the experience-derived know-how that professionals intuitively use. Eraut quotes Oakeshott (1962), following Aristotle, as making a clear distinction between 'technical knowledge' and 'practical knowledge'. Technical knowledge is capable of written codification but practical knowledge is expressed only in practice and is learned only through experience with practice.

If Eraut is right in his analysis, therefore, the relationship between these two is difficult to assess and is called the theory–practice gap.

Similarly, and much later Heath (1998) uses Moch (1990) to compare the knowledge that evolves within research-based practice and the theory that might stem from practice, or is derived separately from it. She suggests that during the reflective process the professional may recognise that the knowledge s/he is identifying has evolved from within *that very* practice.

Meerabeau (1992) draws on the work of Polanyi (1958, 1967) to describe 'tacit knowledge': experts do not use the same pattern of skills as learners but they view situations holistically and much of their knowledge is embedded in practice. It would seem that the embedded knowledge that Meerabeau describes is the intuitive knowledge suggested by other writers. Eraut (1985) draws on the work of Broudy et al (1964), who suggest that this intuitive mode of knowledge (called semi-conscious) often involves metaphors or images that do not derive only from practical experience but also serve as carriers for theoretical ideas. As metaphor can only be articulated in language the argument is carried into the necessary recognition that language use is of considerable importance in espousing knowledge.

Deshler (1990a) suggested that metaphor is the means whereby critical reflection and transformative learning can be recognised and identified. Metaphors can assist us to reflect on personal, popular-cultural and organisational socialisation. Through 'unpacking' meaning associated with these domains, metaphors uncover frames of reference or structures of assumptions that have influenced the way we perceive, think, decide, feel and act upon our experience. Deshler states that metaphors are concrete images that require us to find threads of continuity and congruence between the metaphor and the primary object.

Mezirow (1981) argues that perspectives are constitutive of experience. They determine how we see, think, feel and behave. Human experience is brought into being through language. Restrictive language codes can arbitrarily distort experience so that it gets shoehorned into categories of meanings or typifications. *Meaning perspectives* can incorporate fragmented, incomplete experience involving areas of meaninglessness, and *typification* is the process of categorising our perceptions.

The chapter has so far worked through some major concepts related to learning, reflection, judgement and knowledge and the next step in the process of using reflection in practice is to look at ways in which these concepts might be structured in the thinking process. A number of models of structured reflection have been postulated by writers. This chapter is concerned with three only, the Gibbs (1988) model which is recommended for the early days of learning to reflect, and the two models set out in Boxes 6.2 and 6.3.

The community practice teacher plays an important part in unpacking the reflective journal jointly with the student. Language and metaphor use in the journal requires exploration and checking back with student conceptualisation of the experience articulated. Initially, of course, this process is a shared process during the period of shadowing of the community practice teacher by the student. However, later, when the student is practising alone and articulating the content of the practice intervention, it is essential to explore the meaning of language and metaphor used. This entire process should be normalised to the extent that it becomes totally integrated into the student's subsequent qualified practice. Good health visiting practice should always be managed in such a way that the practitioner deliberately allows time for reflection and this may need to be written rather than just mused upon.

Currently, the purchasing of health visiting practice is based on a quantification of task analysis in those areas of practice visible to the purchasers. As yet unexplored is the entirely new concept of the purchase of reflective practice. If, as is well articulated in the literature, good professional practice is research-based reflective practice, this should be the practice that purchasers

---

Box 6.2   A model of structured reflection (Carper 1978, Johns 1992)

1. Description of the experience
   1. Phenomenon – describe the here and now experience
   2. Causal – what essential factors contributed to the experience?
   3. Context – what/who are the significant background actors in the experience?
   4. Clarifying – what are the key processes (for reflection) in this experience?

2. Reflection
   1. What was I trying to achieve?
   2. Why did I intervene as I did?
   3. What are the consequences of my action for:
      – myself?
      – the client/family?
      – the people I work with?
   4. How did I feel about this experience when it was happening?
   5. How did the client feel about it?
   6. How do I know how the client felt about it?

3. Influencing factors
   1. What internal factors influenced my decision-making?
   2. What external factors influenced my decision-making?
   3. What sources of knowledge did/should have influence(d) my decision-making?

4. Could I have dealt better with the situation?
   1. What other choices did I have?
   2. What would be the consequences of those choices?

5. Learning
   1. How do I now feel about this experience?
   2. How have I made sense of this experience in the light of past experience and future practices?
   3. How has this experience changed my ways of knowing:
      – empirics?
      – aesthetics?
      – ethics?
      – personal?

Box 6.3   The stage model of reflection (Dudley 1994)

This model was devised for students undertaking a course in theatre studies and although apparently a different perspective from health visiting, nevertheless it has a basic structure that lends itself to health visiting practice.

Stage 1. Description
What was the situation, where and when? Who was there? Why?

Stage 2. Analysis
What did I contribute? What did I think – feel? Is this surprising, i.e. what would I have expected or what would others have expected of me?

Stage 3. Skill analysis
What skills/behaviours did I bring to the situation? What skills/behaviours did I notice in others? What skills/behaviours were needed in the situation? What skills/behaviours would I have liked to have been able to demonstrate?

Stage 4. Evaluation
What judgements do I wish to make about my contribution to this event?
How will I measure my performance against my expectations and against standards/criteria set by others?
What views and perspectives will I adopt to evaluate the norms and expectations of other behavioural frameworks?

Stage 5. Research
What resources are available to help me integrate the changes I want to make?
Make lists of people, readings, recordings, courses, other experiences.

Stage 6. Action plan
What steps will I take to avail myself of these resources and use them? Make an action schedule indicating a) what resources, b) how and when I plan to access each one.

---

use for client/patient care. It is really only in the practicum that reflective journals are regularly used. To carry this argument a stage further therefore, it would appear that, to show quality reflective practice a journal-type approach should be the basis of all recording, and yet this is clearly impracticable for everyday documentation. In addition, the quality of reflection of the learning student is probably clearer than that of the practising professional, whose work will be far more contextually and experientially premised.

It is thus more practical to suggest that where there is extensive intervention work with a client(s) then the additional supplementary records should contain a considerably greater amount of reflection, this of course, being shared with the client. This whole discussion is now leading towards the handling of reflection and thinking in everyday practice.

THE DEVELOPMENT OF CRITICAL THINKING IN HEALTH VISITING PRACTICE

Critical thinking has been the domain of philosophers and analysts since humans began to question. Daly (1998) suggests that critical thinking is purposeful, towards an end rather than the routine thought identified by Dewey (1933). Glen (1995) used Gallie's (1955) work to suggest that critical thinking is contested concept. Critical thinking, therefore, can be seen as the art or science of productive thought, and if it is considered as such then it must be identifiable and tangible. Productive thought can be defined as thinking that has an end-product, which could be a decision made, an idea created and processes for action identified, a brainstorm leading to management of a situation. Nonproductive thought is definable and can best be described as rumination or ruminative thought, when our mental processes churn over problems without coming to any end (productive) result. Referring back to Table 6.3, the third level of reflection identified by Boyd & Fales (1983) could be compared to ruminative thought processes.

Critical thinking is seen, in the developing academic processes of the modern nursing world, as necessary for research-based practice and informed care. Many commentators (Watson & Glaser 1964, Glen 1995, Daly 1998) argue coherently that critical thinking must be a taught or guided process; others, including Mezirow (1981), suggest that it should be left to the individual in competency-based programmes, particularly in technical or instrumental learning such as learning to use a computer.

Taking into consideration the discussion above, as health visiting is such an abstract process with problem-solving requirements, it clearly requires guided techniques of reflection and conceptual mapping in order to facilitate the process in the individual learner. Both processes are now discussed, using critical incident analysis, through critical reflection and concept analysis.

Critical incident analysis

The critical incident technique is described by Dunn & Hamilton (1986) as a sophisticated method for collecting behavioural data about the ingredients of competent behaviour in a profession. They cite Ingalsbe & Spears (1979) as proposing that the strategy of critical incident analysis, when compared with other methods of performance evaluation, is a more objective and efficient method of determining performance effectiveness. Critical incident technique was devised by Flanagan (1947) as a method of training air pilots – by collecting information based on first-hand observation. Flanagan constructed a short questionnaire to distribute to the instructors:

Think of the last time you saw a trainee pilot do something that was effective/ineffective.

What led up to this situation?

Exactly what did the man do?

Why was it effective/ineffective?

These questions required answers based neither on intuition nor on opinion but on fact.

As a result of this work Flanagan (1954, 1963) made a clear statement of definition of a critical incident:

By an incident is meant any observable activity that is sufficiently complete in itself to permit inferences and predictions to be made about the person performing the act. To be critical, an incident must occur in a situation where the purpose of the act seems fairly clear to the observer and where its consequences are sufficiently definite to leave little doubt concerning its effects. The main concern is always with the incident, never with the individuals concerned except as a means whereby they might learn from the incident.

Dunn & Hamilton (1986) suggest that the main value of critical incident technique lies in the three areas of competency-based education, priority areas in education and problem-solving material. Brookfield (1990) suggests that the process of critical reflection can be viewed as comprising three interrelated phases:

- identifying the assumptions that underlie our thoughts and actions
- scrutinising the accuracy and validity of these in terms of how they connect to, or are discrepant with, our experience of reality
- reconstituting these assumptions to make them more inclusive and integrative.

Critical incident analysis is a technique that seeks to highlight particular, concrete and contextually specific aspects of people's experiences.

It is often threatening to the learner to ask for their assumptions in response to a direct question on a general issue. For educators to help develop critical thinking in others they must be able to do this for themselves and this often works well with a small group of educators and learners. In practical terms it is often useful to describe an incident or set of circumstances in relation to your work with a client, and then analyse and examine the assumptions underlying the intimate relationship with the client. Once this is done it can then be thrown to the group to take up particular points and learn to challenge assumptions made. It is interesting to look for commonalties and differences in the assumptions that each person identifies. If there are commonly held assumptions, do they represent what passes for conventional wisdom in your field of practice? If there are major differences, to what extent might these signify divergent views in the field at large? Or might the differences be the result of contextual variations? As this is done within a climate of trust which has been engendered by the initial self-exposure of the educator, student response is often relaxed and perceptive.

Benner (1984) uses critical incident technique to identify the difference in the behaviour of nurses with different levels of experience within the acute field and it translates easily to community health care, where many assumptions are made and the working time with clients is generally irregular and often sporadic.

Dunn & Hamilton (1986) used critical incident technique to ascertain and identify the competencies of the pharmaceutical profession and much depended on the ability of the interviewer to gain the trust of the professional so that the interview itself became more of an anecdotal dialogue but one containing concrete examples of carefully described detailed incidents. The interviewee was then asked for any incidents they had observed or participated in when the pharmacist could have done a little better. In this way, the interviewers were able to identify important competencies of the profession and in compiling something like 700 incidents were able to say that these were the competencies of the profession.

It can be seen therefore, that critical incident analysis is a basis for two strategies – an objective and efficient method of determining performance effectiveness, and contributing towards determination of the competencies of a profession. However, critical incident analysis can also be valuable to explore the assumptions of the student in relation to their knowledge – see Table 6.5.

Watson & Glaser (1964) developed a list of abilities that comprise critical thinking:

- the ability to define a problem
- the ability to select pertinent information for the solution of the problem
- the ability to recognise stated and unstated assumptions
- the ability to formulate and select relevant hypotheses
- the ability to draw valid conclusions and to judge the validity of inferences.

The student health visitor is approached by the GP, who has been visited by a mother with a 15-month-old child with apparent sleep problems. The community practice teacher has previously tried to help the family with this problem. The student health visitor suggests to the GP that she spend some time with the mother, who is still in the waiting room. Private and gentle discussion with the mother gradually took her back to preconception life, pregnancy and the early postnatal period following a caesarean section. The mother said that the child's sleeping problem was creating big difficulties in her family life.

The ability to define the problem

Later, using Watson and Glaser's abilities list and guiding the student through this critical incident analysis, the initial process was to determine and define the problem. The student was encouraged to consider the behaviour of the mother as a result of actually questioning her problem. In many situations a client comes with a problem and is not well known to the health visitor whom she is consulting, who initially can only work with the client on the expressed problem.

The ability to select pertinent information

The student has encouraged the client to consider what would be an acceptable solution. Within her own knowledge framework the student is encouraged to consider whether what the mother wants is achievable. The student would be encouraged to explore a more in-depth history of the problem. She would ask about support, beliefs, attitudes, significant other family members, family routines and so forth.

The ability to recognise stated and unstated assumptions

Using this incident the student would be encouraged to question the presenting problem and consider whether beginning some work on it is the best way forward at this stage. Is it better to go along a management path, aware that in time more relevant information may be revealed and the basic problem exposed, or not to initiate anything immediately, except the maintenance of a sleep diary, which would precipitate further exploration?

The ability to select relevant and promising hypotheses

The use of a sleep diary could lead to: non-completion of the diary; completion revealing a very disturbed sleeping pattern; completion revealing infrequent waking patterns; completion showing extended daytime sleep; completion showing unsettled family rhythms; and others. On the basis of these suggestions the student is then guided into selecting several hypotheses. Noncompletion could suggest that the child's sleep problem is not the main difficulty; very disturbed sleeping patterns may mean that it is the prime problem and needs sleep management techniques; extended daytime sleep may reveal little or no parent–child interaction; unsettled family rhythms may suggest discussion of parenting skills and their relationship to settled child rearing, etc.

The ability to draw valid conclusions

The student will recognise that she will be unable to draw valid conclusions unless her knowledge level is appropriate to the incident. The application of reflection processes and techniques will facilitate this conclusion. The student will also recognise where her own thoughts about the origin of the problem are in relation to those presented by the client, and any mismatch between cause and effect. Using a reflection process on evaluating her own potential communication processes, the student is guided to recognise the validity of the inferences she has drawn in relation to the original incident experienced by her community practice teacher and used as a teaching tool to guide the whole analytical reflecting process.

Using a phenomenological approach there is the assumption that specific responses to critical incidents often have the generic embedded within them. In other words, critical incident analysis does not necessarily mean that general conclusions can be made from one analysis. Critical incident responses alone as primary data sources give insights into learners' assumptive worlds in expressions that are indisputably the learners' own and have not been taken from other sources.

CRITICAL REFLECTION

Mezirow et al (1990) suggest that critical incident analysis challenges the reflecting practitioner to question the presumptions that are brought to the process. Are the assumptions the analyst is beginning from appropriate to the critical incident situation? They may have been acquired in a different context and therefore do not 'fit' the present situation. This suggests that the reflecting practitioner then has to go back to stage 5 of the reflective judgement model (Table 6.5) and realise that knowledge (and thus assumptions) must be placed in context. The context must be ascertained in critical incident analysis before reflection can really take place.

Critical incident analysis is therefore an important prerequisite for valid and accurate critical reflection processes.

The process of critical reflection can be viewed as comprising three interrelated phases (Brookfield 1990):

• identifying the assumptions that underlie our thoughts and actions

- scrutinising the accuracy and validity of these in terms of how they connect to, or are discrepant with, our experience of reality (frequently through comparing our experience with others in similar contexts)
- reconstituting these assumptions to make them more inclusive and integrative.

Central to the process of critical reflection is the recognition and analysis of *assumptions*. An assumption is one of those taken-for-granted ideas, common-sense beliefs and self-evident rules of thumb that inform our thoughts and actions.

Before asking others to be critically reflective of their assumptions and meaning perspectives, practitioners must be able to do this for themselves. To do this, model the kinds of critical reflection that students might be asked to explore by taking something you have written or said and analysing it publicly for its distortions, inaccuracies, oversimplifications, contradictions and ambiguities. The focal point behind this exercise is to teach recognition of the ways in which assumptions become distorted within the contexts of situations. This is not particularly easy to do, but the very process will enable students to move forward in their critical reflection methods.

CONCEPT ANALYSIS AND CONCEPTUAL MAPPING

Conceptual analysis and conceptual mapping are tools used not only to consolidate and develop critical reflection, but also to develop creative thought. The use of conceptual analysis and conceptual mapping in relation to reflection will be considered first. Conceptual analysis has been defined from a number of perspectives, two of which will be considered here. Norris (1982) used a definition: 'Concepts are abstractions of concrete events. They represent ways of perceiving phenomena. Concepts are generalisations about particulars, such as cause and effect, duration, dimension, attributes, and contunua of phenomena or objects'; and Meleis's (1985) definition adds the following: 'Concepts are a mental image of reality tinted with the theorist's perception,

experience and philosophical bent. They function as a reservoir and an organisational entity and bring order to observation and perceptions. They help to flag related ideas and perceptions without going into detailed descriptions.'

There is a close relationship between this and the use of metaphor in reflective learning as suggested by Deshler (1990a) in the earlier discussion on knowledge. Both metaphor and concepts help to classify and distinguish between ideas and primary and secondary subjects, by a process of highlighting the primary subject and suppressing the secondary and less important features, recognising the congruence between them. Thus in critical reflection the community practice teacher guides the student to identify and tease out the apparent merger of several different threads of thought. The difference between using metaphor and concept analysis is that concepts classify and organise and metaphor articulates this.

The use of the concept analysis has enabled health visitors to articulate and disentangle information that comes from several different sources during one single incident (observation, sensory, knowledge, assumptions and intuition). The community practice teacher assists the student to interpret metaphors used to illustrate meaning. These will include the assumptions, values and beliefs of the student. For example, in discussing mothers' uses of the descriptors 'diarrhoea' and 'constipation' the community practice teacher helps the student to see that these are metaphors (concepts) for apparent bowel dysfunction. Once unpicked, the student can then work to enable the mother to understand that for her child not to have a daily bowel movement does not necessarily signify constipation, or that breast-fed babies tend to have either frequent or infrequent bowel movements, which might be caused by the mother's diet.

Carrying and guiding the student into these advanced areas of critical, analytic reflection, is aided by the use of *conceptual mapping*.

Conceptual mapping is a practical technique that can be used to reflect critically upon our concepts, their relationship to each other and our underlying assumptions and values about the matters under consideration. This technique can be applied to a broad range of subject matter to assist in making explicit to ourselves the taken-for-granted frameworks, propositions and structures of assumption that influence the way we perceive, feel, and act upon our experience.

Our critical reflections on these maps reveal new pathways we may take to connect meanings among concepts in propositions. (Definition of proposition: statement, suggestion, statement of a theorem or problem.) Also revealed to us may be omissions and missing links, inconsistencies, false assumptions and previously unrecognised relationships.

A concept map is a schematic device for representing sets of concept meanings embedded in the framework of propositions (Novak & Gowan 1984). Flow charts or other organisational charts are not really concept maps because their key words are usually not concepts with meanings. Concept maps are holistic, spatial, hierarchically constructed representations of the relationships among essential concepts.

Concept maps can be read as compound sentences that visually depict subordinate concepts and operations. Thus, complex multiple relationships can be displayed. Written or spoken concepts usually come to us in the form of linear propositions. Conceptual thinking, on the other hand, is more hierarchical or holographic (Novak & Gowan 1984). Concept maps assist us in transforming linear material into more holistic visual imagery and therefore help us to evaluate, synthesise and perceive new ways.

The process of creating concept maps, critically reflecting upon them and reconstructing and validating them can contribute to transformative learning and emancipatory education.

Using the same sleep example, a simple analogy here is the concept of an infant's sleep. The patterns of infant sleep vary and although they may be dependent on management, for this example we are interested only in the concept of sleep. A mother comes to the health visitor concerned that her infant has a sleep problem. On enquiry the mother states that infant wakes several times during the night. The mother wakes with her infant and worries that the infant is not sleeping, therefore he must have a sleeping problem and she is concerned. The health visitor suggests that the mother keeps a sleep diary for several nights and they then discuss the situation again. When they analyse the diary together the infant appears to wake twice during the night but is not distressed or crying. The health visitor then analyses the concept of sleep with the mother and she realises that sleep does not necessarily mean unconsciousness but may include restful waking. In addition, waking actually only occurs twice a night and the infant appears even-tempered and happy most of the time. He does not appear fractious from lack of sleep. The mother then realises that the problem was hers and arose from her understanding of what sleep meant. In using this type of concept map the health visitor and mother work together to appreciate the understanding of sleep behaviour as a pattern and not a problem (Figs 6.3 and 6.4).

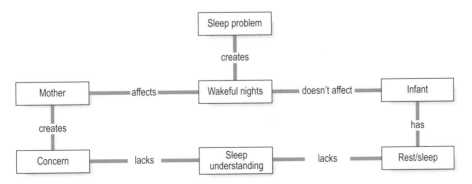

Figure 6.3   A concept map of a sleep problem (based on an original idea in Deshler 1990b)

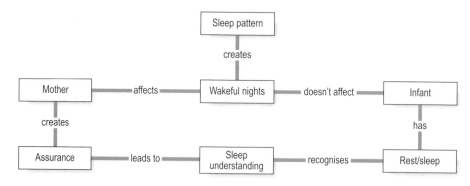

Figure 6.4   A concept map of a sleep pattern (based on an original idea in Deshler 1990b)

The use of the above as an example is to help change concepts or assumptions within them. Some mothers may understand the process of concept mapping but it is more likely that the community practice teacher will use this tool with the student to enable the student to recognise the conceptual changes that need to be made in order to cope with events that challenge assumptions.

Creating initial concept maps

The purpose of an initial concept map is to confront ourselves with the current structure of our knowledge about the subject under discussion. It is not, at this point, an attempt to be critical about what we know but to describe our ideas and assumptions as they are.

To introduce conceptual mapping, we should begin with content of concern to students:

- concerns with which students are personally struggling
- concerns about what other people think about them, which may have an unrecognised influence on their behaviour
- concerns about theory/practice
- concerns about professional decision-making.

We can introduce current dilemmas that will provoke the need to reflect critically through the creation of concept maps. Transformative learning (Deshler 1990b) is most likely to occur through concept mapping when the focus is on concerns that we as learners recognise as:

- *Important*, so that learning central to our

future situations, environmental conditions, lifestyle or ethical behaviour can occur
- *Puzzling or cognitively dissonant*, so that learning can result in new synthesis of knowledge, ideas or feeling
- *Constraining*, so that learning can result in the expansion and emancipation of choice.

Deshler (1990b) suggests that, after the focus of concern has been identified, the procedures for creating initial concept maps include the following steps:

- write or talk about the subject of concern
- understand the difference between concepts, names and linking words
- make lists of the key concepts
- select the one concept that is most general
- arrange the other concepts underneath the general concept
- draw linking lines between concepts and write linking words
- consider the maps as temporary, pliable, in-process and never finished.

The concept map of a sleep problem/pattern shows evidence of transformatory learning resulting from critical reflection on the initial map, which led to a more specific step for critical reflection.

Here is another example of a concept map in relation to student health visitor education. In this example the student in possession of a good honours first degree elected to undertake health visitor education at postgraduate diploma level. The community practice teacher was concerned

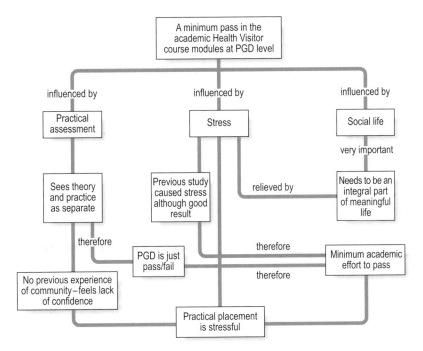

Figure 6.5   Concept map of a student health visitor's academic progress

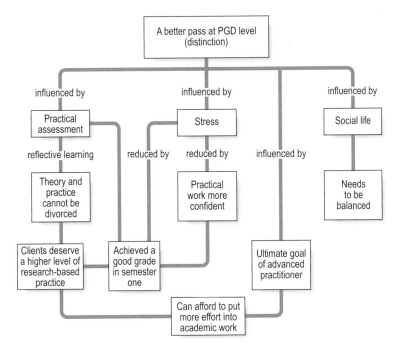

Figure 6.6   Reconstructed progress map of the concept of academic work effort

that, although the student was functioning well in the practicum, it was apparent that a minimum of effort was being put into academic work – merely sufficient to scrape a pass. The community practice teacher brought this up in discussion and suggested a concept map approach, and the student complied by producing Figures 6.5 and 6.6.

What the student had not been aware of was that the academic level achievement could be raised to distinction and not just pass/fail. The student had also failed to see that practice could only be enhanced by academic comparability, and therefore had not realised that a bare pass in academic level could be reflected by a bare pass in practice. As it happened, the student did well in the first part of practice, but having recognised that it was possible to achieve without becoming too stressed, it was also possible to work harder at academic work without becoming too stressed. The student's confidence level received a boost at the first practice assessment and

thus a PGD distinction was within the bounds of possibility.

CONCLUSION

Health visiting has always used reflection, but originally in a cruder form. A criticism made of health visitors practising in the 1960–70s was that they were always contemplating their navels – the premise being that health visitors were very good at evaluating themselves but much less able to evaluate their work. Formalisation of this process by using reflection to both teach and learn health visiting has meant that there has been a forward movement into linking the evaluation of professional self to the evaluation of effective practice. The processes of understanding reflective practice in health visiting as critically discussed throughout this chapter must now be carried into a formal logging of the process so that discerning purchasers can recognise the value of purchasing health visiting.

7

Health visiting in child protection

Jane McKears and Margaret Reynolds

INTRODUCTION

Child protection has become a major concern of health visitors and social workers since active campaigns brought the death of Maria Colwell in 1973 to public attention, resulting in a public enquiry. Maria's unhappy death thus became a political issue and resulted in strengthening and restructuring of the roles of those professionals such as health visitors and social workers who were involved. Child protection became more firmly defined as identification of neglect and abuse and the subsequent handling of situations where this had been highlighted. Parton (1981) particularly traces the change from child protection according to a disease-prevention model to child protection according to a social–prevention model stemming from the early 1970s. Health visitors were involved in child protection according to a disease-prevention model from the early part of the 20th century, with gradual sophistication of their methodology from improved nutrition and sanitation to the development of psychometric testing in the early 1960s. The Hall Report (Hall 1996) formally reviewed and restructured developmental screening and proposed developmental surveillance linked with health promotion as a child protection programme. The social–preventive model of child protection had became progressively more formalised and this culminated in the Children and Young Person's Act 1969, which, however, failed fully to cover the social perspective of child abuse.

The 1969 Act allowed the state to intervene

and enforce child-rearing standards and it was possible for child protection orders to be made to protect children from abuse in an increasingly violent society. The Children Act 1989 strengthened the social response and clearly acknowledged the role of health visitors, among other professionals, as case-finders of children who need protection. This chapter shows the two aspects of the macro and micro approach to child protection. The first (macro) approach is about the need to really understand child protection methodology and the focus is from a viewpoint of overt abuse – physical, psychological/emotional and sexual – looking at the structures in place to support health visitors in their roles, and making suggestions to facilitate health visiting practice. The second (micro) approach explores the dimensions of child protection from a developmental screening perspective. The tools used for a sensitive screening approach focus on the child through the Schedule of Growing Skills and the mother/carer through a self-efficacy measurement tool, which in its pilot stage shows immense promise in the area of identifying a deficit in parental knowledge which may lead to child neglect or abuse.

CHILD PROTECTION IN HEALTH VISITING

Jane McKears

Child protection is only a small part of most health visitors' workload but can be disproportionately stressful. While trying to respond to all the current NHS changes, and often with a large caseload, the health visitor needs to be constantly vigilant and aware of the possibility of child protection issues arising within any of the families she visits.

Working Together (Department of Health/Department of Education and Science/Welsh Office 1991) defines child abuse as having four categories: neglect, physical abuse, sexual abuse and emotional abuse. A child must be suffering from 'significant harm' within these categories to warrant inclusion on a child protection register.

'Significant harm' is not clearly defined in the document and is open to interpretation, but harm is generally considered to mean that it impacts considerably on a child's well-being. It is possible that there is disparity across the regions as to when a child's name should be added to the register, depending on the local interpretation of 'significant harm'. Staff working in areas of high social stress might change their yardstick about when children are suffering harm if they are exposed to widespread deprivation over a long period of time.

In practical terms, neglect can range from children's 'failure to thrive' to failure of parents to take children for medical appointments, which impacts seriously on their health. Physical abuse encompasses injuries such as bruising and shaking, or more rarely (and often more sadistically) burning and scalding. Sexual abuse includes any kind of sexual activity with young children, who are unable to give informed consent, and incest. Emotional abuse is included in all forms of abuse – it is not possible, for instance, to physically abuse a child without also emotionally abusing them. If a child is subjected to physical harm, not only is there an injury but there is also the accompanying fear of repetition of the incident. Because physical punishment is an expression of power over someone more vulnerable, there is accompanying humiliation. A child may then be afraid to behave in a certain way and become timid if she fears she will be hit. This is sometimes aggravated by threats to her if she discloses the abuse to anyone, with the result that she may have to put up barriers between herself and other people who might help her. Children have been known to repeat false accounts of how they became injured, which were eventually discovered to have been concocted by the perpetrator. The emotional abuse category is used when it is the only (or most important) form of abuse. It is the category in which children are least likely to be registered and yet can have long-term damaging effects.

Prevention is a key task for health visitors and child protection is no exception, If vulnerable families are identified, health visitors can target their extra visiting and plan care accordingly.

PROFILING

Profiling of families to assess their vulnerabilities includes using a list of factors that are sometimes associated with child abuse. Profiling families for child protection is different from community profiling which tends to be more quantitative; for example, that 50% of the community smoke cigarettes is a hard fact supported by statistics that show a relationship between lung cancer and heart disease. However, child protection profiling is related to 'Stop and think factors', which prompt a health visitor to increase the visiting pattern and consider mobilising other resources. There is not necessarily a cause and effect relationship, however. Many public inquiries into the deaths of children as a result of abuse show that the families were isolated. This might prompt a health visitor to encourage families to attend parent and toddler groups or family centres; however, some isolated families never need the services of the Child Protection team.

Profiles are often decided upon locally, and will vary slightly in different areas.

The following tables suggest that health visitors may find it relatively easy to acquire this information. However, experience shows that it is often as a retrospective discussion following an incident that this information emerges. Nevertheless the factors listed in Boxes 7.1–7.3 have been recognised by researchers (e.g. Browne et al 1988, Parton 1990) as being important in the profiles of abusers and abused children.

Where there are several factors present, a

Box 7.1 Factors that may make parents abusers

- Parents previously abused children
- Parents themselves abused as children
- Parent has severe mental health problems
- Parent has severe physical health problems
- Parent has drug-related problems
- Parent has alcohol-related problems
- Domestic violence
- Parent has learning disabilities
- Parent has low stress threshold
- Parent has unrealistic expectations of children
- Parent has no support network
- Parents are isolated

Box 7.2 Factors that may make children more vulnerable to abuse

- Short gaps between the birth of children – this can result in the mother becoming physically depleted through repeated pregnancies and childbirth with little time to recover in between; it also means that she has highly dependent children to care for as they have not had long to grow up before the next one is born
- Child was low-birthweight, which often results in the need for more regular feeding accompanied by parental anxiety about whether there will be any other associated complications
- Child has feeding difficulties
- Child has disabilities
- Child is the 'wrong' sex
- Child reported to cry a lot – this can be a reflection of the parents' (negative) perception of it or, if accurate, probably means extra stress and less enjoyment of the baby for the parents

Box 7.3 Social factors that may precipitate child abuse

- Poor housing
- Overcrowding
- Racial harassment
- Financial problems
- Poor provision of community facilities, e.g. playgroups

(This list is not exhaustive!)

family may be considered vulnerable. However one factor alone would produce a similar response, if it was serious enough; for example, if a parent had a severe drug-related problem that impacted badly on the family.

If using such a profile, health visitors need to consider carefully the impact of these factors on the child and on the family. There is usually a complex interaction between factors that results in the abuse of a child yet many families suffer from some of the above factors and manage to successfully raise their children. A large percentage of children in the UK are living in poverty and yet, as far as we are aware, most of them are not abused.

However, profiling is not universally accepted as being helpful. Appleton (1994) describes how health visitors expressed concern at the lack of definition of vulnerability, which led to disparity in identification of such families due to differences in perceptions. Her study acknowledges the sometimes transient nature of vulnerability but showed that health visitors had difficulty removing families from their vulnerability identification system once they were on it.

Others (Dingwall 1989) have highlighted pitfalls in identifying families as being vulnerable: staff have overreacted in some situations but failed to react in others because of the family's vulnerability status. It is possible that people seeing a bruise on a child whose name is on the child protection register might be more likely to believe that it is as a result of abuse than if the family were believed to have a very low vulnerability scoring.

Roberts (1988), however, does show that there are still some influences that are frequently associated with violent or neglectful behaviour in parents. At the present time most trusts use a system of vulnerability identification and this is still a useful tool when used advisedly with an awareness of its pitfalls. It is necessary to remember that it is usually an accumulation of interacting stresses that predisposes to the possibility of child abuse, but ultimately it is the parents' individual response to those stresses that leads to abuse.

Having identified vulnerable families, the health visitor needs to be resourceful, imaginative and sensitive in producing a tailor-made service for them.

THE CONCEPT OF PARTNERSHIP IN CHILD ABUSE

Health visitors are required to work in partnership with parents, ensuring that parents have every opportunity to share their point of view. The concept of 'partnership' implies an equal relationship and in practice this might not be possible. Perhaps a more honest description would be 'working towards partnership'. Practical steps that health visitors can take to achieve this goal might include only visiting by appointment but, even so, in some chaotic families (where they have repeatedly not been at home when appointments have been made to see them)

opportunistic visiting might be a compromise that needs to be made following repeated 'no reply' visits.

Partnership also includes supporting parents in setting realistic goals for their families and helping them to achieve them through support, encouragement and advice. The value of the Personal Child Health Record, which is kept by the parent, is that of information sharing through partnership. However, health visitors should be aware of the power imbalance that can exist in some relationships with clients, and need to address these issues. The following are examples.

- Families may believe they are being 'watched', particularly if there have been previous child protection issues.
- Parents may feel socially inferior or may fear covert racism or homophobia.
- For some families there may be educational disadvantages.

Health visitors need to be honest with themselves about where they are on the journey towards anti-oppressive practice and consider the impact this will have on their clients. Sensitive use of vocabulary and body posture as well as good listening skills are essential.

Pound (1992) suggests that the main focus of preventing child abuse must be the promotion of positive parenting, which includes the promotion of the rights of children and discourages the use of physical punishment. This presupposes that health visitors value these principles, for there would be tension for staff whose private values were in conflict with this. The Children Act (1989) did not challenge the legality of the physical chastisement of children. Few people will have missed the irony of the fact that if they hit someone of their own size they might be charged with assault but if they hit their child it is legally sanctioned.

While many people agree in principle that children should have 'rights', what these rights actually are is usually decided on by individual adults in society. Laws require that children attend school (or at least receive an education) and yet truancy rates show that many of them find formal education irrelevant to them. Children should have a right to a reasonable home environment and yet many children today are living in bed and breakfast accommodation or in cramped hostels where their mothers have fled to escape domestic violence. There would appear to be no formal system monitoring whether the rights of children are being met.

Having targeted vulnerable families by observation and identification of problems, the health visitor assesses how these problems impact on the parents and on the child. The health visitor works with the family to try to improve the situation and the care plan they agree between them should be recorded and a copy made available to the parents.

The care plan will address issues that need to be discussed and also other identified health needs, including developmental surveillance as recommended in the Hall Report (1996). Other specific health visiting inputs might include a baby massage group, which could improve parent–child interaction and might even produce the spin-offs of reducing crying and colic.

ALTERNATIVE METHODS OF REACHING FAMILIES

Some health visitors are employed in family centres and work with social services staff to try to reduce stress in families that might result in child abuse. Group work, perhaps bringing women together to discuss coping strategies, which could include assertiveness training, have been found to be very useful, as have groups to understand child development, which might result in improved home safety. Groups should include member participation as a major factor. Whenever possible, parents should be given lead roles in stimulating discussion and sharing knowledge and ideas. Videos and games are often more enjoyable than 'lectures', and working through a leaflet together can be quite effective. All these might help to reduce the incidence of physical abuse inflicted as a response to unrealistic expectations of children. For instance, McKears has personal experience of working with families where a child has been quite badly assaulted for wetting the bed at 2 years old

because the parents thought the child was doing it deliberately to provoke them.

Postnatal groups at clinics can reduce stress if parents can share their feelings and worries and support one another by discussion, and these can sometimes be more empowering to parents than a health visitor-led group. McKears has run antenatal groups and the most successful ones were where local mothers led the discussion. One talk on breast-feeding, led by a 'Hell's Angel' mother who had breast-fed her own child, resulted in all the group members choosing to breast-feed – an uncommon occurrence in that area at that time. This highlights the advantage of using a credible group participant to promote good practice.

By addressing specific problems facing the family the aim is to prevent the situation from escalating until it becomes a child protection issue. The health visitor might be the only professional person involved with the family at this point and needs to be keenly aware of any deterioration in the family situation that would warrant referral to social services.

It is, of course, essential that health visitors are honest with their clients, and explain the reason for referral to social services. If it is a case of neglect, the health visitor needs to explain clearly to the family what the concerns are – e.g. insufficient food may have led to low infant weight gain – and let the parent know what they are aiming for, such as regular clinic weighing, use of a food diary, providing the parents with a centile chart. If there is insufficient progress the parents will realise why it is necessary to refer to social services.

Careful use of vocabulary is essential. If a parent is told, 'I am reporting you to social services because you haven't done as you were told,' there is unlikely to be a positive response. Phrasing it, 'I am referring you to social services because I feel you need more help and support than I can give you to bring about changes in your baby's health and weight gain,' may be more acceptable This needs to be followed by an honest and open discussion on the role of social services. If a child protection conference is convened, the parents will usually be present and there should be no surprises for the parents about the health visitor's views of their parenting skills.

SAFETY ISSUES RELEVANT TO HEALTH VISITORS WORKING IN CHILD PROTECTION

A formal procedure to ensure staff safety as far as possible should be the responsibility of trusts. However, health visitors are also responsible for their own safety.

As health visitors work for much of their time in isolation, it is essential that they discuss a worrying family situation with colleagues to ensure an even perspective and prevent them from getting 'stuck'. The public inquiry into the death of Paul (Department of Health and Social Security 1994) highlighted this issue. Here a health visitor worked in isolation with a family and did not appreciate that slow, insidious deterioration in the family had led to an unacceptable situation that resulted in Paul's death by neglect.

Health visitors should have regular formal child protection supervision, as recommended by the UKCC (1996), where guided reflective practice can help health visitors who have become 'stuck'. Supervision should also be a time of increasing knowledge by dissemination of research and articles, and also a time for reducing stress by sharing responsibilities. Supervisors need to ensure that health visitors have an up-to-date knowledge of child protection procedures and access to multiagency training with regular updates, as recommended in *Working Together* (Department of Health/Department of Education and Science/Welsh Office 1991).

Supervisors also need to be aware of the attitude of health visitors to this area of work. They may have suffered childhood abuse themselves, but the impact of this is not always understood or respected. Staff have changed jobs or needed to take extended sick leave after child protection cases triggered memories of their own childhood abuse that they had never previously shared.

Professionals can behave dangerously by un-

wittingly colluding with abuse and neglect and staff need to be challenged on this area in supervision. Finkelhor (1984) showed how perpetrators 'groom' adults – including professionals – to make it unlikely that they would suspect abuse. For instance, a health visitor may become involved in the client's problems to the extent of feeling such empathy for the mother as to 'turn a blind eye' to the child's neglect. Equally, health visitors can be so overwhelmed by their own personal problems that they have difficulty in identifying with the client's situation.

THE CHILD PROTECTION ADVISOR

Most trusts employ a Child Protection Advisor, who is usually a specialist health visitor although one trust at least has a social worker in this post. The role varies geographically but generally includes providing formal child protection supervision. The advisor often provides multiagency and single-agency training and advice and support for staff, including help with report writing and attendance at Court.

The advisor may be a member of the Area Child Protection Committee (ACPC) and its subcommittees and of the primary care group. In the event of a child dying as a result of abuse, the Child Protection Advisor will make the agency contribution to the Part 8 review, which involves securing the records immediately so that no alterations can be made. These records are examined so that a picture of the service given becomes apparent. The advisor then interviews the staff working with the family to expand on and clarify the history given in the records. A factual chronology is then produced, with the advisor making comments at each stage on whether the interventions were appropriate and whether procedures were followed. There is a summary by the advisor, making recommendations, which could include training needs, policy change, etc. This report is then sent to the ACPC, which makes a report from a composite of all agency reports and its own recommendations, which is finally sent to the Department of Health.

Having a Child Protection Advisor means that staff have access to someone with specialist knowledge – however, there is a possibility that this could be disempowering for the staff if the advisor sits on all the ACPC subgroups personally and fails to cascade information. The ACPC is a multiagency body with overall responsibility for child protection services within the area. Usually, there are subgroups for training, procedures, practice and serious cases. It is a useful experience for health visitors to be members of these groups, and spreads knowledge further.

It is essential that information is passed on to staff and one way of doing this is by multidisciplinary Child Protection Interest Groups. These can be a forum for cascading new information and research and building on the knowledge gained in multiagency training.

DOMESTIC VIOLENCE

The recent understanding of the impact that domestic violence has on children has resulted in many trusts producing guidelines about concerns that health visitors may have about a potential domestic violence situation.

Messages from Research (1995) presents a challenge in which the emphasis is firmly placed on prevention of abuse and the identification of children in need. Their warning of 'low warmth, high criticism' as being a potentially dangerous environment for children should be heeded by health visitors working with families of this type. It is believed that children who live in families where there are few cuddles and little praise but much criticism may suffer more harm than children who live in generally loving homes with occasional 'overchastisement'. Health visitors should concentrate on positive parenting and the importance of cuddles and have an appreciation of the position of insecure parents who fear the disapproval of others if their children misbehave.

CULTURAL FACTORS

Racial issues are not new, but increasingly we are becoming aware of the impact of racism on children's lives. Clinics should be welcoming places that reflect a diversity of cultures.

More recently, with the advent of artificial insemination, the numbers of lesbian and gay parents have increased and health visitors need to provide a sensitive and caring service. There have always been lots of different types of family – it is just that we are becoming more aware of them!

Interagency working remains vital, with sadly repeated inquiry reports showing failures in the system. Unfortunately multiagency training does not always effectively improve professionals' knowledge of one another's roles and this is an issue that needs to be addressed (McKears 1994). Staff need to work in partnership for the good of children. This might include acknowledging and discarding stereotypes they may have about workers from other agencies.

In the future, as a result of the introduction of primary care groups, special consideration must be given to the support provided to staff on child protection issues. Two health visitors working in a pilot scheme for primary care groups found that there was confusion and lack of planning in this area and waited 6 weeks to find out who should be providing supervision for them. With the expansion of primary care groups from April 1999, staff need to ensure that provision is made for child protection.

Now at the millennium, we can cast our minds back to the past and see that much has changed and some things have improved, but there will always be challenges. The recent increase in the incidence of Munchausen's syndrome by proxy and paedophilia on the Internet are just two examples of the need to be constantly alert in the changing world. One thing will always remain the same – the need of vulnerable children for adults who are willing and able to act on their behalf (Children Act 1989).

PROTECTION BY DEVELOPMENTAL SCREENING – HISTORICAL OVERVIEW

Margaret Reynolds

Developmental screening was first introduced in Britain in the 1950s and 1960s (Lancet 1986).

However, interest in child development can be traced back more than 200 years. The first known account is that of Tiedmann in Germany, who published a detailed account of the developmental progress of one child in 1787 (Illingworth 1987).

Little interest was shown until nearly a century later, with Charles Darwin's account of the development of the eldest of his 10 children in 1877, followed by Shinn publishing one of the most complete accounts of a young child's development in 1893 (Illingworth 1987).

Possible reasons for more interest in children and their development may have been a drop in the infant mortality rate as a result of advances in medical science and changes in the economy, which was previously dependent on child labour. Parents were in less danger of losing their children so could afford to have fewer of them and to become more emotionally involved with them (Kessen 1965).

An example of the social and economic climate in 19th-century Britain concerning young children is that as late as the 1840s one in five children died before their first birthday. The Prudential Mutual Insurance, Investment and Loan Association (now the Prudential Corporation) refused to insure the lives of children under the age of 10 for fear of them being murdered so that the insurance could be collected (Dennett 1998).

Pioneering work in developmental testing was carried out mainly by child psychologists, who were interested in designing pass/fail systems to establish 'norms' of intelligence or behaviour. An example is Gesell, who, while studying mentally defective children, began thinking about the early signs of mental deficiency. He set up studies of the normal infant that led to the establishment of 'norms' (Gesell 1925, Gesell & Amatruda 1947).

Others who developed developmental testing scales included Stutsman (1931), Buhler & Hetzer (1935) and Cattell (1940) for children under 2 years of age. Binet scales of various types were available for children over 2 years of age (Binet & Simon 1915). Work by Bayley was concentrated on children under the age of 3 years (Bayley 1933,

1940). The Denver Developmental Screening test (DDST), developed in Denver, Colorado (Frankenburg & Dodds 1967), was later revised and abbreviated. The age range covered is 2 weeks to 6.4 years.

A British psychological scale of note produced by Griffiths, a paediatrician, consists of five subscales initially for use with children aged 14 days to 24 months, later extended to 8 years (Griffiths 1954, 1970). These scales were subsequently revised in 1992. In her work, Griffiths changed the emphasis to devising testing procedures to aid in paediatric diagnosis, management of young handicapped children and guidance for parents.

In Britain further work was carried out by Sheridan in development of the psychometric test Stycar developmental sequences (Sheridan 1960). This work drew on the developmental testing scales available in the late 1930s and 1940s (see above; Sheridan 1975). Reasons for this work were that none of the previous scales were British, they did not agree among themselves and there was a lack of graded tests for visual and auditory acuity, necessary for paediatric assessment of young handicapped children. Additionally, the available scales did not cover signs of communication disorders, unstable personality or social maladjustment.

It is from the Sheridan Stycar sequences that the Schedule of Growing Skills (SGS) was developed. Initially it was developed as a research instrument, covering children up to 3 years in the National Childhood Encephalopathy study. This was set up in response to alleged neurological reactions to pertussis vaccine (Bellman 1984). It was later developed further up to the age of 5 years, together with the use of the Reynell language scale, as Sheridan was weak in identifying speech and language delay early (Reynell 1969, Bellman & Cash 1987; Table 7.1).

The tool has been shown through research and validation to be applicable to ethnic minority groups as well as the indigenous population. This is an important issue considering the composition of the child population in the UK today. No child fails, which was a criticism of older tools with a rigid pass/fail system. Nine skill

Table 7.1   Stycar areas and schedule fields

Stycar areas (Sheridan 1975)	Schedule fields (Bellman & Cash 1987)
Posture and large movements	Passive postural skills
	Active postural skills
	Locomotor skills
Vision and fine movements	Manipulative skills
	Visual skills
Hearing and speech	Hearing and language skills
	Speech and language skills
Social behaviour and play	Interactive social skills
	Self-care social skills

areas are covered, a breakdown of the original Sheridan Stycar areas creating a much more sensitive tool, yet still quick and easy to administer. The screening results highlight a child's strengths and weaknesses and can be used for health promotion, working in partnership with parents (Bellman & Cash 1987). A copy of the screening results is given to the parent, other copies being available for the GP, the health visitor and for referral if necessary. An example of SGS paperwork is shown in Figure 7.1.

Prematurity is taken is taken into account at the interpretative stage. Subsequent minor revision of SGS was carried out, together with the introduction of a cognitive scale (Bellman et al 1996).

THE SCREENING DEBATE

The screening debate has been ongoing over many years, influences upon it including research and moral and ethical considerations, as well as cost and cost-effectiveness. In considering this issue, child health surveillance, child health promotion, screening and developmental screening will be considered.

Child health surveillance

This is a broad term including developmental screening and surveillance, immunisation, growth monitoring, detection of child abuse and management of chronic and acute illness (Lancet 1986). It is a preventative programme aimed at improving all aspect of children's health, which should be carried out in partnership with parents or carers (Birmingham Health Authority 1990).

Hall (1991) broadly agrees with this, also stating that surveillance involves a set of activities initiated by professionals and including oversight of physical, social and emotional health, monitoring of developmental progress, offering and arranging intervention where necessary, and health education. The relationship between primary healthcare professionals should be one of partnership rather than professional supervision, with parents being enabled to make use of services and expertise in a way most appropriate to their needs.

An example from the health visiting perspective could be where delay in speech and language development has been identified through developmental screening and the professional and parent discuss together possible reasons for this and ways to help the child. It could be that attending play group is the initial agreed course of action: mixing with other children of a similar age could help to stimulate speech and language development. If after further review it is found that satisfactory progress has not been made, parent and professional might then agree that the best course of action is referral to a speech therapist at a venue convenient for mother and child. A satisfactory outcome for the child is far more likely if parent and professional work in partnership.

Child health promotion

In order to emphasise that preventive health care for children involves more than the detection of defects (implied in the concept of surveillance), Hall (1996) proposed the term 'child health promotion'. 'Child health surveillance' would be retained but would refer specifically to activities designed to achieve early detection (secondary prevention).

The following key principles are included in child health promotion: work based on need, partnership between client/carer and professional, primary prevention, a public health approach and teamwork.

When applying these two concepts in practice

The top section of the Profile acts as a referral or information note to a specialist practitioner

Three extra copies of the Profile are generated for use when referring a child on to a different specialist.

The total scores in each field are transferred from the Child Record Form to the Profile. The appropriate age band is then blocked in to give an overall visual summary of each child's developmental status.

The Profile provides a visual summary of the child's development, allowing the assessor to identify areas that need further investigation

For example, this child's developmental age within the fields of Hearing and Language and Speech and Language is 18 months, which is 2 intervals below his chronological age. Suggested action would be assessment by a speech and language therapist preceded by a hearing assessment.

Concern about the quality of performance within a skill field can be marked at the bottom of the chart with a cross.

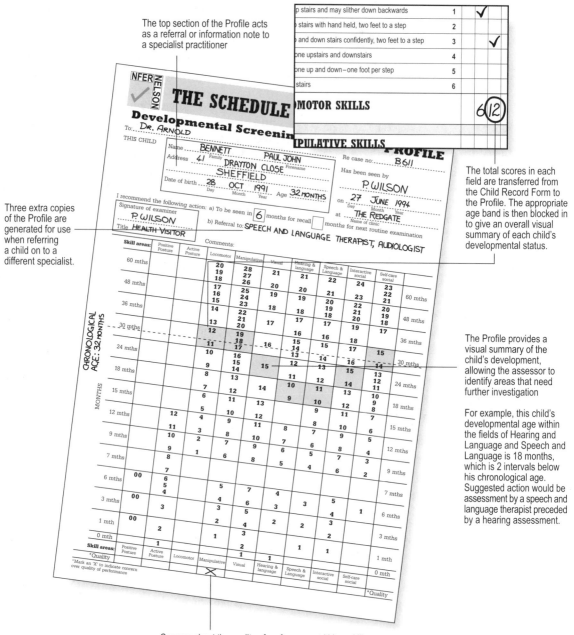

Figure 7.1 A sample child profile from the Schedule of Growing Skills ©1987 Martin Bellman and John Cash. (Reproduced by permission of the publishers, NFER-Nelson, Darville House, 2 Oxford Road East, Windsor SL4 1DF, England. All rights reserved)

– the core programme for child health surveillance and recommendations on child health promotion (Hall 1996) – the first should be continued and the second used selectively in the light of locally defined need and outcomes (Department of Health Specialist Clinical Services Division 1996).

An example of child health promotion in health visiting practice is anticipatory guidance given to a mother with an 8-month-old child just starting to get around by rolling and squirming. It would be pointed out that soon the child would be crawling, then walking and taking every opportunity to explore the world within his/her reach. Accident prevention in relation to the child's age and stage of development would therefore be a particularly important topic to discuss. Enabling the mother to understand why, for example, a fireguard and safety gate was needed, with assistance given in obtaining these items through a local scheme if the family was on a low income, would be more likely to be effective in promoting child safety in the home than simply telling the mother to purchase them.

Debate on the value of screening in general

There is ongoing debate about various types of screening relating to child health. Specific examples and conclusions from recent screening research are included here, together with questions raised, in order to explain more clearly why there is debate. The value of continuing research into screening should be recognised, with its potential to add to and improve health care.

We need to question continually what we are doing in relation to screening; not only why we are doing it, or whether we need to do it, but also, if we do, is there a better way?

In many areas these questions are continually being raised, as the following research examples show. As some questions are answered, still others are raised, opening up further debate. It may not simply be a question of whether a particular type of screening is right or wrong but what is best practice in giving value for money.

This may conflict with what is considered to be ethically or morally right or wrong.

In developmental screening, as knowledge increases this should be used to inform and change practice. What is important is to use the best tool available but to acknowledge the importance of continuing research. Older tools need to be subject to ongoing evaluation and changes made as research indicates. The limitations of a screening tool, however good, need to be acknowledged, as the professional's judgement and expertise are of significant importance in interpreting results. A simple example could be where a child is not able to walk alone by the age of 20 months. If the child has been kept strapped in a pushchair for much of each day and not allowed the opportunity to develop gross motor skills, the reason for delay could be environmental rather than medical. This is an important factor that the health visitor may be aware of, and would be an important consideration when making a medical assessment of the child.

Screening for Hearing Loss (Davis et al 1997), which looked at neonatal screening in detection of congenital hearing loss, shows the complexity of the issues that have to be considered. The research was carried out because of doubt concerning the efficacy of existing programmes – a health visitor distraction test at 7–8 months – in identifying early, permanent hearing impairment. There was growing evidence that new technology available was a more effective option.

Although examples of good practice were found, it was concluded that the health visitor distraction test had poor sensitivity, the median age of identification being 12–20 months. This compared with neonatal screening, which showed high test sensitivity and high specificity, median age of identification being 2 months. However, it was noted that the number of universal neonatal hearing screening programmes being implemented was limited at present.

In terms of cost, universal neonatal screening was approximately half as expensive as the health visitor distraction test (HVDT), with targeted neonatal screening approximately 20% as expensive as universal HVDT. Targeted screening included neonates in whom 'at risk' factors had been identified. Issues here included the high initial cost of equipment for neonatal screening and whether neonatal screening should be universal or targeted, the latter carrying the risk of failing to identify all 'at risk' children, or whether HVDT should be continued, with its comparatively poor rate of early identification of deafness and high cost.

An Evaluation of Screening for Speech and Language Delay (Law et al 1997) again raises questions as well as providing some answers. It was found that there was insufficient evidence to support formal universal screening for speech and language delay. However, early speech and language delay should be viewed with concern by those undertaking child health surveillance, i.e. health visitors and GPs, because it may indicate both minor and major disabilities. Parents need to be aware of language development in young children and to share any concerns with health visitors and GPs, to allow access to specialist services (Law et al 1997).

Questions that need to be asked here are: how do we ensure that health visitors and GPs have the skills to identify speech and language delays early, and how can parents be educated in language development in young children? Once identified, what happens if there are insufficient resources to cope with identified children in need?

There is a danger in thinking that researchers must always be right: this may not necessarily be the case. Absence of conclusive evidence that a particular type of screening should be stopped when there is some evidence that it is beneficial can be an argument for its continuation, as the following example shows.

Research into *Pre-School Vision Screening* (Snowdon & Stewart-Brown 1997) found that little is known about the natural history and treatment of amblyopia and no treatment trials have been identified using a nontreatment control group, which would have been precluded on ethical grounds. Research indicated lack of evidence to support preschool vision screening in a small-scale trial, but screening by the orthoptist was found to be more effective than screening by a health visitor or GP. In spite of the

research findings, Fielder (1997) argued that preschool vision screening should continue on the grounds that research was small-scale. It should have opened up the debate about screening, and the community had in effect been bypassed. Research evidence on the treatment of amblyopia should be obtained and the child with visual defect should not be ignored.

Issues here, besides dissension about continuing screening while acknowledging the need for early intervention, are effectiveness of a service in ethical terms and cost-effectiveness. Uptake for preschool vision screening by the orthoptist was poor and more children were seen by the health visitor. Would more children with possible visual defects be identified if health visitors were given specific training in this area, then referred on for specialist assessment and treatment when necessary?

The research detailed in *Population Growth Analysis Using the Child Health Computing System* (Hulse et al 1997) showed not only how important it is to use the appropriate tools for a particular type of screening but also the importance of training in their use and accurate recording and interpretation of results. Without these simple safeguards, not only may a particular research project founder and its potential value to child health be lost, but inaccurate measurements may result in inappropriate referrals being made. This may result in unnecessary parent/child anxiety as well as failing to identify children in need of specialist treatment.

The research discovered errors in the way a tool was used, which affected the outcome of the study. It found that there was increasing agreement that children with height below the 0.4th centile or above the 99.6th centile should be evaluated for possible growth disorder. However, there was less agreement about the value of assessing children where height velocity was abnormal, particularly where height was within the normal range. However, at that time there were too many errors on growth data on the child health computing system for it to be of value for screening (Hulse et al 1997). This research was carried out using information from child health records in Kent.

Training for professionals in accurate growth measurement and completion of centile charts, for information to be meaningful, has been long advised by the Child Growth Foundation.

There is a danger in assuming the value of a particular type of screening without its effectiveness having ever been evaluated, as *Screening for Congenital Dislocation of The Hip: A Cost Effective Analysis* (Dezateux et al 1997) indicates. A national policy for universal neonatal screening for congenital dislocation of the hip (CDH) had been introduced in 1969 but not formally evaluated prior to introduction. Results of the research indicated that the effectiveness in reducing false negatives of universal ultrasound screening, which had been introduced in some European countries, was uncertain. It was the system used in two-thirds of maternity units in this country but was not the primary screening test. It was used to assess babies with clinically detected hip instability or with high risk factors for CDH. In this case research did not provide a definitive answer but indicated the need for ongoing evaluation of current and alternative primary screening strategies. The best approach was not yet known.

A further example of where research can highlight the need for ongoing research is the national study *Cost Analysis in Child Health Surveillance* (Sanderson 1997). Results indicated that the majority of local policies followed the recommendations of Hall (1996). There was little variation in the number of checks and the ages at which they were undertaken, but two, hearing screening and routine vision checks, were performed in a variety of ways. Ongoing study into the cost of providing child health surveillance and costs to parents, including follow-up visits and referrals, was incomplete.

Neonatal Screening for Inborn Errors of Metabolism (Thomason et al 1997) again indicated that research should be ongoing rather than accepting the effectiveness of a screening method for all time. Findings were that universal screening for phenylketonuria is worthwhile and should be continued. Screening for biotinidase deficiency and congenital adrenal hyperplasia should be introduced, with co-ordinating evaluation to

ensure that the programme is cost-effective and review in 5 years' time. Screening for cystic fibrosis should be encouraged but there was no evidence to support a newborn screening programme for galactosaemia.

From the research examples above, it is evident that screening procedures may be less than perfect and that what was once the most appropriate procedure becomes outdated or is superseded by a more effective method. In practical terms, it is essential to be prepared to change the tool/procedure used in the light of current research. Also, where there is some evidence of its usefulness, a tool should not be dismissed as ineffective without sound research-based evidence to support this.

Developmental screening

Developmental screening is the process of checking the development of a child whose parents believe it to be normal (Illingworth 1987). It is a rapid application of a test or other tool for the purpose of separating those who have or are very likely to have developmental delay (Hall 1986, Lynn 1987). Bellman et al (1996) agree with this view, adding that its aim is to check children are developing normally for their age when measured against prescribed criteria, failure to meet these indicating developmental delay or defect.

The prime purpose of a developmental screening tool is to identify children with possible developmental delay early, so that they can quickly be referred to a specialist for the problem to be confirmed or refuted (Frankenburg et al 1973, Bellman & Cash 1987). If it is confirmed, a diagnosis can be made and, where possible, appropriate treatment given to enable the child to achieve his/her potential. In many cases, this can prevent development of special educational needs.

Debate has arisen in recent years as to the value of routine developmental screening of all 0–5-year-old children, which was introduced in the late 1950s and early 1960s. The Working Party on Child Health Surveillance (Hall 1989) did not recommend this, nor did it recommend any particular developmental screening tool. It was of the opinion that trained professionals, by using their observational skills, can satisfy themselves in the majority of cases that the child's development is within normal limits. Professional judgement, local policy and needs and wishes of parents should be taken into account when deciding how much time should be spent on developmental screening. Macfarlane (Macfarlane et al 1990, personal communication 1991) endorses this view. The Working Party did not, however, recommend developmental screening (Hall 1991, 1996), although the 1991 report does acknowledge its place in child protection work.

There are a number of people who feel that routine screening of all children is of value in early identification of children with possible developmental delay. These include Frankenburg & Dodds (1967), Bellman & Cash (1987), Illingworth (1987) and Bax et al (1990). Bernice (1986) and Bolton (1986) highlight the importance of hearing and language screening: as delay is often indicative of other disorders, it is also an important part of child health surveillance (Court 1976). Bernice and Bolton's observations are also emphasised by Law et al (1997). Bellman et al (1996) view routine developmental screening as an ethically acceptable part of child health surveillance and promotion provided that appropriate action is taken in terms of prevention and support. While supporting developmental screening for all children, Cash (1991) warns against putting the onus back on parents to report problems, as not all do and the child may suffer as a result. In the Muslim culture, for example, the feeling is that problems are the will of God. In Cash's experience, intervention is allowed if the professional identifies the problem, although there is ambivalence about the result of treatment.

Additionally, when working in partnership with parents for the good of their children, it is important to take their views into account. There are indications that they value developmental screening (Sutton et al 1995, Fagan 1997).

The problem of what is normal development and the dangers of assessment by people ignorant of what they are doing and how to do it is discussed by Illingworth (1987). A wrong diagnosis can cause immense trauma to parents and children, yet parents have a right to know as soon as possible if their child is handicapped.

Is routine developmental screening effective? *The Lancet* (1986) argues that studies of children have shown failure to identify physical and developmental problems relating to the preschool years, but no statistics are given. Aukett (1990) found that the experience of health visitors in a West Midlands area was that about 10% more children with speech and language delay, including Asian children, were identified using SGS than previously with DDST. While studying preschool children over a 7-year period in Dundee, Drillien & Drummond (1983) found that 9% had moderate to severe developmental delay and 73% were identified through screening. Early intervention reduced the numbers needing special education.

A study in one West Midlands area found that only one child of school age, who had moved into the area, had been missed in the preschool years, and the two children missed by the doctor were subsequently identified by health visitors through developmental screening (Humphries 1989).

Although it is felt that more children with developmental delay are being identified early, overall there is a paucity of statistics to prove conclusively the effectiveness of routine developmental screening in the preschool years (Griffiths 1970, Hall 1989). Yet as Cash (1991) points out, in spite of a lack of research in this area, no research has been carried out to show the difference between two groups of children referred, for example, for speech therapy, where one group was treated and one was not. However, to attempt this would create a moral dilemma.

Views can change over time, as shown by Hall (1991), in which although routine developmental screening is not supported for all children, support is given to its use in child protection work. Hall (1996), while not advocating the use of any developmental screening tool, noted that SGS and DDST were the most widely used. The report goes on to state that developmental reviews should be aimed at disadvantaged children and those with disabilities. Children who have been subject to abuse can fall into either or both of these groups. The lack of research is again highlighted. It is this issue that research by Reynolds (1992, 1999) has sought to address by implementing small-scale studies in order to open the debate further and stimulate further research.

RATIONALE FOR THE USE OF THE SCHEDULE OF GROWING SKILLS IN CHILD PROTECTION

The health visitor's role in child protection

Health visitors have a key role in the promotion of children's health and development in child protection (Department of Health/Welsh Office 1995, Department of Health Specialist Clinical Services Division 1996). Health visitors are in a unique position, working with children and families on an ongoing basis. They have knowledge and prior information that may give valuable insight into why crises have occurred. This has implications for ongoing work (Birchall & Hallett 1995).

A fundamental principle of the Children Act 1989 is that the child's welfare is paramount. Accurate, contemporaneous records, including a child's developmental status, that can be clearly understood are likely to be of particular importance in cases of child abuse, which involves working on a multidisciplinary/multiagency basis. All professionals working in partnership and finding effective ways of working together in practice to serve the child's best interests is a key issue in child protection work (Department of Health/Department of Education and Science/ Welsh Office 1991).

Developmental screening in the context of child protection

Hall (1996) supports developmental reviews for disadvantaged children and those with disabilities. Cash (1991) supports developmental screen-

ing, considering it to be vital, when assessing children in need, to have a yardstick by which to measure their progress or lack of it. In this context, it is important to use the most appropriate developmental screening tool available. Knowledge of a child's developmental status is viewed as important by social services, hence the inclusion of information relating to child development in the social work assessment guide (Department of Health 1995b).

Research by Reynolds (1992) sought to identify the most appropriate developmental screening tool to use with 0–5-year-old children in one Midlands area. Tools considered were, first, a very modified form of Griffiths with no recorded research or validation, which was currently being used within the area, and second, the Denver Developmental Screening Test (DDST), with well recorded research and validation but with a rigid pass/fail system in common with other older tools and criticised for limitations in its ability to identify speech and language delay early (Lynn 1987). Research by Greer et al (1989) also indicated its failure to identify developmental delay in preschool children. The third tool was the Schedule of Growing Skills (SGS), a newer tool with well recorded research and validation, in the development of which health visitors had been involved. Findings indicated that this last was the most appropriate tool for the identified age group in the area. Further research was then carried out to explore its usefulness in the context of child protection (Reynolds 1999).

A literature search revealed a paucity of information linking child protection with developmental screening in either general or specific terms. Curtis specifies the SGS screening tool for child protection (Curtis 1993, 1995), but no further literature linking the two issues was found. Information from Cainey (1995) indicated that the tool had been used by social workers with 'at risk' children in West Lothian, but no formal evaluation of this work was available.

Current thinking in relation to child protection advocates a change in emphasis. It is being argued that it would be advisable to transfer some of the effort put into investigating child abuse to child and family support. The focus should be on the child's needs, then seeing if there is a protection issue within them. It is by meeting the wider needs – offering the family support services on a multidisciplinary basis following assessment (which includes developmental screening results) – that the risk of abuse to the child can be reduced (Birchall & Hallett 1995).

Parenting skills can profoundly affect the parent–child relationship and the child's social and emotional development (Bowlby 1953). Bowlby is particularly concerned with the importance of the mother–child or mother-substitute–child bond in this respect, as well as acknowledging the importance of the father figure and siblings. Ainsworth (1965) points out that subsequent research supports this view. Psychological learning theory, psychoanalytical theory and theories based on the concept of 'sensitive phase' all indicate the potential damage of maternal deprivation to the child's development. Both the child's age at the onset of deprivation and the age at which relief occurs influence future development. The earlier relief occurs the more likely it is that subsequent development will be normal. All areas of development, not only social and emotional, may be affected (Lewis 1988).

Government concerns in relation to parenting skills have initiated a *Sure Start* programme in which health visitors are heavily involved (Turner 1998).

SGS covers all areas of development, including social and emotional. Results from screening using this tool shared in the multiagency child protection forum can therefore highlight areas of need at an early stage. Addressing those needs, by professionals working with the family as a whole, as well as specific help for the child if required, can help to protect the child from further abuse.

Research project: the use of the Schedule of Growing Skills in child protection

The project did not seek to establish support for continuing routine developmental screening for all children but to explore its usefulness in child protection work. How reviews of young children are carried out in the light of Hall (1996) is a matter for each area to decide in line with local policy. For the purpose of this study, the original version of SGS was used, as three routine screenings of children in the comparison group were required, at 8, 18 and 30 months, which meant drawing on screening information prior to the introduction of SGS II.

Preliminary work

Prior to the main study, the views of those most likely to be affected by the proposed change were sought. These were all health visitors within the local community trust, 68% of whom responded, and a small sample of convenience of GPs, parents and social workers. The aim was to establish their views on developmental screening of 0–5-year-old children and their likelihood of accepting a change of tool to a new, research-based one, results of which could be shared with parents and other professionals if necessary.

Results indicated that a change to SGS would be acceptable to health visitors, and the small sample groups of parents, GPs and social workers, the majority of the last group perceiving it as beneficial in child protection work. Developmental screening of young children was acknowledged as being of value. It was crucial to establish this before considering possible change or continuing developmental screening at all.

Once all health visitors had been trained in the use of SGS and the tool had been introduced across the trust, a questionnaire was sent to all health visitors 6 weeks and 10 months postintroduction to find out their views about its use in practice and whether there were any problems.

Overall findings indicated an increasing acceptance of the SGS tool, familiarity with its use and perception of its value in general use, as well as a reduction in screening time. Children responded well to it, both parents and professionals generally viewing it favourably. From the professional viewpoint comments included its thoroughness, objectivity, being visually graphic and giving a clear picture of a child's developmental status. It was useful for referral and sharing results with parents/other agencies. Additionally, in the second questionnaire comments indicated that it was a good tool to use with children on the child protection register and was useful to teach students about developmental screening.

Main study

Here the overall aim was to explore the usefulness of SGS in child protection work. Evaluation took place over a 6-month period. Routine practice was that screening information was brought to the initial case conference and screening was carried out again prior to the review case conference.

Health visitors whose caseload included a child on the child protection register at the commencement of this stage were identified.

Quantitative data were obtained from SGS scores of subject children and those in the comparison group. Qualitative data were obtained by carrying out semi-structured interviews with participating health visitors at two points: after the initial case conference and after the first review. These two points were chosen because the literature indicated that the greatest volume of work by all agencies was achieved following the child's initial registration. The purpose was to determine:

- health visitors' views about the ability of the tool, in child protection work, to identify need
- how need identified by health visitors fitted in with that identified by other professionals at case conferences
- the success of the child protection plan (anticipated after initial registration and actual after first review)
- whether the system was working in relation to the health visitor contribution
- perceptions as to whether improvements could be made to the health visitor contribution.

Data were collected by interviews with health visitors and from routine anonymous health visiting SGS profiles. There was no access to written health visiting records. Verbal consent was obtained from each health visitor before participation in the study and there was no compulsion to participate.

Children included in the study

In all, six children, boys and girls aged 0–5 years within the trust on the local social services child protection register formed the subject group. The comparison group consisted of 10 children, five boys and five girls, from the caseloads of each of the six health visitors who participated in the study. This was a sample of convenience, matched in terms of age group, social class and ethnicity with each subject child. Additionally, the children in the comparison group were not on the child protection register, were not born prematurely and had no known developmental delay. Three routine screenings were required, at 8, 18 and 30 months, prior to the start of the study. This was so that an estimated SGS score could be calculated that matched the age of each child in the subject group, by a process of statistical regression.

Combination of the qualitative and quantitative approach

Although some continue to argue that qualitative and quantitative research are incompatible, increasingly it is believed that many areas of inquiry can be enriched through the combined approach, using more than one method of data collection in a single investigation (Polit & Hungler 1995). Both numbers and words are needed to understand the world (Miles & Huberman 1994). Miles & Huberman view quantitative and qualitative research as a continuum in the process of enquiry and not as separate entities. In linking quantitative and qualitative data, the four broad reasons described by Rossman & Wilson (1991) were all appropriate to this particular research. These were: to enable confirmation or corroboration of each other via triangulation; to elaborate or develop analysis, providing richer detail; to initiate new lines of thinking through attention to surprises or paradoxes; and to turn ideas around, providing new insight.

With this in mind, the combined approach was used in this study. Qualitative data were obtained by discussing what health visitors felt about the success of the child protection plan after initial and first review case conferences with SGS scores before initial and first review case conferences.

Quantitative data were obtained in two ways. Firstly, scores for each child before initial and first review case conference were discussed to find out whether there were differences and if so in what areas. In SGS, a score for each skill area is obtained. Health visitors' perceptions of the effectiveness or otherwise of the child protection plan were then compared with the screening results. Secondly, screening results of the two groups, children on the child protection register and those who were not, were discussed. This was to find out if there was a difference in the rate of development between the two groups and where such differences were. Lack of research in this area indicated the need for exploration.

Discussion of results

All health visitors involved in the study valued using SGS in child protection work in identifying need and felt the needs they had identified fitted in with those identified by other professionals at the case conference. They felt that ways of meeting those needs were incorporated into the child protection plan.

Perceptions of the effectiveness of the child protection plan indicated that other issues besides content were important. These included the importance of professionals working together, co-operation from the parents and worker planning meetings between case conferences. These could, in effect, provide ongoing monitoring of the plan. The co-operation of parents and professionals was necessary to meet the child's needs, including protection from and prevention of further abuse.

All study participants felt that the SGS tool was of value in child protection and in sharing that information at the case conference. However, the comment was made that although in their view it was the best tool available, as with any

tool it had its limitations. The health visitors interpreted the results in the light of their professional judgement, based on experience and expertise; knowledge of the family and child was also very important. This was borne out by their response to the question: Did they feel the child was achieving his/her potential? It was generally felt that the answer was no, apart from the period of time one child was in foster care. This response was given even where children's development appeared to be age-appropriate, or even above the chronological age. This was an important finding as, if a child's development appears to be age-appropriate, the case conference may conclude that it is satisfactory. The health visitor needs to put forward her/his view, with reasons as to why this may not be so, in order to look at ways in which the child could be helped further.

One participant experienced difficulties in identifying emotional problems. This linked with a difficulty identified in the pilot study, where a participant felt that an additional tool could be used to identify social and environmental issues. It was acknowledged that the health visitor's knowledge of the family could identify many of these issues but that perhaps more weight should be given to them initially. It is likely that only the health visitor will have this information at the initial case conference stage.

Another participant drew attention to the fact that there was a quality issue in respect of interactive social skills. The level of achievement in this area was not consistent: it was dependent on family circumstances and who was present in the home. The child's behaviour could regress, reflecting the level of emotional instability experienced, which identified a need for planning to provide the stability that such children need.

A further comment from participants was concern about parenting skills and the need for improvement in this area.

Comparison of SGS scores of register children and non-register children

These indicated progress relating to the health visitors' perceptions of the effectiveness of the child protection plan. Progress, where it took place, was more rapid than in the general population. Areas where delay was indicated in the subject group included hearing and speech, speech and language, visual comprehension (the child's ability to verbalise and indicate understanding of what they see), interactive social skills and self-care skills. One child had delayed locomotor skills, which proved to be environmental in origin. One child's development was above the chronological age initially. Acknowledgement of the child's needs and subsequent foster placement resulted in further progress being made.

All respondents felt that participating in the study had enabled them to reflect on their work with SGS in child protection and to value it. At the same time, they recognised the limitations of the tool, or any tool. It was the best available that they were aware of, four having used a number of others previously. They were very positive about its use, commenting on its clarity and simplicity when sharing results with other case conference participants. It was useful when working with parents to identify needs and areas of progress. On reflection, one participant felt that she would have valued the actual information generated when giving evidence in Court on a previous occasion. Most participants felt that with time a more appropriate tool might be identified through research.

THE FUTURE

Health visiting is a preventive service in which proactive work is of vital importance. A topical example is the government's parenting skills initiative, in which it is anticipated that health visitors will play an important part. The reason why this is important to the health of children is indicated in research by Barlow (1997). Her research indicated that parent training programmes were effective in improving behaviour problems in children aged 3–10 years. This is particularly important as the most important health problems in childhood and adolescence are behaviour problems and mental health problems. If programmes were set up on a preventive basis, not only where problems have already

occurred, this could be an effective way of improving children's health.

Consideration, then, needs to be given to not only teaching those skills but also to giving positive feedback to parents. They need to know how their child is progressing, in what areas they need further help and how to promote further development if their child is to achieve his/her potential. This is another possible area where SGS could be usefully used. In conjunction with this, the parent's level of self-esteem could be assessed as a means of promoting positive parenting. The same approach could be used in a first parenting programme, with assessments taking place at intervals deemed helpful by both parent and professional, as well as with vulnerable families.

Bandura (1977b) felt that people's perceptions of their capabilities affected how they behaved and their level of motivation. In relating this to children and their development, Roter (1977) pointed out that it was acknowledged that, when a mother felt confident in her ability to help her child, the child picked up those feelings and was likely to do better than a child whose mother had a low self-efficacy level and had difficulty coping.

The partnership approach between client and professional is acknowledged as being particularly important (Billingham 1991). The professional provides expert knowledge, enabling and empowering clients to make informed health choices as individuals and for families as a whole, including young children. This concept can be particularly useful when working to enable parents with poor coping ability and poor parenting skills to change their behaviour and have confidence in themselves. The likely effect would be an improvement in their parenting skills, increasing the potential for their children to grow and develop to realise their potential. Attributes in parents that encourage children's progress include realistic expectations of their child, meeting their need for love and security, provision of an appropriate learning environment and providing opportunities for appropriate socialisation (Luker & Orr 1992). Bellman & Cash (1987) and Illingworth (1987) broadly agree with this view.

Table 7.2   Scale to measure the self-efficacy of a carer

Scale subarea	Direction of scoring	Question
a	+	1. I find it easy to believe that children have different competencies at different ages
a	+	2. I know how to choose toys appropriate to my child's age
c	−	3. I find it difficult to accept when my child does not do what I expect him/her to do
a	+	4. I know what games to play with my child to help development
c	+	5. I am able to express my love for my child by cuddling and kissing him/her
b	−	6. I find it difficult to decide on a proper diet for my child
c	−	7. I have trouble getting my baby/child into a routine
c	−	8. I find it difficult to be patient with my child
a	+	9. I find I have the skills to guide my child to give appropriate activities to encourage development
d	−	10. I find it difficult to make opportunities for my child to mix and play with other children
b	+	11. I am confident in my ability to keep my home warm and clean for my child
d	+	12. I make opportunities to talk to my child and read to him/her
d	−	13. I find it difficult to find time to take my child out to places of interest to him/her
d	+	14. I encourage my child to help me when I am doing household chores
b	−	15. I find it difficult to decide what clothes to dress my child in
c	+	16. I know when to say 'no' to my child when he/she goes to do something which will harm him/her
b	+	17. I am confident in my ability to look after my child's health

Key: + = scoring direction strongly agree 5, strongly disagree 1; − = scoring direction strongly agree 1, strongly disagree 5.

A suggested scale measuring the mother/ carer's level of self-esteem (Reynolds 1992), based on the Diabetes Self-Efficacy Scale (Padgett 1991) is given in Table 7.2. It is acknowledged that further useful work could be carried out in validating this scale.

The scale is divided into four subareas. These are items directly related to: (a) developmental progress, (b) general health (including diet, warmth and appropriate clothing), (c) love and security (including behaviour management and establishment of a routine), (d) provision of an appropriate learning environment (including opportunities for play, socialising and outings to places of interest for the child).

Questions in the scale that relate to each of the four subareas are: (a) developmental progress – questions 1, 2, 4, 8, and 9; (b) general health – questions 6, 11, 15 and 17; (c) love and security – questions 3, 5, 7, 8 and 16; (d) provision of an appropriate learning environment – questions 10, 12, 13 and 14.

A five-point Likert scale was used, ranging from strongly agree to strongly disagree, with a similar number of positively and negatively worded questions.

The purpose of the tool is to gain knowledge of the mother/carer's self-efficacy level and insight into their strengths and weaknesses. The raw scores can be converted into a percentage score overall, as well as one for each scale subarea. The scale could be used as a useful starting point at the commencement of teaching parenting skills and later on to ascertain the level of achievement. If it were used in conjunction with SGS, it could positively reinforce the concept that improved parenting skills can aid a child in achieving his/ her potential (Fig. 7.2).

The scale was used with mothers in a small-scale study. It was used initially and then 3 months later following input from the family health visitor in teaching parenting skills. In results shown in Box 7.4, Mother 1 had good parenting skills, a high level of self-esteem and her child appeared to be developing satisfactorily. Mother 2 had low self-esteem, less understanding of parenting skills and her child was exhibiting behaviour problems.

Results after 3 months showed the first mother's improvement in parenting skills and her child's development continued to progress age appropriately. Results for the second mother indicated a marked improvement in parenting skills, improved level of self-esteem and her child showed improvement in development, particularly in behaviour. Both mothers stated

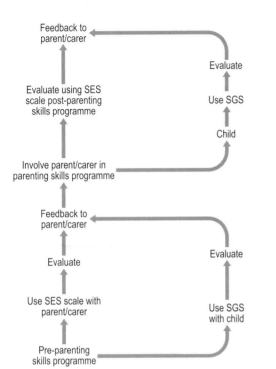

Figure 7.2   How the self-efficacy scale (SES) and SGS could be used in evaluating a parenting skills programme

that they appreciated a simple written indication that they had benefited from the programme and the effort they had put in had had beneficial results for both their child and themselves.

Summary

Interest in child development dates back more than 200 years. Work on developing developmental tests and scales was mainly carried out in the 20th century, with DDST and SGS being the most commonly used in this country today. Debate continues as to whether developmental screening should continue as part of child health promotion/surveillance.

SGS was found to be effective in enabling health visitors within a Midlands Trust to fulfil their role in child protection work, but its limitations were acknowledged. Health visitors' professional judgement and interpretation of results in the light of their knowledge of family circumstances was deemed to be of great importance. Even when a child's development appeared to be normal, this may not mean that the child is achieving his/her potential. This should be acknowledged when considering the child protection plan.

A further possible valuable use of SGS could be in teaching parenting skills. This could be of particular importance in view of the government parenting skills initiative. It could be used in conjunction with a self-efficacy scale, as a positive reinforcement to parents of the benefits to their child following baseline assessment.

As with all screening tests or tools, professionals should use the most appropriate and reliable tool

Box 7.4 Self-efficacy scale results					
Maximum score = 85					
Total score Mother 1	First time Second time	= 73 = 85.88% = 80 = 94.11%			
Total score Mother 2	First time Second time	= 41 = 48.2% = 62 = 72.94%			
Score Mother 1	First time	a 17 (20) = 85% b 17 (20) = 85% c 21 (25) = 84% d 18 (20) = 90% (86% overall)	Second time	20 (20) = 100% 19 (20) = 95% 22 (25) = 88% 19 (20) = 95% (94% overall)	
Score Mother 2	First time	a 9 (20) = 45% b 9 (20) = 45% c 16 (25) = 64% d 7 (20) = 35% (48% overall)	Second time	15 (20) = 75% 14 (20) = 70% 18 (25) = 72% 15 (20) = 75% (73% overall)	

but acknowledge that, with time, existing tools may be improved or be outdated as a result of further research. Prior to using a developmental screening tool thorough familiarisation with its use in practice is extremely important if it is to be effective and offer a standardised service in the area in which it is used.

The small-scale study undertaken (Reynolds 1999) could have a valuable role to play in opening the debate further concerning the developmental screening of young children, leading to an increase in the body of knowledge and the development of even more effective tools.

CONCLUSION

The two sections of this chapter have discussed in depth the health visiting role in relation to child protection. McKears, in the first section has traced situations and factors of child abuse and analysed in detail the part that health visitors play in its prevention and detection. Reynolds has taken this a stage further and discussed the use of two tools in the prevention of child abuse or its identification. The Schedule of Growing Skills is clearly a sensitive and accurate tool for this type of work and has led to a deepening of knowledge among the health visitors who use it. Reynolds's second tool, for parenting skills assessment, shows some very interesting results and clearly could be used in the measurement of health visitor effectiveness. In a climate of clinical governance this tool has a very positive part to play.

8

The economics of health visiting

Jane Powell

INTRODUCTION

In health-related matters economists are often perceived as preoccupied with costs, cutting services and saying no. This perception has probably arisen as a result of the monetarist brand of health economics that has predominated in the NHS since 1991. However, as this chapter will demonstrate, health economists are also concerned with the efficient use of limited resources, testing the quality of evidence, providing information on the cost-effectiveness of treatments and reporting on implications for policy (CHE News 1998). Furthermore, it is probable that the techniques of economics can be applied usefully in appraisal of and priority setting for health visiting activities.

In this chapter, the first section defines economics and traces the development of the health economics discipline and its application both as a way of thinking and a set of tools and techniques. In the second section two key concepts in health economics are explained and techniques of economic appraisal are outlined. These two sections provide the background for the next section, in which published economic appraisals in health visiting are reviewed critically. The role of health visitors looks set to develop further given New Labour moves towards a primary care-led health service (Department of Health 1997a). It seems likely that health visitors will contribute to debates concerning priority setting and purchasing in primary care groups (PCGs). In view of this eventuality, the principles of priority setting and purchasing in health economics are outlined in the fourth and final section of the chapter.

WHAT IS ECONOMICS?

'What are you studying at University, Jane?' asked my sister's ex-boyfriend some years ago.

'Economics,' I replied.

'That's how to make your dole money stretch out over the week, isn't it?' he retorted.

An amusing exchange and illustrative of lay views about the discipline of economics and what is perceived as a preoccupation with costs or prices.

A definition of economics by Paul Samuelson (1976) provides a broader summary of the main concerns of economics than in the above 'definition'. Economics is:

the study of how men and society end up choosing with and without the use of money, to employ [allocate] scarce productive resources, [which may have alternative uses] for production and distribute them for consumption [efficiently and equitably], now and in the future, among various groups and people in society. It analyses the costs and benefits of improving patterns of resource allocation.

Economics is a discipline or a way of thinking (Cohen & Henderson 1988). A number of tools and techniques, such as economic appraisal, are associated with economics as a discipline. Orthodox economics can be applied to any system in which inputs have to be converted to outputs. Orthodox economics views all systems as subject to scarce or finite resourcing, which is therefore limited. Economic agents or people in systems have unlimited wants or infinite demands. The combination of scarcity of resources and unlimited demands creates a need to make choices about allocating resources. Alternatives for allocating resources are weighed up by taking account of opportunity costs. Efficiency and equity are the two criteria for choice in allocation and distribution of resources.

Why is economics relevant to health visiting?

We can relate the function of health visiting directly to this definition of economics. Resources are scarce or finite. Health visitors cannot do everything for patients they would wish to as resources will not allow for this. Therefore, health visitors have to make choices about how to allocate the scarce resources at their disposal. Efficiency is one criterion for sharing out or allocating resources among all competing uses in health visiting. Resources should be allocated in order to obtain the maximum 'health improvement' from the finite amount of resource. However, most health visitors would be concerned to allocate resources equitably as well. Unfortunately, it is very unlikely that an efficient allocation of resources will also be an equitable one. However, this fact does not detract from the potential usefulness of economic techniques in any activity where scarce resources have to be employed and distributed efficiently.

The development of health economics as a separate branch of economics

Adam Smith made the first published contribution to economic theory in 1776 with his book *The Wealth of Nations*. Although Smith was also concerned with the welfare of society, his work later formed the basis of the monetarist ideology concerning free markets, competition between businesses and privatisation of state-owned monopolies. Monetarist ideology is particularly associated with Margaret Thatcher's time in government and was at the forefront of the creation of the internal market in 1991. Monetarist economic theory is particularly concerned with efficiency, as opposed to equity, as the criterion for allocation of scarce health care resources. In the health service, the proliferation of monetarist theory has created a false and damaging impression that health economists are the same as accountants and concerned merely with costs.

At the end of the 19th century, the basis for orthodox modern economic theory was developed. Mathematical developments in the physical sciences were used by economists with science training who sought to lift economics to the same status as the physical sciences. These early mathematical economists viewed the world as a smoothly functioning machine (Ormerod 1994). The introduction of mathematics using Walras's methodological framework, resulted in, among other things, the development of 'marginal economics'. The 'margin' is a key concept at the core of modern orthodox economics and health economics. Later economists, most notably Alfred Marshall, contributed in various ways to the development of 'marginal economics' (Marshall 1936).

The subdiscipline of health economics developed around 26 years ago from the main discipline of economics. Health economics is rooted mostly in micro (small) as opposed to macro (large) economics. As a branch of microeconomic theory, it is concerned with the behaviour of individual people and businesses as opposed to the behaviour of aggregate, macro or whole economies. Both the way of thinking and tools and techniques of health economics are borrowed from the mother discipline. At present, mother economics is in a state of flux as a consequence of the collective inability of the profession to predict economic events from economic models of economies, grounded in orthodox economic theory. Some commentators (Ormerod 1994) have openly criticised the ideologies of leading monetarist and Keynesian economists of the past as fundamentally flawed and too orthodox to explain the operation of complex economies. In addition, criticisms of microeconomic theory have been directed at its shortcomings. In particular, the assumption of rational behaviour on the part of economic agents or people, pervasive in microeconomic theory, has been questioned forcefully. These criticisms have important implications for health economists as health economics is firmly rooted in orthodox microeconomic theory. The issue of rationality is considered further in the last section of this chapter.

KEY CONCEPTS IN HEALTH ECONOMICS

Orthodox economic theory is founded on numerous principles and is full of jargon. Fortunately for those in health visiting who have not had a thorough grounding in economic theory, explanation of a few key concepts covers a substantial amount of what is needed to get by.

Opportunity cost

This is the value of a good or service as measured by the next best alternative foregone. Resources are limited and if they are used in one way they are not then available to be used in another way. Very few activities are costless and costs can be incurred without money changing hands. For example, if a health visitor foregoes the opportunity to take a day's leave in order to attend to an urgent case then there is a cost, which is the benefit foregone in not enjoying the day's leave. The value of the best opportunity foregone as a result of undertaking an activity or the sacrifice involved is the opportunity cost. Usually, money is used as a means of measuring opportunity cost. Definitions of cost in economics and accounting are different. Economists' notions of cost extend beyond the cost falling on the health service. All sacrifices involved in pursuing a particular policy are relevant, including those of other agencies, patients and their families.

The margin

Marginal analysis is used to evaluate the change in costs and benefits produced by a change in production or consumption of one unit. Less formally, it is often used to refer to the change in costs and benefits produced by increases or decreases in resources under consideration.

Efficiency

Allocative efficiency is concerned with objectives to meet and to what extent to meet them when not all of them can be met. Technical or X-efficiency is about how best to meet a given objective at least cost.

Equity

Equity is the criterion concerned with the fairness of the distribution of resources. 'Fairness' is a value judgement and so greater equality may not mean greater equity.

Quality-adjusted life year (QALY)

QALYs are indicators of the benefit or outcome of a treatment or service. They are/can be calculated by multiplying the changes in subjective, patient ratings of their quality of life with and without treatment by the number of years of life for which the change is experienced. Quality of life can be measured by presenting patients with a scale, where 0 is equivalent to being dead and 1 equivalent to perfect health or well-being. Patients can indicate where on the scale they perceive their current quality of life to be. Therefore an improvement of 0.1 on the quality of life scale, measuring patient quality of life ratings before and after treatment, for 1 year is equal to 0.1 of a QALY gained.

Economic appraisal

Let's imagine that all activities undertaken by health visitors are under review in order to increase effective use of resources. A number of techniques from the same family can be applied in order to view systematically the costs and benefits of alternatives ways of allocating resources. The technique chosen would depend on the precise objective of any review of health visiting activities. The units in which outcomes of the different alternatives are measured must relate to this objective. If this is not the case, it is not possible to make comments about effective use of resources. There are three types of economic appraisal.

Cost-effectiveness analysis (CEA): the evaluation and comparison of the relative costs of treatments and services (in money terms) and the relative effectiveness of treatments and services (in terms of units of effect, e.g. number of children with learning difficulties identified). A strict CEA requires all costs for different alternatives to be similar and the outputs or benefits of all alternatives to be similar. In fact, this requirement is not often met because of practical difficulties of quality and availability of data. CEA allows projects with similar outputs to be ranked in terms of their efficiency.

Cost-utility analysis (CUA): the evaluation and comparison of the relative costs of alternatives (in money terms) and the relative output of programmes. CUA always contains QALYs as the measure of output or utility. CUA differs from CEA in this respect only.

Cost benefit analysis (CBA): the evaluation in like terms (usually money) of all or as many as possible of the costs and consequences or output or benefits of a project. CBA attempts to evaluate all the gains and losses in resources associated with competing activities even when these attempts are imperfect. As such, it is the most complete method of economic appraisal.

ECONOMIC APPRAISAL AND OTHER EVALUATION STUDIES IN HEALTH VISITING
What sort of questions can economic appraisal help with?

Drummond et al (1997) have produced a very comprehensive guide, to which readers are referred. In this section a more brief explanation of economic appraisal is attempted.

Many health visitor interventions take place every day. Some of these interventions are more beneficial than others and it is vital to appreciate the status of health visitor interventions, particularly when resources are cut or expanded.

There is no point in attempting to establish the economic effectiveness or efficiency of an intervention that is not beneficial clinically. Non-efficacious interventions consume resources in the same way as efficacious interventions and so clinical appraisal of interventions must always precede economic appraisal. All interventions with positive outcomes are of course beneficial, but in economic evaluation we wish to establish through clinical evaluation the most efficacious interventions.

By making some assumptions with a hypothetical example, the above points can be clarified. Let us assume that two health visiting interventions, rehabilitation of elderly stroke victims in their homes and advice to the elderly to prevent fractures in the home, are rated similarly in a clinical evaluation. Furthermore, assume that a later economic evaluation based on these findings reveals that the benefits of both interventions are not large, but of similar size, and that the cost of advice from health visitors to prevent fractures in the elderly is much lower than rehabilitation of elderly stroke patients. An economic evaluation would conclude that prevention of fractures is a more efficient intervention (technically) than rehabilitation of elderly stroke victims, as the ratio of benefit to cost is larger for the former intervention than the latter.

Cost-effectiveness analysis in health visiting

Cost-effectiveness analysis (CEA) and cost-utility analysis (CUA) are applied to questions of how to allocate scarce resources among competing treatments or services when either the objective of treatment or the budget for treatment is fixed, but not both. In these circumstances questions of technical efficiency, or X-efficiency in economic jargon, are being asked. The focus in CEA is mostly on relative costs of treatments and services and so it is more usually applied to questions of resource allocation within programmes, e.g. discovering the most cost-effective intervention for screening infants for hearing loss. In CEA studies, in which benefits are listed, these are not usually quantified nor are the relative benefits of the opposing treatments or settings compared. Conversely, in CUA benefits can be quantified in terms of QALYs and these can be compared with costs. There are no published CUAs in health visiting.

Cost benefit analysis in health visiting

Cost benefit analysis (CBA) is applied to questions of whether and to what extent scarce resources should be allocated when objectives and budgets are both variable. In order to answer questions of allocative efficiency a full range of direct and indirect tangible and intangible costs and benefits to individuals, families and society should be considered. In CBA the concept of cost is that of opportunity cost where the cost of a resource is equal to the value of its next best alternative use. Direct costs include the resources involved in the interventions and the costs, such as travel, to the patient. Direct costs will also fall on other agencies or organisations and these

should also be included in economic evaluation studies. Indirect costs of interventions include patients' possible loss of income from working or loss of leisure time during health visitor intervention. Intangible costs include stress, anxiety, pain and suffering. All of these are difficult to quantify but are likely to vary in size depending on the nature of the intervention. The intangible benefits of health visiting interventions to individuals, families and society are often very large. Naish & Kline (1990) recognise that what counts can't always be counted in health visiting activities and outline some alternative measurements to recommended performance indicators in the community. It is well worth considering very carefully the magnitude of intangible costs and benefits in economic evaluations of health visiting interventions.

In CBA a societal perspective of all costs and benefits is taken. A societal perspective acknowledges that the opportunity costs of decisions to reallocate resources made by an individual organisation often impact on third parties. For example, health visitors may wish to calculate all the resource implications for their organisations if they stopped visiting mentally ill people in the community. However, an organisation perspective would ignore the costs falling on the police, local authorities and voluntary agencies. A societal perspective in economic evaluation guards against cost-shifting to other agencies.

It is not possible to measure the full range of benefits using single-dimension outcome measures, but multidimensional quality of life instruments can come much closer than these to doing so. Economic evaluation can aid the process of establishing not only which interventions are beneficial in terms of positive outcomes but which are the most effective or efficient. When resources are scarce such knowledge is vital to produce as much benefit as possible from existing resources.

What do cost effectiveness studies in health visiting reveal?

Economic appraisal can be applied to allocate resources among competing treatments, and settings. A search of the Health Management database of Data, Helmis and King's Fund databases (HMIC database) revealed 28 studies with health visit/or and cost-effectiveness as key words. Only one of these studies is a full cost-effectiveness analysis (Brown 1992). The methodology and findings of this study are reviewed in this section.

A cost-effectiveness study of a district programme for screening infants for hearing loss was conducted by Brown (1992). Three main alternatives were costed using the methods of decision analysis (Gravelle et al 1982) in one district health authority. These were no screening, the current, conventional policy or a change nothing option and one alternative option. The conventional policy included health visitor screening at 8–9 months plus development assessment and hearing screen if necessary at 10 months by a clinical medical officer. The alternative option was to miss out health visitor screening and offer screening by a clinical medical officer at 10 months only if concern was expressed or if clinical indications emerged during developmental assessment. The introduction of a clue list or check list of the general signs indicating that a baby is hearing normally during the first year of life, to be issued to families at the initial health visitor visit, was considered (Brown 1992).

According to the author, the annual expected cost per unit of output was £20.57 for the conventional policy, between £11.13 and £11.23 for the alternative and £11.27 for no screening. Introducing the clue list under the alternative policy was likely to raise the cost per unit of output, but the effects were uncertain. Consequently, it appeared that the alternative option, which removed health visitors from the screening of infants for hearing loss, was more cost effective than the conventional policy but also had little advantage over not screening at all (Brown 1992). How much reliance can be placed on this study? Are there any methodological shortcomings that limit its findings?

Critique of Brown's 1992 study

Use of CEA in principle. The objective of Brown's study was to investigate how resources should be allocated for the screening of infants for hearing loss. The study objective is not clear. Is the purpose of evaluation to identify what should be done to identify more infants with hearing loss? Is the budget for this programme variable? If the answer to both of these questions is yes, then CEA was not the appropriate technique to use in this instance. CEA can help with how to allocate resources when either budget or objective is fixed. Otherwise, CBA should be used. Furthermore, economic evaluation is an appropriate methodology for considering efficiency in the method of provision of screening infants, but does not allow for questions of equity or fairness. Units of measurement used in the study should correspond to the study objective, but because this is not clear it is not possible to comment on their relevance.

Data problems. The probability estimates used in the decision analysis are estimates and so are uncertain. Arbitrary weights from 0 to 1 were used to reflect the value of health outcomes under the different options considered. In addition, the health service costs of audiology and treatment were based on crude data. Hypothetical situations had to be considered in order to estimate the health service costs of referral, the clue list and private costs associated with the respective events under the options appraised. However, data problems are very common in economic evaluation and this study has been thorough in its coverage of costs and provision of data.

Measuring benefits. The lack of a method for measuring the benefits of early detection of hearing problems limits this study. Problems of defective hearing in infants can affect speech and learning if not identified and remedied. Evaluation was made difficult by the absence of any quantitative measures of benefits or effects of early diagnosis and treatment of hearing problems. More research is needed in this area, with the development of quality of life instruments being one potential solution to measuring the consequences of nondetection of hearing problems in infants. There is no requirement in cost-effectiveness studies to quantify the benefits of treatment in terms of money. Consequently, it can be argued that this study has focused too much on relative costs and not enough on the full range of benefits to individuals, families and society from health visiting. It may be the case that additional benefits of health visitor intervention outweigh costs to such an extent that additional costs are worthwhile.

Consideration of opportunity cost and the margin. Unit or average costs are used in the study instead of marginal costs. This is common in CEA as unit costs are more readily available. However, marginal costs should be used as these are more relevant to decisions to expand or contract services.

Use of discounting and sensitivity analysis. The discounting (at a suitable discount rate) of costs that occur in the future back to the present is fastidious in this study. Discounting allows expenditure that occurs at different times to be valued in like terms and means that costs are not then overestimated. However, the fastidious discounting of crude data has to be questioned. The study includes a very comprehensive sensitivity analysis to compensate for some of the data problems in the study. Sensitivity analysis is used to test the sensitivity of the results to changes in underlying assumptions. The results of the study that health visitors screening at 8–9 months is less cost-effective than other options including no screening has to be viewed with a great deal of caution. This conclusion is likely to be affected by data problems and by the arbitrary nature of the health outcomes used in the study.

Plus points. The study is rigorous and systematic, but suffers from data problems common in economic evaluation in practice. Given the qualifications in the study its conclusions do not seem robust, despite the views of the authors.

Other cost-effectiveness studies in health visiting

A study evaluating the first 7 years of a health visitor intervention programme in Sheffield to prevent unexpected infant death (Carpenter et al 1983) concluded that home visiting by health visitors was highly cost-effective in comparison

with paediatric cancer therapy, but no cost data were presented to substantiate this conclusion. A comparison of a wider range of interventions would have been more revealing and useful.

Randomised controlled trials (RCTs) in health visiting (including reviews of RCTs)

One of the long-standing challenges for the health visiting profession has been to justify the additional cost of achieving and maintaining itself as a separate profession compared with other home visitors. Presumably, a rationale for the existence of a separate group of highly trained home visitors known as health visitors is the additional benefit the profession confers in the practice of home visiting over other health-care professionals with some client groups.

The aim of this section is to consider the evidence of gold-standard RCTs of health visitor interventions in relation to these questions. The methodological rigour of each study needs to be assessed when drawing conclusions concerning the relative effectiveness of health and home visiting.

A search of the Cochrane Database Controlled Trials Register (CCTR) revealed 18 randomised controlled trial evaluations with health visitor/ visiting broadly defined to include other home visitors other than health visitors. The Cochrane Reviews Database contained two reviews relevant to health visiting. Evaluations of health visiting and home visiting are categorised. There were no RCTs concerned with the comparable performance of specialist and generalist health visitors with different client groups.

The first section below considers reduction in health inequalities between socioeconomic groups. Other RCTs are discussed by client group category. These categories have been ordered to reflect the evidence from RCTs of greatest benefit in health visitor interventions. The second section discusses evidence concerning the family, including young mothers and children. The third contains evidence about health visitors and adults (after acute intervention). The elderly are considered in the fourth section and mental health issues in the last section. Categorisation of the evidence can help to focus on areas of priority in health and home visiting and which group of health and social care professionals should take the lead in providing interventions for each group. However, quality of findings is dependent upon quality of research methodology and this has to be considered. All RCT studies included below applied random allocation of subjects and controls.

Reductions in health inequalities (RCTs)

That health visitors are the professional group of healthcare experts in the community most able to reduce health inequalities has long been suspected. Gephens & Gunning-Schepers (1996) conducted an international review of interventions to reduce socioeconomic health differences (SEHD) and found evidence to support this view. Specific interventions related to health visiting were included in this review, which contained 405 studies. Interventions aimed at specific age groups, prenatal care, infant care, preventive care for young children, child development, nutrition, tooth decay prevention, child safety at home, general health promotion, licit and illicit drugs, adolescent mothers and adult women were reviewed. In addition, 25 publications concerning cardiovascular disease, cancer in adults and smoking screening were included in the review. A further 26 publications concerning interventions aimed at unemployment, healthcare accessibility, general, financial and cultural were also included. Finally, 31 interventions described in grey literature were reported in little detail as they related to local health education interventions. MEDLINE was searched and recent journals consulted and experts in the field of SEHD were approached for published and unpublished material.

The number and brief and incomplete reporting in most studies made only a narrative review possible. However, some clear findings emerged from the collective evidence. Interventions were classified into three groups and these were effective, ineffective and dubious. An effective intervention demonstrated positive outcomes

and was at least as effective for the lowest socio-economic social groups (SES groups), as for the highest. In most of the studies included in this review, efficacy was assessed in terms of the targeted outcome of the intervention (performance indicator) over social groups and not in terms of the reduction in health inequalities.

The findings of this review demonstrate the effectiveness of the health visiting profession in reducing socioeconomic health differences. Interventions to reduce inequality in health can be effective if they either address structural determinants of health or include both information and personal support. Provision of information alone is not likely to reduce socioeconomic differences in health (Gephens & Gunning-Schepers 1996). Health education approaches in the community that provide only information seem to be effective in higher SES groups, but are not as effective as interventions by health visiting professionals, providing information alongside personal support, in reducing socioeconomic health differences. These findings suggest that the input of health visitors may be crucial to government programmes such as Sure Start. Sure Start is aimed at supporting families and one of its aims is to reduce social inequalities in health. On the basis of this wide-ranging review, it appears that health visitors are the professionals uniquely placed to reach all groups in the population with a similar degree of effectiveness.

These findings suggest that information and personal support are very important factors in the reduction of health inequality. This implies that health inequalities can be further reduced with better information and more personal support. It is unlikely that any other group of healthcare professionals is better placed than health visitors to play a role in the further reduction of health inequalities.

These are favourable findings for health visiting, but this review has a few limitations. Firstly, the authors have not searched the Social Sciences Citation Index and PSYCLIT for suitable RCTs to include in their review. Inclusion or exclusion criteria for RCTs in the review have not been stated and intervention designs have not been described. Nevertheless, this review contains suitably presented data in narrative form and clear results and implications for each study (Cochrane Reviews Database).

Families, parents and children (RCTs)

The findings of all RCTs concerning the family, except one, are positive for health visitor interventions. Health visitor interventions of the information and support variety have been recognised as beneficial in reducing health inequalities. In the one RCT study in which the findings were negative the health visitor intervention was provision of information on smoking behaviour in families with preschool children (Eriksen et al 1996). Interventions concerned with information only were argued to be less effective than those employing information and support (Gephens & Gunning-Schepers 1996). Consequently, the balance of evidence from RCTs reflecting positive outcomes for health visitor interventions with the family seems to indicate this area as a priority for health visiting.

Roberts et al (1996) investigated home visiting in prevention of childhood injury and abuse in the UK by conducting a systematic review of RCTs. 3433 subjects included in the review were the parents of disadvantaged children. The follow up period was between 8 months and 4 years in this study. Extensive searching of MEDLINE, EMBASE and BIDS was conducted. In addition, the reference lists of all relevant articles and textbooks were reviewed and the *Journal of Child Abuse and Neglect* was hand-searched from 1977–95 using the terms social support, family support, home and health visitors, home and health visitations, child abuse and child neglect. Experts in the field were contacted and asked about published and unpublished work they were aware of. The quality of trials was assessed independently by two reviewers and agreement on methodological criteria was evaluated. Disagreements were settled by collaborative review. The review concludes that home visiting programmes have the potential to reduce significantly rates of childhood injury. However, the use of self-reported abuse as an outcome instrument in RCTs of home

visiting has questionable validity. Nevertheless, the relative effectiveness of professional versus nonprofessional home visits is a question that remains unanswered on the basis of this study.

Deaves (1993) assessed the value of health education in the prevention of childhood asthma. Subjects were three groups of children examined over 2 years. Both groups demonstrated a good improvement in knowledge of asthma and its treatment. Health education has a significant positive impact on morbidity indicators related to night symptoms and restricted activities. Qualitative analysis also highlighted the value parents of asthmatic children place on counselling.

A study of risk status and home intervention among children with failure to thrive by Hutcheson et al (1997) highlights the importance of follow-up assessments in the evaluation of home intervention services by lay home visitors. The results suggest that home visitors are most productive among mothers with low negative affectivity in families of low socioeconomic status with children demonstrating failure to thrive. Differences in motor development, cognitive development and behaviour during play among children of mothers who reported low negative affectivity was demonstrated at 1 year.

A study supporting home visitor programmes by community health nursing professionals was conducted by Starn (1992). Support for community health visits for at-risk women and infants was established by allocating 30 subjects to one of three groups. The Barnard Model of parent–infant interaction was used in the study. A third of participants were under 19 years of age and 20% abused alcohol, cigarettes or illicit drugs during early pregnancy. Counselling and supportive interventions established rapport and encouraged women to develop and maintain healthy lifestyles. Results indicated that substance abuse stopped or substantially decreased during intervention. Mothers in the intervention groups had fewer perinatal complications and better parent–infant interaction scores than controls. Healthy pregnancies and improved child development were the main outcomes of the study.

A study by Oehler & Vileisis (1990) demonstrated the effect of early visitation of siblings whose new brothers and sisters were in an intensive care nursery. The intervention group demonstrated a significant decrease in negative behaviours on a specific subset of Missouri Behavioural Checklist (MBCL) items.

Larson (1980) demonstrated in a longitudinal follow-up study the efficacy of prenatal and post-partum home visits on child health and development in working class families. Significant differences between subjects and controls were established for accident rates, assessments of home environment and maternal behaviour, lower prevalence of mother–infant interaction or feeding problems and of nonparticipant fathers. The results support the efficacy of home visits, but only if a prenatal visit is included. Furthermore, the authors suggest that the relationship between mother and home visitor is sensitive to the timing of the initial encounter between them.

Eriksen et al (1996) examined the effect of information on smoking behaviour in families with preschool children. 443 consecutive families with one or two smoking parents attending mother and child health centres in Oslo, Norway were allocated randomly to an intervention group ($n = 221$) and a control group ($n = 222$). Communication between the health visitor and the family was prolonged at one well child visit with a brief session on smoking and the parents were given three brochures. There were no significant differences between the groups with respect to change in smoking behaviour.

Adults

The context of studies in this category is variable and it is not easy to establish the positive effects health visitors might have in interventions with adults. The evidence seems to suggest that the rehabilitation of stroke victims with remedial therapy from health visitors is of limited benefit (Smith et al 1981). The findings of this study must be qualified as only a few stroke patients are suitable for intensive outpatient rehabilitation and so other professional healthcare groups might have achieved similar outcomes in this instance. Other professional groups are more suited to interventions with adults in need of

rehabilitation. A study by Mor et al (1983) of the impact of follow-up surveillance by a friendly visitor on discharged rehabilitation patients indicates that the need to alert the medical system to impending patient problems occurs rarely. These findings suggest that informal support systems and regular use of medical services may be sufficient to monitor rehabilitation patients' progress.

The elderly

Burridge (1988) canvassed health visitor opinion concerning priorities in urban and rural areas. Her small study sample demonstrated that health visitors considered visiting the elderly a low priority. Health visitor opinion supported strongly the employment of specialist health visitors as a more appropriate way of fulfilling the needs of the elderly in the community. These findings are supported by the balance of evidence concerning the outcome of health visitor interventions with the elderly.

A study by Dunn et al (1994) considered health visitor intervention in reduction of unplanned hospital readmission in patients recently discharged from geriatric wards. 204 subjects were allocated randomly to normal follow-up services and normal services including a health visitor on the third day after discharge. Findings indicated that a visit by a health visitor to elderly patients after discharge from geriatric wards was unlikely to be of sufficient benefit to the patients for the service to be funded from a saving in unplanned readmissions.

Vetter et al (1992) investigated the ability of health visitors to prevent fractures in elderly people. Their subjects were 674 patients aged 70 plus on general practice records in a market town. Subjects were interviewed, and 350 were assigned to an intervention group and 324 to a control group. Health visitor intervention over 4 years concerned nutrition, referral of medical conditions, correction of environmental hazards in the home and fitness. The fracture rate over 4 years was measured. The incidence of fractures was insignificant at 5% in the intervention group and 4% in the control group. Health visitors were concluded to have no significant effect on the incidence of fractures in the elderly (70 years and over).

Williams et al (1992) evaluated the care of people over 75 years by health visitor assistants (HVAs) after discharge from hospital. A group of patients were allocated randomly to a programme of visiting and compared with an equally sized group of controls having no visits.

A process evaluation examined the actions taken by health visitor assistants during their visits and related the actions taken to patients' measured health status and other characteristics. No overall benefit from the programme of visiting was found in the outcome evaluation. There was a wide variation in the numbers of actions recorded for different patients. Numbers of HVA actions were related to patient health status and sex with more actions being initiated for those in poorer health and women. Neither age nor whether the patient lived alone were found to be related to numbers of HVA actions. It was concluded that the lack of demonstrated overall benefit and the wide variation in actions suggests this type of service cannot be recommended for all discharged patients over 75 years.

However, a few studies have demonstrated positive outcomes in health visitor interventions with the elderly. Runciman et al (1996) evaluated health visitor follow up in discharge of elderly people from an accident and emergency department. 222 intervention patients and 192 controls were compared. Intervention patients received more services and were significantly more independent at 4 weeks. Consequently, health visitor assessment was seen as helpful.

Vetter et al (1984) considered the effect of health visitors working with elderly patients in general practice. A random sample of patients in general practice aged 70 and over were investigated. Independent assessments made at the beginning and end of the study showed that the health visitor in an urban practice has some impact on patients. More services were provided for them, their mortality was reduced and their quality of life improved, though the last measure just failed to be statistically significant. The health visitor working in a rural practice, however, had no such effect.

A study by Hendriksen et al (1989) of co-ordinated contributions of home care personnel in admission to and discharge of elderly people from hospital in Denmark demonstrated improved outcome for home visits. An intervention group ($n = 135$) had an average hospital stay of 11 days compared with 14.3 days in the control group ($n = 138$). The total number of bed days were 1490 and 1970 respectively. No differences were observed with respect to number of diagnostic procedures during hospitalisation, number of deaths, diagnoses on discharge and functional capacity.

The influence of a 'friendly visitor' programme on the cognitive functioning and morale of elderly persons was studied by Reinke et al (1981). 49 nursing home residents were assigned randomly to a group focusing on conversational interaction, a group in which the playing of cognitively challenging games supplemented conversation, or a no-treatment control group. Each subject was visited by a student twice per week for 8 weeks. Subjects were given four tests of cognitive functioning (vocabulary, matrices, memory, problem solving) and three tests of morale (Life Satisfaction Index A, Philadelphia Geriatric Center Morale Scale and self-perceived health). They were rated by nursing home activity directors on morale, programme participation, alertness, sociability and physical condition. A multivariate analysis of covariance in which age, education and length of nursing home residency were covariates revealed a reliable overall effect for the treatment. Subjects in both groups demonstrated improved performance relative to control subjects. Furthermore, subjects in the conversation plus games condition demonstrated the greatest improvement. The findings above, particularly in the last study (Reinke et al 1981), support the notion of home visiting as opposed to health visiting conferring relatively greater benefit in the elderly when compared to other categories above.

Mental health

The area of health visitor interventions for families and clients with mental health problems is very underresearched. There is only one RCT included in the Cochrane database for health visitor interventions and this has a positive outcome.

Holden et al (1989) investigated whether counselling and support by health visitors was helpful in managing postnatal depression. 60 women identified as depressed by screening at 6 weeks postpartum and by psychiatric interview at 13 weeks postpartum were allocated randomly to an intervention and control group. Eight weekly counselling visits by health visitors were conducted. After 3 months 18 (69%) of the 26 women in the treatment group had fully recovered compared with nine (38%) of 24 in the control group. The study concluded that counselling by health visitors was valuable in managing non-psychotic postnatal depression. However, as these results were not compared with those for other health and social care professionals, the findings cannot provide a benchmark for service provision.

ECONOMIC PRINCIPLES FOR PRIORITY SETTING AND PURCHASING IN PRIMARY CARE GROUPS

The size and complexity of healthcare services illustrate both the necessity for and the difficulty of allocating resources effectively. The main role of the newly formed primary care groups will be to plan strategically health improvement programmes (HImPs). PCGs will purchase some healthcare services with due regard to a systematic assessment of local needs. PCGs may decide to carry out formalised needs assessments but there are a variety of possible approaches to priority setting. Orthodox health economists have criticised persuasively certain of these approaches, advocating instead the techniques of programme budgeting and marginal analysis.

In this section, studies of health authority purchasing are reviewed. These studies suggest that there has been some movement from incremental to more formalised methods of decision-making. These studies, however, do not deal with issues of organisational politics and lack of integration in the needs assessment process, which

are likely to be particularly problematical in the multiagency context of healthcare.

A number of studies are also examined that report on the implementation of projects aspiring to implement the orthodox health economics approach. In practice, these projects have been carried out pragmatically, partly because of behavioural aspects that are not accommodated in the theory underpinning conventional health economics. This seems somewhat ironical in the light of the criticism of other approaches as theoretically unsound, although the studies themselves do contain undoubted insights.

The inability to implement comprehensively rationalistic procedures echoes the failure of earlier attempts at 'rational' methods of resource allocation in the public sector. A modified version of the health economics approach, however, could be compatible with Lindblom's concept of strategic analysis and give valuable results. The conclusion that more studies of resource allocation and performance evaluation by healthcare commissioners, examining both quantitative and qualitative factors, are needed to gain further insight into the dynamics of decision-making is difficult to avoid.

Approaches to priority setting in general

Priority setting is an area of much controversy. There is a lack of agreement, however, in public health policy circles concerning the setting of priorities for purchasing overall healthcare services. Evidence both from the literature and practical experience (Mooney et al 1993) indicates a range of different practices in health authorities for setting overall priorities.

It is suggested that there are a range of approaches including incremental, total needs assessment, target setting, social audit, programme budgeting and marginal analysis. In practice, these approaches are not necessarily encountered in a pure form and purchasers may adopt an eclectic approach. Orthodox health economists favour the programme budgeting and marginal analysis approach and have criticised other approaches forcefully.

Empirical evidence concerning differing approaches may be helpful to PCGs as they begin to organise themselves to plan HImPs for local areas. Some health visitors will become members of PCGs and so it is important they familiarise themselves with priority setting approaches in theory and in practice.

Incrementalism

This approach follows broadly historical patterns of expenditure.

Needs assessment

Nearly all health authority purchasers carry out 'needs assessment' (Obermann & Tolley 1997). A form of needs assessment is 'total needs assessment'. Here the total needs of a client group are established and expenditure is allocated according to the size of those needs pro rata. For example, if 30% of the client group of maternity patients consisted of antenatal patients then 30% of the budget for maternity services might be allocated to services supporting them. Another type of needs assessment is of the rapid appraisal variety. Rapid appraisal of needs is based on many different sources of research and information of all types. This is assessed and graded and an overall picture is formulated very quickly.

Target setting

'Target setting' aims to incorporate central government targets for health promotion and reduction of disease, cited in policy documents, into local priority setting. Most purchasers respond to these directives and combine them with their current methodologies for priority setting. For example, targets for the reduction of CHD and drug and alcohol use were set out in the White Paper *The Health of the Nation* (Department of Health 1992).

Social audit

Social audit can be seen as a complementary approach to needs assessment. Hawtin et al (1994) state that 'the term social audit encapsu-

lates the relationship between needs on the one hand and resources on the other ... a social audit attempts to reveal the "health" of a community which results from the interplay of public services, housing, employment, the natural and social environment and many other factors'.

Unfortunately, however, the term has a number of different uses, many of which stress reporting activities rather than assessment of need (Cotton et al 1997).

Orthodox health economics approach

Orthodox economists do not tend to favour these approaches, for a number of reasons. The usefulness of total needs assessment is limited in that allocation of resources according to the size of a problem can be very misleading. Not all needs can be met, so merely measuring need gives no guidance about resource allocation. The total needs assessment approach offers no useful guidance by which resources can be allocated across programmes and subprogrammes.

Specifically, in total needs assessment no attention is given to potential costs and benefits of treatments, but only to the size of problems. Need is a dynamic, multidimensional and changing concept, so how can purchasers incorporate data on total needs into their decision-making? In addition, needs assessment generates much information, some of which is of questionable usefulness and time-consuming to handle. These distractions take decision-makers away from key aspects as they become immersed in the quantity and detail of information. Similarly, setting targets in itself gives no guidance as to how targets may be achieved, or ranked and traded off against each other.

Orthodox health economics is said to provide a way of thinking logically through the problems of setting priorities as well as offering the techniques of 'programme budgeting' and 'marginal analysis' to support decision-making concerning resource allocation. Furthermore, the orthodox economist's approach is said to allow purchasers to move their attention away from the mass of NHS statistics and focus on key data and decision-making criteria.

Programme budgeting can be used as an information framework (Cohen & Henderson 1988) to allow health services to be disaggregated into programmes that have relatively homogeneous outputs. The information in any programme budget will include cost or expenditure data together with some sort of indicator of the output from the programme. Marginal analysis (Cohen & Henderson 1988) then provides rules for deciding how resources should be moved between subcategories of a programme to achieve a more effective allocation of resources. Services are then ranked on the basis of ratio of marginal benefits to marginal costs. The concept of opportunity cost figures prominently in these techniques.

Many studies in the literature referred to below have been carried out by teams of orthodox economists. In most of these studies no critical appraisal of the orthodox economics approach is offered. Given that orthodox health economists have become influential in the debate about priority setting, it is important that a critical view is presented.

Priority setting – empirical studies

Klein & Redmayne (1992) analysed the purchasing plans of 114 health authorities. They argue that 'rhetoric is not always matched by funding'. In purchasing plans for 1992/93, health authorities emphasised mental health and handicap, for example, as service priorities. Nevertheless, of the total resources allocated to new developments in 1992/93, greater extra expenditure than expected was spent on acute services. According to the authors, misallocation of resources is the consequence of previous spending commitments. The authors further report 'priority overload', with health authorities being swamped by national, regional and local shopping lists of priorities. A response to this and to finite resources is to pursue a strategy of 'spreading the money around'. On average, each purchaser funded 15 priorities, with relatively small amounts often going to many different services.

Only 12 authorities in the survey rationed priorities explicitly by denying or limiting the availability of specific forms of treatment. However, the authors expected that significant moves away from implicit to explicit rationing would take place when the purchaser/provider split had been in place for longer. Tools for assessing health gains and measuring need would then increase in importance.

Obermann & Tolley (1997) reported the results of a more recent survey of 121 health authorities in England, Wales and Scotland between September 1995 and January 1996. The authors examined the extent to which these health authorities perceived themselves as involved in setting priorities for health service resource allocation and the nature of public participation in priority setting. Only four claimed noninvolvement in priority setting. High numbers of very important/important ratings were given for equity, health gain and cost-effectiveness criteria in priority setting. The survey also demonstrated that the pursuit of explicit priority setting in resource allocation is generating needs for more information on key decision-making criteria. The authors conclude that achieving these information requirements is likely to be fraught with difficulty.

A comparison of the results of these two quantitative surveys demonstrates changes that took place in priority setting in health authorities over a 5-year period. Priority setting appears to be a more formalised, evidence-based process than previously and variables such as equity, cost-effectiveness and health gain are more important. However, quantitative research methodologies preclude the investigation of variables such as lack of integration in the priority-setting process and the impact of 'politics' and 'product championing'. Investigation of these qualitative variables requires a different methodological approach (Watt & Freemantle 1994).

Evidence – orthodox health economics

A number of papers addressed the development of an overall structure and process for priority setting and rationing within the commissioning process (Mooney et al 1993, Craig et al 1995). Mooney et al (1992) stated that choices should be related to objectives. While a number of objectives may be identified for the NHS, they are generally agreed to include efficiency and equity. Other approaches to priority setting are regarded as theoretically unacceptable compared with the orthodox health economics approach of programme budgeting and marginal analysis. The orthodox health economics approach is supported by tools such as QALY league tables, which rank treatments and services on the basis of marginal cost per QALY gained. Mooney et al (1992) regard the QALY approach as theoretically acceptable with respect to allocative efficiency, although they acknowledge there are practical difficulties with data. Furthermore, the objective of equity is difficult to handle using the orthodox economics approach.

The well known Oregon experiment attempted to use both QALYs and public participation, but is regarded as disappointing in both respects (O'Neill 1990, Dixon & Welch 1991). It is claimed that QALYs can help in priority setting provided their conceptual and measurement limitations are recognised. This approach is said to work best when QALY measures are location-specific.

Mooney et al (1993) described an attempt to use programme budgeting and marginal analysis to set priorities in North Mersey Health Authority. The group set out to produce a programme budget for client and disease groups. This necessitated describing all the services or subprogrammes within a programme. An incremental wish list was produced from which resources could be switched at the boundaries of subprogrammes. The information in a programme budget, according to the authors, included cost or expenditure data together with an indicator of the output of a programme. The problems of having to use limited and unreliable data and making subjective value judgements were highlighted during the study. However, the authors commented on the importance of adhering to the agreed principles of priority setting because quality, availability and reliability of data is a problem whichever method of priority setting is used. Furthermore, they suggested that the values of the local community should be used to make judgements in a priority setting context, despite the difficulties associated with doing so.

The authors criticised health authorities for not adopting at the outset what they considered to be the correct principles of the priority-setting process. They emphasised the importance of being clear about the objective of the service, which is very often allocative efficiency, and measuring the outcome of the service in units directly relevant to that objective. In theory, it is essential to maximise the social benefit from whatever resources are available and to use the decision criteria giving priority to those treatments where the ratio of marginal benefit to marginal cost is greatest. Moreover, this perspective does not take into account the realities of organisational politics whereby resource allocation decisions are determined, to some extent at least, by issues such as power and prestige (North 1997). Thus, in practice, a more pragmatic approach must be adopted and this is also acknowledged by other orthodox health economists (Donaldson & Farrar 1991).

Donaldson & Farrar (1991) have shown how a modified mainstream economics approach can be used in priority setting. Although this approach can apply to all areas of health provision, Donaldson & Farrar concentrated on the area of dementia services for elderly people. The results of this project demonstrate that it is possible to reorientate resources so as to produce greater benefit for all. The results of this study coincided with the views of the consumers, although this is not always the case. The logical conclusion is that contracts should be based, as far as possible, on assessments of the marginal costs and benefits of changes in the service mix. This will make it more likely that the welfare of the community is maximised, given the healthcare resources at its disposal.

Craig et al (1995) described work being undertaken in Tyneside Health Authority. The authors believed that programme budgeting and marginal analysis could be used to give focus to needs assessment and to create explicit links between individual contracts and a health strategy. However, this approach needs to overcome some constraints such as the transferability of data across different settings and contexts and shortcomings in local epidemiological information.

The main issue highlighted in this paper is the process by which purchasers make overall priority-setting decisions. The authors comment on the lack of integration of needs assessment within priority setting and the organisational political processes that seem to override explicit principles and rules for decision-making in resource allocation.

Are priority setting processes rational?

The orthodox economist's approach is a variation of CBA, which has been widely applied previously in public sector management. CBA is based on the 'rational model' in which decision-making is a sequential, feedback loop process going through the following stages.

Firstly, determine the objectives of an organisation and identify a need, problem or opportunity. The next step is to consider all alternative ways of meeting needs identified and evaluate options in terms of all the costs and benefits associated. Select and implement the option that gives maximum net benefit in relation to organisation objectives. Lastly, review and evaluate the impact of the option chosen and modify activities, objectives, etc. with respect to the review.

Thus, it is held that decision-making is, or should be, a formalised and structured process of matching means to ends.

However, the rational model has been much criticised, both on practical grounds and because it is said to ignore behavioural, organisational and political realities that decisions are made by people (van Gunsteren, cited in Jones & Pendlebury 1992, p. 77).

In the public sector much more than in the private sector, organisational objectives are often multiple, vague and perhaps confused. Outcomes may well be difficult to define and costs and benefits have significant nonfinancial aspects. Moreover, processes are just as important as outcomes. Politicians may see budgeting, therefore, primarily as a way of financing commitments derived from the electoral process rather than of solving problems that are in any case multilayered. 'Political' approaches may be biased

towards stability and continuity and narrow the area for controversy while remaining flexible at the margins of expenditure. 'Budgeting is incremental, not comprehensive ... attention is focused on a small number of items over which the budgetary battle is fought' (Wildavsky 1964, p. 15).

From this perspective, it is necessary to focus on marginal changes in expenditure, with only a small number of options considered and increases and decreases in resources allocated being relatively small. It is argued that directing attention to marginal changes in expenditure gives a more realistic chance of altering spending patterns, while accommodating political values and policy preferences.

However, large changes in public expenditure will need to be considered from time to time (Tomkins 1987). Incrementalism, while a necessary corrective to the comprehensive, rationalistic approach, is broadly descriptive. It is of little use in improving the resource allocation process. Tomkins argues for a 'negotiated order' perspective, from which public sector decision-making, etc. is seen as allocating scarce resources among competing actors who build coalitions and 'cut' deals. The budget can then be seen as a legitimisation device, giving an apparently rational and objective form to political decisions.

Incrementalist theory containing the notion of 'bounded rationality' is often associated with the work of Lindblom (1959, 1979). According to Lindblom human beings attempt to be rational but are constrained or bounded in doing so by numerous factors. Lindblom criticised rationalism as being overly ambitious in claiming that all options and future outcomes could be known. Moreover, despite the apparent logic, it is nearly always impractical to set objectives before making decisions. In practice, policies and objectives are set simultaneously (Lindblom 1959, 1979).

CONCLUSION

Economics is relevant to all health visiting practice. In the first section of this chapter the link between economics and the commodity 'health visiting interventions' is explained. Economic thinking and techniques can help whenever resources are scarce and demands are unlimited. All health visitors are familiar with these constraints from their everyday work. Often the need to extract better outcomes from dwindling resources can become overwhelming and economics can help with the process of deciding how priorities for purchasing should be established. In common with other areas of health care, some health visiting activities confer more benefit for a given cost than others. Economic evaluation studies can help to identify these activities to achieve efficient allocation of resources. Naturally, the incorporation of economic thinking and techniques in this areas is conditional upon overcoming the jargon barrier. This chapter has attempted to clarify the meanings of the key terms and concepts necessary to get by as a practising professional.

The value of information and support from health visiting professionals so vital in reducing health inequalities seems to be clear from review evidence. In addition, the role of economic factors such as growth, inflation, unemployment and income in health outcomes in conjunction with health visiting interventions needs to be better understood. More economic evaluations of health visiting interventions are recommended. The quality of the current stock of clinical evaluations of health visiting interventions, apart from a number of reviews of RCTs, is poor. A number of areas, e.g. mental health, have been neglected badly. In addition, the distinction between the benefits of health visiting and those of other home visiting activities and the relative benefits of specialist and generalist health visitors with various client groups have not been adequately researched. More research to quantify the benefits of health visiting for individuals, families and society is needed for the true worth of the profession of health visiting to be reflected in future economic evaluations.

9

Corporate and clinical governance and the health visiting service

Anne Robotham and Jane Harvey

CORPORATE GOVERNANCE

Corporate governance is the necessary means by which companies in general function effectively, both competitively and for their own survival. Survival is less important in the public sector, but the assurance of effective accountability is essential where public money is used to fund a service. There have been failures of financial governance in the NHS in recent years that were due to financial mismanagement (Wessex and West Midlands Regional Health Authorities). Subsequent investigative reports about this mismanagement collectively highlighted a common link as a loss of control and accountability by the RHA board over the RHA management. In addition, the NHS management executive was also slow to realise that something was wrong because there were weak accountability links from the health authorities to the Department of Health. As a direct result of these failures, the organisation of the relationship between the authorities has improved, with the reduction of the number of authorities and transfer of members of the NHS Executive into the regions. It was also clear from the failures that there needed to be a clarification of the balance of accountability and influence between executive and nonexecutive directors. Thus it becomes essential to seek clarity about the role of nonexecutive directors if they are to be both supportive and 'independent scrutineers', for it is not possible to do both effectively.

The reforms at board level following *Working*

for Patients (Department of Health 1989b) mean that nonexecutives, who are all independent of the organisation, now comprise just under half of RHA board members. The chair is now taken by a nonexecutive who is appointed by the Secretary of State, and the position of the chief executive is entirely separate. Thus implementation of government policy and accountability directly to the Secretary of State is undertaken by two powerful figures who function separately. Healthcare professional influence was minimal at board level and more by integration of clinical practitioners into the management hierarchy and decision-making processes. However, the model, which was based on the private-sector board accountability approach, meant a predominantly director/medical clinician membership with little direct public, nursing or paramedical accountability. This weakness has now been addressed through the development of primary care groups (PCGs), which have, at board level, representatives of nursing, paramedical services, lay public/community health councils and social services. The balance of professional, lay and nonexecutive representation may not necessarily be correct in the early days to ensure equal division of accountability between the professional groups (GPs still dominate numerically). However, the potential strength of these boards is that here is the opportunity for point-of-delivery/need to be working in tandem with the overall management of the authority.

The methods by which primary care groups are run at board level, including terms of reference, chairing, committee procedures and the education of members in organisational management and decision-making processes are all important. The effectiveness of boards is about the ability of individual members to understand issues across all its functions and take a corporate view. Killoran et al (1998), discussing the effective deployment of management, point out that where there are several PCGs to a district there may well be repetitive costs linked to the devolution of functions. The probable development in these cases is for supra-PCGs to have an umbrella function across and above PCG level. Indeed, Smith et al's (1999), research in Birmingham involving GPs, the health authority and the local medical committee found support for this idea. Clinical governance and strategic city-wide planning emerged as particularly suitable for such arrangements. They will include local public health and strategy development, service specifications, definition of clinical pathways, negotiation of service agreements, public information, quality assurance, organisational development and local performance management. Health visitors who have been elected to primary care boards are in an excellent position to influence policy and decision-making but they will need to be supported by a strong nursing forum who are in a position both to respond quickly to requests for information and to feed through ideas and proposals for improvement in clinical effectiveness.

CLINICAL GOVERNANCE

The term 'clinical governance', used in *The New NHS – Modern, Dependable* (Department of Health 1997a), means: 'a framework to ensure that all NHS organisations have the proper processes for monitoring and improving clinical quality' (Department of Health 1998b). The principles of clinical governance apply to all those who provide or manage patient care services in the NHS. The principles supporting quality improvement are the same for large and small organisations. In practice, clinical governance locally needs to take account of the needs, complexity and size of individual NHS organisations. The emphasis is on processes that are simple to use and, above all, produce results. The requirements of clinical governance are backed by the new statutory duty of quality which is placed on NHS trusts and primary care trusts. In essence, the three aspects of clinical governance are:

- setting quality
- delivering quality
- monitoring quality.

As part of the arrangements for clinical governance, chief executives of NHS trusts are legally responsible for clinical quality and the various components that come together under the governance umbrella. The government requires all professionals involved in healthcare organisations to work together in multidisciplinary teams, if necessary across organisational boundaries, to provide quality care. There is a requirement to develop local information and organisation information systems to aid standard-setting and to collect data to demonstrate improvements in the quality of care and services (see Chapter 3).

The National Institute for Clinical Excellence (NICE), which came into existence in April 1999, has the responsibility of developing standards that will go towards a national service framework to specify the way that particular services are to be provided. The first framework in place provides a national approach to and standards for coronary heart disease, which was originally brought to public attention when Townsend et al (1988) demonstrated the inequality of service provision between the north and south of England. Estimates at that time were made of the potential for complete recovery from coronary thrombosis for sufferers in the south as against the north, including such variables as: economic equality; dietary equality; emergency care, including ambulance service response; and subsequent clinical care and aftercare. It was clear as a result of these estimates that there was a marked inequality in delivery and care, and epidemiological studies of noninfectious disease show clearly that coronary heart disease is one of the most preventable and treatable diseases.

The expectation of NICE is to draw up and issue 10–15 scientifically based guidelines to doctors and other health professionals each year, setting out the best treatment options for patients. For health visiting this could entail effectively evaluating approaches to preventive health measures and publishing these findings to share expert practice. Once this information is available to the profession then NICE will be appraising results for the benefit of effective evidence-based practice. Two concerns may find support – firstly that NICE may be too influenced by economics to provide the most purely clinical evidence for effectiveness, and this may be unacceptable to a caring medical profession. The second consid-

eration is that if NICE is given such power to impose 'best treatment options' there may be punitive measures for those members of the medical profession who choose, for clinical reasons, to pursue a treatment in the best interests of the patient. It remains to be seen what will be considered to be the minimum standard for equality in medical care.

This whole concept is a massive undertaking and culture change. Indeed, although quality assurance mechanisms and healthcare quality standards have been in place for 15 years and more, imposing the legal responsibility on NHS trust chief executives requires the setting up and maintenance of effective systems and standards of care management and measurement. When setting standards there are always concerns about what their underlying basis will be and the underlying motives of those setting them. Economic constraints have been cited as reasons for deliberately setting standards that are easily achievable, and this should be minimised by ensuring that all interested parties, professional and consumer, have a voice to ensure that appropriate targets are set and met.

The Commission for Health Improvement (CHI), set up during the period 1999/2000, will conduct a rolling programme of visits to each organisation in the NHS to check that the systems for ensuring quality are in place. The CHI will also be responsible for monitoring the implementation of standards, especially those set nationally through national service frameworks for specific areas of care such as mental health. Each healthcare organisation will be required to produce an annual clinical governance report, the first of which will be due in April 2000. As with other government measurement mechanisms, the appropriate department, i.e. the Department of Health, is likely to use these to publish 'league tables' for different aspects of care quality. Despite criticism from commentators this approach is likely to continue as the only visible means by which the Department of Health can show quality and effectiveness. The main problem is that it will tend to concentrate on short-term successes and, as the health visiting profession is well aware, most of the value of preventive work is long-term. Yet again, this points to the need for health visiting to explain and demonstrate the effectiveness of long-term preventive healthcare and to be party to devising its own standards and measures/indicators of quality.

STANDARDS IN CARE DELIVERY AMONG HEALTHCARE PROFESSIONALS

Nursing, midwifery and health visiting professionals

It is a requirement of every practising professional to ensure that their registration with their professional organisation is current. Primarily, this requirement is aimed at protecting the client and all recognised professions have their appropriate regulatory committee to whom representations can be made where professional conduct or performance is below acceptability level. The need to protect the public from the poorly functioning professional has always been at the heart of the function of the United Kingdom Central Council for Nursing, Midwifery and Health Visiting (UKCC) and its predecessor, the General Nursing Council (GNC). To this end standards have been set in relation to professional practice in documents such as the *Code of Professional Conduct* (UKCC 1992a). Registration with the professional body also ensures that, where it is written into the regulations, the required amount of professional updating and development is undertaken within a prescribed period of time. With the important implicit need to promote lifelong learning within postregistration education and preparation for practice (PREP; UKCC 1994a; see Chapter 1), it is also important that nurses, midwives and health visitors show evidence of continued learning through courses and study days. A minimum standard of the number of days required is set down for each re-registration period. As specialisms and specialist areas of practice have grown in keeping with the development of modern medicine and healthcare, so also has the need to ensure that practitioners do not take on areas of practice for which they are not trained. To attempt to ensure that practice is maintained at a level commensurate with the development of the role, the UKCC developed a position statement on the scope of professional practice (UKCC 1992b). There are two sections that are very relevant to health visitors and form part of this profession's involvement in clinical governance (Box 9.1).

To ensure standards of quality within professional practice the above principles identify the safeguards that should be taken by professional organisations who have any responsibility for the health, safety and care of others. It is also interesting to recognise that codes of conduct or standards for practice are not always constraining by reason of setting boundaries and limits. In some instances they also help practitioners to develop their roles within wider boundaries where previously there have been impediments to such developments. A clear example of this is the Scope of Health Visiting Practice section set out in the larger document (UKCC 1992b), and this bears direct quotation in the same way as the 'Principles' above (Box 9.2).

Box 9.1 Principles for adjusting the scope of practice (from UKCC 1992b)

The registered nurse, midwife or health visitor:

- must be satisfied that each aspect of practice is directed at meeting the needs and serving the interests of the patient or client
- must endeavour always to achieve, maintain and develop knowledge, skill and competence to respond to those needs and interests
- must honestly acknowledge any limits of personal knowledge and skill and take steps to remedy any relevant deficits in order effectively and appropriately to meet the needs of patients and clients
- must ensure that any enlargement or adjustment of the scope of personal professional practice must be achieved without compromising or fragmenting existing aspects of professional practice and care and that the requirements of the Council's Code of Professional Conduct are satisfied throughout the whole area of practice
- must recognise and honour the direct or indirect personal accountability borne for all aspects of professional practice and
- must, in serving the interests of patients and clients and the wider interests of society, avoid any inappropriate delegation to others which compromises those interests.

Box 9.2 Scope of health visiting practice (from UKCC 1992b)

The position of health visiting differs from that of nursing and midwifery, as there are frequent occasions when the full contribution of health visitors may not find expression where it is most needed. There is, for example, often a concentration on the role of the health visitor in relation to those in the under five age group at the expense of other groups in the community who need, or would benefit from, the special preparation and skill of health visitors. These circumstances have the effect of constraining practice and limiting the degree to which individuals and communities are able to benefit from the knowledge and skills of health visitors. There is merit in allowing health visitors, where they judge it to be appropriate, to use the full range of their skills in response to needs identified in the pursuit of their health visiting practice. To single out any aspect of practice would be unwise but, where health and nursing need is identified, the health visitor is well placed to determine what intervention may be necessary and able to draw on both her nursing and health visiting qualification.

The community setting of health visiting practice, the relationship between numerous agencies and services and the health visitor's professional relationship with clients and their families are factors which must be taken into consideration. The health visitor, in all aspects of her practice, is subject to the Council's Code of Professional Conduct.

Although *The Scope of Professional Practice* was issued in 1992 its principles made very little difference to the way in which the majority of health visitors work. This is a sad reflection on the ability of the profession to make the most of its opportunities. The reasons why practice has changed so little to meet emerging needs are twofold: the nature of health visitor education and the lack of opportunity for continued professional development. As part of clinical governance the government has stated a clear need for 'lifelong learning' and is committed to ensuring that such programmes are set up.

The medical profession

In a briefing paper (February 1999) the King's Fund discusses the methods by which the performance of doctors and other healthcare professionals will be monitored. It is clear from the above section that the nursing, midwifery and health visiting professions have good systems in place in order to ensure standards in existing practice and conduct, as well as guidelines on professional development. The medical profession also has procedures for investigating complaints against doctors, through their regulatory body, the General Medical Council.

In contrast to nurses, midwives and health visitors, who now have to prove professional updating, no such system is in place for doctors, and this has led to the consideration of a similar type of re-registration for doctors. The King's Fund suggests that this would require a system to monitor each doctor's performance and the likelihood of deregistration until such time as education has improved competence to acceptable performance levels.

The CHI will also have a part to play in that they will endorse a national review of all hospital doctors, producing data on performance against a national standard. This will require a system of appraisal similar to that used for nurses, midwives and health visitors and will be part of each hospital's clinical governance programme. For general practitioners, primary care groups will take responsibility for ensuring that systems and guidelines are in place for dealing with suspected poor practice among GPs within their locality. Where necessary, however, the CHI will act as an investigator of outcomes that may be pointing to poor medical practice, either in individual doctors or organisationally in relation to protocols.

Assessing the performance of a doctor or other healthcare professional is a complex procedure and higher mortality rates for one surgical operating team than another may not be due to inadequate performance of any of the team members. It could be that the team is a victim of its own success and receives an increasing number of referrals of patients who are a greater surgical risk.

Social services

In a White Paper, *Modernising Social Services* (Department of Health 1998c), radical changes were made to ensure that standards in social services were brought into a new regulatory framework to mirror those being introduced in the healthcare services. For adults, a long-term care charter will enable easier use of services, with more individual tailoring to need. For children accommodated by the local authority, the Quality Protects programme will improve inspection standards in all homes, independent fostering agencies and residential family centres.

For vulnerable adults and children, the eight regional commissions for care standards will regulate the entire range of care services.

With the continuing development of national vocational qualifications (NVQs) throughout the health- and social-care services, a new body, the General Social Care Council (GSCC), has been set up to raise standards in the social-care workforce. This will set practice and ethical standards and training levels across all social-care support staff.

HEALTHCARE PERFORMANCE MEASURES

These measures form part of government strategy to press for a system based on partnership, driven by performance. This approach will help ensure equal access to services and quality of care across the country. The new national performance framework will focus on six areas of care and these have 37 high-level performance indicators to assess whether healthcare is in line with the expectations of *The New NHS – Modern, Dependable* (Department of Health 1997a). The six care areas, with a commentary reflecting health visiting are:

- *Health improvement*: overall health of the population reflecting social and environmental factors and individual behaviour; appropriate care provided by NHS and other agencies.

  Health visiting can support this area by setting up good alliances with social agencies such as social work departments and voluntary and charitable organisations and with environmental agencies such as housing departments. The value of these alliances is that they are drawn into the partnership processes that health visitors set up with clients.

- *Fair access to services*: the fairness of provision of services in relation to need with the following variables: geographical; socioeconomic; demographic; care groups.

  The importance of health visitors working to reflect the needs identified through active and passive caseload and area profiling (Chapter 2) cannot be overemphasised. The organisation of health visiting processes should allow quick movement of professional practice to respond to identified need. However, this must be without withdrawal from the previous needy groups and this may require alternative methods of organising health visiting, e.g. using a corporate caseload approach.

- *Effective delivery of appropriate health care*: services should be clinically effective with evidence-based care packages; appropriate to need; timely; in line with agreed standards; provided according to best service organisation; delivered by appropriately trained and educated staff.

  Health visiting will continue to develop practice that is totally evidence-based. There is a developing body of evidence to support the statement that ultimately all practice will be evidence-based. However, this evidence needs constant dissemination by publication and also a means whereby a database is set up to which all practising professionals have access. Health visiting particularly needs to develop electronic information networks to underpin quality practice. A number of databases are now available and health visitors should be in a position to access these.

- *Efficiency*: the extent to which the NHS provides efficient services, including cost per unit of care/outcome; productivity of capital and human resources.

  Health visiting must be able to demonstrate that effective practice is not necessarily cost-effective. Cost benefit analysis (Chapter 8) should show overall health improvement (often in the field of mental health) but this may well not be achievable without spending time with clients on a one-to-one basis in their homes. If clients can cope and develop with this type of support and advice without any resort to acute services, this is positive cost benefit.

• *Patient/carer experience*: patient/carer perceptions of service delivery, including responsiveness to individual needs and preferences; skill, care and continuity of service provision; patient involvement, good information and choice; waiting and accessibility; organisation and courtesy of administration arrangements.

Chapters 5 and 11 particularly focus on health visiting skills and methods of practice that respond to client need and provide positive client experience. In preventive practice responsible response to need is about working closely with clients to enable them to develop their own preventive skills and positive health behaviour. This may be carried out in a variety of settings to provide evidence of cost benefit practice and cost-effective practice.

• *Health outcome of NHS care*: NHS success in using resources to reduce levels of risk factors; reduce levels of disease, impairment and complications of treatment; improve quality of life for patients and carers; reduce premature deaths.

Health visiting through preventive practice will continue to develop positive health outcomes. The aspects of practice detailed in Chapters 7 and 10 show how levels of unhealthy situations can be improved by a wider development of practice. It is also important that health visitors concentrate on the epidemiology of noninfectious diseases when using data as a baseline for their work on health outcomes. This is suited to their model of work and may help to concentrate the measurement of outcomes away from more easily measured infectious diseases data and immunisation levels as the only clear measurement of effectiveness.

These six categories will require careful monitoring with good support initiatives to underpin their efficiency. They will be part of national standards set through national service frameworks and NICE. National service frameworks spell out how services can best be organised to cater for patients with particular conditions and the standards that services have to meet. They indicate which services are best provided in primary care, in hospitals and in specialist centres.

Proposals to undertake these initiatives will be threefold.

The NHS Research and Development Programme will continue to be used to assess clinical and cost-effectiveness of various aspects of healthcare. It is currently providing access to a rapidly expanding evidence base on healthcare interventions and services. However, because the evidence provided has lacked in local guidance as to how it should best be used, NICE and the CHI are required to assist.

The National Institute for Clinical Excellence (NICE), as mentioned earlier in the chapter, is to promote the use of clinical guidelines derived from evidence-based practice with inbuilt advice on clinical audit criteria and evaluation. It will have a role in the assessment of prime research and systematic reviews and appraisal of clinical guidelines. Alongside these roles there will also be the requirement to ensure the dissemination of information on clinical and cost effectiveness and sharing of best practices.

There are six stages to the work of NICE:

• Stage 1: Identification a) for new health interventions, for example, new drugs devices and procedures that may benefit patients and clients in the NHS; b) for existing interventions in relation to variation in use, clinical effectiveness or cost-effectiveness

• Stage 2: Evidence collection – undertaking research to establish clinical and cost-effectiveness of interventions

• Stage 3: Appraisal and guidance – carefully considering the implications for clinical practice of the evidence on clinical and cost-effectiveness and producing guidelines

• Stage 4: Dissemination of the guidance and supporting audit methodologies

• Stage 5: Implementation at local level through clinical governance

• Stage 6: Monitoring the impact and keeping advice under review.

It will be some time before NICE will be in a position to move its focus from clinical issues to public health, health promotion and screening programmes, but in time these will also come into its orbit. One of the most influential aspects of NICE is its mechanism of work, which will be to draw on as much published evidence as is available to identify effective measures and programmes. This makes it all the more important for health visitors to ensure that they disseminate evidence of effective practice through publication and conferences.

The Commission for Health Improvement (CHI) will be a statutory body to support those who are developing and monitoring local systems and multidisciplinary standards for clinical quality. The chair and officers will be appointed by the Secretary of State and there will be a new appointment – that of Director of Health Improvement. The Commission will offer an independent guarantee that local systems to monitor, assure and improve clinical quality are in place. It will have the capacity to offer specific support on request when local organisations face particular clinical problems. It will also investigate and identify the sources of problems and work with organisations on lasting remedies to improve quality and standards of care (Wilson & Tingle 1999).

The Commission's core functions will be to:

- provide national leadership to develop and disseminate clinical governance principles
- independently scrutinise local clinical governance arrangements to support, promote and deliver high-quality services, through a rolling programme of local reviews of service providers
- undertake a programme of service reviews to monitor national implementation of national service frameworks and review progress locally on implementation of these frameworks and NICE guidance
- help the NHS identify and tackle serious or persistent clinical problems; the Commission will have the capacity for rapid investigation and intervention to help put these right
- over time, increasingly take on responsibility

for overseeing and assisting with external incident enquiries (Department of Health 1998b).

CLINICAL QUALITY IN PRIMARY CARE

The New NHS – Modern, Dependable (Department of Health 1997a) considers the characteristics of a quality organisation to be as listed in Box 9.3.

The following sections will discuss each of these characteristics in relation to health visiting practice within primary care. It is clearly important to emphasise that health visiting is not working in isolation within primary care but that the focus of this book is on health visiting in context and that context may include integrated team approaches.

Quality improvement processes – clinical audit and integrated quality programme

Clinical audit

Quality mechanisms and total quality management have been part of the NHS for several years

---

Box 9.3 The characteristics of a quality organisation (Department of Health 1997a)

- Quality improvement processes in place, e.g. clinical audit, and integrated with the quality programme for the whole organisation
- Leadership skills developed at clinical team level
- Evidence-based practice in day-to-day use with infrastructure to support it
- Good practice, ideas and innovations (which have been evaluated) systematically disseminated within and outside the organisation
- Clinical risk reduction programmes in place
- Incidents detected and openly investigated and lessons promptly applied
- Lessons for clinical practice systematically learned from complaints made by patients
- Problems of poor clinical performance recognised at an early stage and dealt with to prevent harm to patients
- All professional development programmes reflect the principles of clinical governance
- The quality of data collected to monitor clinical care is itself of a high standard

and systems for the installation and maintenance of these are already in place. Kogan & Redfern (1995) draw together some of the aspects of the early work of Donabedian in analysing healthcare quality, quality of medical care and a system-based framework for quality. They quote Donabedian (1980), defining health care quality as:

- *goodness of technical care*, which refers to the effectiveness of healthcare, its ability to achieve the greatest improvement in health status possible within the conventional wisdom of medicine, i.e. of science, technology and clinical skills
- *goodness of interpersonal relationships among those involved in healthcare*, in particular the relationship between the user (patient/client) and the provider (therapist, nurse, doctor, other healthcare professional); thus an important aspect of high-quality care is that patients are treated with respect and their autonomy and interests are safeguarded
- *goodness of amenities*, which refers to creature comforts and aesthetic attributes of the healthcare setting. These can be difficult to distinguish from interpersonal care because privacy, courtesy, acceptability, comfort, promptness and so on are relevant to amenities as well as to interpersonal relationships. Donabedian emphasises the inextricable intertwining of his components, thus demonstrating his appreciation of quality as a whole entity.

They quote Donabedian (1980), giving four definitions of quality of medical care:

- his *individualised* definition judges quality with reference to patients' values, means, wishes and expectations
- his *social* definition recognises that there must be a net benefit for the population and effective social distribution of that benefit
- his *absolutist* definition requires care to achieve an optimum balance between health risks and benefits, and thus relates closely to scientific and technical aspects of medicine; thus, useless or redundant care is equivalent

to poor care because it wastes money and resources
- his *primary function of medical care is to advance the patient's welfare* definition emphasises patients as the judge of their own welfare and the importance of patient and doctor sharing the responsibility for balancing risks and benefits and defining objectives.

Finally Kogan & Redfern (1995) quote Donabedian's (1988) application of a system-based framework to inputs, processes and outcomes of health care:

- *structure* refers to organisational factors that determine the conditions under which care is given, e.g. the physical environment, management style, staffing levels, support services
- *process* focuses upon the complexity of interactions, transactions and activities between healthcare workers and their patients
- *outcome* is not simply a measure of health, well-being or any other state. Rather it is a change in status confidently attributable to antecedent care.

Other quality systems have been developed since Donabedian's original work but mostly they are adaptations and modifications. One such development of Donabedian's ideas was put forward by Maxwell (1984) and this probably comes closest to the ideas now contained in *A First Class Service – Quality in the New NHS* (Department of Health 1998b):

- *relevance*: the service or procedure is required by the individual or population
- *accessibility*: time, distance and structural access are within accepted norms
- *effectiveness*: the service achieves proper benefit for the individual or population
- *acceptability*: reasonable expectations of the patients and community are met
- *efficiency*: resources are well used
- *equity*: there is a fair share for all the community (Maxwell 1984)

and the Department of Health (1998b) quality statements are:

There should be three continuing objectives:

- to continually improve overall standards of clinical care
- to reduce unacceptable variations in clinical practice
- to ensure the best use of services so that patients receive the greatest benefit

and care provided should be

- appropriate – to people's needs
- effective – drawing on the best clinical evidence
- efficient and economic – to maximise health gain for the population.

A simple quality audit in health visiting

In its simplest form, clinical audit is about assessment, planning, implementing and evaluating (APIE) and most health visitors will recognise that this was the basis on which the nursing process was first premised. Indeed, readers of the record-keeping section in Chapter 10 will note the quality process in the SOAPIER mnemonic that Charles uses in her record-keeping standards. The nursing process was originally devised as a problem-solving cycle but in addition lends itself to an audit process, as in Figure 9.1.

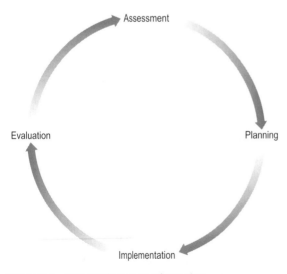

Figure 9.1 The nursing process/care plan

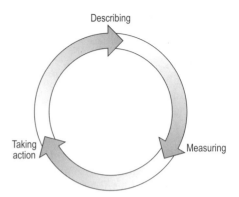

Figure 9.2 The Dynamic Standard Setting System

This is insufficiently rigorous to act as an audit tool as it stands because there are no standards identified and it assumes an ability to identify a problem, so that it is not possible to measure any quality performance.

To set quality standards many health visitors have been involved in a process called quality circles, which has as its basic steps:

- select a topic of relevance
- select indicators of quality for the care
- develop criteria and a level of acceptable performance
- identify standards for each criterion.

In 1990 the RCN published the Dynamic Standard Setting System (DySSSy) which is a cycle consisting of three elements (Fig. 9.2).

However, the process is not as simple as Figure 9.2 suggests because each of the elements has components that must be achieved before the element can be completed (Table 9.1).

Audit is a critical element of the quality cycle and is the catalyst for dynamic growth and changing practice.

It is essential that planning for improvement, taking action and evaluating the results of that action must follow the audit process (Fig. 9.3).

A trust in the West Midlands was required as part of its purchaser/provider contract with the health authority to set breast-feeding rates as an impact measure of health visiting (i.e. a clinical audit of the effectiveness of health visiting in relation to breast-feeding advice and support). The authority required quarterly information on the percentage of babies breast-fed at the time of the primary visit and 6 weeks after birth. The baseline

Table 9.1   Components in a quality cycle (RCN 1990)

Element	Component
Describing	Select a topic for quality improvement
	Identify a care group
	Identify criteria in relation to Donabedian's
	structure, process and outcomes definition
	Agree the standard
Measuring	Refine the criteria
	Select or design an audit tool
	Collect data
	Evaluate the data
Taking action	Consider action to be taken
	Plan the action
	Implement the plan
	Audit

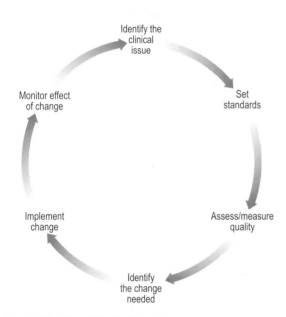

Figure 9.3   The clinical audit cycle

measure set was for the last 6 months of 1996 when the breast-feeding rates were 44% at the primary visit and 33% at a 6-week check. Breast-feeding rates have since been collected quarterly and include all breast-feeding even if mixed feeding has been introduced. Since the commencement of the audit little change has been seen in the rates at the primary visit but the breast-feeding rates at the 6-week visit have improved slowly from the initial 33% to a current 40.5%. In real terms this represents 95 more babies benefiting from breast-feeding and their mothers decreasing their risk of premenopausal breast cancer.

Since 1996, alongside the increased awareness among the staff of breast-feeding rates by caseload, clinic locality and trust, many other activities have taken place. A significant number of staff have undertaken nationally recognised breast-feeding training. The trust is currently a pilot site for the UNICEF Baby Friendly Initiative in the Community.

Audit tools

It is not the intention of this chapter to critically analyse the wide range of audit tools available to management but mention of the mechanisms of one or two of the more common tools that are more suited to health visiting audit is felt to be useful here.

Qualpacs was developed in the US for both research and quality-assurance purposes and has been used in the UK by several health authorities. It works by assessing the quality of care delivered to specific groups of patients/clients using a 68-item scale divided into subsections: psycho-social/individual, psychosocial/group, physical, general, communication and professional implications. Each item is accompanied by cues designed to assist the user of the scale in interpreting the item and is scored on a five-point rating scale. Observers should work in pairs to reduce the possibility of bias and are required to observe care over a period of 2 hours as it is delivered to 15% of the total patients on a ward or to five patients, whichever is greater. After a 2-hour period of observation a further hour is spent examining charts and records. This is a tool that could be used for auditing health visiting, although it would require modification to suit home visiting with the client's permission or, alternatively, the clinic situation.

Rush Medicus Nursing Process Quality Monitoring Instrument was again developed in the US and it is suggested that this is the instrument most widely used to measure the quality of nursing care. Like many of the nursing quality audits it is based on the 'nursing process' and has six main objectives of care:

- the plan of nursing care is formulated
- the physical needs of the patient are attended
- the psychological, emotional, mental, social needs of the patient are attended
- achievement of nursing care objectives is evaluated
- procedures are followed for the protection of all patients

- the delivery of nursing care is facilitated by administration and managerial services.

Each of the objectives has a subset that links across the initial range and also takes into account medical care. Observers are experienced nurses not directly involved in the ward/department, who work with the nursing staff to feed the results into a computer package that generates a set of criteria questions directly relevant to the patient information input. The system is used randomly across a sample of 10% of 1 month's admissions but has not found real support in the UK because it is seen as a top-down management tool rather than a local professional quality tool.

Monitor was developed in the UK (Goldstone et al 1983) and is a modification of the Rush Medicus tool. It was originally designed for acute care nursing but subsequently modified for a wide range of special care groups, including health visiting. It was championed in health visiting by Barker (1988), who developed it to run alongside the early childhood health and development programme, and it became the Early Health and Development Monitor (EHD). The objective for EHD was to assess the effectiveness of health visiting as a support service focused on prevention and development goals for the parents of 0–4-year-old children. The tool consists of detailed questions relating to the health and development of the child and views these against the socioeducational environment of the family. It is used at 1 month, 6 months, 12 months, 24 months, 36 months and 48 months and should take 15–20 minutes to complete. Barker (1991) considered it the most effective tool to measure outcomes of health visiting interventions but critics have considered that the number of visits calculated for a 400-family caseload (500 visits in any one year/approximately 11 visits per week in a 45-week year), to be too time-consuming to be cost-effective. Nevertheless, pilot studies in two West Midlands community healthcare trusts provided a wealth of evidence over many fields – epidemiological, socioeducational, maternal and child health, nutrition and developmental progress. As with most audit tools, the commitment of the professionals using the tool must be 100%

and good electronic systems should be readily available for the information to be quickly downloaded and easily accessed for future consideration.

The Edinburgh Postnatal Depression Scale (EPDS), in its original design, identified the presence of postnatal depression in women and used a scoring system to measure the intensity of depressed moods and feelings. A study undertaken in the West Midlands has shown that it is possible to use the EPDS tool to measure the effectiveness of different types of health visiting and other clinical interventions by scoring women after a period during which the client-determined intervention has taken place. The development of this study into using the EPDS tool both as a focus for identifying level of mood and feeling and to audit the effectiveness of a variety of interventions is currently being explored.

The majority of audit tools are designed to elicit quality information in connection with planned patient/client-centred interventions. In health visiting, some of the more common audit tools are effective when exploring, for example, breast-feeding or immunisation uptake rates and quality control mechanisms. It is for the profession to challenge auditors to use mechanisms whereby the quality of the intervention is set in context against the long-term effects of support and working in partnership with clients.

Clinical leadership skills developed at clinical team level

Clinical leadership

Leadership is a dynamic process whereby the leader influences others in order to achieve a common objective. The goal of leadership in health visiting terms is to actively practise using the four principles of health visiting:

- the search for health needs
- the stimulation of awareness of health needs
- the influence on policies affecting health
- the facilitation of health-enhancing activities

outlined in greater detail in Chapter 5. Leadership is where someone takes the initiative, showing others direction, by caring and sharing but not dominating. The skills of health visiting have been discussed in considerable depth in Chapter 5 and differ little from the skills of leadership. In essence, the main skills are:

- two-way communication: the ability to talk and to be understood, and to listen
- to give encouragement to people who need it, to make them feel that their contribution is wanted.

Girvan (1998) explores leadership through three interpretations – as a personal quality, as a behavioural style and as a contingent approach.

Leadership as a personal quality. Girvan suggests that the usual characteristics of integrity, lateral thinking, intelligence, enthusiasm, ability to make decisions and self-confidence are often present in the individual leader but on their own do not necessarily mean that an individual possessing them is a leader. Girvan suggests that these characteristics need to be explored in the context of the situation and that to them should be added 'the ability to use power effectively'. It is important when exploring the meaning and characteristics of leadership not to confuse these with management skills. Leadership and management have similar ends but very different means, and teaching people management skills will not necessarily produce good leaders, or indeed leadership skills. As a personal quality, leadership emphasises the promotion of shared values and the desire for change, being facilitative rather than directive, mutual rather than authoritative, empowering rather than coercive.

Leadership as a behavioural style. This was studied by Lewin (1935), who identified two main styles of democratic and autocratic leadership and found that the former was the more effective for teamwork and good morale while the latter was more productive in terms of work done. However, Girvan's (1998) exploration of research evidence shows that the more effective behavioural style is the one that uses Lewin's two approaches in the optimum circumstances for effective results. In clinical leadership it is more likely that the behavioural style is leading from the front while at the same time giving the impression of truly empowering others and a democratic approach to decision-making.

Contingency for leadership. Fiedler (1967) proposed contingency theory based on the premise that people become leaders not because of their characteristics or personalities but because of situational factors and interactions between the leader and group members. Girvan (1998) builds on these ideas of contingency by linking path–goal theory in group work. In other words, if a leader wants the group to perform well the group members must know how to achieve goals and also how to achieve their personal goals in the process. Girvan thus postulates the idea of choosing a leadership style once the leader has considered:

- the personal characteristics of the group members
- the environment in which they are working
- the understanding that leadership is about relationships and working together.

Clinical leadership may have interpretations such as those outlined above – personal qualities, behavioural style and contingency – but to these should be added other dimensions such as educational, political and strategic/managerial skills. The clinical leader, as suggested above, will use styles suitable for the situation and will move fluently in and out of these as a matter of contingency, and again Girvan (1998) adds to the picture by suggesting that styles cannot exist without a portfolio of skills from which to draw.

1. Having and achieving goals
2. Initiating and implementing change
3. Having and using influence
4. Having and using power
5. Taking responsibility for the growth of self and others
6. Mentoring
7. Having and articulating a vision
8. Forging and sustaining relationships.

The 'having' components in this list of necessary skills do not have to be innate, i.e. the effective clinical leader may develop them as a result of the circumstances in which clinical practice is taking place. Of the numbered list above, skills 1, 3, 4 and 7 may well all develop within the situation. Skills 2, 5 and 6 tend to be the result of continued education and the opportunity to develop personal strengths. Skill 8 tends to result from personal charisma and the experience of developing healthy alliances.

Clinical supervision

Clinical supervision is defined by Butterworth & Faugier (1992) as: 'an exchange between practising professionals to enable the development of professional skills'. Bond & Holland (1998) suggest that there are 'core' elements to the clinical supervision process and these are listed as:

- Modification and empowerment of skills
- Critical debate about practice authority through reflective processes
- Protection towards independent and accountable practice
- Clinical supervision education should commence after qualification as part of professional development
- Clinical supervision must be seen as 'active' time and energy on the part of the developer.

Clinical supervision has been in place in midwifery for some considerable time now but with a disciplinary element attached to the process. The comparison with the models used in mental health nursing, clinical psychology, social work and counselling shows these to be developmental for staff concerned. Quality in midwifery practice is statutorily linked to the supervision process in that where poor practice is identified the midwife is not allowed to practise alone until a professional standard is re-established.

However, if clinical supervision is used as intended in the nursing and health visiting professions, it serves to enrich practice and becomes a tool for professional growth and development. Primarily, clinical supervision is where two practising professionals meet regularly to discuss their practice and identify effectiveness and less productive practice. The clinical supervisor should be an experienced practitioner and the most favourable scenario is likely to be where

the supervisee has chosen the supervisor and an informal contract is drawn up by them to clearly identify their roles, the purpose and ground rules.

The Open University (1998) suggest that the clinical supervisor should have skills covering the following:

- To develop and maintain the relationship:
  - by practising empathy
  - by attending and active listening
  - by reflecting back and paraphrasing
  - by self-disclosure.

In health visiting this approach is an everyday occurrence both within the active process of health visiting and also during the education of student health visitors when the community practice teacher (CPT) carries out a similar role. It is important in the supervisory process that health visitors recognise that they are not in the student/CPT relationship and that this a more professionally mature approach, which uses these valuable and essential skills to maintain and nurture a professionally therapeutic relationship. Situations where a health visitor is concerned about any aspect of work with a client are explored through challenge and support. The more these skills are used at the beginning of the supervisory relationship the more fruitful such a relationship will become.

- To manage the process:
  - by monitoring
  - by managing time
  - by using intuition
  - by reviewing and evaluating
  - by summarising and integrating
  - by decision-making and action planning.

Monitoring, in clinical supervision, refers to monitoring those aspects of practice that are explored within the session rather than actual health visiting work. An experienced health visitor supervisor possesses the ability to use intuition as an extension of the skill practised in working with clients. Within the supervisory relationship, familiarity with the complexities and contexts of health visiting will allow thoughtful reflection on the totality of practice in relation to the individual practitioner's perceptions and self-awareness. It is also important that the ground rules related to the timing of each session do not allow it to over-run, enabling both practitioners to remain focused. The most effective sessions are those when, at the end, the supervisee comes away with a clear idea of their own capabilities (restorative), support for the practice under discussion (normative) and an enthusiasm for exploring alternative strategies (formative) for similar working circumstances.

- To carry out the supervision processes:
  - by questioning
  - by focusing
  - by using silence
  - by giving constructive feedback
  - by informing
  - by confronting.

Chapter 11, discussing the skills of health visiting, showed the value of Heron's six-category intervention model in health visiting practice. The use of the same model in the clinical supervision process allows for both the authoritative and facilitative aspects to be used within the supervisory process. Clinical supervision is about using intervention strategies to promote discussion, reflection on and analysis of practice, and the Heron model facilitates this as well as promoting positivism and support within and for the supervised practitioner. Implicit within this is the capacity for effective reflective skills in both supervisor and supervisee.

Clinical supervision places an emphasis on personal and interpersonal aspects of supervision and encourages self-actualisation. In health visiting it encourages practice feedback at times when the isolation and autonomy of the role make this otherwise difficult. Clinical supervision encourages interpersonal regard and the development of trust, caring and interdependence between practitioners. Properly organised and set up it manages tension between practitioners and helps the supervisee deal with uncertainties, fostering clinical autonomy. Clinical supervision facilitates the recognition of practice

boundaries and limitations in skill and competence. When carried out in a positive environment it enhances morale in order to inspire and motivate towards excellence. Supervisees are helped to recognise the service delivery functions of their role in relation to the ethical and moral values of the profession.

The West Midlands Clinical Supervision Learning Set led to a network being established that has produced a guide to clinical supervision. This is based on the experience of implementing clinical supervision in various trusts, with a view to identifying good practice, particularly in audit and evaluation. The combination of the learning set pack with Open University (1998) and the Royal College of Nursing's pack (RCN 1998) gives a comprehensive overview of the methodology and implementation of clinical supervision which is still in its infancy in many areas. The Learning Set Guide (Brocklehurst 1998) has a useful section on case studies of implementation within several trusts in the West Midlands. Box 9.4 lists pointers to success – recommendations and what to avoid and are extracted from each trust case study.

A pilot project in clinical supervision set up in a West Midlands community healthcare trust in 1998 yielded the following response. Of the 16 respondents, 14 said that clinical supervision significantly improved job satisfaction and 15 said they would be influenced in applying for a new post if it provided access to clinical supervision. When asked if they had benefited from their clinical supervision sessions 15 respondents had benefited but one was uncertain; 14 respondents had made changes to their practice as a result of receiving clinical supervision. One supervisor felt that with the development of primary care groups they needed clinical supervision more than ever and another felt that the process was vital for ongoing development. In discussing the question of whether supervision should be from someone from the same discipline or another discipline, eight respondents had same-discipline supervisors and eight had supervisors from a different discipline. Comments from supervisees with a supervisor from the same discipline were: the person is more important than the discipline; s/he understands the problems; it's wonderful/most appropriate. Comments from supervisees with a supervisor from a different discipline were: discipline not significant; 'with me it's better, I have more freedom to talk and have to be more objective'; positive decision that worked well; advantages and disadvantages – helpful to have a different perspective; difficult to discuss certain issues, they need explaining rather than reflecting.

Box 9.4 Pointers to success in setting up a clinical supervision system

Recommendations for success

- Involve the practitioners in the planning stage as early as possible
- Allow a long time for planning, consultation and marketing
- Arrange the best training that can be afforded for supervisors or group leaders
- Allow clinical supervision to be practitioner-led and confine managerial input to support only
- Plan the project carefully in line with current issues within the organisation
- Carry out a comprehensive evaluation
- Set ground rules in all clinical supervision settings, including confidentiality
- Make sure that there is management/stakeholder support at all stages of the development and implementation of clinical supervision

What to avoid

- Avoid excluding management when trying to encourage a practitioner-led approach to the development of clinical supervision
- Do not overemphasise the mandatory nature of clinical supervision
- Do not assume that once people are trained that they will necessarily start providing supervision without encouragement
- Avoid making claims for clinical supervision that are hard to substantiate or fulfil ('this will change the world!')
- Avoid planning the detail before practitioners have had a chance to influence the development
- Do not begin with a group of practitioners who do not appear motivated to try clinical supervision.

The education of effective supervisors requires a nonthreatening setting where potential supervisors come with a desire to be educated. The basics of supervisor education hinge on an ability to further develop personal self-awareness and to work on the Heron (1986) six category intervention skills. A contract between the participants in the supervisory relationship and clear guidelines of responsibility for supervisor and supervisee are essential tools for a purposeful relationship. Written records are kept about issues discussed during supervision, their confidentiality being part of the contract.

Evidence-based practice

The requirement to bring research into practice has become increasingly important with the development of quality and measurement of outcomes within practice. The setting up of NICE to give a strong lead in clinical and cost-effectiveness by drawing up guidelines has created a momentum within all the professional disciplines working in the NHS. In ensuring consistent access to services and quality of care right across the country, the national service frameworks will bring together the best evidence of clinical and cost-effectiveness, with the views of service users, to determine the best ways of providing particular services.

The work of Sackett et al (1997) has raised awareness of the importance of recognising different levels of evidence and Table 9.2 defines the grading likely to be used by NICE for all professions.

In a summary of a systematic review of health visiting (discussed in Chapter 11) Robinson (1998) consistently found weaknesses in studies available for meta-analysis using randomised controlled trials (RCTs). This was mainly due to the small of size of the studies giving them insufficient research power, poorly documented randomisation, insufficient reported detail to allow meta-analysis, and nonblinded assessment of outcomes. Controlled trial research deals only with outcomes, whereas much of health visiting work is associated with processes and this results

Table 9.2 Definition of levels of evidence

Level	Descriptor
Level Ia	From a meta-analysis of randomised controlled trials (RCTs)
Level Ib	From at least one RCT
Level IIa	From at least one well-designed controlled study without randomisation
Level IIb	From at least one other type of well-designed quasiexperimental study
Level III	From well-designed nonexperimental descriptive studies, e.g. comparative studies, correlation studies, case-control studies
Level IV	From expert committee reports or opinions and/or clinical experience of authorities
Level V	From a meta-analysis of observational studies (an observational study is classified as level III but where the research question is best addressed by a cohort study then systematic reviews of valid, relevant cohort studies match level I evidence)

in many studies being inappropriate as evidence unless they are more rigorously constructed and better documented.

A glance at Table 9.2 shows the obvious medical underpinning for graded evidence and the science of the medical research approach is clearly acknowledged. However, as level III shows, well-designed studies rooted more in the field of sociology are also important additions to research evidence. Health visitor students typify much of the nursing profession approach by using survey methods to collect attitudinal, biographical and demographic information and the tools are usually questionnaires, interviews or observation. However, quantitative analysis is frequently applied to the data collected. Qualitative methodology is of great value provided that the sampling techniques are rigorous. There is little problem in accepting surveys as a methodology providing that the randomised (if possible) sample is compared with a controlled sample drawn from a similar population. It is essential that the aims are clear from the outset and that the study design is focused in every stage of the methodology, including decisions about sampling, size, the techniques by which subjects will be allocated to a group, how the intervention will be introduced, statistical applications required and the methods for evaluating the outcomes of the study.

Clinical trials in medicine almost always embrace a drug or equipment trial but there is no reason why clinical trials in health visiting should not embrace a supportive or educational procedure. An example of this is a health visitor who offers intervention to a group of fathers who have postnatal mood-lowered partners and compares the EPDS scores against a control group of similar postnatal mothers whose partners have not elected for/been offered health visitor support. It is not necessary for any of these studies to include very large sample sizes because the use of meta-analysis can combine the populations and findings of many trials provided that the design and documentation have been meticulous.

It is important at this stage of the discussion to differentiate between evidence-based medicine and evidence-based practice. Sackett et al (1996) define evidence-based medicine as 'the conscientious and judicious use of current best evidence in making decisions about the care of individual patients…. [It is] a process of integrating individual clinical expertise with the best external clinical evidence from systematic research'.

Nursing, midwifery and health visiting professionals aspire to deliver research-based knowledge, information and advice to patients and clients and there is probably considerable justification for these aspirations. However, many practitioners and commentators would give credence to the comments of Burrows & McLeish (1995), Hunt (1996) and Kitson et al (1996) that many nursing practices in the 1990s were based on experience, tradition, intuition, common sense and untested theories. French (1999) argues coherently that evidence-based practice needs to be evaluated and validated in the practitioner's own context whenever possible, therefore undertaking 'small-scale' rigorous research projects in the practice setting.

Upton (1999) considers it difficult to achieve evidence-based practice if there is a theory–practice gap in nursing, but French (1999) suggests that a significant attribute of the concept of evidence-based practice is the focus on the practitioner's own experience and the practice context and that this is important in minimising the theory–practice gap. In essence, he says, the 'evidence-based practice' approach to research is determined by the practitioner researcher's personal judgement regarding the aims, relevance, feasibility, constraints and significant variables associated with the particular research issue. Much of the blame for the difficulty that nursing has in using evidence-based practice Upton (1999) places firmly at the door of education programmes. There may be some substance in this and it has been discussed in Chapter 1 in the context of processes of problem-based learning.

Action research has become more commonly used in nursing and health visiting research and has its theoretical basis in experimental design, in that the practitioner undertaking the research makes a change and then sees what happens. Much of this happens in direct work with clients when the health visitor and the client work in partnership by making a change and observing the results. This particularly occurs in behaviour modification of a young child, when various approaches are tried using a quasicontrolled approach to find which one is the most effective. As with any partnership, the recording of changes is of great importance, both from the viewpoint of communication and also as an essential feature of action research. Action research involves working closely and actively with groups to identify problems, implement solutions and evaluate their effectiveness as part of a cyclical process. DeVille-Almond in Chapter 2 shows how well she has worked in partnership with the community in an action research style. She also shows the value of documenting her work, although her contribution is written more as a descriptive study than from an action research perspective. Action research requires clear, insightful recording of changes, results and potential links. It must include negative as well as positive outcomes, which may be the reason why it is underused.

Clinical effectiveness

The essential essence of clinical effectiveness is to improve patient care by better use and translation of evidence. If the skills and components associated with clinical effectiveness are mastered it can help all health visitors to achieve more effective practice. The NHS Executive defines clinical effectiveness as 'the extent to which specific clinical interventions, when deployed in the field for a particular patient or population, do what they are intended to do, that is maintain and improve health and secure the greatest possible health gain from the available resources' (NHS Executive 1996). The origins of clinical effectiveness lie in evidence-based medicine as described by Sackett et al (1997).

In nursing disciplines the most commonly quoted definition of clinical effectiveness is that of Kitson, 'Clinical effectiveness is about doing the right thing in the right way and at the right time for the right patient' (RCN 1996). To the above definition can be added 'at the right price'. Health visitors, like other health service professionals, are aware of the negative results

of rationing of healthcare. It is, however, unrealistic to remain in the fantasyland of unlimited resources and an awareness of cost-effectiveness is an undeniable part of clinical effectiveness.

Clinical effectiveness has three main approaches:

- **Inform** describes the sources of information available and what is being planned for the future to make information more readily accessible
- **Change** describes and suggests ways in which changes to services can be encouraged based on well-founded information about effectiveness
- **Monitor** describes ways in which changes to services can be assessed to show that change results in improvement.

If evidence-based healthcare is to dominate then it has to combine evidence for intervention with client preferences and clinical/practitioner expertise.

Evidence for intervention may come from a variety of sources, including research publications, and guidelines of protocols. Good quality guidelines, recommendations and policy for good practice should all indicate the source of the evidence on which they are based and who agreed it. Client preferences can stem from a variety of experiences and influences in context and are the least controllable of the three factors. Clinical and practitioner expertise comes from best-practice information and experience but skilfully modified to the context.

Clinical audit may identify areas where practice needs to be altered to improve clinical effectiveness and the original practice can then act as a baseline against which change is made. If areas of practice require examination then the issue becomes a researchable question and action research in practice becomes the reality. This reality is then a clinical effectiveness cycle (Fig. 9.4).

The close similarity between the clinical effectiveness cycle and the clinical audit cycle will not go unnoticed but the main difference is that within the former there exists the research process and this should be founded on a well-designed

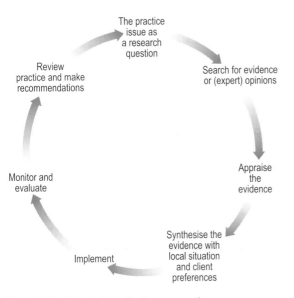

Figure 9.4   The clinical effectiveness cycle

and well-documented small-scale research process as proposed above. This lends itself to the rigour of the evidence-based medical model.

Good practice ideas disseminated

Many health visitors today are becoming involved in outreach programmes and activities that are proving exciting and effective and are fairly easily evaluated. A major problem is that very few colleagues outside the immediate area ever get to hear about what a particular health visitor or group of health visitors has achieved. This could be considered negligent to a certain degree because clients or health visitors working in similar circumstances in other areas are being denied the opportunity for improved care arising from innovation or good practice. It is therefore essential that health visitors recognise that they have a responsibility under clinical governance to disseminate their results. The most common argument put forward is that there is not enough time to do this and that it would inevitably come out of the health visitor's own time. This argument should be challenged on the basis that to disseminate good practice and innovation is part of working time and thus allowances should be made for such work.

There is evidence that health visitors assume that management would not allow time away from day-to-day work for study/writing/library time in order to prepare a report or paper. In reality, this is probably far from the truth because managers see the value of the good practice and innovation by their staff and how it reflects on the organisation. People want to work for employers who have forward-looking and innovative staff: thus job vacancies are fewer in trusts where staff are allowed to develop their dissemination skills. The development of information technology through electronic means should be recognised as an important mechanism whereby dissemination of evidence-based effective practice can take place. Many health authorities are recognising that by developing and using their own website they are in a position to act as role models for other authorities and thus save time and prevent 'reinvention of the wheel'.

Forward-looking health visitors should ask their trusts about the possibility of developing a well-resourced library with electronic searching facilities for staff use, for three main reasons:

- to keep up to date with journal articles and new texts, particularly electronic journals
- to access important sources of material such as nursing databases, PubMed or the Cochrane database
- to access Department of Health command papers, health service circulars, health service guidelines and local authority circulars.

Clinical risk reduction programmes in place

A health visitor should know the main tools for risk identification within their organisation and should have a responsibility for ensuring that the procedures are followed accurately and professionally. Indicators that ensure a good clinical risk programme is in place include the following:

- use of incident reports, including reports for near misses
- criteria for clinical audit, effectiveness or quality control

- reports and minutes available for any planning meetings held
- a speedy system for dealing with client complaints
- adherence to the appropriate service agreement charter in relation to visiting times and schedules
- policies and procedures for all aspects of care and surveillance
- client-held records, supplementary records, computer data entry systems
- channels of communication, especially to the Child Protection Advisor.

It is important that not only are these systems in place but that they also work effectively and where there seems to be substandard quality in any of these areas it is the responsibility of each health visitor to make representations to the appropriate manager, both verbally and in writing. Effective practice means effective risk management strategies.

Clinical risk management

Risk in its simplest clinical definition is 'the potential for unwanted outcome'. Risk in the Penguin English dictionary is defined as 'hazard, chance of injury, harm, loss' and is the reason for complaints of suffering, delay, lack of communication and many other concerns that may be experienced by patients and their relatives. Clinical risk modification provides the best service for patients and clients by the establishment of multidisciplinary standards of care and best practice guidelines to enhance professional development of nursing, medicine and other therapy professions. The changes in healthcare delivery, with much higher expectations from patients, greater clarity of roles and responsibilities of clinicians and the emphasis on devolving decision-making as close to the patient as possible, are meant to affect the entire performance of healthcare delivery. The focus of healthcare risk management is very much on the systems and practices that affect patient care in order to proactively manage overall cost and appropriateness of care delivered.

Wilson & Tingle (1999) make the following important statement:

Risk management is the systematic identification, assessment and reduction of risks to patients and staff:

- through providing appropriate, effective and efficient levels of patient care
- by prevention and avoidance of untoward incidents and events
- by learning lessons and changing behaviour/practices as a result of near misses, incidents and adverse outcomes and
- through communication and documentation of care in a comprehensive, objective, consistent and accurate way.

The risks that apply to health visiting differ in many ways from those of acute nursing and midwifery and may not appear so immediate. However there are various ways in which health visitors should ensure that risk is minimised. Clearly, communication and documentation is the category of practice where risk may occur. Decision-making by the client can be difficult in the light of limited knowledge and an immensely important aspect of health visiting practice is in ensuring that clients have all the knowledge they wish. However, as Rose points out in Chapter 12, how much knowledge can a client be reasonably expected to cope with and how does the client know the legitimacy of that knowledge?

The health visitor, Kate, is discussing with Jane the impending immunisation session to which her daughter Lizzy has been invited. Kate makes the following record in the parent-held personal child health record:

Date and time of immunisation

Immunisation discussed and reference made to the immunisation leaflet that Kate has given to Jane. Any concerns regarding Lizzy's health at the time of immunisation to be notified to the health visitor present at the time or the doctor giving the injection.

Kate also reminds Jane verbally to bring the child health record to the immunisation clinic so that a correct record can be made.

This is where documentation is all-important because clear recording of what has been said will ensure that, should there be a question in the client's mind, scrutiny of the records should prompt memory. Equally, should there be a complaint against the health visitor for the advice given, records should show the principle of what was discussed. It is important not only to record but also to tell clients what is being recorded and why. It is also important to have previously checked that the parent can read or that there is someone who can read records to them.

Clearly, recording detail of discussions would be time-consuming and result in cumbersome records; nevertheless it is important that notes include such statements as in the vignette above.

This type of detail does mean that should there be an untoward complaint about possible lack of information from health visitor to client, the record can give a clear outline of the original discussion content.

Incidents detected and openly investigated and lessons promptly applied

Incidents tend to be related to patients or clients on health centre or GP practice premises or to health visitors while out on home visits or in public places. There should be clear guidelines and protocols to follow should an accident occur to a patient or client. The transfer of many child health clinics to GP surgeries sometimes means that they are being held in a less than appropriate setting. There are two major issues:

1. The well baby is being brought to a building in which there are people with communicable diseases, because the health visitor is running a well baby clinic at the same time as the GP has a normal surgery. This is because the GP wishes to organise his surgery attendance in one single session and thus undertake the child surveillance at the end of the session.
2. The only room available is a treatment room. The surgeries are being used, the practice nurse has her own office and so the health visitor is using a room that is too clinical with many movable pieces of equipment and an uncovered floor.

The problem is that a mother attending the clinic with a small baby and an inquisitive toddler or two is an accident waiting to happen. GP surgeries are still primary care centres and as such should be safe for all primary care clients to attend. Health visitors involved in working in general practice where such situations are common have a responsibility to try to change matters to improve safety. Child health clinics held in GP surgeries should be held at a time when ill patients are not attending. The rooms which mothers, young children and toddlers are using must be fit for the purpose or alternative arrangements must be made.

There are situations in practice where the health visitor is likely to be working alone and at as much risk of an accident as any other member of the general public. There are also certain situations where health visitors may find themselves in potentially violent circumstances and these mean that they must ensure their own safety as well as the safety of any particularly vulnerable person present at the time. It is not possible to provide guidelines for every set of circumstances but there are general safety strategies that should be used by every health visitor. These include:

- If the client or partner/family has a history of violent behaviour then find out, if possible, the circumstances in which such episodes have occurred
- If the client or partner/family has a history of violent behaviour or have been abusive in the past, a health visitor should always visit with a colleague who either comes in to the house with them or waits in the car for a predetermined length of time
- Health visitors should be aware of the fact that in most violent circumstances it has been a move on the part of the victim that has precipitated a violent response. Such moves may be:
  - the use of assertive language or behaviour
  - moving too close to the perpetrator – invasion of space
  - appearing to threaten the perpetrator by representing 'officialdom'
  - appearing frightened or failing to maintain eye contact
- Health visitors should ensure that they don't unwittingly, for example, pass the perpetrator a weapon such as a cup of hot tea
- A health visitor should always tell colleagues

or the clinic receptionist when they are going to visit a client about whom they are concerned

- If visiting a client about whom they are concerned health visitors should always go back to their base at the end of the day and should never go directly home without ensuring that someone knows that the visit is ended.

Barbara, a health visitor, is notified that a family has moved into her area. She checks to find that only the mother and two children have registered with the practice and writes to make an appointment to visit. On arrival at the house Barbara introduces herself to the mother and children but the man present ignores her. Conversation about the family and the children ensues and gradually the man gets drawn into the discussion. It eventually emerges that he is the father of the two children and he tells Barbara that he has a history of schizophrenia, and because of his violent behaviour towards GP receptionists he cannot find a local GP who will accept him on the practice list. As he explains, he does not like to be kept waiting in an appointment system.

This type of situation is not uncommon. Information can be very slow in catching up with mobile families and therefore there are times when health visitors may come unwittingly into potentially dangerous circumstances.

Lessons for clinical practice systematically learned from complaints made by patients

In the past, health visitors had few complaints from clients about clinical tasks. However, this appears to be changing as a result of public litigation awareness and advertising by law firms. It is possible that health visitors could be sued for failure to screen for a hearing defect, a mobility problem thought originally to be late walking, missing developmental delays and so forth. There is also the possibility of complaints from clients where the health visitor is intervening in potential cases of child neglect or abuse, particularly if the health visitor has not worked openly in partnership with a family where there are suspicious circumstances. The most important factor to be remembered is that accurate and contemporaneous recording is essential in these situations. It is also important that the

health visitor does not appear to be defensive when a complaint is made but has a clear explanation as the result of careful listening to the client's concerns.

An incident occurred because a father telephoned the health visitor to seek advice over how much formula milk his 2-month-old daughter should be taking. The health visitor was surprised that the baby was on formula milk because she had recently seen the baby at home with its mother, who was breast-feeding the baby. Apparently the father, who was separated from his wife, had found the child left on its own the day before, and had since taken parental responsibility for the baby. The health visitor could not answer the question because she had to find out from the mother what the feeding arrangements now were. The father took objection to this last response and made a formal complaint to the health visitor's manager saying that she was unhelpful and would not give him the advice he sought.

In this vignette the health visitor had taken the telephone call at a time when she happened to be alone in the office. She immediately logged the content of the call so that when she was summoned to explain to the manager there was a clear record of what had happened and her subsequent actions between the phone call and her meeting with the manager. Incidentally, the events that followed were that the mother began to give expressed breast milk in order that the father could continue feeding the baby.

Problems of poor clinical performance recognised at an early stage and dealt with to prevent harm to patients

The section on standards among all healthcare professionals that deals with accountability contains guidelines on dealing with colleagues whose practice is causing concern to either clients or peers.

Four health visitors share an office. Two of them, Doris and Ann, work with the same practice, the other two each work for a different GP team. The office acts as a good forum for sharing work-based experiences, brainstorming ideas and generally supporting one another. Gradually over a period of time, Doris becomes more withdrawn, less sociable and ceases to join in office discussions. She still attends in-service training days but there is no noticeable improvement in her practice. Questions directed to her elicit monosyllabic responses. This situation slowly develops over about 3 years. Ann, from the same practice, becomes

increasingly concerned because not only do the GPs seek her out in preference to her withdrawn colleague but clients are also asking for Ann rather than Doris. Periodically the three health visitors quietly discuss what they can do to help Doris, but find it increasingly difficult even to get her to come to any social occasions they are involved in. Some 18 months from the beginning of this period the advice of the manager is sought but no changes are made. Managers come and go, some with health visitor qualification, some without, but the situation continues to deteriorate until finally a GP in the practice writes a letter to the current manager, detailing his concerns and itemising instances where he feels Doris has been practising particularly ineffectually. Doris is seen by her manager and it is decided that she should take sick leave and seek help from her family doctor.

This is a not unfamiliar situation. It took a long time to develop and no-one closely connected with Doris in her workplace felt in a position to act. Management felt trapped: there was little direct evidence of dangerous practice but clearly it was ineffective. However, when does one intervene? Most of the managers approached by the three health visitors asked for a statement in writing but none of the three felt that she had sufficient evidence to make any accurate or detailed statement. Even if client records were subject to an audit procedure poor practice might only become evident if an entry made by a colleague on behalf of Doris proved to have a substantially different content. Educational courses that Doris was asked to attend were completed but this did not contribute to a change in practice. All the health visitors felt guilty, but disabled; they knew that something should have been done much earlier, they felt sorry for Doris, who lived in difficult circumstances, but they lacked the mechanisms to allow them to intervene.

This type of situation is probably best coped with through clinical supervision and this was discussed earlier in the chapter. However, there is a fine line between ineffective practice and dangerous practice. It can be argued that if a health visitor gives inappropriate advice a client need not take up that advice and thus client choice may act as damage limitation. If a health visitor fails to notice developmental delay or an obvious physical defect in a baby, is this dangerous or merely unfortunate? The profession has perhaps an even greater need to ensure that systems are in place to prevent or deal with poor

clinical performance. The main mechanisms open to health visitors that could anticipate this occurrence, particularly when there is an insidious onset, are regular use of a reflective journal, clinical supervision and appraisal. However, like many systems, unless they are well taught, well maintained and well supported by management they are only as good in action as the performance of the weakest participant.

Professional development programmes reflecting clinical governance

Professional development programmes, in the spirit of clinical governance, follow the pattern of 'lifelong learning', a phrase introduced to the nursing, midwifery and health visiting profession with the advent of PREP (see Chapter 1). In *A First Class Service* (Department of Health 1998b) the point is made that continuing professional development programmes are best managed at local level to meet service needs and those of individual professionals. Under the new statutory requirements for periodic re-registration with the UKCC, nurses, midwives and health visitors are required to show that they have undertaken a minimum of 5 days' study since their last registration, and must produce a current portfolio of their professional development. *A First Class Service* (Department of Health 1998b) suggests that individual health professionals should have a personal development plan (PDP) as part of their professional development. There are a variety of ways in which learning takes place and clearly 'on the job' or 'with the working team' are two such opportunities. However, there will need to be exploration of other alternatives, and universities and trusts will need to be creative in enabling learning to take place without attending courses away from the workplace. The other aspect of creativity is in relation to financing of learning opportunities. The Department of Health (1998b) makes the statement that:

Continuing Professional Development (CPD) is currently financed in a variety of ways (for example, local training and development budgets, charitable and educational trust funds and industry sponsorship).

Arrangements vary among the different professions and there are clearly significant inequities. Most health professionals share financial responsibility for their own professional development. The total resource (including opportunity costs) devoted to CPD is substantial but we believe this investment can, and should, be targeted more effectively.

The government is working towards having training and development plans in place for the majority of health professional staff by April 2000. It is likely that primary care groups will be responsible for ensuring the funding for such programmes and this is possibly where there may be greater opportunity for equity between medical and nursing staff with the combination of the original separate training budgets. There is also opportunity for joint learning between health and social service staff, which has been quietly taking place for several years now since the consolidation of NVQ programmes in, for example, health and social care, and other initiatives.

Funding from both the health and social care budgets will be planned under the guidance of education consortia, which bring together key health and social care stakeholders. Regional educational development groups will have a key role in facilitating and delivering this strategy and related developments, ensuring that they take account of best practice, and NHS and social care regional offices will monitor implementation. The national training organisations for the health and social care sectors have been required by government ministers to co-operate fully and report annually on their proposals for securing joint training initiatives among groups of staff working with clients with multiple needs (Department of Health 1998d). There are many ways in which learning opportunities may take place – through distance learning, the use of learning sets, self-directed learning through journal learning-articles, project work and so forth.

A locality action forum in a multicultural area of the West Midlands had been concerned for some time about the amount of adult violence occurring in the area. Key workers decided that a day conference might be helpful to raise awareness of concerns and bring together many of the agencies working in the area. Funding was provided by the social services department and invitations were sent to police, social workers, healthcare workers (health visitors, practice nurses, district nurses), health co-ordinators, local religious leaders and community development workers. The community health council sent a representative. The local university provided a keynote speaker from the public health degree course. The entire day was spent exploring the problem and learning about the underlying theoretical causes for adult violence.

This type of education initiative is very much in the spirit of clinical governance, in that it is focused on the problem and all the disciplines involved gain education and information in a problem-based learning approach. It means that key workers can understand the thrust and perspectives of the other workers and recognise the reasons for varying approaches. As discussed in Chapter 13, research (Bennett et al 1997) shows that social workers perceive psychological abuse and neglect as more common than physical abuse, police, lawyers and mental health workers perceive verbal abuse as more common than physical abuse. Community psychiatric nurses report more physical abuse whereas social services staff report more financial abuse. As a result of these factors the studies found that in approaching intervention social workers sought to change the situation or behaviour, police sought to detect or prevent crime and nurses attended to health needs. Problem-based learning allows for understanding and consolidation of the different approaches, particularly in consultation with the local community leaders. This approach to education crosses old boundaries between disciplines and will clearly be a more effective use of funding to the benefit of the community.

Problem-based learning can also be very effective in single-discipline learning as part of updating and continuing professional development. Chapter 15, on pharmacological knowledge, shows the advantage of this approach in transforming theory into practice and is very much in the spirit of clinical governance.

Quality of data collected

Wain and Shuttleworth, in Chapter 3, discusses the enormous importance of the role of information technology in healthcare practice today. Clinical governance also stresses the importance of information and particularly highlights the necessity for good data collection. Data about the health needs of a community or particular population group provide information on the scope of services that need to be provided: financial data allow health-care systems and programmes to determine whether they are within budget and provide accountability for resource expenditure; and baseline programmes allow a service to evaluate and assess whether it has met required standards or their stated aims and objectives.

As part of *The New NHS – Modern, Dependable* (Department of Health 1997a), the White Paper states the aim of replacing the internal market with a system called 'integrated care' based on partnership and driven by performance. There is a particular commitment to more investment in better technology and this was followed up by the paper *Information for Health* (NHS Executive 1998b) setting out the strategy for modernising the collection, storage and use of information. There are two main beneficiaries of quality data – the staff who are to access and use these and patients/clients whose records will be instantly available whenever there is a need for access, no matter where they happen to be. There are two main concerns that also exercise staff and patients/clients alike – for the patients/clients confidentiality is the main priority, for staff the accuracy of data is the chief concern.

Data are only as good as the person who uses a methodological tool to collect data and the person who enters information onto a database. It is therefore essential that the systems used are effective and the collection tools equally sound. This means that, as has been discussed above, the design of research is such that the correct/appropriate information is collected using the most effective tool. It is also necessary for data to be entered quickly on to a spreadsheet/database so that in the event of a time lag between data being collected and analysed the aims and objectives of the research are not modified and data are not, in effect, 'manipulated' to fit an alternative research question. It is equally important that those practitioners who collect data continuously as part of their intervention processes also have the opportunity to access the information systems to which they are adding data in order to best inform their practice, not only on a qualitative basis but also on a quantitative economically analytical basis. This then allows the true spirit of clinical effectiveness cycles to be brought into play and the information is made available to inform best practice.

Waters & Oberklaid (1998), studying child health systems in Australia, comment on the information gaps in data collection systems that inhibit reliable information concerning progress towards achieving policy objectives or monitoring individual children or population subgroups who may be at risk. They reinforce the argument that the development of community-based health monitoring and tracking programmes will also be increasingly important as community-based integrated systems of care emerge that link primary care services in the community with secondary and tertiary services in hospitals or academic medical centres.

CONCLUSION

Clinical governance will be part of the performance-driven NHS for some time to come and health visitors have a proactive and responsible part to play in ensuring quality practice. As autonomous practitioners it is essential that health visitors are well up to date and at the head of the field, not only because of the work they do but also because they work closely with primary care groups and will have much to offer the effective running of these bodies. This chapter has explored many of the aspects of clinical governance that will directly involve health visitors as well as the alterations in practice that new quality approaches will bring about. The most important factor that is running through this whole chapter is the recognition that effective practice is practice designed in a responsible and responsive way for the benefit of public health, and the health visiting profession is a discipline best equipped by education and reflective practice to deliver research-based interventions.

Leadership stems from the practice and knowledge base of health visiting but this is only achieved by virtue of hard work through a flexible, responsive practice in line with the health needs assessment of the population. Leadership also offers the opportunity to determine the pathway down which a profession moves and health visiting has been criticised in the past for not taking up its opportunities. To leave leadership of health visiting to a few more erudite individuals, on the basis that one is too busy doing the job, is inappropriate in the clinical governance climate and all practitioners should be in a position to write about good and effective practice. Clinical governance is not for the few: all health visitors are accountable and none is more accountable than another.

10

Issues in practice

Randa Charles, Janice Frost, Jean Glynn, Joan Leach and Anne Plant

INTRODUCTION

This chapter was written by practising health visitor community practice teachers in North Staffordshire. The issues discussed are current and pertinent to community practitioners in the 'new NHS'.

Public health is firmly on the agenda, with the focus on equality in health. Glynn explores some inequality issues and applies these to sexual health.

Practitioners must look critically at the information they collect and how they use it. Charles discusses the issues around records and offers suggestions on how they can be adapted to meet the changing needs for information in practice while meeting professional requirements and accountability.

Current policy recognises the need for parents to have timely advice about child health issues. Plant highlights the child health surveillance programme, with its main focus on child health promotion. Parenting and supporting families is high on the policy agenda. Frost offers practical interventions to assist health visitors to work with parents and children in the management of behaviour problems. Leach focuses on work previously published in relation to accidents in children and enlarges on her research.

INEQUALITIES IN HEALTH

Jean Glynn

When profiling for health needs in Stoke on Trent

health visitors are mindful of the fact that Tones & Tilford (1990) found that people in the north of England had poorer diets than those in the south despite being aware of healthy and unhealthy foods. Individuals are prevented from making healthy choices because there is sometimes a conflict of priorities between paying for food or rent. Low income may therefore prevent women from purchasing a nutritional diet for their family, but this is further compounded by geographical factors. Local shops are more expensive and sell fewer healthier foods compared to the larger, more distant supermarket where food is cheaper but more difficult to access.

Gender differences have also been noted in health. Women are three times more likely to smoke in the lower classes than in professional households and smoking is increasingly linked to poverty and disadvantage (Roberts 1990, Blackburn 1993). Nonattendance at child health clinics has also been found to be related to maternal smoking (Pitts & Phillips 1991). In addition to influences of gender, class and geography, health is also determined by an individual's behaviour. The likelihood of an individual performing a behaviour is dependent on privately held attitudes about behaviours and whether positive outcomes can be achieved from performing them (Becker 1974, Broome 1989). Smoking is not always seen by the individual as a negative behaviour because it can give mothers a break from caring, enabling them to cope by resting, and gives positive reinforcement in that psychologically they feel less tense and stressed (Blackburn 1993). Adolescents may seek peer approval and therefore engage in 'risk-taking' behaviour, such as unprotected sex, drug and alcohol abuse (Broome 1989). Individuals may not be interested in future disease prevention if they have other priorities, such as poor housing, unemployment and financial problems (Tones & Tilford 1990). Poor self-esteem, low confidence and lack of self-empowerment are also factors that inhibit individuals from making positive health choices (Ewles & Simnett 1992). The decision to carry out preventative health behaviours may be possible for the individual, but the ability to perform the desired behaviour can therefore be seen to be constrained and limited by social, physical, environmental and emotional factors.

In 1994 the RCN outlined key activities in public health work for nurses and health visitors to address some of these problems. Two of those activities included:

- assessing the health needs of the local population
- increasing the uptake of services by ensuring they are accessible, offered appropriately and effectively targeted.

This fits in with the health visitor's public health role in using epidemiological data to underpin practice, communicating with the local public health departments and networking with other agencies to maintain healthy communities (North Staffs Combined Healthcare Trust 1996).

Health visitors are able to target families with greater health and social care needs and offer flexible services, like choice of clinic times, drop-in and evening sessions (North Staffs Combined Healthcare Trust 1996). The flexibility of the health visiting service is an advantage, because health visitors can respond to clients' needs and be accessible because they work in the community in general, in public, the workplace and other settings. Health visiting 'is a unique non-discriminatory professional service', and health visitors are therefore accessible to those who might not otherwise seek health advice (North Staffs Combined Healthcare Trust 1996, p. 3).

IMPACT ON SEXUAL HEALTH

Young girls, once grown out of the childhood infections stage and assuming they have no chronic illness, rarely come into contact with the NHS until they move into the reproductive stage of their lives. It is at this point that many aspects of a female's life are medicalised. The male is seen as the 'norm' in medicine and he is not subjected to the same number of screening programmes, such as cervical smears, breast examination and mammography (Coney 1995). Women have become sought after 'commodities' in the health service; this may be because some women are now in a position to pay to improve their health and well-being because they are in paid employment (Coney 1995). Also, many research programmes are now focused on women and their fertility is often determined by medicine (Coney 1995, Roberts 1990). Choice of treatment may also be determined by health economics. The cost of some contraceptives and fertility treatment may limit choices for women. Richardson & Robinson (1993) offer an alternative view: they consider that woman are prescribed pills so that they remain sexually available to men at all times. Oral contraception can have health risks for some women. Concern has been expressed that injectables may lead to osteoporosis due to amenorrhoea, and there is an increased risk of arterial disease with the combined pill (Guillebaud 1993). So all women need adequate information, access to appropriate contraceptive services and health promotion clinics in order to feel empowered and in control of their health.

A survey of young people found that half had experience of sexual intercourse before they were 16 (Department of Health 1993a). Of particular concern to the government and health professionals was the number of teenage pregnancies resulting from this. *The Health of the Nation* (Department of Health 1992) aimed to reduce the number of unwanted pregnancies by reducing the conception rate in under-16-year-olds from 9.5 per 1000 in 1989 to 4.8 by the year 2000 (Department of Health 1993a). However, the Green Paper *Our Healthier Nation* (Department of Health 1998a) has not continued this sexual health target, choosing instead to seek targets that were felt to be more achievable. The UK has the highest pregnancy rate among 15–19-year-olds in Western Europe and with this is a high percentage of terminations. Half of all conceptions in under-16-year-olds and one-third in 16–19-year-olds end in termination (Fullerton et al 1997). This high termination rate may be due to poor information and low uptake of emergency contraception or, as suggested earlier, be part of the risk-taking behaviour of adolescents (Broome 1989, Fullerton et al 1997). Jones (1996), however, found that teenage pregnancy continued to be a problem

despite the availability of reliable contraceptive methods.

Some improvements have been achieved in reducing the number of pregnancies. Recent figures show there has already been a reduction to 8.3 conceptions per 1000 in under-16-year-olds (Fullerton et al 1997). Programmes that combine sex education with access to contraceptive services have been found to be effective in increasing contraceptive use and have contributed to the lower rate of teenage pregnancies (Fullerton et al 1997). Pregnancy remains higher in socially deprived areas where, for some adolescents, there are positive outcomes despite the risk of adverse health, education, social and economic outcomes (Fullerton et al 1997). To improve the accessibility of services and information for young people it is necessary to take into account local need and circumstances. The compilation of a local profile that includes current service provision and health data provides the basis for a comprehensive needs assessment of the local population. A needs assessment is a complex process involving the determinants of physical, mental, social and environmental factors that may impact on health. It therefore identifies individuals and groups at risk, as well as identifying gaps in the provision of services.

Services need to attract the young, give both males and females confidence to attend and ensure confidentiality, while working within the Gillick principles (Department of Health 1986). The type of clinic is an important factor and there are many examples of good practice where a variety of approaches and venues have been used by health visitors and other health professionals. Initiatives have included:

- drop-in clinics
- after school clinics
- information packs for young people attending their general practitioner
- roadshows
- Saturday clinics (Department of Health 1995c).

High rates of teenage pregnancy in Tayside Region in Scotland and the demand from the young for more accessible healthcare led to the development of drop-in clinics, open days and condom initiatives (Goudie & Redman 1996). Issues of confidentiality and a positive attitude from the staff, as well as better information given on how to access the services, were found to be important for young people in improving attendance at family planning clinics (Jackson & Plant 1996). Similar findings were noted near Glasgow during the development of a teenage club by a health visitor (Little 1997). The service was developed in conjunction with the teenagers, who selected topics about healthy lifestyles, including contraception issues. The teenagers wanted a clinic that was easy to get to, with no appointments, welcoming, somewhere they were able to bring friends, confidential and providing a range of services (Little 1997). Young people's clinics established in general practices found that individuals attended mainly for information on safer sex and contraception. Overall studies have found that attendance is higher and pregnancy rates lower when contraception is provided by clinics specifically for the young, where there is improved access, a relaxed atmosphere achieved through staff attitudes, and where refreshments and music are available (Jackson & Plant 1996, Boston 1997, Little 1997).

Individual support is also needed for young women who find themselves pregnant, so that they are able to make their own decisions, as they usually experience less emotional and practical assistance than other pregnant women (Nolan 1996). Often they are given poor information about their care and are treated as stupid or it is implied that they should be ashamed of their situation, but teenage mothers should not be stereotyped as they are not all unsupported, single or come from abusive backgrounds (Nolan 1996). Causes of pregnancy in teenagers may include social influences, limited access to appropriate health services, socioeconomic factors or individual characteristics, but improvements can be made to reduce pregnancies with good education and access to family planning services developed to meet local need, and the poor socioeconomic and health outcomes associated with pregnancy can be reduced with support.

Health visitors can help to alleviate some of the negative health and social outcomes by devising special antenatal programmes for young expectant mothers, which may include future contraception, sexual health, healthy relationships, women's health in general and parenting. Home visits can support the pregnant teenager and her family, while parenting skills can improve the mother–child interaction (Fullerton et al 1997). Domiciliary services can also help to meet the needs of ethnic minorities and individuals with disabilities (Dwivedi & Varma 1996). Language and cultural barriers, as well as lower expectations and lack of knowledge of services, can compound the problems of accessing services. The current emphasis on improving quality of services may address some of these issues, with the focus on health improvement, fair access, effective delivery of service, client/carer experience and health outcomes (Department of Health 1998b).

RECORD KEEPING IN PRACTICE

Randa Charles

With an increasing demand for health related data, practitioners must examine the issues to get the balance of the need for information right. There are many different types of record used by practitioners in different trusts and healthcare settings. It would be unrealistic to assume that a standard universal record might emerge to suit the information needs of all. However, basic principles of good record keeping should underpin the development of records used by practitioners, focusing on an accurate account of the interaction with the client. The driver for the interaction should be not the need for information but keeping a record of the relevant information upon which professional decisions are made.

Practitioners must be aware of the potential of professional records to collect other information. The public health agenda and developments of primary care groups put the focus on assessing the health needs of the population. Practitioners must look critically at existing records and decide if current documentation does assist practitioners to assemble relevant data from which these health needs may be identified.

THE PURPOSE OF RECORDS

The purpose of a record developed for and written by nurses and health visitors is to document the professional interaction between client and professional. The UKCC (1998) maintains that this record must provide 'accurate, current, comprehensive and consistent information' about the assessment of the client. This would lead to the practitioner identifying the health needs of the client and recording the action taken in response to those needs. The record should be written in such a way that the 'chronology of events' is clear to anyone looking at the record. This suggests that it is good practice for records to be written contemporaneously and for the practitioner making the entry to sign and date it at the time.

Record keeping should be supported by locally agreed standards developed by health visitors and their managers around the types of record issued and how they are used in practice. This standard setting process considers quality issues and audit to ensure that local standards are being met responding to developments in practice. Audit of the records and the processes for using them allows practitioners the opportunity to share good practice and to identify problems in using the documentation. For example, the change to parent-held records identified a need to review health visiting documentation to meet changing practice and need for information (Charles 1996).

Working in partnership with clients indicates a change in fundamental practice towards records being written with clients. Both parties are then clear about their role within the partnership and what the problems regarding healthcare may be. This type of working creates the environment in which inaccuracies can be corrected – this may be factual information contained within the record but equally it may be inaccurate views the client may hold about the service offered. There are training issues about using appropriate language, clarifying that documentation records interaction, issues about sharing other information and writing about difficult issues if practitioners are concerned.

Practitioners not only assemble information but must be skilled in managing the data they gather. This management of information is a function critical to both practitioners and their managers in the current climate of NHS reforms. The collection and presentation of these data assist practitioners and managers within the organisation/practice with three main functions (Torrington et al 1989, p. 338):

- planning
- control
- decision-making.

Planning

From a practitioner perspective, this can mean recording the assessment of a client using a structured approach from which a health visiting care pathway emerges, e.g. the need for additional support for a mother with postnatal depression, reflecting the agreed intervention with the client, the time committed to offer counselling and a measure of outcome – a repeat Edinburgh Postnatal Depression Scale Scoring. For managers, the data about health visiting activity form a part of the information for strategic planning of the nursing service for the organisation. This can only be achieved by looking at activity data of community practitioners and setting these against local and national policy. Currently, the focus on inequalities, parenting issues, accident prevention and mental health gives tremendous opportunities for health visitors and managers to link practice to research evidence reflecting positive outcomes. Records developed to assist data collection on an individual and collective basis can provide managers and health visitors with powerful information on which to base a case for service development. An example of this could be health visitors developing a means of recording the identification, intervention and outcome measures of supporting women with postnatal depression and measuring this against referral patterns to secondary services. Practitioners must therefore be aware of the planning process and use opportunities proactively to present 'good' information to managers on positive health outcomes for clients arising from health visiting intervention.

Control

Torrington et al (1989) also suggest that controlling (or evaluating) information influences operational issues and how the overall strategy is carried out. Managers must therefore ensure that information collected reflects the need of the organisation to demonstrate to those purchasing the service that the contracts are being met.

Ensuring quality is a major factor here and audit may identify poor performance – possibly due to covering vacant caseloads or unequal distribution of workload among staff. From a practitioner's perspective, evaluation must reflect how identified client health needs are being met; for example, have the child surveillances due been identified, completed and documented? Practitioners can use these statistical data to identify unmet health needs, excess demands within a workload or innovation in response to demand and articulate this case to managers and colleagues.

Decision-making

This is concerned with 'the day to day execution of activities' – the action of delivering a service (Torrington 1989). Practitioners must keep an accurate account of their interactions with clients as an *'aide memoire'* so that these can be reviewed at the next contact and progress can be measured. This professional record would be part of any investigation of a problem or complaint about professional practice.

Good practice in record keeping is essential and critical in terms of accountability and 'is not an optional extra' (UKCC 1998).

The UKCC *Guidelines for Professional Practice* (UKCC 1996) state that 'as a registered nurse you are personally accountable for your practice and in the exercise of your accountability'. It is therefore essential that local records, policies and standards reflect this professional accountability

by focusing on documenting clinical decisions related to patient care and raising the awareness of responsibilities in terms of record keeping.

TYPES OF RECORD
Professionally held records

These may take the form of manually or electronically held records. The type of record is determined by local agreements within organisations. Whatever the type of documentation developed, communication must take place between managers and practitioners to address the needs in terms of documentation. This ensures that the organisational need for information and practitioners' needs for information are both taken into account as well as reflecting professional accountability requirements and developments in practice.

The UKCC makes it clear that the prime importance of nursing and health visiting records is to communicate factual data to team members and others – what has been observed or done. In a court of law 'if it is not recorded it is not done'. Completing professional records with clients is good practice giving them an opportunity to correct inaccuracies (Baldry et al 1985, Naish 1991). Information is power and working in partnership implies equality, which must include health information. Clients must have access to information about their health on which to make informed choices about their healthcare and behaviour.

There are several formats used when documenting in records (Fischbach 1991, Iyer & Camp 1991). The narrative and problem-oriented approaches are possibly the most common methods used in health visiting.

The *narrative* technique is the most traditional method of recording information in health records. The information is recorded in a chronological order but the style will differ depending on who is recording the information. Fischbach (1991) suggests that the advantages are in chronology and sequence of patient events and allowing practitioners to determine how the information is recorded. The disadvantage in this type of recording is in quality of information, which may be disjointed, with 'buried information' and time-consuming. In addition there are difficulties in information retrieval, such as in determining and tracking the health status of the client. As can be seen from the vignette below, hidden information may surround areas of concern about the child – poor parenting, lack of routine, safety issues. There may be a tendency with this format to record less factual information and record instead opinions, which are less likely to be shared by clients.

Claire and Ben are a very young couple with their first baby. Claire does have some contact with her mother but Ben resents her 'interfering'. Baby Rebecca is 8 weeks old and the health visitor has concerns about her: her feeding pattern is erratic, she is not gaining much weight and she has nappy rash.
Claire had not brought Rebecca for her check-up because the surgery was fully booked. The surgery had sent an appointment but the baby did not attend.

The *problem-orientated* system – the most familiar to many practitioners – is the SOAP/ SOAPIER method of recording data relating to client interaction.

SOAP is a process of recording that focuses on:

S subjective information, and
O objective information, forming the basis of the

A assessment; a problem list is developed from which a
P plan is developed for the client. The extended SOAPIER documents the planned/agreed intervention, and
I implementation recording the actions taken by practitioners to carry out the plan. This approach also makes the practitioner focus on planning
E evaluation of the interaction and future
R reviews.

A simple adaptation of this format applied to the vignette appears in Table 10.1.

A benefit of this format is the focus on the patient's health need/concerns, and details of the interaction to address the need. The agreed actions of both client and health visitor are explicit, and realistic outcome measures have been put in place. This type of record also helps to define the professional role and explain to others how the job is done at a micro level – something that is often difficult or perceived as too complex to attempt.

Fischbach (1991) acknowledges that focusing on problems can 'foster a negative approach to treatment', but this must not overshadow the benefits in recording in such a way (Table 10.2).

Table 10.1 A problem-orientated system

Actual/potential need (subjective/ objective data)	Agreed action (action planning/implementation)	Date of review of plan	Evaluation/outcome of agreed plan
For Rebecca to have regular feeds	1. Claire and Ben know how to sterilise bottles and make feeds 2. To offer feeds to Rebecca every *n* number of hours 3. Parents to keep a feeding diary 4. HV to visit and talk about progress on (enter time and date) 5. Weigh baby at (time and date) 6. Claire and Ben have HV contact number	 Enter date of action 4 Enter date of action 5	 3. Diary sheet discussed with parents 4. Plan amended if necessary 5. Baby has gained weight 6. Claire contacted HV for advice re night feeds
For Rebecca to have her check-up and receive treatment for nappy rash	1. Parents contact surgery to make appointment 2. Claire's mother willing to drive them to surgery 3. HV to remind Claire about appointment 4. Go over previous advice about cleaning skin and nappy changing	Enter date of action 1 Enter date of action 3	1. Rebecca attends appointment 4. Nappy rash treated and improving

Table 10.2 The value of problem-oriented system records

Professional requirement in record keeping	Does the problem-oriented system fit?
Identifies problem/need	Yes
Focus on intervention	Yes
Records action/plan	Yes
Measures outcome/progress	Yes
Information easily retrievable	Yes
Factual, concise, consistent information	Yes
Involve/share with client	Yes

This method of documenting care does require a change in the way we think about practice and recording care. It requires a corporate approach to documentation to reduce the risk of confusion in record keeping.

The public health agenda and health needs assessment within the primary care setting could have an impact on community practitioner documentation. Profile information about the health of the community/caseload, together with a system for recording an effective outcome of interaction, helps practitioners to demonstrate the health needs of clients and communities within their specialist area and the effectiveness of their clinical intervention. The changing need for different data should encourage professionals to review existing documentation, developing or testing modifications to existing systems. Any review in terms of data collection must be underpinned by two factors. First, the information must be realistic, meaningful and inform individual practice, and second, it must be realistic in quantity. We must consider the extent to which the information we collect can contribute to the issue of clinical governance within primary care groups. The evidence to meet this agenda is grounded in the information assembled by practitioners and is much more meaningful than 'the focus on achieving a maximum number of contacts' (Health Education Authority 1997a).

Health Visitor Index Card

One such innovation in record keeping was the development of the *Health Visitor Index Card* in North Staffordshire Combined Healthcare NHS Trust (Fig. 10.1). The index card was developed by practitioners and was built on work within the trust by health visitor colleagues developing a tool for profiling (Watts 1992) and performance outcomes (Plant 1992).

The catalyst for change was the successful pilot of *child-health parent-held records* and planned implementation across the district. This meant a change in practice towards an overt partnership with clients and this included documentation. This ran alongside the development of a personalised health visitor computerised information system to help health visitors manage their data. Practitioners identified a need for a record that would assemble meaningful data on an ongoing basis in a format ready for input, allow updating and reduce clerical activity. The record also had to meet practitioners' needs concerning accountability. What a challenge!

Within the process of developing the index card, consultation took place with managers, health visitor colleagues, child protection advisors and the school health service. This was to ensure that the need for information from all perspectives was taken into account. It was also anticipated that change in health visitor documentation might have an impact on other nursing records used within the trust.

Profile and outcome data

Both health visitor profile and outcome data are assembled on the front of the card in a coded format for easy computer input. This information is confidential and used for providing baseline information, planning of services, measuring impact on health and access to health visiting and other services. Breast-feeding is an example

	Address		GP	
LABEL	1		1	
	2		2	
	3		3	
	4		4	
Reference Address	Health Visitor		Clinic	
1	1		1	
....	2		2	
2	3		3	
....	4			

IMMUNISATION

			1	2	3	4	B	BCG

LABEL

PROFILE

A/N	Breast fed	Breast 3 mths	Hand M/P	S/C	CPR	Inc. visits	Un-supp	Cult diff	Lang diff	Hosp feed prob	Unsuit accom T/U		

CHILD HEALTH SURVEILLANCE: SPOTRN

Prim	6 wks	HT	8 mth	18 mth	3 yr	Orth	

S – Satisfactory   P – Problem   O – Observation
T – Treated   R – Referred   N – Not examined

CONTINENCE MATERNAL

Advice given	
Problem	Y or N
Referred	

SMOKING

No. of carers who smoke	ADVICE GIVEN
1	
2	
3	
4	

REVIEW DATE

1		7		13		19	
2		8		14		20	
3		9		15		21	
4		10		16		22	
5		11		17		23	
6		12		18		24	

ACCIDENT PREVENTION

	ADVICE GIVEN	ATT. A & E
1		
2		
3		
4		

DENTAL HEALTH

DATE PACK GIVEN ....

MENTAL HEALTH

EPDS	SCORE	DATE
5–8 Weeks		
3–6 Months		
Repeat		
Referred		

Figure 10.1   The health visitor index card developed by North Staffordshire Combined Healthcare NHS Trust (reproduced with kind permission of the Trust)

of one performance outcome developed by Plant. Research supports our practice that there are major health gains from breast-feeding for both mother and child. Baseline data are collected at first health visitor contact. Health visitors offer an intervention to breast-feeding women, possibly in terms of additional advice and support, and are able to measure the prevalence of breast-feeding at 6 weeks and 3 months as an indication of the efficacy of this interaction. Data can be compared against previous individual figures and local, regional and national statistics. This represents a potentially powerful tool in actually being able to demonstrate health gains linked to health visitor intervention. It is recognised that there may be other variables that could influence this health gain.

Information on contact data and forward planning is recorded on the back cover of the record card. The record is reviewed annually and is supported by trust health visiting standards on record keeping.

Evaluation of the index card showed that it was successful in recording contacts with clients, assisted in collection of profile and outcomes data and was useful as a forward planner for intervention (Charles 1996). Clients were asked for their views and said that the index card was acceptable.

Personal child health records (PCHR)

These were launched in 1990 by the British Paediatric Association with the support of other professional nursing and medical associations. This record is intended as the main record of the child's health, initially developed for the period between birth and 5 years of age.

The PCHR serves two main functions: first as a resource containing information and advice given by professionals, outcomes of health checks and details of immunisations, weights and measurements. Information for parents, observations and checklists are also included. This sharing of information facilitates working in partnership as a two-way process. Secondly, the record can be used as a teaching tool using the basic health education material contained within it. This information may be tailored to identified local health needs and be a means of universally targeting health messages to all parents.

Parents need information on which to make choices about the health of their children. This process cannot be achieved by issuing a record alone but must embrace the concept of working in partnership with parents in an open and participatory way (HVA 1991). This change means that parents are more involved in decisions about the health and well-being of their children. Professionals with experience of parent-held records are in favour of parents holding the main child health record and suggest that they are less likely to lose them than health professionals (Macfarlene & Saffin 1990, Pearson & Waterson 1992, Charles 1994)! From the professionals' perspective, use of the record enhances communication, is a comprehensive record of immunisation and surveillance and may improve uptake of screening and immunisation by opportunistic review and offer of such services (Charles 1994).

The PCHR can be a means to promote mutual trust and respect between parents and professionals. For this to happen, professionals must actively encourage parents to bring the PCHR when attending the child health clinic, ask to see and read parents' entries and observations, and record the advice given at this contact. Parents have highlighted the benefits, e.g. helping them to remember advice and 'important things' and feeling more actively involved in their child's healthcare; parents value the record and have no difficulty in remembering to bring it to child health clinics (Charles 1994). Booking-in procedures at clinics and surgeries that include the PCHR in the process are one way of raising their profile and importance. Health visitors and school nurses can affect the use and value of the record by including the use of the PCHR in standards and protocols related to child healthcare. Advice given to parents should be recorded using appropriate language so that the carers then have the opportunity to review advice given and this advice is also available to other professionals who may be involved.

When issuing the PCHR to parents and carers, the time spent by health visitors promoting the importance of the record and their responsibilities in keeping it safe is a valuable investment and directly affects the importance the parents place on it and its subsequent use (Charles 1996).

Additional documentation

The type of information and record will differ from organisation to organisation depending on interpretation of guidelines and local and national policies.

Occasions may arise when more detailed documentation is needed for some clients. Health visitors and managers should work together to develop guidance criteria for the introduction of additional records, in order that practitioners can feel safe in practice and also to reduce the risk of informal and unofficial records being kept.

Some issues to consider may involve children with multiple or chronic health needs, and complex needs due to socio-economic factors or child protection concerns (Charles 1996). This additional documentation helps to clarify for the client, and other professionals, the nature of the intervention and a measure of outcome from the health perspective among sometimes complex multi-agency intervention.

This documentation should also be completed with parents. The UKCC (1998) suggests that supplementary records kept without access by the client or family members should be the exception rather than the norm. A way forward may be to use a carbon-duplicated care plan with a copy each for professional and parent. An agreed action between client and practitioner is written and any dissent is recorded. The document must be signed and dated and a copy kept in the professional's record. The client also has a copy of this detailed plan, which they may keep. The difficulty for some practitioners lies in setting out and writing care plans that act as a working document (Charles 1996) and training may be required.

LEGAL ISSUES

Professional records are legal documents and can be required before a court of law.

It is essential that practitioners recognise their responsibility for accurately recording not only care given but 'deviation from the norm' or 'the need for more intensive intervention' (UKCC 1998). Practitioners must be aware of local policies relating to the retention of records.

Confidentiality should be broken only in exceptional circumstances and should be considered carefully. Practitioners do need to obtain the consent of the client before specific information is disclosed and there are only exceptional circumstances when this rule does not apply (UKCC 1996).

The Data Protection Act 1984 was introduced to protect members of the public from the misuse of personal data held on computers and electronic processing systems. Within the healthcare sector, there is a nominated manager who is responsible for registering the system every 3 years and practitioners are acting as agents for this person (Gastrell & Edwards 1996). Clear local protocols are necessary to guide staff who have access to computer-held records (UKCC 1998). The introduction of computer technology should not compromise the confidentiality of records. Professional accountability extends to ensuring security, whatever system is used including fax (UKCC 1998).

The Access to Health Records Act 1990 gives patients/clients the right to see and receive their written health records and all practitioners who create or use records must be aware of this right (UKCC 1993). The change in practice towards writing professional records and reports with clients should reduce the incidence of clients needing to proceed along this legal avenue.

Parent-held records (parent child health records) are the property of the issuing trust or health authority, although held by the parents. Confidentiality about the information held within the record therefore rests with the parent. They choose with whom the record is shared. Access to the record can be requested and enforced by law if necessary and health professionals are not liable if the record is lost by parents or 'otherwise unavailable' (HVA 1991).

In relation to child protection issues 'the best and most effective defence … is to remain within procedures' developed within individual trusts (Clark 1994). Clark suggests that where there are no child protection issues there is no problem. He strongly advises that when a child is placed on the child protection register there is a need for additional documentation. Professional judgement must guide practice in the grey area of 'cause for concern' and follow advice to record deviation from normal, more intensive care/intervention and cause for concern (UKCC 1993).

CONCLUSION

This contribution has attempted to raise some of the issues around the records and record keeping from a practitioner's perspective. Records are not static but must be the subject of review and be developed to respond to innovation and developments in practice. Health visitors and community practitioners must look critically at the documentation kept. Does it reflect the patient's outcome? Can it contribute to research evidence of practice? Is it acceptable to both clients and practitioners? Has it considered professional accountability? Does it measure quality in a meaningful way? Is the information collected used?

THE CONTRIBUTION OF HEALTH VISITORS TO CHILD HEALTH PROMOTION PROGRAMMES

Anne Plant

CHILD DEVELOPMENT – A HISTORICAL OVERVIEW

The earliest record of an individual child's

development was published by Tiedemann in 1787; more famously, Charles Darwin (1877) kept notes on his first child's progress from its birth in 1839. Some 50 years later Arnold Gesell established the first series of 'norms' in child development and went on to describe the technique of developmental testing (Gesell et al 1930, Gesell 1948). Others (Cattell 1947, Griffiths 1954, Illingworth 1975) followed with manuals dedicated to infant development screening, based heavily on Gesell's work. From the 1960s almost every child in the UK was subjected to a battery of tests at regular intervals in the belief that early identification would substantially improve health outcomes, although Illingworth himself accepted that it was 'probably never possible to draw the line between normal and abnormal'.

THE CHANGING AGENDA

Hall (1996) noted an increasingly critical approach to all forms of child health surveillance, citing health authorities' inability to justify their value (Butler 1989). The view that screening activities could be not only financially wasteful but also unethical gradually gained ground. Hall strongly advocated a move away from the process of actively seeking defects and disorders – secondary prevention – to providing primary prevention through child health promotion.

Evidence for effectiveness in health promotion is difficult to measure. Speller et al (1997) believed that the UK overemphasised the role of health promotion in developing personal knowledge and skills to provide outcomes at a client level. In order to redress this individualistic approach and adopt a more European and community approach, recent attempts have been made to target interventions at neighbourhood, school and workplace level (Department of Health 1998a).

That aside, the government remained committed to providing a service to individuals to ensure that each child 'should enjoy the highest attainable standard of health, with access to treatment and rehabilitation' (UN Convention on the Rights of the Child, 1991, Article 24).

Parents are the gatekeepers for children's access to health, with around 90% of children's

minor illness episodes diagnosed and treated at home without recourse to professional intervention. Some parents are more successful at this task than others. The 'cradle to grave' National Health Service resulted in many carers presenting simple illnesses or injuries to doctors because they lacked the confidence and/or knowledge to manage them with simple remedies. Anecdotal evidence also abounds of parents not seeking help, either because they were unwilling to accept that something was gravely wrong or because they were ignorant of normal child development. The introduction of the personal child health record in the 1990s actively encouraged parents to participate in monitoring their child's' development by informing them about what to expect at specific ages while simultaneously providing basic health education and promotion advice.

THE PLACE OF THE HEALTH VISITOR IN THE PROVISION OF CHILD HEALTH PROMOTION PROGRAMMES

Health visitors are well placed to educate and support parents in the task of parenting with the best results achieved by working in partnership relationships, e.g. supporting mothers to maintain lactation or promoting 'positive smoking', where carers smoke in a room other than where the child is nursed. Such collaborative interventions require a 'specialist practitioner' approach, with high levels of knowledge of the physiology of child development and well developed interpersonal skills.

A further important strand of their work relates to participating in public health initiatives. The data that health visitors routinely collect from individuals contribute to compiling community profiles, which can be used to identify needs, stimulate awareness at personal and political levels and encourage individuals, communities and providers to engage in health-enhancing activities.

SUGGESTED MINIMAL UNIVERSAL CORE PROGRAMME (HALL 1996)

Hall (1996) devised a minimal universal core

programme to ensure that all children achieve their full health potential. To be effective the members of the primary healthcare team must train and work together. Standards, protocols and procedures should be clearly laid down and outcomes measured. Specialist support practitioners, such as speech and language therapists, audiologists, child psychologists, physiotherapists, dentists and podiatrists, need to be easily accessed and appropriately provided.

All interventions should provide the parent with the opportunity to discuss concerns and the professional to review the past history and offer age-specific health promoting advice and information.

The practitioners carrying out the surveillance must:

- listen to the parents. It is only in recent years that professionals have come to accept that parents are the experts on their own children and actively involve them in the surveillance programmes.
- observe the child over time in their social context. Even very young children employ play and nonverbal communication skills to transmit messages to attentive adults.
- proffer age- and client-specific health education advice. Health education has been defined as 'any activity which promotes health through learning' (Hall 1996)
- perform screening tests for those defects or diseases that are unlikely to be recognised by either parents or professionals in the presymptomatic stage without the application of tests, examinations or other procedures. Although the terms 'screening' and 'surveillance' are often used interchangeably, clarity is essential in order to provide meaningful child health promotion programmes.

Wilson & Jungner (1968) devised a set of essential criteria that must be applied to all screening programmes (Box 10.1).

Cochrane & Holland (1971) added the following essential characteristics:

- simple, quick, and easy to interpret and

Box 10.1   Wilson & Junger's criteria for screening programmes

- The condition sought should be an important public health problem
- There should be an accepted treatment
- Facilities should be available for diagnosis and treatment
- There should be a latent or early symptomatic stage
- There should be a suitable test or examination: it should be simple, valid for the condition in question, reasonably priced, repeatable in different trials or circumstances, sensitive and specific, the test should be acceptable to the majority of the population
- The natural history of the condition should be understood
- There should be an agreed definition of what is meant by a case of the target disorder
- Treatment at the early, latent or presymptomatic stage should favourably influence prognosis
- The cost of screening should be economically balanced in relation to expenditure on the care and treatment of persons with the disorder and to medical care as a whole
- Case finding may be a continuous process and not a once and for all process
- The incidental harm done by screening should be small in relation to the benefits from the screening/assessment/treatment
- There should be agreed guidelines on sharing the results and the provision of supportive counselling
- Regular reviews to take into consideration changes in demography, culture, health services and epidemiology of target conditions
- Costs, effectiveness and benefits must be considered

---

capable of being performed by paramedics or other personnel
- acceptable to the public, since participation is voluntary
- accurate and repeatable
- sensitive and specific.

The reviews should take place at key stages of the child's life and be framed around the acquisition of motor, social, emotional, behavioural, fine manipulative, visual, auditory and linguistic skills.

If personal child health records are used, age-specific surveillance and screening checks are recorded on developmental examination records using a standardised SPOTRN format. SPOTRN is a nationally accepted abbreviation, used in the clinical situation to denote 'satisfactory' (a normal result); 'problem previously identified' (no new action needed); 'continue observation' (recall arranged); 'treatment' (advice given at this consultation); 'referred' (to any community or hospital service) and 'not examined' (for this item). Three copies are made. One is retained in the record for the parent, one is sent to the child's GP and the final copy is kept by the health visitor in the child's index card, after the computer department has logged the result for Korner and performance indicator purposes.

1. The neonatal examination

The neonatal examination is usually performed by a paediatrician, the general practitioner or the midwife. These results are not documented in the PCHR because in most areas the record is not presented until the health visitor's first visit.

Hall (1996) recommends that the professional reviews the family history, the pregnancy and the birth before performing a physical examination of the infant including length, weight and head circumference, testicular descent (if appropriate), heart, eyes and hip check. Universal neonatal screening for congenital dislocation of the hips was introduced in 1969 without a formal evaluation (Dezateux et al 1998). Currently, two-thirds of children requiring surgical correction are not detected by screening and the numbers remain at the same level as before screening was introduced. Some European countries have introduced universal imaging of the hips of newborns, but its effectiveness in reducing false negatives is uncertain.

Hall strongly advocates offering age-specific advice and information about prophylactic vitamin K, reducing the risk of cot death, infant feeding and transport in cars, and an explanation of the Guthrie Screening Test at 6 days for phenylketonuria, thyroid test (and in some areas, haemoglobinopathies). This population-based screening programme is applied to infants around the sixth postnatal day to reduce the morbidity, severity and mortality of certain biochemical disorders using blood samples. Current moves are afoot to extend the screen to detect a wider variety of metabolic or genetic diseases.

2. The health visitor's first visit

The Patient's Charter states that all parents will be visited within 14 days of delivery by the named health visitor.

Often, written documentation of problems detected at the neonatal examination is not available when the health visitor conducts this first visit and verbal reports from the parents vary in accuracy. Most publications of the PCHRs contain an examination checklist to be completed with the parent to encourage discussion about normal child development (Fig. 10.2).

An explanation of current infant feeding and weaning practices, and the need for a final dose of oral vitamin K may be offered, with age-specific accident prevention and immunisation advice.

This review affords the health visitor the opportunity to assess the physical and emotional well-being of the mother as well as the physical health of the infant.

Health Visitor initial assessment		
Date		Comments
Fontanelles/sutures		
Eyes		
Mouth		
Breasts		
Umbilicus		
Skin		
Muscle tone		
Bowels and bladder		
Genitalia		
Feeding		
Immunisation		
Comments		Signature
		....

Figure 10.2 An example of examination checklist

3. 6–8-weeks surveillance check

This is usually performed by the child's GP, with the health visitor in attendance, at the surgery.

This physical examination is the last that Hall recommends. It should include weight, length and head circumference, with recheck for congenital hip dysplasia, undescended testes (if appropriate) and jaundice. Findings should be documented using the developmental examination record in the PCHR if available.

The topics for health education may include: nutrition, with an explanation of current weaning practices and information about iron-deficiency anaemia; immunisation; age-specific accident prevention, including cot death; the recognition of illness in babies; home treatment; and how to access assistance.

In many districts the mother is offered the opportunity to complete the Edinburgh Postnatal Depression Scale. The results, treatment and referral options should be discussed in full.

4. Immunisation – 2, 3 and 4 months

This is performed by the practice nurse, health visitor or GP in the surgery.

At these ages the baby should receive the primary immunisation course to protect against diphtheria, tetanus, pertussis, polio and some strains of meningitis. No specific checks are required but the parents should have the opportunity to discuss concerns and use the PCHR fully. Regular weighing of healthy normal babies is of uncertain value, but parents value the procedure. Hall believes that there is no reason why parents should not be encouraged to weigh the baby themselves.

5. Review – 6–9 months

This can be performed by the GP and health visitor together, or it can be regarded as primarily the health visitor's responsibility.

This age was selected because it is the ideal time to perform the health visitor distraction test. Parental concerns about the child's health, development, vision and hearing are discussed. The

weight and length can be measured if requested or indicated. Visual evidence of congenital hip dysplasia or squint should be sought (Fig. 10.3). Topics for health education might include accident prevention – anticipating the child's increased mobility – nutrition and dental prophylaxis.

The health visitor distraction test (HVDT)

This is performed either by two health visitors or by one health visitor and a trained assistant. It should be performed in protected time by adequately trained staff. Strict procedural guidelines should be in place to ensure that the specificity and sensitivity of the test are high. The child is presented with two high (4 kHz) and two low (500 Hz) tone sounds at 35 dBA and must respond bilaterally by turning towards the sound source. Currently, only half the children with significant permanent hearing loss are detected before 18 months, and only three-quarters by 3½ years of age (Davis et al 1997). It is probable that, in the next few years and taking into consideration the accompanying technological advances, a universal neonatal screening test for hearing will be implemented. In many districts, high-risk children (Box 10.2) are tested using otoacoustic emissions (OAE) or auditory brainstem response (ABR) in the neonatal period.

Children with the last four predisposing conditions listed in Box 10.2 should also be tested

---

Box 10.2 Risk factors associated with sensorineural hearing loss.

- Weighing less than 1500 g
- Less than 32 weeks' gestation
- Ventilated for more than 24 h
- Required exchange transfusion
- Given high levels of aminoglycoside antibiotics
- Meningitis
- Hypoxic ischaemic encephalopathy
- Family history of sensorineural loss in a first-degree relative
- Chromosomal or other dysmorphic syndrome, particularly if it involves the head and neck
- Mother infected with rubella or cytomegalovirus during pregnancy
- Parents closely related

NAME ....

Date of this contact .... Weight ....

Examiner .... Length ....

Centre .... Head circumference ....

Item	Guide to content	S	P	O	T	R	N	Comment
Physical	General health							
Vision	Squint visual							
	Behaviour, parental							
	Concern							
Hearing	See separate review							
Locomotion	Sits alone, weight bearing							
Manipulation	Passes toy hand to hand							
Speech/lang	Babble							
Behaviour	Sleep							
Hips	Symmetrical abduction							
	No leg shortening							
Testes/genitalia								
Heart	Not tested							

Figure 10.3 A typical developmental examination record for the 6–9-month review

but unless they have been admitted to the neonatal unit it is unlikely that the audiological scientist will be made aware of them. It is the responsibility of the health visitor or GP to refer them at the earliest opportunity.

6. Immunisation – 13 months

The practice nurse, health visitor or GP gives the measles, mumps and rubella vaccine (MMR).

7. Review – 18–24 months

This is performed by the health visitor – possibly in the family home. As before, parental concerns are elicited with particular regard to behaviour,

vision, hearing and comprehension. A child should be walking with a normal gait and Hall suggests that the child's standing height should be checked. Later research doubts the value of growth monitoring (Hulse et al 1998) but parents have strong views about continuation of this facility. Topics for health education should include: age-specific accident prevention; the child's changing developmental and social needs, with emphasis on language and play; and avoiding and managing behaviour problems.

8. Review – 39–42 months

This is performed by the doctor or health visitor and may be combined with the preschool booster.

The purposes are to ensure that the child is physically fit and has no disorders, defects or developmental problems that may have educational implications. Hall suggests that this review should be targeted at those children who are not in any nursery facility, attend a child minder or persistently default for immunisations.

Health education topics should include: road and water safety; preparation for school; nutrition; and dental care.

Many districts also offer a vision screening test around this age. Hall suggested that 'vision screening (for amblyopia and refractive errors) was of little value unless performed by a trained person'. Snowdon & Stewart-Brown (1997) found little evidence to recommend even orthoptists performing the task and offering treatment.

EVALUATING THE EFFECTIVENESS OF A CHILD HEALTH PROMOTION PROGRAMME

After each intervention, information – usually copies of the Developmental examination record – should be sent to the appropriate authority to facilitate monitoring at individual and district level. Data collection of this type actually measures efficiency, i.e. what percentage of the population was screened or surveyed. Efficacy can only be truly evaluated retrospectively. For example, was the child with sensorineural deafness detected before the age of 18 months, as recommended by the National Deaf Children's Society in 1995?

Multidisciplinary standards for each intervention should be agreed at district level and regularly audited. This has severe cost implications but ensures that high standards are maintained.

Recently, systematic reviews have been conducted to evaluate the efficacy of child health programmes, and their findings have radically altered our belief in the value of many interventions – vision testing, the HVDT and hip checks. What must be borne in mind is that 'no evidence of effect is not evidence of no effect'. The findings of national reviews have been disseminated through the NHS Centre for Reviews and Dissemination and published in the Effective Healthcare Bulletin series.

Continuing research is important. Many interventions in health promotion do not lend themselves to 'hard' quantitative methods. Well constructed qualitative research can often be used just as effectively.

CHILD BEHAVIOUR PROBLEMS

Janice Frost

The most common questions parents ask their health visitor concern the behaviour of their child, whether normal or abnormal. Issues relating to the management of sleep problems, toilet training, feeding or tantrums can cause parents much anxiety.

Health visitors' role in teaching parenting skills and behaviour management of children, particularly the under-5s, encompasses assessment, recognition, prevention and intervention. Hall (1996) states that 20% of children have significant psychological problems, of whom approximately one-quarter need psychiatric assessment; the remaining 15% have emotional, behavioural or psychological abnormalities that may benefit from healthcare. Health visitors are at the front of this delivery of healthcare. Health visitors knowledge regarding the 'normal development' and expectations of child behaviour enable the assessment of individual children and their families to commence. Recognition and referral of children with abnormal development due to congenital conditions or abuse forms part of the health visitor's initial assessment. However, before health visitors contact families it is important to have an awareness of the extrinsic factors that could influence the child, and influence the parents in their handling of the child's behaviour.

INFLUENCES ON PARENTING AND BEHAVIOUR

Modern parenthood is too demanding and complex a task to be performed well merely because we have all once been children (Pringle 1975).

Memories of our own childhood and the way our parents handled our outbursts influence how we handle our children: the example given by parents and grandparents and how individuals interpret their memories may influence their own parenting style. Health visitors have to be able to challenge familial and cultural parenting practices and offer updated research-based advice. Recent changes within society have had a lasting effect on how parenting must develop in the future: working mothers, child care, the reduction in the role of the extended family and the enlargement of the father's role in child rearing have implications for the management of children. Social trends, including increasing numbers of single-parent families through higher divorce rates and lower marriage rates, influence child management; increased stress caused by lone parenting and reduced extended family support add to the burden and pressures of modern life.

Much research has been done on the needs and characteristics of children from homeless families and those living in poverty. Poverty influences the growth and development of the child through undernourishment (Pollitt 1994) and also by its effect on parenting. The stress caused to parents by poverty can lead to detrimental parenting practices, which adversely affect the child's well-being and behaviour. High levels of unemployment in turn increase the levels of poverty (Bassuk et al 1997).

Postnatal depression has been identified as a factor in externalising and internalising problems in the preschool and school-age periods (Downey & Coyne 1990). Shaw & Vondra (1995) suggested that early maternal depression interfered with the mother's ability to respond contingently to the infant's cues, thus affecting the infant's attachment.

Parental expectations and perceptions of their child will also have an effect upon how a child's behaviour is handled. 'Normal' toddler behaviour may be seen by some as characteristics of a difficult child; parents who identify their child as particularly difficult may respond to the child with less sensitivity, which in turn may intensify the behaviour problems as the child strives to gain parental attention. Perception of behaviour and expectations are also gender-linked: what is acceptable boisterous 'boy' behaviour is not deemed correct for a little girl. In educating parents health visitors can address these gender issues as well as giving accurate expectations of age-related behaviour.

ADDRESSING COMMON BEHAVIOUR PROBLEMS

What is seen as a problem by one parent is not a problem to everyone. It is important that the parents identify what the problem behaviour is and that the health visitor enables them to address the behaviour in a way that is suitable for the individual child and family. The parents' full co-operation is needed to enable a programme of behaviour modification to be developed and completed successfully. There are many books and views available to assist health professionals and parents in the management of child behaviour. Try to select a text that is parent-friendly to reinforce your messages. Before selecting particular management techniques it is important to obtain a full history of the behaviour causing concern and the methods already tried by the parents in order to maximise the effect of a chosen technique.

Behaviour problems such as sleep problems, tantrums and faddy eating often benefit from keeping a diary of the problem behaviour prior to and during the management programme. Keeping a diary enables accurate assessment of the problem, records the progress of failure and highlights the true nature of the problem for the parents.

Basic steps of a child behaviour modification programme

- Take a full history, including birth history, medical history, previous medication, help sought relating to the problem and social background. Include specific details pertaining to specific problem behaviour, e.g. sleeping arrangements/room availability for the family for sleep problems, family eating patterns for feeding problems.

- Complete a diary for a minimum of a week prior to dealing with the problem. This will help to identify the problem and highlight the parental difficulties relating to it.
- The parent should identify the 'long-term aim' of the programme.
- Devise a structured 'plan of action' in partnership with the parents, which is achievable, not too demanding and takes a step-by-step approach. Basic written instructions for the programme on a week-to-week basis are often needed.
- Review the programme at regular intervals, using diaries to monitor progress, and adjust the plan.
- Remember – the child's behaviour has not developed into a problem overnight but has often taken months or years, so do not try to resolve the problem overnight – take time and aim for steady progress.
- Let the parent decide when the problem has resolved to a manageable level for completion of the programme, but offer open access back to the programme if necessary.

Sleep problems in the under-5s

A child who sleeps only for short periods can cause many problems within the family: tired parents and children become irritable, miserable and less able to cope with everyday life and routines. Expectations of how soon a young baby should sleep through the night vary greatly among parents, but a meeting between parents with a wakeful child and parents with a child who has slept through the night since birth is almost guaranteed, thus exacerbating the former's problem. A sleep problem is only a problem when identified as such by the parents, not the professional. Once approached by the parents, follow the basic steps of a child behaviour modification plan.

A sleep diary is a useful tool in the development of a programme (Fig. 10.4).

Behavioural sleep problems can generally be classified into those associated with nonsettling, those with a sleep pattern that consists of frequent waking throughout the night and those

with both settling problems and frequent waking. Health visitors are ideally placed to help the parents of children with disrupted sleep patterns. Many parents have already turned to sedatives to force the child to sleep and have found that, if sedation has been successful, the problem often recurs once it is removed. A planned programme of behaviour modification often helps.

Key strategies include the following.

- 'Cue' the child before bedtime, telling them what is expected – what bedtime is
- Develop a structured approach to bedtime, e.g. bath, pyjamas, drink, teeth brushed, story and bed
- Take the child to bed awake – confusion arises in the night if they wake in a different room from the one they went to sleep in
- Sort out the settling first: this may require a programme in itself, e.g. sit by the bed, move towards the door, leave the room, call, etc. (all the tactics are detailed in many texts); once the settling is sorted the night-time waking often resolves
- If settling is not the problem but night waking is, find out why, using the diary – what is the parent doing when the child wakes? Giving drinks, getting into the child's bed or taking the child to the parent's bed, putting on the television and taking the child downstairs to play are all rewards for undesirable behaviour.

Helping parents who have a child with a disruptive sleep problem can be time-consuming, challenging and very rewarding. Many texts have been written offering guidance on handling sleep problems and must be used as resource material for both professionals and parents.

Children whose sleep problems are medical in origin, e.g. nocturnal epilepsy or sleep apnoea, must be referred on to the medical profession.

Eating problems in the under-5s

Many parents get extremely anxious when their child refuses to eat or has a very limited dietary intake. The child who lives on spaghetti hoops only is not uncommon. Often this situation can

	Monday	Tuesday	Wednesday	Thursday	Friday	Saturday	Sunday
Time of waking and mood							
Time of daytime naps							
Daytime activities							
Evening bedtime							
Time to sleep in evening							
Time(s) of night waking. What you did. How long to settle							
Parent bedtime							

Figure 10.4   An example of a sleep diary

develop into a battle of wills between parent and child, with the parent finally turning to the health visitor in desperation. It is important that, prior to any intervention with behaviour modification, the health visitor is able to eliminate any failure to thrive or physical reason for the child's behaviour, and must liaise closely with medical staff. In-depth knowledge of the nutritional requirements of children is important (Ministry of Agriculture, Fisheries and Food 1989, Department of Health 1995d). This information, when shared with the parents, offers a basis for adjusting the toddler's diet to incorporate their needs. Again, the use of a diary often helps to identify actual problems or highlight unreasonably high parental expectations (Fig. 10.5).

Key tactics include the following.

- Make feeding time a fun and sociable activity; eat family meals together if at all possible
- Let the child eat what the family eats wherever possible – 'what is on your plate must be nicer than what is on mine'
- Independence is a trait of most toddlers: they like to feed themselves no matter how messy it is – messy eating is not abnormal
- Many sweet snacks can be nutritious: if the only thing a child will eat are sweets, then put popular cereals in little bags and offer as sweets – most cereals have added vitamins
- Remember, children do not do the shopping, parents do – if it is not there it cannot be eaten
- Do not make a big issue of faddy eating: it is usually what it says, a fad that will soon pass if played down.

	Monday	Tuesday	Wednesday	Thursday	Friday	Saturday	Sunday
Breakfast (a.m.)							
Morning							
Lunch							
Afternoon							
Evening meal							
Supper							
Snacks							

Figure 10.5   An example of a food diary

Tantrums and behaviour problems in the under-5s

Tantrums and antisocial behaviour in young children often lead to the parent versus child battle of wills. It is health visitors' knowledge of the 'normal developmental stages' of children that enables them to offer advice and reassurance to parents caught in the trap of conflict with a toddler, in order to redress the balance. Biting and kicking, tantrums, head-banging and clinging are all behaviours experienced to a greater or lesser extent in normal children. Often, it is the parents' approach in handling these behaviours and high expectations of children to behave as 'little adults' that exacerbate the problem. Use of a diary helps in the recognition of factors associated with the 'bad' behaviour (Fig. 10.6).

It is important to identify what happens immediately before the undesirable behaviour, what exactly the behaviour is and what the parents do about it before any programme of change can be formulated. Many texts are available as resources to help create specific programmes of behaviour management tailored to the individual child and family, as well as professional help from behavioural psychologists in difficult cases. Techniques such as distraction and positive or negative reinforcement may be used in such behaviour-modification programmes.

Key tactics include the following.

• Share information regarding normal child development and behaviour with the parents

Day and date	Child		Parent	
	What happened before behaviour?	Behaviour	How did you respond?	Effect of what you did

Figure 10.6 An example of a behaviour diary

- It is often a change in parental behaviour that brings about change in the child's behaviour
- Encourage the parents to respond to good behaviour and to look for the positive aspects of their child – even an extremely naughty child has some good points
- Convince parents of the importance of consistency; they should work as a team, applying the same rules of discipline to the child and not giving out confusing and conflicting information.

Groups versus individuals

The advantages of a support-group approach or an individual approach when dealing with child behaviour problems can be discussed at length; both approaches have benefits and drawbacks.

The group offers release from isolation – often parents feel they are the only ones in the world with a child with a behaviour problem – peer support and the sharing of management skills, which many parents find useful. Parenting groups set up locally by health visitors offer access to a large number of clients in a cost-effective way.

Individual programming in the home is often time-consuming for the health visitor but offers continuity to the client. Change in behaviour can be monitored over a long period of time, thus giving the family ongoing support.

An alternative to individual management of behaviour problems in the home is the setting up of clinics aimed at specific behaviour problems, such as sleep clinics. This offers the client access to health visitors who have a special interest in child behaviour and, because of their involvement in the clinics, have developed increased experience and expertise in dealing with the problem.

Health visitors are equipped with the knowledge and communication skills to assess and offer assistance to parents and families experiencing difficult childhood behaviour problems. All behaviour problems can be assessed using a process similar to those discussed above.

CHILD ACCIDENT PREVENTION

Joan Leach

Health visitors are the most appropriate community-based health professionals to promote accident prevention with families. Health visitors' long-term professional association with all families with preschool children, their community base and detailed knowledge of their clients, the community and local facilities, and their interest and skills in profiling, all place them in an ideal position to be the community's prime workers in the field of child accident prevention.

The principles of health visiting (CETHV 1977) form the conceptual framework for the process of health visiting and have been used to illustrate the role of the health visitor in child accident prevention.

THE SEARCH FOR HEALTH NEEDS

The literature shows convincingly that every area has its own problems in relation to childhood accidents. There are no national statistics that are actually representative of any particular area. Research findings for a socially deprived urban area cannot reflect the same problems as a middle-class rural area.

It is therefore suggested that every area should conduct its own research to enable identification of the needs, trends and problems specific to that area with regard to accidents to children. Collecting local information about accidents is imperative if health visitors are to stand any chance of influencing plans for service provision or initiatives to meet local need.

If a system does not already exist to inform health visitors of accident victims, then communication with other health professionals and departments needs to be addressed.

Setting up a health visitor liaison service with local accident and emergency (A&E) and minor injury hospital departments would inform the health visitor of every hospital attendance for children who have sustained an injury. It must be recognised that this information would only provide a partial glimpse of the overall picture because not every child who has an accident is necessarily taken to hospital, particularly if the injury is minor or the family lives outside easy travelling distance from a hospital. McKee et al (1990) found that the distance from a patient's home to an A&E department was an important factor in the rate of attendance. Appropriate use of A&E departments is also a fact to consider when identifying local need: Ingram et al (1978) found that patients living nearest to an A&E unit tended to use it as a substitute for general practice.

Initiating communication systems within GPs' surgeries (if not already in existence) would also be useful to identify children who are seen or advised within the primary care setting following an accident. This would be particularly helpful in rural settings or wherever the nearest A&E unit is not within easy travelling distance.

Many minor injuries are dealt with by the family, either because they feel confident and competent to treat minor injuries themselves or because they choose not to seek medical advice or intervention. Unless accidents are specifically asked about, the health visitor is usually unaware that these children have sustained an injury.

The health visitor must try to find ways to gain more knowledge about the local area and so help to establish a fuller local picture of the 'accident problem'. Caseload profiling should have accidents as an indicator. This would enable the health visitor, exercising statistical expertise, to record data in such a way as to allow meaningful interpretations of hard facts and in time permit monitoring of trends on a caseload, geographical, primary care group or health authority area basis.

STIMULATION OF AN AWARENESS OF HEALTH NEED

Having searched out and identified a health need in relation to child accident prevention, it is important that the health visitor has an action plan to address the need.

In the past, health visitors have not been seen in a very positive light in this respect. Laidman (1987), the Child Accident Prevention Trust (1991) and Carter et al (1992) all highlight the shortfalls in health visitors' knowledge, training and delivery of safety advice to clients.

Hall (1991) tried to address this issue to a certain extent by including child accident prevention topics to be discussed at each child surveillance contact. Although better than nothing, it could be argued that surveillance contacts are not the ideal time to be doing specific accident prevention work. It could be seen as being 'slotted in' and so loses its emphasis and importance, particularly if conducted in clinic or surgery surroundings where the child is not being seen in his/her normal home environment. Home is where potential hazards would be identified more easily and more meaningfully by the health visitor.

Health visitor training was identified as having shortfalls over 10 years ago and Laidman (1987) recommended ways of teaching child accident work as a specific topic rather than linking it with other course work. Qualified health visitors need to request regular updating and training to improve and update their local knowledge and to improve their skills in delivering this specialised area of care.

It is important that each employing NHS trust and/or primary care group encourages health visitors to work in collaborative groups, as opposed to working in isolation, to address the issues of child accident prevention. When working in groups, ideas can be shared, schemes of work can be piloted and strategies can be formulated more easily. These groups need to be able to monitor their work in a recognised, recordable way so that their outcomes can be readily measured and audited. It is hoped that working collaboratively will not only raise and stimulate awareness of this particular health need but will also result in evidence- and research-based methods of working.

INFLUENCES ON POLICIES AFFECTING HEALTH

The influences on policies which affect health tend to be at macro level, as most are government-generated.

The Health of the Nation (Department of Health 1992) aimed at reducing ill-health, disability and death caused by accidents. Its main target was to reduce the death rate for accidents among children aged under 15 years by at least 33% by the year 2005. Nurses were encouraged to influence this policy by submitting work they had done that either changed behaviour, changed practice or changed the environment. These initiatives were published in *Targeting Practice – The Contribution of Nurses, Midwives and Health Visitors* (Department of Health 1993b). Although most of this work was done at a micro level,

it was hoped to influence the macro problem. An example of these initiatives is given in the following vignette.

The health visitor attached to two general practitioners in the North Staffs area, concerned by the number of children who were sustaining head injuries, set up a research project. The objective was to examine whether providing parents with information on how to prevent accidents that result in an injury to the head, and giving them concrete guidelines as to when to seek medical help or advice should their child sustain a head injury, reduced the number of children presenting at the local accident and emergency department. All children on the GP list for the health visitor's practice were subjects of the study. The method used necessitated establishing the number of children from the district and the study practice who had attended the A/E department following an injury to the head for the period 1991/1992. This was achieved through the information supplied by the A/E liaison health visitor. In April 1992 every family on the study caseload was sent a special 'head injuries to children' leaflet. Families joining the practice after that date also had the same leaflet given to them and the contents explained. Every child on the study caseload who presented at the A/E department between May 1992 and April 1993 was followed up with a home visit and a questionnaire was completed.

The results were that the total number of children who attended the A&E department during 1991/92 was roughly the same as previous years, with only a 1% reduction in the total number of children who presented with a head injury. Following the intervention there was a reduction of 17% of children presenting with a head injury for the period of May 1992 to April 1993 on the study caseload when compared with the previous 12 months.

The majority of families interviewed found the head injury leaflet informative and helpful. Some parents said it was instrumental in their decision actually to attend the A&E department with their child. However, overall there was a 17% reduction in attendance with head injuries, allowing more appropriate use of A&E services.

The recent Green Paper, *Our Healthier Nation* (Department of Health 1998a), also targets accidents. The aim is to reduce the rate of accidents – defined as those that involve a hospital visit or consultation with a family doctor – by at least a fifth (20%) by 2010 from the 1996 baseline.

Identifying the needs locally and developing strategies to stimulate an awareness of the need should result in local policies being influenced. If local policies are influenced and actioned, this in turn will affect the national situation. Collaborative working must be the key issue if we are to stand any chance of influencing policies that will affect the incidence of accidents to children.

THE FACILITATION OF HEALTH-ENHANCING ACTIVITIES

Most research on childhood accidents states that children from economically deprived backgrounds have a markedly higher death rate from accidents. The Child Accident Prevention Trust (1989) believes that the social-class gradient for deaths due to accident is far steeper than for any other cause of child death; the incidence of nonfatal accidents may also be related to social class. The cause of this relationship is probably a combination of many factors. A fatalistic attitude to accidents among parents in the lower socio-economic groups arising from lack of control over many other aspects of their lives has been suggested as a causal factor.

The Child Accident Prevention Trust illustrates that families in social classes IV and V are likely to be more at risk because of less satisfactory housing in terms of location, overcrowding, space, property maintenance and the lack of money to maintain potentially dangerous equipment and to buy safety equipment such as fireguards. The lack of access to adequate play facilities is frequently associated with poor housing. All contribute to the level of risk.

The recent government document *Our Healthier Nation* (Department of Health 1998a) reiterates the health divide: childhood injuries are closely linked to social deprivation. Children from poorer backgrounds are five times more likely to die as a result of an accident than children from better-off families – and the gap is widening. Health needs assessments and caseload profiling will help to identify the vulnerable and will enable the health visitor to concentrate her accident prevention work on families and communities known to be vulnerable.

The introduction of the parent-held record system has resulted in health visitors being able to work much more effectively with families. Being able to work in partnership with clients helps the health visitor to have a deeper understanding of their health beliefs and knowledge base.

Using a model when working with families would ensure the health visitor has a framework on which to base accident prevention work. Becker's health belief model (1974) would be an appropriate choice, because it identifies the key issues needed in this area of work:

- *Individual perceptions*: identifies client knowledge base and beliefs
- *Modifying factors*: identifies what the client believes they must do to make a child's environment safer
- *Likelihood of action*: clients would have a greater understanding of the possible consequences of their actions or nonactions.

This particular model fits comfortably into the conceptual framework of most care plans. Care plans are a useful tool to use with families where a safety issue has been identified.

Increasing parental knowledge about preventing childhood accidents would seem a sensible route to take when considering facilitation of health-enhancing activities. Health visitors would, at all times, use their professional expertise when delivering this to clients, in a way that has been proved to be most effective with the particular client group. Health visitors are notoriously holistic, and never miss an opportunity to raise preventative health issues when interviewing clients.

It is feared that a lot of accident prevention advice is 'slotted in' with other topics under discussion and families and clients may underestimate the importance of the message. To make accident prevention a specific topic for discussion during appointed home visits to individual families proved to be the most effective way during the Play it Safe campaign (Colver 1983). To discuss and inform during group activities with parents, or to hold special health promotional events dealing specifically with child accident prevention are other examples of facilitating health-enhancing activities to reduce the accident rate among our child population.

CONCLUSION

The issues identified by the writers of this chapter are fundamental to the work that health visitors regularly undertake and thus are the 'bread-and-butter' of health visitor support and advice. However, behaviour problems and childhood accidents are also areas of practice that are most likely to be underused when overwhelming social problems are to the forefront of the client agenda. As has been mentioned on several occasions throughout this book, records and record keeping are essential to safe practice and will become even more so under clinical governance. It is also important to recognise that records can form the basis of meta-analysis for evidence-based practice.

Child health surveillance is the basis of the health visitor working with families and is essential to improving inequalities in health.

The debate between surveillance and screening is heightened when Plant's section is compared with the work of Reynolds in Chapter 7.

That health visitors are essential to reducing inequalities in health and Glynn's work with adolescents to reduce unwanted pregnancies remains in the forefront of preventive health care.

Accident prevention and child behaviour management challenge parents and health visitors equally. The need for constant vigilance in parents is as important as the need for health visitors to constantly raise awareness of accidents. Caring parenting is also learning about how to handle changes in behaviour that with little prompting turn into intolerable problems.

11

Domiciliary health visiting and some intervention strategies

*Anne Robotham and
Doreen Sheldrake*

INTRODUCTION

This chapter examines the theory and effectiveness of health visiting in the home, exploring some of the major concepts that health visitors use to facilitate home visiting. The concepts are not exclusive to visiting in the home and apply equally to other areas. Not to have included them here would have been a grave omission, to reiterate them in the other spheres in which health visiting is discussed in this book means repetition. Therefore the reader is asked to transfer these concepts:

- partnership
- empowerment
  - locus of control
  - self-efficacy
- advocacy in partnership and empowerment

into other areas of health visiting practice.

Health visiting within the family is where health visiting began, because it was to work with families in their homes that the forerunners of health visiting came into being. Later when health visitors were required to be nurses, they nevertheless focused their main concern on the family in the home. In the early days of health visiting, work with the family was public health work, communicated through hygiene, family nutrition, health teaching and promotion. Health visitors became accepted as professionals who worked with families, following on from the midwife once delivery and immediate aftercare were completed. Goodwin (1988), discussing the reorganisation and refocusing of health visiting, commented that there should be no question of throwing the baby out with the bathwater – health visitors are good at working with families and should definitely retain that aspect of their work.

In her seminal work on evaluating health visiting Robinson (1982) collated the research evidence available on the effectiveness of health visiting in relation to the reduction of infant mortality. She cites a study by Ashby (1922), which attempted a controlled trial of health visiting in Birmingham where the Medical Officer of Health found that infant mortality in a selected ward where health visiting was carried out was below the average for previous years, whereas in the other wards it was above average. This Ashby considered to be a result of health visiting interventions, but other variables at the time – wet summer, improved sanitation, mild winter and so forth – must not be ignored.

This expressed caution over the effectiveness of health visiting has been repeated time and again in relation to variables both in the ambience in which the family is living and the type of intervention practised by the health visitors concerned. It is thus important that work that health visitors undertake with families is evaluated for effectiveness before any further examination is made of health visiting and families.

RESEARCH ON DOMICILIARY HEALTH VISITING

We are grateful for the work of Robinson (1982) in detailing the activities undertaken by health visitors in four studies: those of the Jameson Committee (Ministry of Health 1956), Jeffreys (1965), Marris (1971) and Clark (1973). The important points from these early studies on health visiting were that although they had a research methodology basis they were concerned about what health visitors did in practice rather than the effectiveness of health visiting. No two of the methodologies for the four studies cited were similar: Jeffreys provided a picture of the work of staff in social welfare services, Clark examined

the work of a health visitor in the home, the Jameson Committee focused on the range of health visiting tasks and Marris looked at a 2-week diary of health visitor activities. Only Clark's (1973) study looked at the characteristics of visits to the home and concluded that the greater number (62%) were initiated by health visitors compared with 12.2% by the client and 5.3% by the general practitioner. All four studies looked at the content of home visits and quantified the time spent on various topic areas. It is interesting to note Robinson's (1982) comment that the shorter visits tended to be those initiated by the health visitor where no particular topic/general advice on practical matters of child rearing was the main concern. Clark particularly commented on the stereotypical health visitor of the day with the didactic authoritarian approach. However, she was able to show that, as there had been a syllabus change during the data collection, there was already a difference in the approach of younger, more recently qualified staff from those of older education status.

Dobby (1986), exploring an assessment of health visiting, used Barker's (1985) comment on the Körner recommendations for data collection to show that process evaluation has little meaning without outcome evaluation. Luker (1978) had also explored this in an earlier discussion and considered that individual interventions with clients when set against their goal attainments could provide a way of looking at outcomes and thus at the effectiveness of health visiting. Again, she urged caution in assuming that health visitor interventions alone were responsible for changes in client behaviour, because of other uncontrollable variables. In a later discussion (1985) Luker revisited this point of measuring effectiveness of health visiting. She used the principle of the nursing process, with its goal-setting, evaluation and problem-solving approach to care, as appropriate to health visiting. To overcome any criticism that health visitors work with families or individuals who have problems, Luker differentiated between actual problems, which precipitate or arise during a home visit, and potential problems, which are about the preventive aspect of health visiting, such as preparing the family for the mobility of the growing infant in the interests of safety.

In analysing home visiting practice by health visitors While (1986) demonstrated that during the first year of infant life health visitors made more visits to families from lower social classes, living in local authority accommodation and with social security benefits (family income support). She found a weak link between increased visiting and single parenthood, unplanned pregnancies, paternal unemployment and increasing family size. No other factors appeared to precipitate increased visiting patterns. In the second year of the infant's life, While (1986) found again increased visiting where there was social disadvantage, a single parent, unemployment, lower social class, families on income support and unplanned pregnancy infants. She found that few families received regular contact during the first 6 months of the infant's life and that during this period any visits undertaken were more likely to be on the basis of a medical model of health, such as an illness problem. In the later months of the infant's first year, While found that health visitors began to move away from a medical model of health towards a more socially adjusted model of the infant's family life and circumstances. At the end of her study she questioned whether health visiting could be effective. She concluded that such a limited contact by health visitors in the home (once or twice in the second year) would support the belief of the government of the day that child health could be achieved through education of parents.

Moving forward from the valuable work carried out in the late 1970s and early 1980s to more recent evidence of the effectiveness of domiciliary health visiting, Robinson (1998) demonstrated the difficulty of using published studies on the effectiveness of home visiting because of the quality of the research evidence. However, Robinson's study group showed home visiting effectiveness results:

- in relation to parents and children
  - improved parenting skills and quality of home environment
  - amelioration of child behaviour problems

  - improved child intellectual and motor development, especially in low-birthweight children and failure to thrive
  - increased immunisation uptake
  - reduced use of emergency medical services
  - reduced unintentional injury and, to a lesser extent, the prevalence of home hazards
  - improved detection and management of postnatal depression
  - enhanced quality of social support to mothers
  - improved breast-feeding rates
  - initiatives limiting family size
- in relation to special needs, chronic and terminal illness
  - improved psychological functioning of families
  - increased knowledge of asthma and its treatment
- in relation to elderly people and their carers
  - reducing carers' coping stress
  - enhancing carers' quality of life
  - reducing mortality among elderly people
  - reducing hospital admissions.

Robinson (1998) drew on research studies mainly from outside the UK to reach the above conclusions because she was using random controlled trials as the methodology. There is little evidence of this research methodology in relation to either nursing or health visiting studies in the UK literature. What Robinson did find was that the UK literature tended to concentrate on process rather than outcomes. However, as Barker (1985) mentioned, process will lead to outcome. On the basis of the application of this to the UK literature Robinson (1998) suggests that:

- health visitors are remarkably successful in gaining acceptance by a wide range of individuals and their families, who appear to value their interventions highly
- health visitors are most successful in working in a nondirective, supportive way, encouraging clients to set their individual agendas
- the health visitor is the only professional who has been trained to integrate successful parenting, biopsychological and

socioeconomic factors and the wider environment into the assessment of health need and the planning of appropriate interventions

- health visitors reach the 'unreachable' – Travellers, the homeless, poor, depressed mothers
- the health visitor is the linchpin in a network of professional and voluntary agencies
- historically, health visiting has shown effectiveness in the prevention of sudden infant death syndrome and is still modifying advice, on the basis of recent research findings, to further positive effect.

Although Robinson has demonstrated the effectiveness of health visiting in relation to the above topic areas, other aspects of current work appear to be less well demonstrated in the literature. These include:

- the effect of home visiting on the physical development of children
- uptake of other child health services
- incidence of childhood illness
- use of inpatient child-health services
- mothers' use of informal community resources
- the size of mothers' informal network
- mothers' return to education or the workforce, or use of public assistance
- reducing child abuse and neglect
- in- and outpatient service use for asthma
- school absenteeism
- admission of the elderly to long-term institutional care
- elder physical health or functional status
- elder psychological status
- elder well-being or quality of life.

Robinson's (1998) work clearly shows that the effectiveness of health visiting practice is not well illustrated by the scientific positivist approach to research. The basis of medical, and some health and nursing research is on random controlled trials and the difficulty for health visiting research is that the random controlled trial is inappropriate for analysis of any large-scale interventions. This is because of the very nature of trying to combine a biopsychological and socioeconomic approach to health need and intervention cannot be managed on a large scale and lends itself to small, focused research studies. The other important factor is the ethical dimension in attempting to evaluate effectiveness while manipulating any variable such as intervention processes.

To complete this section it is worth noting that Wright (1998) showed that to develop health visiting practice the use of action research in a small-scale study led the researchers to certain conclusions. While it was appropriate for influencing the development of health visiting practice, the problems were nevertheless very great in relation to the outcome analysis if a researcher (health visitor) moved on and the study was unable to demonstrate whether the desire for change remained. Action research, while recognised for its influence during practice and thus on practice, nevertheless would not be recognised for the science of its methodology or control of variables.

The home

Domiciliary health visiting is concerned with working with client groups or individuals in the social setting in which they live as opposed to the medical ambience of the clinic or health centre. Where people live can reflect their wider environment, or indeed stand above and beyond their wider environment. Home is also a concept that distinguishes where we live from the nature and nurture of family life, which we call home. Developmental psychologists consider that the home (our home life) is the single most important influence on our lives and is a major contributor to the development of attitudes and personality in the individual.

In considering 'a home' Roberts (1996) uses Carboni's (1990) description of a home as:

being more than a physical environment – it is also an experience that emerges from many complex relationships between the individual and his environment. The concept of the home has a particular meaning for each individual, which will vary with the person's experience. The concept of home should be considered as a whole, and cannot be broken down into parts without losing some of the sense or meaning of the whole. Home is unique to each person, and is not necessarily consistent with the physical surroundings.

If the concept of home is important for early growth and development, laying down of values and beliefs, inculcation of relationships and the fostering of perceptions and caring, it is not surprising that both psychologists and sociologists in general recognise the tremendous influence that home has on individuals and families.

The earliest organised systems of health visiting began with home visits from women of the Ladies Sanitary Reform Association, and this is hardly surprising given the influence of the 'home' on young and developing families. The earliest measures for family support within the home were to do with health and hygiene and later this moved into advice on child nutrition and child rearing. Commentators on the effectiveness of health visiting at this time indicated that there was some improvement in general health and a reduction in morbidity and infant mortality statistics. However, many writers on health visiting have shown their concern about the way in which domiciliary visiting developed into advice and 'telling' (oppressive) and this spread of the paternalistic approach led to concerns that health visitors were social police. Mayall & Foster's (1989) research quoted a number of comments from mothers who approved of the 'watchdog role to safeguard children' (p. 84) and recognised and valued the support that health visitors gave them. Other mothers in the same study, however, were critical of their health visitor telling them what to do – 'especially if they have not got any children of their own' (p. 69).

Domiciliary health visiting intervention was traditionally professional-led. Clients had little say in when and why the health visitor came to see them. Many health visitors in the 1960–1980s argued cogently for opportunistic visiting, because it allowed them to see families at their potential 'worst'. It was argued that if women had time to clean up the house then the health visitor possibly could not see the circumstances in which children were being reared. There is little wonder that the term 'policing' was used and many health visitors felt uncomfortable with the situa-

tion in which they found themselves. Coupled with this was the way in which the professional took her own agenda to the client, with objectives already predetermined, often on a superficial analysis of how the family lived. It is hardly surprising that there was confusion among both health visitors and their clients over their apparent role. Clients saw health visitors in the traditional role of maternal and child health, working with clients in an authoritarian and directive manner, promoting health and preventing ill-health by advising and informing in a manner that precluded client participation.

It was during the 1980s that health visiting hit a crisis of confidence over the way forward. Health visiting practice was challenged by the Early Childhood Development Unit (Barker 1984), Goodwin (1988) and Mayall & Foster (1989) to consider what they were doing in relation to changes in society and the family unit. It was also clear that moves towards a revision of education for general nurses (Project 2000), the raising of academic standards for health visitor education to diploma and ultimately degree level and a number of government reports (Department of Health 1987, 1989a, b) all combined to show health visitors that a fundamental change in the delivery of their work, particularly in homes, was necessary.

Of the changes cited above, the Child Development Programme (Barker 1984) was probably the most influential in changing the way health visitors practised in the home. The aim underpinning the programme was to offer support to families, particularly new-parent families. Although they were often in disadvantaged circumstances the programme was offered to all new parents – arguably a nonstigmatising intervention. It focused on preparing a parenting programme relevant to the needs of child and parents, using concepts and strategies that were simple and realistic, delivered via a cartoon approach that all parents could relate to, whether highly educated or illiterate. The programme still relied on home visiting as the most effective ambience for health visitors and their clients to work together on an equal basis. It concentrated on changing the immediate caring environment of the child by working with carers to seek their own solutions to problems of child rearing, using health visitors as resources rather than instigators.

The programme was well evaluated and showed considerable improvements in child health through a reduction of the numbers of child protection issues and increased immunisation uptake, to name but two measures. It was, however, expensive relying on materials and organisation of health visitors that were seen to be untenable in a cash-strapped, human-resource-limited NHS. In addition, the universality of the programme meant that it was felt by some health visitors to be unnecessary to some populations, demanding as it did the need for extended regular visiting, which some clients did not require.

The Child Development Programme is still used widely across the country. However, the advent of GP fundholding spelled its demise as a universal programme because GPs were unable to see its value as opposed to other ideas for the employment of health visitors. Barker (1984) published extensively in health visiting and community health journals but felt no need to publish in the medical press, and it was probably this factor that reduced the impact of his programme.

However, two outcomes of the methodological change in health visitors' intervention styles that was required by the programme were a new way of working truly in partnership with clients and families and a way of raising self-esteem through client empowerment.

The White Papers *Working for People* (Department of Health 1989c) and *The Patient's Charter* (Department of Health 1991) influenced some community trusts to advise health visitors on visiting patterns. Trusts in parts of the West Midlands required that health visitors should visit families with new births for up to 6 weeks minimum in the first instance. Other trusts encouraged midwives to extend their visiting patterns to the length of their traditional remit of 28 days. The fundamental premise behind these directives was that domiciliary visiting was more effective than other ways of delivering support to mothers and new babies. It also took into account ethnic groups in the area, especially Asian mothers who are unable to leave the house for 6 weeks after delivery (see Chapter 16).

Universal versus targeted home visiting

To promote health visiting as a public health service it must be available to the public in general. Traditionally, health visiting was available universally but to one sector of the population only, namely mothers and babies, although the argument was that by visiting mothers and babies in the home health visitors gained access to all other family members. That this left a considerable part of the population outside the reach of health visitors was recognised but not responded to except in small pockets, where health visitors began to work with older age groups.

The debate over a universal or a targeted health visiting service continues to rage from the standpoint of cost benefit analysis and human resource management. In Chapter 8, Powell shows how economic evaluations support domiciliary visiting. Robinson (1998), evaluating the effectiveness of domiciliary visiting, particularly focuses on the need to understand the debate and consider how, within public health, the service can seek to reduce health inequalities and improve health status.

Goodwin (1988) proposed a targeted service following a universal initial contact whereby the client is contacted in person or by telephone and the benefits of the service are outlined. Goodwin particularly proposed this in relation to new-birth visits and suggested that clients who wished to take up the service would become the domiciliary caseload of health visitors; others would meet the health visitor through the child health clinic. Many health visitors have difficulty in accepting this programme, arguing that vulnerable clients will be missed: circumstances change and if health visiting is not solidly in the background these clients will forget where to turn to for support. This argument seems to contain similar sentiments to those put forward by health visitors wishing to retain their social policing role, albeit disguised by the notion of advice and support.

Targeted health visiting was also behind the use of the dependency rating scales used during the late 1980s and early 1990s and it must also be recognised that health needs profiling is also, in effect, a targeted service. Dependency rating scales for children and their immediate families were based on an objective scoring system against certain criteria. One such scoring system is given in Box 11.1.

This type of system 'scored' the child at the new-birth visit or the next visit and the 'score' changed as situations improved or deteriorated. There was no intention for this to replace normal health visiting practice: it was used as a scoring of extra dependency. Health visiting management thus had an extra tool to use when arguing for resources. This type of dependency rating

mirrored the medical/public health approach to population need, which used the Jarman Index (Jarman 1983) or Scott-Samuel score (Scott-Samuel 1984) and was in many ways an important means of obtaining resources. It was also a way for health visitors to score their caseload in terms of intervention strategies, which could be evaluated depending on score improvements.

At one stage this type of tool was used to measure the effectiveness of targeted visiting. However, it soon became clear that it was simply another subjective means of profiling using criteria whose validity in relation to parenting and child rearing practices could be challenged. Many of the factors identified were present in families about which there was no concern, and indeed it would not be possible to use this tool without the 'universal' approach, reaching every family.

Universal visiting is still not practised by health visitors. It is practised with targeted groups, i.e. antenatal women, the under-5s (and their families) and, in some areas, older people. It is therefore incorrect for health visitors to say that they are a universal service, or indeed that they reach clients that other professionals do not. For domiciliary health visiting to be effective, it should remain a universal service to at-risk groups.

To reach other groups in the population health visitors practise in a different way, using health promotion group methods to work with the chronically sick, e.g. asthmatics, to minimise deterioration and maximise potential health gains. Other ways of working include targeting communities through users' groups, liaising with acute units and working in child protection.

Box 11.1 Child dependency rating (the points scored for a positive answer are given in brackets)

Physical health (minimum 0 maximum 15)

- Abnormal delivery (1)
- Preterm/low-birthweight (1)
- Multiple birth (1)
- Low Apgar score – below 3 at 1 minute (1)
- Minor abnormality (1)
- Major abnormality/chronic illness (5)
- Developmental delay (5)

Family factors (minimum 0 maximum 11)

- Parental mental/physical ill-health (1)
- Mother under 18 years or over 35 with first child in the household (1)
- Three or more children under 5 in the household (1)
- Chronically sick or handicapped sibling in the household (1)
- History of stillbirth, sudden infant death or other significant bereavement (1)
- Lack of basic amenities (1)
- Unsatisfactory hygiene (1)
- Social isolation (1)
- Unemployment (1)
- Other agencies involved with family (1)
- Inadequate understanding of English language by mother (1)

Other factors (minimum 0 maximum 10)

- Known family violence (1)
- History of child neglect or abuse of siblings (1)
- This child – known or suspected neglect or abuse (5)
- Registered – yes (3)

Professionals and nonprofessionals in domiciliary visiting

Health visitors were the original nonprofessionals in domiciliary visiting until the time of their regularisation and qualification. This has meant that for a period of over 50 years child care in the UK has been the domain of mothers and families and professional health visitors. It was only in 1983 that a scheme was set up in Ireland (in

Dublin) as part of the Child Development Programme pilot study. Because of lack of resources the intervention programme hitherto run by health visitors could not continue. Experienced volunteer mothers in disadvantaged areas were recruited to implement the programme instead of health visitors and underwent 4 weeks of training. They aimed to support five to 15 first-time mothers each under the guidance of the child development programme advisor. Later, a random controlled trial (Johnson et al 1993) was set up to examine the effectiveness of these volunteer community mothers against a control group of general health visiting (public health nursing). The trial concluded that the child development programme could be delivered effectively by nonprofessionals, but effectiveness was not compared with health visitors working in the Child Development Programme.

Jackson (1992) discussed two projects pioneering community mothers in England, each with a slightly different focus. One project trained community mothers to visit families with more than one child who, although not experiencing serious difficulties, would in the view of their health visitor benefit from extra ongoing support. If further problems arose during the community mother's work with a family then this would be reported back to the health visitor, and there were guidelines over what community mothers should report on without losing their credibility with client and health visitor. One of the comments about the effectiveness of community mothers in this project was that the support they offered often helped to defuse family crises before they exploded. The second project reported on by Jackson was in a programme that aimed to offer a community mother to all mothers in the city's Asian community for whom English was not the first language. It began because the routine health visiting service was failing to meet the needs of Asian women, largely because of the language and cultural divide.

Since these pilot projects in the early 1990s there have been further developments in other parts of the country. The original notion of community mothers arose, as has been mentioned, from shortfalls in the health visiting service.

However, more recent projects have been set up for the more esoteric reason of avoiding the language and cultural divide and addressing the higher rates of perinatal mortality and low birthweight that occur in Asian babies. Criticism has been levelled at the potential for breaking of confidentiality and relationship difficulties when mother and community mother meet outside the home. However, with a good selection and training process and with fairly average rates of pay, it is likely that the right women are employed in this position. Well-structured ground rules and good working relationships between health visitors and community mothers ensure that the beneficiaries are the families and children.

Suppiah (1994) uses evidence from one such research-based community mother programme to show benefits in three areas:

- facilitating empowerment
- bridging the client/professional gap
- costs and benefits.

In the first area the training encouraged community mothers to discuss with families a range of options to enable them to find solutions to their own problems, enabling parents to raise their self-esteem and avoid dependency on the community mother because they could make their own choices. In the second area, community mothers were able to bridge the gap between professional and client, being seen as 'street-credible' because of similarities in background and experience. In the third area, although some health visitors found community mothers a threat to the notion of professional expertise, others described a sense of shared endeavour and increased job satisfaction. As one community mother wrote in *Health Visitor* in 1992, 'one of my mums said, "I like you, Donna, 'cause you're just like me – dead common."'

The nonprofessional position of community mothers employed by the NHS differs little from the position of auxiliaries employed in community units or acute units. They are given a minimum training and are part of a team, whether a district nursing, ward or health visiting team. It is therefore difficult to understand why some health visitors (Jackson 1992) are so threatened by community mothers. In the same way, skill mix in health visiting was initially seen as equally threatening. The major question thus arises of whether health visitors are so inflexible or didactic in their work that they cannot see that partnership and support is the main benefit of any domiciliary visiting.

Health visiting teams in domiciliary visiting

On the whole, development of health visiting teams has included the involvement of community staff nurses (i.e. a registered staff nurse employed in the community but with no extra training) and, more commonly, community nursery nurses. Nursery nurses are skilled workers in child care whose initial professional education includes an understanding of primary education as well as child health and development. They do not make initial assessment visits to families in the home, but they follow up where the health visitor considers that there is a need for development of child care skills in the parent and other forms of education and support. In addition, they are able to teach simple cookery skills, play development and suggest appropriate toys for children. Once the need for the nursery nurse is identified then a joint visit by the health visitor and nursery nurse is undertaken and a programme of intervention is agreed, including time scale, evaluation of objectives and finally termination of the intervention, all on the basis of the mother's expressed needs. This means that the health visitor can reduce her/his involvement in the knowledge that, if a situation arises that the nursery nurse cannot handle, the health visitor will intervene again. Nursery nurse and health visitor meet regularly, possibly even after each nursery nurse visit, to report progress. The nursery nurse has the same access to the parent-held child record as the health visitor and the mother. Other domiciliary work that nursery nurses can do is to relieve mothers who need time out and the opportunity for a rest. The nursery nurse occupies the children for an agreed period of time – provided the mother remains in the home.

Where there are families with multiple births, nursery nurses can be involved to help the parents learn to cope with the sudden extra family. Other ways they have been used in the home involve speech and language development in the young child, play therapy and behavioural therapies.

Interpreters may be used in domiciliary visits and can facilitate two-way communication between the health visitor and client where English is not the client's first language. It is inevitable that there will be some distortion of information but good interpreters keep this to a minimum. This mode of communication involves non-linguistic features such as body language and eye contact. The quality of voice tone and cultural nuances all come into play. All good practice regarding ethnic minority service provision indicates the need for interpreters. According to the national Health and Lifestyles survey (Health Education Authority 1995), Johnson (1996) reported that six out of seven people from India said they spoke English, although less than half of women over 50 years old did so. For Bangladeshi communities this fell to less than 60% speaking English. This shows that interpreting services are an essential form of communication and access channels in health work.

INTERVENTIONS IN HEALTH VISITING

We now move on to discuss a number of terms, some of which may be considered almost hackneyed through repeated use, others relating more to health psychology. Phillipson (1992) argues coherently for the professional to work with the client through a process of advocacy, enablement and empowerment, particularly when a client is marginalised, and health visitors' education should prepare them for this. The exploration of these terms will enable the reader to relate a more theoretical basis to important intervention strategies.

Partnership in health visiting

Health visitor education has embraced the introduction of advocacy, enablement and empowerment into client interaction and these lend themselves well to reflection on intervention outcomes. The traditional paternalistic approach to health visiting precluded any use of partnership because health visitors were ill-equipped to working with confident, questioning clients, choosing to leave them to manage alone because they clearly needed no direction. Partnership requires professional and client to be on the same level; when health visitors chose to undertake domiciliary visits unannounced this put the client/family at a disadvantage – one way of creating a imbalance between the authority of the professional and the recipient family.

A simple but effective way of initiating partnership is for health visitors to make appointments to visit clients in the home, and this really emerged as the result of *Working for Patients* (Department of Health 1989b), *The Patient's Charter* (Department of Health 1991) and, to a lesser extent, the Children Act 1989 (HMSO 1989). Visiting by appointment not only puts the health visitor into a position of seeking client invitation but also allows the client time to prepare by thinking about what is wanted from the health visitor, whether objectives set from previous visits are effective and appropriate and how these should be developed. Health visitors have their own agenda of objectives based on child health and child development needs, and these are introduced if and when appropriate. The true partnership approach, however, involves the client setting the agenda on the basis of an understanding of the health visitor's role. This is established at an introductory visit, described by Chalmers (1992) as giving and receiving of information, when the health visitor explains her/himself as a resource for the client and the client gives whatever background personal information they wish. Empirical evidence shows that health visiting is ineffective if the role is not clearly understood either by clients or by other professionals, for example GPs.

Thus a partnership begins on the sound footing of clearly established professional and client information exchanges. The transaction is entirely nonjudgemental and allows communication to flow uninhibitedly between health visitor and client. Once unconditional regard is established then true partnership can function, with the client bringing their own unique personal situation and the health visitor bringing knowledge based on education and experience. This knowledge is offered for client selection when prompted by the agenda, with the client in the position of making an informed choice to suit the needs of the topic/agenda. Health visitors may select knowledge from experience but their professionalism is in being able to recognise the client's perspective and offer information or knowledge appropriate to their situation. Clients may reject the practical knowledge/know-how that the health visitor is suggesting but it should be offered with information about the research underpinning its effectiveness, presented in a meaningful way, and if there are conflicts between modern and traditional practices, the partnership aspect is to acknowledge traditional practices and their value, but then to show the differences that new research and methods can make to healthcare issues.

Partnership also embraces the concept of mutual esteem, which is determined by unconditional regard. To ascertain whether the information/knowledge offered is acceptable to the client the health visitor will check out by questioning whether their needs are suited. This puts the health visitor in the position of possible rejection by the client and this can be uncomfortable unless they have developed the type of relationship in which mutual respect plays a prominent role. Similarly, clients may have to be challenged by health visitors about an apparently dangerous practice in relation to the health or safety of a family member. Challenge is not necessarily aggressive or even assertive but requires an ability to speak plainly without offence in order to modify behaviour – on the basis of research evidence.

Partnership is also based on client and health visitor using the same record, as shown in Chapter 10. This system resulted from national concerns about the freedom of information in relation to databases held by the NHS. Charles discusses the value of client-held records from several perspectives, but one of its prime uses is to serve as an agenda for each domiciliary visit while remaining the property of the trust; this difference between client *access* and trust *ownership* makes the partnership approach questionable. It is acknowledged that the red book is only a record of the child. Any records on other family members are kept on supplementary records, of which the client should have a copy; their content is usually based on care pathways mutually agreed by client and professional.

The term 'care pathways' is used deliberately in opposition to the more common nursing use of 'care plan'. A care pathway belongs to the idea of universal home visiting, in which all clients are offered the same structured visiting which they can take up or reject as they choose. Nursing care plans tend to be more specific to the needs of individual patients with medical or nursing problems.

A challenge to the concept of partnership can arise in relation to parents and their children's development. Health visitors are educated in normal and abnormal child development and first-time parents in particular may have little knowledge or experience about child growth or care. Many parents themselves come from small nuclear families and have not gained the experience of sibling rearing that was the rule in large, early-20th-century families. The Child Development Programme (Barker 1984) offered parents the opportunity to focus on the continued developmental achievements of their children and other health factors such as diet, and to develop their own ideas for care and stimulation. This gave health visitors a flexible approach, based on parental knowledge and observation, where an idea for anticipatory safety guidance, for example, is fostered through an analysis of developmental progress. The health visitor may say, 'Belinda is beginning to move so fast now that she will probably be crawling before long. How do you think that will affect the way you look after her?' This allows the parent to suggest stair gates or fireguards without the need for 'telling' by the health visitor. In everyday life our own ideas are more productive than other people's.

Partnership has been discussed in relation to home visiting but it also involves working with communities. Twinn (1991) uses Drennan's (1985) and Hennessy's (1985) earlier work to show health visitors sharing their knowledge and expertise openly with community groups to create emancipatory care, which they consider fundamental to working practice. It is also argued on this basis that emancipatory care belongs as much to domiciliary visiting as to community work. The outcome is freedom of choice to a client liberated from traditional practices. First-time mothers may be overwhelmed by advice from well-meaning family members that they find difficult to challenge. Discussion with a health visitor bringing research-based information allows the client to balance this new knowledge against traditional advice and make a truly informed decision about her child healthcare. To retain good relationships with influential family members is important in reducing the stress experienced by mothers in this vulnerable position. The Marcé Society (1994) has shown in published articles that this need to retain a harmonious balance between the knowledge she would like to take up and the knowledge forced on her can frequently lead a mother into a downward spiral of depression over child healthcare management. Chapter 16 illustrates the same dilemma in first-time Asian mothers, where care may be delivered by the mother-in-law and the new mother has knowledge that she would like to use if traditional practices did not prevent her.

Fagan (1997) looked at a partnership approach to child health surveillance as recommended in the Hall Report (1991), using a pre-Child Health Surveillance questionnaire sent out prior to each session at 9 months, 18 months and 3 years. This showed that clients responded to requests for their own surveillance linked to the major areas of child development discussed in the parent-held child health record. This small-scale study suggested that there was an improved attendance at child health surveillance sessions and that, even if they did not attend, parents completed the questionnaire, indicating their interest in the process. It also gave the health visitor a chance to applaud parents on their vigilance and care about child development and maintain the positive regard between professional and carer.

Empowerment in health visiting

Empowerment is a term overused in health visiting practice and yet it has an important place in the health visitor–client relationship. In health visiting practice, empowerment means giving clients the means of exerting their own authority over the circumstances in which they find themselves. Authority is based on confidence and knowledge: knowledge is gained in partnership, as discussed above; confidence-giving is another skill of health visiting. It begins by using processes to improve clients' self-esteem. In Chapter 4, Carnwell discusses the use of Twinn's (1991) model supporting roles and paradigms in health visiting and this is an important link in recognising self-esteem as a fundamental need.

A criticism of empowerment in health visiting is that there has been insufficient exploration of the psychological perspectives underpinning the process. Tones (1991) takes a psychological perspective whereas other writers (Blaxter 1990, Blackburn 1991, Gibson 1991, Twinn et al 1996) all consider the sociopolitical perspective to be the root cause of lowered self-esteem and advocate empowerment and education as a solution. Education has an important part to play in reversing a loss of self-esteem but it is by no means the only answer. Taking a psychological perspective requires investigation and understanding of theoretical concepts. Several may be helpful and relevant but the most useful are *locus of control* and *self-efficacy*.

Locus of control with relation to health

Rotter (1966) particularly focused on enabling people to understand whether they had an *internal* or an *external* locus of control. He described people who believe they have control over their own successes or failures as having an internal locus of control, whereas people who believe that their lives are controlled by forces outside themselves – fate – have an external locus of control. For example, in the health field, patients

who prefer doctors and specialists to make decisions about their treatment and don't want to know the details, 'just tell me what to do' could be seen as having an external locus of control. Patients who want to know exactly what their condition is and what treatments are available before they make decisions as to which they want have an internal locus of control. Some commentators (Blackburn 1991) have argued that personal circumstances such as lack of education and social deprivation override this notion of locus of control. However, health visitors have noted that although clients appear to have the same set of reduced sociological circumstances, some appear to be more able to cope and rise above their difficulties, and it is argued here that it is due to their having an internal locus of control. Health visitors who are aware of this theoretical perspective can fairly easily identify whether their clients have an internal or an external locus of control. This gives the health visitor more insight into the way the client can be empowered. If the client has an internal locus of control the more education and information they have the more they are enabled (empowered) to use their internal locus. Clients with an external locus can also use education and information but to a far lesser extent and need support primarily through advice and encouragement.

A family has an autistic child of about 5. The mother had a minimum education and left school at 16. None of the specialists to whom the child was referred was able to give a diagnosis of his behaviour. It was only when the mother saw a television programme on autism that she realised that that was her child's problem and subsequently persuaded the professionals of the diagnosis. She has constantly asked for her child to be statemented but the education authority in the borough in which she lives refuses to comply. The mother has asked questions and explored the situation, discovering that the education authority in the next borough are willing to statement her child, who as far as they are concerned lives at an address in their borough. To all intents and purposes the family now live in the next borough. The father of the family became very depressed by the whole situation and was unable to see any way forward. He was so stressed by the circumstances and the battle they were having that he ultimately lost his job and the family now live on income support.

This vignette is useful in exemplifying the difference in the parents – the mother has an internal locus of control, the father has an external locus of control. The mother responded to education via a television programme and sought as much information as she could from her health visitor; the father has required antidepressants to be able to cope with the stress the situation has created within him. Interestingly, the mother later confided to the health visitor that when her husband began to feel better he stopped taking his medication. His wife knew that he should continue until he became more stable, so she crushed the daily dose up and, unbeknown to him, mixed it into his breakfast cereal! An amusing anecdote and not to be interpreted too literally because it takes us into a whole new scenario.

The locus of control theory highlights a dilemma in health visiting – the control element. If a health visitor recognises that their client has an external locus of control then they may offer their services from a benevolent motive that may be interpreted by others as a means of taking control. Mayall & Foster (1989) use the following interpretation (p. 146):

It is particularly where the work is interventionist that [this] conflict comes to the fore. For instance, when a health visitor visits with the benevolent intention of supporting and educating a mother, her visit on private territory can be perceived both by herself and the mother as a move towards assuming some power over activities in the home; this will be especially so if she takes the initiative in proposing and developing topics of conversation. Doctors in the preventive child health services avoid the problems because they offer a responsive rather than an interventionist service.

The interpretation above is part of a discussion on the possible powerlessness that professionals can feel when practising interventionist work, particularly in domiciliary health visiting. The dimension of a theoretical perspective of health locus of control can be an explanation of why health visitors feel powerless – they recognise an external locus of control in the client and thus wish to satisfy client need; indeed the client may push the health visitor into an advising/ apparently control-taking position. In a sense, the client who has an external locus of control, if unable to take control of their lives, can drift into the condition that Seligman (1975) called

learned helplessness – which he described as a principal characteristic of depression.

It can be easier for health visitors to work with a client with an internal locus of control. They appear to respond better to information and rarely ask for advice. The fact that in a fairly brief encounter health visitors may have insufficient time to gauge locus of control in the client may be the reason for clients criticising their approach – information giving or advising – as inappropriate for that particular client.

The apparent anomaly in responses to personal control can be explained by an alternative theory – that of self-efficacy.

Self-efficacy

Bandura (1977a) suggested that self-efficacy is the belief that we can succeed at something we want to do. People gauge their chances of success and failure by their observation or knowledge of the success or otherwise of others in the same circumstances. Bandura showed that people would attempt to do something if they thought that they could succeed or that the circumstances were favourable enough for them to do so. Bandura et al (1985) showed that people with a strong sense of self-efficacy experienced less psychological and physiological strain in response to stressors than those with a weak sense of efficacy.

This could explain why clients who make even small improvements in their personal circumstances despite negative situations cope more effectively. Bandura (1977a) suggested that self-efficacy came about through social learning theory, i.e. we learn from observing the behaviour of others. In early development the significant others are members of the family, who serve as models of behaviour and standards for comparison. Parents who are caring, encouraging and consistent in their standards of behaviour tend to have children with an internal locus of control and a strong sense of efficacy (Harter 1983). Health visitors, particularly in the domiciliary setting where there is more time to focus on client ability, will recognise that those parents who have reached adulthood with poor intellectual and social skills and many self-doubts tend to find life events and parenthood stressful.

Health visitors recognise that knowledge is not the only need that many clients have: their circumstances play an important part not only in how they see themselves but also in their self-efficacy.

Jane is aged 16 and pregnant and is working with Annette, her health visitor. Jane is tearful at the antenatal visit. Her mother is present and is very disappointed in her daughter, whom she sees as shameful and deceitful. She is angry with the baby's father, whom she knows, and embarrassed by the shame brought upon her and her husband, Jane's father. She had such high hopes and expectations of her daughter's life, which she now sees as shattered. Jane says nothing at all. Annette listens to Jane's mother and after a while things quieten down. At this point, Annette asks Jane how she feels about the situation and acts as a mediator to give her an equal right of reply. Giving Jane permission to hold centre-stage in the same way as her mother helps her to begin the long haul back to self-esteem.

This vignette above is a mere skeleton of the knowledge that Annette has about why educationally underachieving 16-year-olds become pregnant, repeat the same patterns that Annette knows their mothers went through, living in council-owned property in a deprived area of the city and never achieving their hopes and ambitions. Health visiting work here is long-term, based on a comprehensive knowledge of the socioeconomic influences on biopsychological development in the individual. To enable Jane, her mother and ultimately the baby to achieve their potential calls for a subtle use of empowerment through support and education. It is also important that health visitors in this situation do not make assumptions: this is a set of circumstances that many will recognise but while it may seem classic it is still unique.

Empowerment is also about helping people to reflect on ways to change their circumstances, by enabling them to recognise their own potential and achieve their aims. This is carried out at the client's own pace: for example, the health visitor may be in a position to give the client information on how to communicate with community leaders or agencies. Client confidence is boosted by positive support that is nonpatronising and based on enabling clients to recognise their own achievements, encouraging them to unravel the process

and reflect on their own abilities within it. Clients often fail to see that where an outcome is only partially achieved they have nevertheless gained immense confidence and can use this to greater effect later in similar circumstances. Reflection is not just a professional practice tool but can be used in partnership with the client to achieve positive outcomes. Guided reflection in this case does not require tools but does require equal partnership with the client to explore situations, circumstances and feelings of self-worth. It is important that reflection is a continuum of action and that the client is helped to explore the process according to their own beliefs and values.

Empowerment is shown by Naidoo & Wills (1994) as an approach to health promotion, helping people to identify their own concerns and health issues and giving them the skills and confidence to deal with them. Naidoo & Wills suggest that there are two main mechanisms: self-empowerment based on nondirective client-centred counselling; and community empowerment through enabling them to challenge and change aspects of their environment.

Advocacy in partnership and empowerment

Advocacy by health visitors on clients' behalf can be viewed as part of empowerment and may be regarded as the beginning of the process. It is not necessarily inhibiting to client development for health visitors to make initial representations on their behalf, and does not reflect the traditional role of the health visitor, putting the client into a passive role. Advocacy is particularly appropriate when health visitors are working with clients from ethnic minority groups who have little or no spoken English and do not understand the healthcare system in general and health visiting in particular.

Mayall & Foster's (1989) research showed that health visitors intervened in the private sphere of the family as advocate for the child and to represent the child on the behalf of society. Discussion with health visitors made it clear that they saw their work as not only protecting the child from abuse but also ensuring that the child was given every opportunity to fulfil its potential. It is interesting that in the study health visitors considered this to justify any amount and type of intervention they thought necessary but saw it as benevolent rather than controlling work because it was for the protection of children. This highlights the need for health visitors to be aware that their work is susceptible to varying interpretations depending on the values and beliefs of the person making the interpretation.

There is evidence from an East London project (Harding & Pandya 1995) that health advocates are used not only as translators, working alongside health visitors, but also for independent home visits. This system was also used in Sparkbrook in Birmingham by Weaver (1996). Comments from health visitors involved in the project to use health advocates as part of health visiting teams were positive and there were clear guidelines on preparation for home visits by the advocates, visiting following an initial joint visit with the health visitor, and subsequent debriefing sessions.

Advocacy is not just about health visitors representing clients' views but, as in the project above, enabling clients to make best use of the health service as well as promoting flexibility in the delivery of health visiting serves to suit different cultures. In Chapter 16 Gogna and Hari make the very clear point that effective health visitors with ethnic client groups must be prepared to listen and learn. The assumption that the Asian family is all-protective and supportive is far from the truth, as is also discussed in Chapter 13.

Intervention strategies with specific client groups in the home

How we communicate is of paramount impor-

tance to health visiting and discussions earlier in the chapter show how misinterpretation of the health visitor's intentions can lead to criticism and rejection of professional intervention. Health visitors are not counsellors but need the counselling skills of listening, attending and reflecting to communicate effectively. Many health visitors use counselling models that they have learned from further development courses and have adapted for use in health visiting, but health visiting is not counselling or casework in the same way as social work or mental health nursing. In Chapter 4 Carnwell shows how health visitors can use adapted models of nursing care pathways and how Twinn used an adapted health-promotion model to provide a structure for health visiting processes. The authors of this chapter strongly feel that health visiting should take up a communication approach that covers all aspects of their work along the bio-psycho-socio-economic continuum and does not leave gaps when health visitors are transferring from one counselling model to another or have to switch to information giving while they are listening.

Heron (1986), using a philosophical humanist approach, has identified a six category intervention analysis, which, he argues, transcends any particular theoretical stance adopted by other counselling models. Heron recognises two basic approaches to intervening and describes these in familiar terms to health visitors as 'authoritative' and 'facilitative'. These two categories are further subdivided into three aspects to each subdivision (Fig. 11.1).

Heron suggested that the two types of intervention – authoritative and facilitative – could be used in a wide range of counselling interventions and he could almost have been thinking

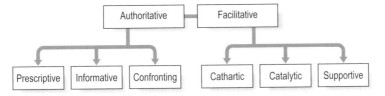

Figure 11.1 Heron's six category intervention analysis (redrawn with kind permission from Heron 1986)

of the range of approaches that a health visitor may have to take on in one domiciliary visit alone.

It is quite easy to recognise scenarios in which each intervention can be used in health visiting.

- *Prescriptive interventions*: a health visitor gives weaning advice to a mother (despite what is otherwise suggested, this is a counselling type of intervention, it is not just telling – mothers have a choice whether to take up the advice or not, so the health visitor takes a directive role and gives advice in a structured way)
- *Informative interventions*: a health visitor shares information on the purpose of HRT with a perimenopausal woman (the position of the health visitor here is not a guided/directive role but one of sharing knowledge to increase the choices open to women)
- *Confronting interventions*: a health visitor says to a mother that she finds it difficult to believe the mother's explanation of her child's bruised face (this is both a challenge and a confrontation – it is stated quietly but with conviction and indicates that the challenge will be repeated if necessary). Heron differentiates between *pussyfooting*, where the health visitor is vague and unclear and skirts around the point; *sledgehammering*, where the health visitor becomes aggressive and the intervention becomes an attack on the mother; and *confronting*, where the health visitor stays calm and keeps to the point.
- *Cathartic interventions*: a woman begins to cry while talking, and the health visitor communicates her empathy (other forms of pent-up emotion such as anger, fear, grief and embarrassment may be dealt with in this way)
- *Catalytic interventions*: a health visitor, approached by 45-year-old Margaret, concerned about her teenage son and daughter's behaviour towards her 70-year-old mother, who lives with them, allows the woman to talk at length about the home situation (the end result is that Margaret, by focusing on her own situation, comes to a decision on what to do next; this is client-centred work – see below)
- *Supportive interventions*: a mother with two bedwetting children brings up an idea as to what else she might do to help her children, and the health visitor empathetically encourages her solutions ('supportive' is a word frequently used in health visiting but there is a difference between facile approval and empathic understanding).

Egan's (1986) three-stage counselling model

This is a structured approach to counselling that involves three stages in the helping process and can, therefore, be modified for health visiting intervention in problem solving. The three stages are:

- *Stage 1: Problem clarification.* This is a collaborative working relationship in which the health visitor 'attends and responds' (Egan 1982, p. 51), i.e. listens actively to what the client is saying, helps the client to focus on the pivotal aspects of all the problem areas and, during the whole process, communicates empathetic unconditional positive regard.
- *Stage 2: Goal setting.* Within this developing helping relationship, the health visitor enables the client to develop new perspectives on the problems identified and the players in the situation, and helps them to establish new goals.
- *Stage 3: Action.* The means of achieving these goals is the focus of this stage, and the health visitor may challenge the client on steps they propose as the way forward. At the end of this process the client, through this intervention method, gains confidence in their own ability to take control in response to problem situations.

Strategies for problem-focused and emotion-focused coping

Sarafino (1994) uses the work of psychologists Perlin & Schooler (1978), Cohen & Lazarus (1979) and Moos & Schaefer (1986) to explore two approaches to coping with stress: strategies to deal with the problem and strategies to deal with the emotions that result from it.

Strategies to deal with the problem include *direct action*, when the client is helped to carry out an activity that may distract them from the problem, e.g. going away, negotiating, consulting. By *seeking information* the client acquires knowledge about how to proceed, e.g. seeking legal advice or approaching alternative accommodation providers. *Turning to others* involves seeking social support from friends and family, applying for a loan or some other means by which other people can help towards solving the stress-creating problem.

In emotion-focused coping the health visitor may help the client in several ways, e.g. helping them to come to terms with the problem – *resigned acceptance*: 'it will not go away, so how can it be accepted in my life?' Another focus is *emotional discharge*; here the client is helped to express their feelings or reduce the tension in such ways as by screaming when angry, crying or using jokes. A third way of emotion-focused coping is to use strategies to re-examine or change the client's view of the stressful situation. A health visitor might encourage the client to talk or write about their problems and negative feelings, which may reduce their stress and benefit their health. Pennebaker (1990) suggests that to write enables the person to organise, consider and assimilate his or her thoughts and feelings more carefully than talking. A comparison of therapeutic approaches is discussed by Cody (1999) and this is complemented by using health psychology to reach the same conclusions, i.e. being with and questioning a person, helping a client to develop personal insight and knowledge.

Rogers's (1951) client-centred approach

This is a model of counselling that is used selectively by health visitors. As with most health visitor interventions, this model involves the client seeking a solution to their own problems. However, when used by health visitors in its original format, one of the main requirements is that there is sufficient time for the client to work through their own situation. It is therefore more likely that health visitors will use it with individuals who have issues in their personal life. Rogers's model concentrates on the process of the relationship between client and counsellor, involving warmth, genuineness and positive regard for the client, leading to a gradual understanding of the client's problems, unfolded at the client's own pace. It is particularly valid in a helping relationship such as postnatal support visits over a planned length of time.

Types of intervention in selected situations

Working with perinatal women

The first introduction of health visiting to the family unit may be in the antenatal period in the home. It is also likely that where pregnant women attend the GP surgery for antenatal care and attend parentcraft classes they will also meet the health visitor outside the home. Health visitors work with women in the antenatal period to establish a relationship, introduce the perspective of health visiting and, if possible, identify any factors in the pregnancy or family history that might create vulnerability in the family. Green & Murray (1994) surveyed literature to assess the extent to which women were found to have depression during pregnancy and from the studies found that the prevalence rates of depression in pregnancy were comparable with those found after delivery. They went on to use the Edinburgh Postnatal Depression Scale to record scores of women in the antenatal period and found a close link between these and the postnatal score. Further pilot studies (Sheldrake et al 1997) have confirmed the increasingly common finding of depression in antenatal women.

Clement (1995) reported on the use of 'listening visits' in the antenatal period, highlighting their value both in helping women to identify early depressive feelings and in ensuring continuity into the postnatal weeks. This is a counselling process under Heron's (1986) facilitative category and can embrace all three interventions under that category – cathartic, catalytic and supportive. The particular counselling structure used would be along the Rogerian lines of client-centred discussion.

Mother's name: ....

Today's date: ....

Baby's date of birth: ....

Health Visitor: ....

I would like to know how you are feeling now, a few weeks after your baby's birth. Please <u>underline</u> the answer which comes closest to how you have felt **in the past week**, not just how you feel today. It has been found that responses are more accurate if they are not discussed with other people, so it is advisable to fill in the form on your own when you have a few spare minutes. Please complete ALL items.

Here is an example, already completed.

I have felt happy:

<u>Yes, all of the time</u>
<u>Yes, most of the time</u>
No, not very often
No, not at all

This would mean: 'I have felt happy most of the time' during the past week.

Please complete the other questions in the same way.

In the past week:

1. **I have been able to laugh and see the funny side of things:**
   As much as I always could
   Not quite so much now
   Definitely not so much now
   Not at all

2. **I have looked forward with enjoyment to things:**
   As much as I ever did
   Rather less than I used to
   Definitely less than I used to
   Hardly at all

3. **I have blamed myself unnecessarily when things went wrong:**
   Yes, most of the time
   Yes, some of the time
   Not very often
   No, never

4. **I have been anxious or worried for no good reason:**
   No, not at all
   Hardly ever
   Yes, sometimes
   Yes, very often

5. **I have felt scared or panicky for no good reason:**
   Yes, quite a lot
   Yes, sometimes
   No, not much
   No, not at all

6. **Things have been getting on top of me:**
   Yes, most of the time I haven't been able to cope at all
   Yes, sometimes I haven't been coping as well as usual
   No, most of the time I have coped quite well
   No, I have been coping as well as ever

7. **I have been so unhappy that I have had difficulty sleeping:**
   Yes, most of the time
   Yes, sometimes
   Not very often
   No, not at all

8. **I have felt sad or miserable:**
   Yes, most of the time
   Yes, sometimes
   Not very often
   No, not at all

9. **I have been so unhappy that I have been crying:**
   Yes, most of the time
   Yes, quite often
   Only occasionally
   No, never

10. **The thought of harming myself has occurred to me:**
    Yes, quite often
    Sometimes
    Hardly ever
    Never

Figure 11.2 The Moods and Feelings Questionnaire (Copyright ©1987 *British Journal of Psychiatry*; from Cox JL, Holden JM, Sagovsky R 1987 Detection of postnatal depression: development of the 10-item Edinburgh Postnatal Depression Scale. Br J Psychiat 150: 782–786)

The introduction of the Edinburgh Postnatal Depression Scale (Cox et al 1987) has created a means whereby health visitors can identify depression in women and gauge the effectiveness of their interventions. The tool is steadily being taken up by health visitors throughout the country and may be used in different ways. In Southern Birmingham Community (NHS) Trust the tool has been modified by a change of title only and is used in both the antenatal and postnatal periods (Fig. 11.2).

The title 'Moods and Feelings Questionnaire' was felt to be less clinical and therefore not to perpetuate an idea that depression belongs to the perinatal period. The tool has become integrated into domiciliary visits aimed at an antenatal period between 22 and 28 weeks and three postnatal periods 1 month, 3 months and 6 months after delivery (following Holden 1994). The tool could, of course, be used at other times when the health visitor and mother wanted to check progress or effectiveness of particular interventions.

The tool is used primarily to give women permission to talk about their negative feelings and to identify low moods. There is also evidence that some women are able to conceal depressive moods and that in others it helped to prevent the spiral of depression (Cox & Holden 1994). The tool is first introduced to the woman and the underlying research is explained; they are given the option to fill it in or not. Women are given space to complete the questionnaire and are encouraged to do it on their own, but it is important that they have a chance to discuss the reasons for their responses with the health visitor or a close confidante. Often underlying issues emerge that have little to do directly with the pregnancy or birth. Evidence (Green & Murray 1994) shows that there is a relationship between low moods and feelings (from any cause) in the antenatal period and postnatal depression. It is not necessarily the scoring system that is important but the ensuing dialogue, which clearly belongs among the cathartic and supportive interventions in Heron's (1986) facilitative category. There is a division of opinion as to where the tool should be offered to women, in the home or the clinic. The pilot project mentioned above (Sheldrake et al 1997) indicated that women preferred to use the tool with the health visitor at home.

Working with mothers and their babies within the family unit

Interventions used here belong more to Heron's (1986) authoritative categories. Here it is essential that there is sensitivity to balance more than one intervention at a time: for example, a health visitor may wish to draw out from a mother her ideas about a particular aspect of child care (exploration) but at the same time will be mindful of the need to ensure safety or hygiene in her practice. Often Egan's (1986) three-stage model serves as a useful structure to facilitate the process by building on existing skills or knowledge. Child health promotion (Hall 1996) is not considered here to be an intervention; however, where lack of stimulation, detected delay or a medical problem is apparent then the authoritative category of intervention – prescriptive intervention – is used. Practical interventions that health visitors may perform within the home will include a variety of initiatives, e.g. immunisation or growth measurements, and could be considered prescriptive.

Fathers in the family unit

Health visitors' interactions with fathers vary with the level of employment in the area. Mack & Trew (1991) quoted research showing that fathers often have different tolerances and attitudes towards child behaviour from those of mothers, both within a normal community and in the event of referral to a psychologist because of behaviour problems. A breast-feeding study (Beske & Garvis 1982) also showed clearly that where fathers were supportive mothers breastfed more effectively and for a longer period of time. Barker (1984) concentrated in the Child Development Programme on raising health visitor awareness of fathers' needs, and produced cartoons to illustrate ways in which men could enhance and maintain their support of both mother and baby. The pilot perinatal study (Sheldrake et al

1997) also showed that fathers could became postnatally depressed alongside their wives. Indeed, one mother asked the health visitor for a scale for her husband and brought the results back to the health visitor; between them, she and the health visitor worked to support the father through his difficult period.

Traditionally health visitors found it difficult to work with fathers, but in recent years attitudes have changed towards men in the parenting role and in many cases, particularly in employment troughs, there have been role reversals, with women working and men staying at home to look after the family. Health visitors need to examine their skills in working with men and recognise that many men have intimate knowledge of child care and development. Intervention categories remain the same as when working with women: authoritative and facilitative approaches are used in context. Barna (1995), focusing on work with young fathers, suggested that one of her main aims was to challenge sexist attitudes and values, ensuring that in so doing she did not compound stereotypical male images but allowed issues of masculinity to be addressed in the context of parenting. Clearly, this type of work relates more to group work in clinics; nevertheless, health visitors may have to challenge men on their sexist attitudes and, if the mother is there, to make sure that this is done in such a way that the father does not feel that 'women are ganging-up on him'.

Health visitors and older people in the family unit

The bulk of health visitor intervention is undertaken with older people who are living on their own. Perceptions and attitudes in health visitors who work with older people are a major factor in determining how best to intervene in potentially deteriorating situations. Health visitors working in these areas of practice should have developed the skills of reflection and should practise these regularly, as well as having a knowledge of systems and policies. It is also important to understand how we develop attitudes towards older people and what creates

bias within cultures. The types of intervention using the Heron (1986) analysis are likely to be skewed towards the authoritative categories, in particular prescriptive interventions, e.g. in encouraging improved nutrition or minimising danger in the home.

Health visitors working with older people and their carers may offer practical support in material terms, obtaining finance or equipment such as a continence service or a laundry facility, respite care in an alternative situation for both the older person and their carer, or a sitting service. Therapeutic interventions require an education approach and the opportunity to see an endpoint, otherwise they may well be considered of little value. They may include strategies such as helping the carer to understand the difference between protection and personal liberty and how to introduce these. Other education approaches include advice and information on a wide range of issues, which may include medical information about health/illness, housing or financial benefit advice, or ways in which the carer can continue in employment. Another major benefit can be gained from multiagency support but this in itself is fraught with difficulties where there is no key worker who can act as co-ordinator to ensure a smooth service.

Domiciliary health visiting and children with special needs

There appear to be two basic models of organisational practice in domiciliary work with children with special needs. In the first model, specialist health visitors are appointed on an outreach scheme and receive referrals from the family health visitor to provide more intensive support and counselling about practical aspects of parental handling of the child with special needs. The second model is where a child has multiple special need problems and is looked after at home by a multidisciplinary team of physiotherapists, speech therapists, possibly the community children's nurse in the case of nursing needs, and available portage helper schemes. In this latter case the family health visitor may act as a co-ordinator for the professionals involved with the special needs child, as well as possibly working with other family members, especially other siblings.

In the first model the typical scenario would be that the family health visitor asks the special needs health visitor to assess the situation. They agree to visit together at a time suitable to the mother and, during the three-way discussion, the special needs health visitor identifies how her involvement may help. It is important that, on this first visit, the mother is clearly party to any decisions made and that the family health visitor is also party to them so that the two health visitors clarify their individual roles and the mother knows exactly where she is.

The special needs health visitor is likely to have a small team of nursery nurses and auxiliaries who can provide regular practical help such as helping the mother to carry out for example, portage tasks or catheterisation in the manner in which she has been taught by the hospital. The individual helpers and professionals involved will depend on the organisational policies of the particular community trust and whether the paediatric unit has a community outreach scheme. If there is an outreach scheme that helps mothers with clinical care then the special needs health visitor has a supportive and planning responsibility to ensure that the overall care pathway is contingent on the family requirements. For example, concentration of services on one child can have negative effects on other children within the family and the special needs health visitor will need to be ever-vigilant in monitoring the developmental progress of the other children. Robinson (1998) shows that

health visitor effectiveness particularly involves improving the psychological functioning of families with a child with special needs.

Where the family health visitor is working in the dual role as a special needs health visitor then her/his situation is likely to be more of a co-ordinator of the other professionals involved as mentioned above. In many ways the health visitor may need to concentrate on supporting the parents – mother, who may be almost overwhelmed with the number of supporting carers that her child needs, and father, who may have to work long hours to bring in money for the extras that the family requires. There is empirical evidence among health visitors that many mothers find it hard to cope with all the attention being focused on the child while their own needs lie buried. These needs may involve feelings of guilt, anxiety, lack of ability to be a 'normal' parent and so forth.

CONCLUSION

The debate will continue to rage about whether health visiting should remain within the home or move into the more economically accessible venues of the health centre or community premises. The argument for the home as the venue is supported by the opportunity to use client-centred interventions that are specific and relevant to the client, and these are therapeutic or strategic as the case may be. Particular client-centred interventions that are more effective in the home are those requiring psychological processes, e.g. listening visits, issues of empowerment and identifying locus of control.

12

Ethical issues in prevention of ill-health and health promotion

Jan Rose

INTRODUCTION

It is the intention of this chapter to raise awareness of ethical issues surrounding the practice of promoting health in its widest sense. Do not expect to be supplied with answers, since ethical dilemmas are intensely personal and there are no right solutions. What is hoped is that this chapter will increase moral reasoning, thus improving the quality of decision-making. Some of the ethical issues germane to the practice of health visiting that carry a potential for harm are health education and health screening, including immunisation.

Ethics is a much used word and as such is open to individual interpretation. Ethical choice is influenced by personal values and personal values are usually learned through the process of socialisation. This means that what may be ethical to one individual could be considered immoral by another. As health visitors you are warned about not imposing middle class values on your clients (at least, I was when I trained back in the 1970s), so can one rely on just one's own personal values and beliefs when faced with a dilemma that impacts on the client? Many healthcare practitioners may take comfort from the thought that they need only comply with the UKCC *Code of Professional Conduct* (1992a) to practise ethically, but the code of conduct is provided for guidance only. The diversity of the various disciplines within nursing means that specific rules cannot be applied. The code of conduct therefore, of necessity, is couched in very general terms and when faced with a particular dilemma it is up to the individual to make the final decision as to the best way to act, or not act, as the case may be. Codes of conduct are therefore of limited value in helping to resolve ethical dilemmas. Consider the guidance set down within the code.

Each registered nurse, midwife and health visitor is accountable for his or her practice.... Each registered nurse, midwife and health visitor shall act, at all times, in such a manner as to: safeguard and promote the interests of individual patients and clients; serve the interests of society; justify public trust and confidence; and uphold and enhance the good standing and reputation of the professions (UKCC 1992a).

This is quite a heavy responsibility and, as Bergman (1981) points out, to be accountable one needs to have the ability to decide and act on a specific issue; ability requires knowledge, skills and values. The knowledge should be research-based and up to date. The responsibility for keeping up to date is the individual's; when workloads are excessive and it is a struggle to get through the day's work, how feasible is it also to keep up with reading relevant literature? As Sieghart (1982) pointed out,

professional codes, if they are to be worth anything, cannot merely confine themselves to asserting that there is a problem and leave it at that – let alone leaving it to individual members of the profession to solve the dilemma as best they can, after consulting their unguided conscience and perhaps a few respected colleagues. At least such a code must say something about how to approach this kind of problem.

The UKCC have gone a long way towards improving the degree of guidance in their publication *Guidelines for Professional Practice* (UKCC 1996) but it is still guidance and does not provide the definitive answer.

The health visitor enjoys more autonomy than other community disciplines. This is a double edged sword since more autonomy means more accountability and more responsibility. As an example of some of the difficulties that may be encountered let us consider a prime concern for all health visitors: child protection. The concept of childhood is relatively new. Up until the latter

half of the 19th century children were regarded as chattels or the property of their parents. When tracing genealogy it is quite common to find the same forename occurring several times within the same family. When a child died the next child born of the same sex was given the first child's name. Thus one supposes that the child was not valued as an individual but merely as an heir or for providing future support for the parents. As Aristotle put it: 'there can be no injustice in the unqualified sense towards things that are one's own, but a man's chattel, and his child until it reaches a certain age and sets up for itself, is as it were a part of himself.'

Children are perceived in the light of cultural values and mores. It is the culture of a particular society that defines the meaning and essential nature of childhood and the length that childhood should last. Children have been subject to abuse for centuries and before children were given recognition through legislation such as the Children Act 1989 the extent of abuse was not documented. Historically, awareness of child abuse came through the writings of social reformers such as Charles Dickens.

With child abuse the abiding decision is when (and how) to intervene. Health visitors may often find that they are 'damned if they do and damned if they don't'. There are horrific examples of the results of failing to intervene, as in the many recent cases where a young child has been killed. Alternatively, the effects on both parents and children of leaping to conclusions with too rigorous an approach, as in the Cleveland case, are still coming to light. In many cases, permanent damage to the family unit may result.

One problem with dealing with child abuse is that once the referral has been made to social services the prevailing attitude appears to be that the parent(s) or abusing adult(s) is guilty until proven innocent. Where there is clear evidence of physical harm to a child, no one would argue that it is imperative to act quickly and either remove the child or the alleged abuser as soon as possible. The issue is not quite so clear when there is suspected sexual abuse without physical violence or actual penetration. As with any form of suspected abuse, if there is evidence of actual harm then immediate action must be taken, but when does a cuddle become covertly sexual in nature? Who can decide this? How much evidence is required before action can be taken? Is there a cut-off age when fathers should stop bathing their daughters or should fathers not be allowed to bathe their female children at all? How practical would it be to impose rules like this when it may be that traditional family roles have been reversed and the mother is the bread-winner? What of male children? Should the same restrictions apply? When do photographs taken by proud parents become pornographic? Incest is taboo in our society but is it necessarily so in other cultures? The ancient Egyptians considered that incest was the only way to keep the royal blood-line uncontaminated.

While not condoning incest, one could argue that it is learned attitudes within the UK towards this practice that colour the healthcare professional's judgement when dealing with a suspected case. It is vital that action should be taken when there is a suspicion that an incestuous relationship with a minor may exist, but potential harm may be done to the innocent victim by a 'shock! horror!' reaction and insensitive probing. The child may perceive what has happened as an expression of love (providing that rape or coercion is not involved); indeed, it may be the only show of love or affection that the child receives. How much damage can be done by rushing in to remove either the child or the alleged abuser because our society abhors the concept of incestuous relationships! As John Harris (1985) puts it: 'There is nothing wrong with sex of any kind.... There is lots wrong with violation, exploitation, the infliction of harm, pain, suffering and so on' (p. 191). Harris goes on to suggest that the sexual preferences of health professionals should not influence their treatment of those whose preferences differ. So it is important not to let distaste colour judgement.

When should the health visitor refer in order to protect the child? Because of an intuitive feeling? Can one take comfort from relinquishing responsibility to the social worker and thus taking no responsibility for subsequent adverse results should the suspicion be unfounded and false?

But what if one fails to pass on concerns regarding a child? Failure to act (an omission) could result in considerable harm being done. Obviously, one should take action if there is anything in the child's demeanour that strongly suggests that a violation has taken place, but if this is not the case then the risk is that reporting your suspicions may adversely affect future relationships within that family unit. This situation is typical of an ethical dilemma where two equally unacceptable outcomes are likely whether an act or omission is undertaken by the healthcare professional. What help is needed in decision-making where ethical dilemmas exist? Is intuition enough? How can we judge when an action is right or good and how do we decide what we ought to do? How helpful is the *Code of Professional Practice* (UKCC 1992a) and the subsequent *Guidelines for Professional Practice* (UKCC 1996)?

Allmark (1992) suggests that the two main approaches to the application of ethics in nursing are to examine the normative philosophical theories or, more commonly, to ignore any insights philosophy may offer and follow a systematic approach based on a form of the nursing process: assess, judge, plan, implement, evaluate. While Allmark admits that the second approach is tempting for nurses, being pragmatic and practical, he warns that nurses who ignore philosophical ideas on ethics are doomed to repeat the mistakes of the past. So before going any further it is pertinent to consider the philosophical basis of what is understood by ethics.

Ethics has been defined as a generic term for several ways of examining the moral life. Originally, 'morals' and 'ethics' were Greek and Roman terms meaning a code of acceptable conduct within the constraints of society. Latterly, morals have taken on more of a religious connotation. When we deliberate about whether a judgement is morally right, we are considering which judgement is morally justified, i.e. which has the strongest moral reasons behind it. Ethics is not one body of thought but a range of different theories from which many other moral philosophies have been derived. There are many books written on ethical theory and it is not the intention to discuss ethical theories in any depth other than to distinguish between two main philosophies and explore ethical principles. (Those interested in studying ethical theory in greater depth are recommended to read Gillon 1986, Seedhouse 1988 and Beauchamp & Childress 1989.)

Deontology is derived from the Greek word *deon*, meaning 'duty' and is sometimes referred to as rights- or duty-based ethics – that what matters most is that a person acts according to a perceived duty and intends that some good should come about. Central to the philosophy of deontology is the idea that to be moral a person must perform his or her ordained duty. In its purest or most extreme form a deontologist would always do what was perceived as the 'right' action, regardless of the consequences. Tell the absolute and unvarnished truth and be damned to the consequences is one example of this duty-based philosophy, which can cause considerable harm.

The best-known proponent of deontology was Immanuel Kant, an 18th-century German philosopher (a devout Christian), who identified what he referred to as the 'categorical imperative' or moral law – categorical because it admits no exceptions and is absolutely binding, and imperative because there are instructions on how one should act. 'To duty every other motive must give place because duty is a condition of will good in itself whose worth transcends everything' (Kant 1964). Kant considered that an action only had moral worth if a person who had a 'good will' carried it out and that a person only has a good will if a moral duty based on a valid rule is the only motive of action. The concept of a valid moral rule was presumably based upon the biblical Ten Commandments; deontology thus has its roots in Judo-Christianity. One should always take the right option regardless of the good or harm it might do.

Deontology aims to establish universal standards of justice and embodies ultimate principles such as truth-telling and promise-keeping. One could not argue that such principles are less than admirable, and deontology has many strengths. Most importantly, this philosophy embraces respect for persons: it is always wrong to treat people as if they were mere objects to be used to further one's own ends. Deontology therefore rejects the concept that the end justifies the means and will not allow minorities to be disadvantaged for the sake of the majority. Deontology also addresses the question of what *ought* to be done. It is very comforting to be able to apply a universal moral rule, but even the right to life is not absolute and who decides, when two Christian countries are at war, which side is right? No doubt priests for both sides send the respective armies off with prayers that good will triumph over evil and God will protect the right side! Which raises the question of which rights are moral rights? How can one trace the route from abstract first principles to determine policies, practices and ways of life? With regard to healthcare practice, how can such rigid principles be adhered to? The process of socialisation and the needs of the society in which we live affect moral codes and ideologies. Is it possible to adhere to a philosophy based on Judo-Christian moral rules in today's multiracial, multicultural society?

The other major philosophy is teleology, derived from the Greek word *telos* meaning 'ends', in other words 'the ends justify the means'. This philosophy is also referred to as consequentialism and ethical dilemmas are resolved by consideration of the consequences of an action rather than its inherent goodness; actions are right or wrong according to the outcome. Consequentialism is based on the concept that value, pleasure, friendship, knowledge or health are the goals of any society. The most prominent consequentialist theory is utilitarianism. Utilitarians maintain that the moral rightness of actions is that they should create the greatest benefit for society as a whole. Utilitarianism does not always assume that there are morally 'right' actions. A person ought always to act in such a way that will produce the greatest balance of good over evil – 'the greatest good for the greatest number' or what is most useful is right, hence use of the term 'utility'. A major strength of this philosophy is that all options can be evaluated and the best outcomes identified.

Decisions are focused on the results of actions so that the philosophy is forward-looking; whatever dilemma presents (and with increasing technological advances there will always be new ethical dilemmas) the results of actions can be set down and the best possible option decided before action is taken. One problem with this philosophy is that it can allow for cost benefit evaluations and one can see the potential for harm in healthcare, which may become routinised, especially when considering allocation of scarce resources. The rule of utility may create an excess of good over evil for the population as a whole but consideration of maximising good for the majority could result in a proportion of the population being disadvantaged, so the potential for discrimination exists.

In order to avoid the pitfalls of advocating either deontology or utilitarianism as providing the answer to all ethical dilemmas David Seedhouse (1988) has devised a tool which he calls the Ethical Grid. This grid uses concepts from both philosophies but also incorporates four well known ethical principles: autonomy, beneficence, nonmaleficence and justice, first espoused by Beauchamp & Childress (1989) and used thereafter by many philosophers and medical ethicists. The principles have been taken from medical ethical codes, notably the Hippocratic Oath; the explanations are therefore couched in terms of doctor–patient relationships but the concepts can be widely applied to all health-professional–client interactions. Before consideration of the ethical grid these four principles will be outlined.

THE PRINCIPLE OF AUTONOMY

Autonomy is derived from two Greek words, *autos* ('self') and *nomos* ('rule, governance or law'; Beauchamp & Childress 1989). So the literal meaning is 'self-rule'. Autonomy is also defined as self-determination. Gillon (1991) defines autonomy as 'the capacity to think, decide and act on the basis of such thought and decision freely and independently and without let or hindrance' (p. 60). Creating and respecting autonomy, Seedhouse (1988) considers, is at the very heart of healthcare. To respect a person's autonomy

means respecting the decisions they make about themselves even though you may disagree with them. There can be no autonomy where pressure or coercion are used to gain consent to a procedure (immunisation, for example). It has been suggested that 'it must be the right of every grown human being to be foolish if that is what he or she chooses to be' (Matthews 1986). Matthews maintains that however foolish a physician considers the decisions of any person to be with regard to their healthcare, the doctor has no right to override those decisions. Matthews uses the analogy of a garage mechanic who may inform him that his car brakes are in a dangerous condition but has no right to take the car away in order to repair it against his expressed wishes. For a person to exercise his autonomy he must be treated with respect. If you feel that you have the right to make decisions for yourself, e.g. what to wear, what to eat, where to send your child to school, where to live, then you should respect others' decisions about their life and how they live it. One problem that health professionals have is that, because they have a certain amount of expertise due to their education and training, they sometimes assume that they know what is best for their patient/client. Provided that there are no defects in autonomy, if full information is given then the decision must rest with the individual, galling though that may be if we disagree.

One problem for the health practitioner is in deciding when autonomy is impaired, or not desired. It is possible to respect autonomy by not disclosing all to the patient/client who has expressed a desire not to be informed. In this case if the patient has autonomously decided to let the doctor make any decision and has expressly stated that s/he does not want to be given distressing news, then health professionals clearly would not be respecting the patient's autonomy if they insisted on telling them all the facts. Harris (1985) disagrees with this opinion and argues that it is doubtful whether the patient possesses a 'right' not to be told; he maintains that there are all sorts of unpleasant things in life that we do not want to be informed about but this does not mean that we have a right not to be informed about them. He does concede that it is a difficult area to discuss, but maintains that it is very clear that people do have a right to be told if they expressly wish it. Harris also considers that consent should not be 'once and for all' and that we have an obligation to keep seeking consent whenever the circumstances change.

Competence, or rather lack of it, is the reason given for overriding patient/client autonomy. But what do we understand by competence? When is a person judged not to be competent? Harris (1985) sets down what he terms defects in autonomy. These he maintains, occur when an individual's autonomy is undermined and diminished by four different kinds of defect. Firstly, there are defects in the individual's ability to control desires or actions, as in mental illness or when under the influence of drugs or medication. A second way in which there may be defects in reasoning is uncritical acceptance of traditional views ('my mother and grandmother told me that the best way to keep the baby from crying was to put a dab of honey on a dummy – and it works'), prejudice or 'gut' reaction, and beliefs that have no foundation in fact ('my grandfather smoked 60 cigarettes a day and died at 95, so why should I stop?'). The third defect is in the information received: it may be false or incomplete, even deliberate deception, or there may be lack of adequate understanding or comprehension. The fourth defect Harris calls defects in stability. He points out that our likes, dislikes and values alter over time and that decisions made when we are young may be regretted later in life. This excuse is often used to overrule autonomy –'you are wrong and I know what is best and you will thank me later when you realise this' – sound familiar? The only true justification for ever overriding autonomy is where there is the risk or likelihood of substantial harm to third persons. Unfortunately, health professionals are often guilty of acting paternalistically. Paternalism, sometimes referred to as parentalism means, as the word implies, behaving like a father or parent. Paternalism, Tschudin & Marks-Maran (1993) maintain, is not only the province of doctors, maternalism is alive and well within the nursing profession, therefore parentalism is

perhaps a more accurate word to use. Parentalism means treating patients or clients like children (for their own good) and so overruling autonomy by invoking the next ethical principle, that of beneficence.

THE PRINCIPLE OF BENEFICENCE

The principle of doing your best for others is embodied in the Hippocratic Oath: 'I will prescribe regimen for the good of my patients according to my ability and judgement ... in every house where I come I will enter only for the good of my patients'. It is easy to see how the desire to do what is best for the patient/client can result in paternalistic decisions. As with the principle of autonomy the principle of beneficence is not absolute. The price of doing good must not be too high and taking the autonomy of the client into consideration is paramount. Doing what is best then depends upon consideration of the principle of autonomy and the next principle, sometimes referred to by the Latin tag *primum non nocere* – 'above all, do no harm'. Perhaps this principle should be given a higher priority, since much harm can be done by the enthusiastic practitioner intending only beneficence.

THE PRINCIPLE OF NON-MALEFICENCE

Like the principle of beneficence, this principle may well have its origins in the Hippocratic Oath, which requires doctors to 'abstain from whatever is deleterious or mischievous'. The first conflict that occurs when considering this principle is that many interventions do harm in that they may cause pain, but the intention is that a greater good will result. An obvious example is public health medicine, where the greater good of society is considered above the needs of the individual (a typical utilitarian standpoint). Take, for instance, vaccination and immunisation, where the procedure is painful and the risk of an adverse reaction is considered to be justified in order to convey 'herd' immunity and protect the population at large. With this principle there is a moral obligation to weigh the expected bad effects of any intervention against the intended good effects. There is also a need to consider autonomy as a component of non-maleficence since the concept of what is harmful is intensely personal.

THE PRINCIPLE OF JUSTICE

There is some controversy as to whether this principle can be applied in ethical debate. Justice implies that there should be fairness or equity; the dictionary states that to be just is to be fair or impartial in action or judgement or awarding what is due. With the current management of NHS provision it is difficult to see how justice can be applied to the population as a whole. There is considerable disparity in allocation of resources and the quality of the service differs according to where you live and sometimes according to the whim of the medical consultant, who decides on the type of treatment on offer (as in breast cancer, for example). The concept of 'to each according to his need' was the principle upon which the NHS was set up in 1948. Since then the cost of healthcare continues to rise, demand is infinite and yet resources are finite, so rationing is a reality. How can there be justice where rationing exists? Be that as it may, it is still incumbent upon all health professionals to treat clients with equity.

DAVID SEEDHOUSE'S ETHICAL GRID

The theories and principles outlined above are by no means exhaustive. There are a plethora of opinions; many of them conflict with one another. It was in an attempt to improve on moral reasoning and aid ethical decision-making that Seedhouse devised his ethical grid (Seedhouse 1988).

According to Seedhouse, we are constantly faced with a range of choice that shape our destiny – we may have our paths limited by what we have done already, by our talents, our education and the historical era in which we exist. But we always have a choice about what to do, what to believe, how to act towards others and what to say. It therefore becomes vital,

Seedhouse states, that health workers not only speak of 'positive health' and 'empowering' but also act according to richer ideas rather than according to the tenets of the old, medically dominated paradigm. A person's actions, he says, are the acid test of his beliefs. It is not enough to believe that individual autonomy should be a major priority for health work – even to the extent that it should be placed above the duty to prolong life – and yet conform in practice to the latter principle.

Seedhouse has developed an instrument, which, he suggests, helps healthcare professionals to develop a powerful health work skill, which is the ability to reason morally. This tool he calls the ethical grid, suggesting that it is not a tool in the same way as a conveyor belt, for example, but rather as a spade that a gardener uses to cultivate his land. As the good gardener knows the best way to use a spade, so, Seedhouse suggests, the healthcare professional will understand the best way to use the grid in order to get the best out of the situation. One needs to understand that the end results are never entirely predictable and that even the most conscientious use of the grid may not produce the most practical results.

There are four different layers to the grid, which Seedhouse has identified by the use of different colours – blue, red, green and black – to aid differentiation. Each of the boxes is independent and detachable. Although each box can stand independently all the boxes have strong relationships with one another.

The grid is an artificial device and is not an exact representation of the mental processes that make up moral reasoning. In order to provide a practical and accessible route into the complexity of moral reasoning, Seedhouse has separated out the layers of the grid and distinguished each layer by the use of colour.

Four distinct layers of the grid are shown in order to show that at least four different sets of elements make up comprehensive ethical deliberation. As Seedhouse maintains, a deliberation that examines only the consequences of actions, or only the law, or only duties, might happen to produce good results on occasion but it will not be a deliberation carried through with integrity. Deliberations made in the context of health work should always acknowledge at least one box from the blue layer, since, according to Seedhouse, the need to create and respect autonomy is at the very heart of healthcare.

Seedhouse maintains that the Ethical Grid can improve moral reasoning, but it cannot take its place. The responsibility, he says, lies with the user and not with the grid. In ethical reflection much depends upon personal values, preferences and mode of thought of each individual and these cannot be represented graphically. Seedhouse states that each box cannot be considered in isolation, inevitably all the other factors listed in the grid will have to be taken into account. To take a box on its own, without considering the boxes in other layers, Seedhouse maintains is both hollow and impractical.

The blue layer

Within this layer appear four boxes. Each box clearly represents the principle of autonomy by the provisos that one should create autonomy, respect autonomy, respect persons equally and serve needs first. These, according to Seedhouse, represent the basic principles behind health work. The blue layer is set at the centre of the grid since it provides the core rationale, the notions that make up the richest idea of health. To create and respect autonomy is essential for the creation of full personhood. To serve needs before wants and respect persons equally is essential for basic personhood. Associated ideas of enablement, personhood and enhancing potential are more likely to produce benefits that can be shared by all than any other option.

The red layer

This layer focuses on duties and motives. It adheres strongly to deontological principles. The layer includes the consideration of duties during moral deliberation. The four boxes are: minimise harm, do the most positive good, tell the truth and keep promises. In addition to a requirement to adhere to moral duties the red layer also invokes the principle of nonmaleficence (minimise harm) and beneficence (do the most positive good).

The green layer

This part of the grid states that one should consider what action will have the most beneficial outcome for the patient, most beneficial outcome for society, most beneficial outcome for a particular group and finally the most beneficial outcome for oneself. This last adjunct allows for consideration of one's personal values. This layer, as can be seen, considers the general nature of the outcome and focuses on various aspects of consequentialism, i.e. the necessity to consider the consequences of any proposed intervention. It encourages reflection about whether the 'good' (specified in advance) is increased for humanity or society as a whole, for a particular group, for an individual or for the agent him/herself. While focusing on outcomes, this layer is not strongly utilitarian in that there is consideration of the most beneficial outcome for oneself and the individual. It adheres almost entirely to the principle of beneficence. It is in this layer that conflicts of interest can arise. Increase of social good will rightly take priority over individual good in cases of danger to others, e.g. the individual with homicidal tendencies or the HIV-positive individual determined to spread the virus far and wide.

An example of conflict when using this layer occurs in cases of child abuse. The boxes 'increase of benefit for self' and 'best outcome for society' may not be considered, or alternatively they may. For example, removing the child to a place of safety may result in family disintegration or the family may benefit by the intervention. Would the best outcome be to remove the abuser? The decision will be affected by many factors, including the family dynamics, and the health visitor is often involved in the case conference to decide which is the best outcome.

The black layer

This is the layer of practicality and contains the pertinent practical features. As such, it is plainly the layer which is the most utilitarian. This layer contains external constraints, which include legal rights. It could be said that in the real world this layer contains the most important factors of all and may effectively take the decision about what to do out of the hands of the healthcare professional. The layer requires consideration of: resources available, effectiveness and efficiency of action, the risk, codes of practice, the degree of certainty of the evidence on which action is taken, disputed facts, the law, and wishes of others. One could argue that, through consideration of disputed facts, effectiveness and efficiency of action, together with the law and wishes of others, this layer also supports the principle of justice.

The ethical grid is simply a tool; used competently it can help make certain tasks easier but it cannot direct the tasks, nor can it help decide which tasks are the most important. The grid cannot replace moral reasoning; the responsibilities, Seedhouse (1988) states, lie with the user and not with the grid.

HEALTH SCREENING

Health screening forms a large part of the health visitor's role. Ethical dilemmas regarding health screening have been, and still are, the subject of fierce debate. The rationale for health screening is that it will be of ultimate benefit to the recipient. It is generally perceived to be 'a good thing to do'. Prevention of ill-health by detecting disease at the early, presymptomatic stage, before the disease process has caused irredeemable damage, is an admirable philosophy and one with which most healthcare practitioners would agree. Advocates of health screening claim that through early diagnosis the condition is cheaper to treat and the outcome more likely to be successful. Another popular belief is that there are only two possible outcomes of screening – benefit or no effect.

This has not always been the case: the earliest recorded health screening was in a brothel in Avignon in France in 1347. This was clearly for the benefit of the clients only – if one considers the lack of effective treatment for venereal disease at that time, this screening certainly could not have benefited the recipients. Early preventative medicine was synonymous with medical policing and screening for disease was initially used as a sieve to separate the healthy and useful from the weak and useless. This latter use, it could be argued, is still a reason for carrying out pre-employment screening, at least as far as the employer is concerned.

In 1973, Sackett looked at motives for carrying out health screening and came up with three: to influence the gamble of life insurance, to protect third parties – as in public health screening – and to do the patient some good. It can be seen from the order in which these are set down that doing good appears to be low on the priority list.

As far back as 1968 Wilson & Jungner laid down a set of principles for presymptomatic screening that are still applicable today: the condition should be serious with a recognisable early stage; early treatment should be available and of more benefit than later; there should be a suitable test that is acceptable to the population; the chance of physical or psychological harm should be less than the chance of benefit; and finally the cost of the programme should be balanced against the benefit it provides. The current literature available would suggest that these criteria are not always adhered to.

Downie & Calman (1989) identify four main areas of concern with health screening: the false-negative test, which could lead to a false sense of security and may lead the practitioner into unjustified reassurance, which will doubly disadvantage the person when the true facts emerge; the false-positive test, which creates unnecessary anxiety that is not always resolved; ineffective treatment for the condition (hence the reluctance among the medical profession to test routinely for HIV positivity, despite pressure from interested bodies such as insurance companies); and the high-risk groups who usually fail to attend for screening. The last group are already disadvantaged as they invariably have low socioeconomic status.

Shickle & Chadwick (1994) point out that, as well as the problems inherent in false-positive and false-negative results, there are also costs with true-positive and true-negative results. A true-positive result is beneficial in that earlier treatment is more likely to be effective and improve the prognosis, usually less invasive and cheaper. There are also advantages of the sick role, for example, being excused social responsibilities. However, the costs could be stigmatisation, anxiety (the worried ill) and the possibility of living longer with the diagnosis. True-negative results, Shickle & Chadwick maintain, may legitimise an 'unhealthy' lifestyle. If a negative result is given without explanation or advice then there is a risk of reinforcing an unhealthy lifestyle, bolstering a pre-existing sense of invulnerability and making participants less likely to return for subsequent testing. Duncan (1990) suggests that it is very difficult to measure the benefits of screening since there is no clear causal link between risk factors and ill-health and no guarantee that screening will lead to health improvement.

What are the unwanted ill-health effects of screening? Should clients be informed that they are at high risk of developing a particular illness or disease? The principle of beneficence might lead one to consider that it should be of benefit, either by more effective treatment through early intervention or by changing to a healthier, less risky lifestyle. Alternatively it could be argued that the increased awareness of mortality and anxieties raised by positive results (false or otherwise) is diametrically opposed to the principle of nonmaleficence. What evidence is there to support this supposition? Stoate (1989) cites an earlier example from Haynes et al (1978) that illustrates 'that the labelling of previously undiagnosed hypertensives, detected by screening in the work place, results in increased absenteeism from work' and argues that detecting abnormalities may have significant costs to the patient. Stoate also maintains that systematic screening may result in making people more aware of their mortality and increase hypochondria, which could lead to greater psychological distress. This viewpoint is also supported by Marteau (1989), who reports that high levels of anxiety are experienced by people participating in many screening programmes. Marteau (1990) states that anxiety is not only an undesirable effect in

itself but also has a 'knock on' effect on physical health, increasing consultation rates while at the same time reducing the patient's ability to recall or act on any advice given. It may also be argued that costs are increased, as many doctors prescribe expensive medication for anxiety, which may not have occurred had the screening not been available. Marteau also discusses a study concerning a group of pregnant women with false alpha-fetoprotein results, who were found to be significantly more anxious 3 weeks later, when subsequent testing had shown the fetuses to be unaffected, than women who had originally received a negative result.

Peter Skrabanek (1990) uses several examples to voice his concern: the tragedy of a trial for clofibrate, a drug that lowers blood cholesterol, in which more healthy men treated with clofibrate died than the controls. It is unlikely that the men were fully informed of the danger from this drug before participating in the trial. Skrabanek also cites the case against screening for hypertension and states: 'The effects of such labelling are serious: they include the erosion of the sense of well-being, lowered sense of self-esteem, marital problems, reduction in earning power, and the adoption of a "sick role" in a previously healthy person' (Skrabanek 1990).

Women are a particularly vulnerable group (Skrabanek 1990): pressure is put on them to undergo regular gynaecological examinations. Cervical cytology is one screening procedure that is considered worthwhile and has been well documented but even so there is disparity in the service offered depending on where you live. Some areas of the country have such poor funding that it can be as long as 3 months before the results are known, with all the attendant worry and anxiety that is incurred until the all-clear is received. Breast screening is another doubtful area: risks include unnecessary surgery and needle biopsy. One claim is that for each woman who benefits from screening, 18 women have to live longer with the knowledge of their incurable disease because of earlier diagnosis (Marteau 1989). There is pressure on women to attend for breast screening and the implication is that if you attend the outcome will be good

(Roberts 1989) – this is by no means necessarily so. There is no empirical evidence that treatment is successful; different surgeons will carry out different procedures and the current strongly implied statement that everything will be all right if women present themselves for screening is therefore unacceptable. Skrabanek (1990) also considers that breast self-examination is unlikely to reduce mortality from breast cancer, because by the time the tumour is palpable it will have been growing for a long time, and that it could be argued that self-examination is actually harmful, particularly for younger women, because it leads to unnecessary anxiety, with surgical and medical intervention.

Developmental screening, one could maintain, is the raison d'être of health visitors. Although the health visitor role has been extended and expanded, historically, it was concern about the neonatal and infant mortality and poor child health of those in lower socioeconomic classes that led to the original inception of the health visitor. The intention of developmental screening, as with all screening procedures, is adhering to the principle of beneficence with early identification of health problems. Hearing tests are of proven value: early identification of hearing problems can prevent communication difficulties, especially with the development of speech. So with this particular test Wilson & Jungner's (1968) principle that effective treatment is available is met. What of other tests? In some areas they are still being carried out routinely despite the Hall (1996) recommendations. Where a mother knows that a screening test is being carried out there is bound to be a certain amount of anxiety and tension that the child will pass.

If there is some slight concern on the part of the health visitor that there may be a problem, what is s/he to do? The Ethical Grid advocates truth-telling, and sharing and openness is vital to ensure trust between health visitor and client. The principle of beneficence and nonmaleficence could be in conflict here. Will more harm result by sharing your concerns and creating anxiety or should you decide not to mention your worries and risk being accused of secrecy (or even negligence) at a later date? Where routine tests are not

carried out but the health visitor remains vigilant and merely observes the young child's developmental progress, when should delays in achieving milestones be shared with the parent? If the parent is not aware that the child's progress is being monitored, does that alter one's responsibilities? Even the most sensitive handling of the situation will be likely to create anxieties. Once the decision has been made that a referral is necessary, then telling the parent is much easier: a problem has been identified and a solution proposed. It is not so easy when the evidence is not clear and the feeling that all is not well is intuitive only. The dilemma is at what stage concern should be verbalised. It has been demonstrated by the literature (Marteau 1989, Skrabanek 1990) that significant psychological harm can occur through false-positive tests. Labelling a child as having slow cognitive development, for example, could impact on that child's future, particularly when starting school. The teaching staff may have low expectations of the child's ability. The health visitor may well keep the information confidential, but the client may be so worried that other family members or friends may be told. The parent may even tell other professionals what the health visitor has told them.

The Human Genome Project, currently being undertaken in several countries, including the UK, will provide data on genetic susceptibility to disease. When genetic monitoring is available, will pressure be put on 'at-risk' groups? Where a history exists of Huntington's chorea, will family members be coerced into taking the test? Will health visitors be encouraged to promote genetic screening in much the same way that they are encouraged to gain consent to immunisations? Which is worse, living with the possibility that you might get the disease, or living with the certain knowledge that you will? Knowledge of carrying the defective gene could lead to eradicating certain conditions within a couple of generations; however the evidence is that the majority would prefer to live with the uncertainty. In a survey carried out in 1990 (Hatchwell 1992), most people (86%) would not take the test and 15% of those studied said that if the test was positive they would consider suicide.

If mandatory genetic screening is introduced, there are considerable resource implications for provision of counselling and support. Health visitors already carry considerable caseloads; what will be the impact on health visiting practice of introducing genetic screening?

Where health screening is offered on a voluntary basis, or even implicitly suggested as beneficial, the uptake will be by self-selection. These individuals are therefore not a representative cross-section of the population and are likely to be of a higher socio-economic status, better educated and more health-conscious that non-participants. This raises the question of whether health screening is 'just' or 'fair'. Clearly, imposed screening procedures are unjust in that they take away an individual's autonomy.

Health screening contains many ethical dilemmas. The principle of justice is not adhered to, particularly when there is a bias towards self-selection, which excludes many within the population who are at risk. Beneficence is often outweighed by the harmful effects of false-positive results, which cause anxiety and fear. Certainly it can be argued that, where research has demonstrated that there is no suitable and successful treatment available, screening for disease is positively detrimental and gives longer 'sickness years'. There is also conflict in respecting the autonomy of the individual. It has been suggested that screening militates against respect and freedom of choice, thus reducing autonomy.

IMMUNISATION AND VACCINATION

One of the most powerful weapons in preventing ill-health and promoting health is vaccination against infectious diseases. Immunisation meets utilitarian principles of creating the greatest good for the greatest number. The more children that are vaccinated the greater the 'herd' immunity. That smallpox has been eradicated from this country has been attributed to successful campaigns for vaccination in infancy. Therefore immunisation is ethically beneficial – or is it?

Even smallpox efficacy is not totally supported by the facts. The Vaccination Act 1871 made smallpox vaccination compulsory, with over 90%

vaccination rates achieved. Because of the strength of the anti-vaccination lobby the compulsory nature of the system was modified in 1898, when subsequent legislation allowed for a principle of conscientious objection, although parents had to appear before two justices or stipendary magistrates and convince them of their belief that vaccination would be bad for their children's health. A further Act in 1907 relaxed the compulsory nature even further by making the parents' declaration before one magistrate or justice of the peace sufficient (Ottewill & Wall 1990). From 1905–18 the rates of smallpox vaccination fell. One might expect that the incidence of smallpox cases would correspondingly rise, but this was not the case. The trend of reported cases was downwards; severe cases were few and the out-breaks that did occur were mainly due to imported cases that had managed to evade port sanitary authorities (Frazer 1950, cited in Ottewill & Wall 1990). It may well be that the fall in smallpox incidence had more to do with improved standards of hygiene and nutrition than smallpox vaccination. However, smallpox vaccination has historically been credited with eradication of the disease from Britain.

Thus vaccination was perceived as a beneficent intervention and opened the door for subsequent vaccines to be developed. Since smallpox vaccination was initiated, vaccination against other diseases followed. Diphtheria vaccination grew in importance during the 1940s and in 1946 the National Health Service Act repealed all previous legislation concerning vaccination and immunisation. Compulsion was removed in respect of smallpox vaccination and vaccination against diphtheria was specifically included. Section 26 of the 1946 Act allowed local health authorities to make similar provisions against any other disease. Thus in 1955 tetanus and poliomyelitis were classified as immunisable diseases and in 1957 were joined by pertussis. Despite BCG being available in the 1940s and, considering the limited treatment options for tuberculosis at that time, it is surprising that it was not until 1956 that this vaccine was given to school children routinely. All these diseases were life-threatening and also had severe complications, leaving those affected with a range of disabilities (provided they survived). So one could argue that vaccination has been one of the most successful methods of preventing ill-health since the Second World War. But since the 1950s vaccines have been developed for diseases in which, while unpleasant, the severe complications of death and disability are comparatively rare. If these vaccines were free from side-effects then there would be little controversy, but unfortunately there are concerns that the vaccines themselves are not without risk. This raises the dilemma for many as to which carries the most benefit and which has the potential for most harm – a direct conflict between the principles of beneficence and non-maleficence. Should one consider the most beneficial outcome for society or the most beneficial outcome for the individual?

The measles vaccine was developed during the 1960s; rubella for 11–14-year-old girls followed from 1970. Since then the triple vaccine, measles, mumps and rubella (MMR) has been developed and is routinely offered to children in their second year.

During the 1970s pertussis vaccine was suspected of causing brain damage in susceptible children. The media attention created a scare that resulted in a dramatic fall in vaccination rates for pertussis, with a corresponding rise in the incidence of whooping cough. Most of the evidence supporting the argument for brain damage was based on anecdotal case studies, according to Nicoll et al (1998). Nicoll et al cite a national study carried out by Miller et al (1993), which found that there was a temporal association with encephalopathy but that the risk of lasting damage was so rare as to be unquantifiable. It is interesting to note, however, that encephalopathy is still listed as a side-effect of the pertussis vaccine in a table produced for the National Vaccine Injury Compensation Program (Health Resources and Service Administration 1997), which presumably means that vaccine-induced encephalopathy resulting in lasting brain damage is recognised in the USA if not in Britain.

Currently, there are concerns regarding the MMR vaccine; most recently the onset of autism has been attributed to this vaccine. Wakefield et al (1998) carried out a study of 12 children who had been vaccinated with MMR, of whom nine had been diagnosed as autistic. All 12 children had developed normally prior to having the MMR vaccine and subsequently all developed intestinal disorders. In eight of the cases the parents or the child's GP said that the changes in behaviour and health followed the MMR vaccination. Wakefield concedes that his research has failed to prove empirically that there is a link, however, he considers that there is sufficient evidence to justify an independent government review. Due to his concern that multicomponent vaccines may overload the immune system of some infants, Wakefield also recommended that the vaccines should be given separately at yearly intervals. The media attention that followed the publication of this article in *The Lancet* resulted in such an increase in parents requesting the separate vaccines that supplies ran out.

Publication of this article released a storm of protest from the medical profession. Letters to the *British Medical Journal* in response to Wakefield's article in *The Lancet* pointed out the value of the vaccine. Young (1998) challenged the methodology of Wakefield et al's research: a cohort of only 12 subjects certainly raises questions about bias and validity. Caldwell (1998) considers that the MMR vaccine has prevented thousands of sick children, thus reducing GPs' workloads, reducing sleepless nights (the GPs', presumably!) and eliminating stress for parents. In a subsequent editorial in the *British Medical Journal*, Nicoll et al (1998) argue that over 600 000 British children receive MMR in their second year, and that since this is the age at which autism typically manifests itself it is likely that some cases will appear shortly after vaccination, and that this is a mere chance association and not a causal link. Kiln (1998) asks why the expert committee convened by the Medical Research Council to investigate Wakefield's findings failed to include general practitioners, health visitors and practice nurses, who have day-to-day experience of the MMR vaccines. Kiln states that what is required is straightforward figures to help parents understand why their child should have the vaccine.

How can parents get accurate information? The medical profession takes a utilitarian stance and encourages immunisation on the grounds of achieving herd immunity. What of other health professionals? In a study carried out in Leeds (Hatton 1990), an audit of the knowledge of health professionals (which included health visitors) of contraindications to the MMR vaccine was carried out. The results were somewhat alarming. Some health professionals, it appeared, would happily give the vaccine to children when it was contraindicated. Other health professionals were applying the contra-indications of the pertussis vaccine to MMR and some would not give the vaccine even when there were no valid contra-indications to its use. How can parents decide when there appears to be confusion and, it would appear, a lack of knowledge among those who should be well informed?

Dyson (1995) argues that infectious diseases such as whooping cough have declined in the context of particular historical and social conditions and persist in the context of particular types of social inequality, and that the respective risks of the vaccine and the disease are still unresolved owing to methodological limitations of studies on both sides of the argument. Dyson also questions the questionable ethics of one-sided health campaigns. This is supported by a letter from a parent to the magazine *Health Matters*, who considers that the decision whether or not to vaccinate a child can only be made when all the information is made available, not just that supplied by the Health Education Authority (Easy 1995).

Sadly, information is difficult to come by: on searching the Internet it is clear that most anti-vaccination information comes from nonmedical sources and as such is denigrated by doctors and epidemiologists. Information from the medical profession highlights the rarity of suspected side-effects and points out the benefits of the vaccine, putting the emphasis on the likelihood of increased death rates and other serious complications should parents stop having their children vaccinated. Begg et al (1998) provide a graph demonstrating how deaths from measles have decreased in the UK (as a result, of course, of increased vaccination rates), as opposed to Italy and France. Total death rates in other European countries may be affected by other socio-economic factors. The graph demonstrates that the death rate from measles fell from 4 during the period 1986–88 and 4 during 1989–91 to 2 for the period 1992–94 but no mention is made of adverse reactions to the vaccine. The Centers for Disease Control (January 1999) list the complications of measles: ear infection, pneumonia, seizures, brain damage and death, with no information as to the incidence of these. Similarly, for mumps the complications of ear infection, meningitis and painful swollen testicles are listed without incidence data. As one might expect from a service devoted to disease control, the benefits of the vaccine are emphasised. On discussing the risks of the vaccines, prevalence figures are provided for all the milder side-effects, e.g. a fever of 103°F or higher 5–15 per 100 doses, but for seizures, severe allergic reactions or coma only the comment that they are rare is made. Surely an official source should provide the actual incidence rates for the more serious side-effects in order that parents may make a fully informed choice?

It appears that vaccination will create the most beneficial outcome for society as a whole but is it the most beneficial outcome for the individual? There is strong opposition from the medical fraternity to the idea that vaccines are dangerous, but it needs to be borne in mind that much of the outcry comes from public health physicians and epidemiologists, who are concerned with controlling epidemics of infectious disease. Calman (ITN News 1998) advocated that it is vital that parents continue to give their consent to vaccinate their children. Calman was the government's Chief Medical Officer and had a wider brief, that of protecting society. No surprise then that he took the utilitarian standpoint of the greatest good for the greatest number and was prepared to risk what is considered to be a small minority of children. General practitioners receive remuneration for every child vaccinated at their practice; a considerable fall in vaccination uptake will essentially result in reduced income. This must be a consideration, however many altruistic reasons are given for encouraging parents into giving consent for vaccination. Pilgrim & Rogers (1995) argue that the financial inducements given to GPs to meet immunisation targets have reinforced suppression of the right to parental dissent and that some families are being removed from GP lists in order to maintain target levels. In terms of financial gain, the pharmaceutical companies that produce these vaccines also have a vested interest in continuing their manufacture. If they could be proved to be safe, there would be no ethical dilemma about advocating their use, but there seems to be a coyness about revealing the actual incidence of brain damage resulting from vaccines.

If the various parts of Seedhouse's Ethical Grid (1988) are applied to the dilemma of vaccination, several conflicts appear. In the blue layer, health professionals cannot create or respect autonomy if they themselves lack sufficient information, and in any case the recipients are young children who are not able to make an informed choice for themselves. The medical profession would argue that they are serving needs first, but whose needs? The red or duty-based layer states, 'tell the truth', but what is the truth in respect of vaccines? Can the health visitor truthfully state that there are no risks from the MMR vaccination? Doctors would maintain that vaccination does the most positive good and that they are minimising harm by reducing the incidence of these three diseases, but would the parent of a damaged child feel the same way? The consequentialist green layer would appear to support vaccination, but then it is the utilitarian layer of the grid. The only conflict could arise when there was an adverse reaction to MMR: then clearly the most beneficial outcome for the patient could not be claimed. Consideration of the boxes in the black layer of practicality highlights the conflicts in using the grid. Disputed facts, the degree of certainty of the evidence on which action is taken, the effectiveness and efficiency of action and the risk all need to be taken into account.

Much of the information about brain damage is accused of being anecdotal, is reported by parents or other nonprofessionals, and therefore lacks scientific validity. If this is the case, then why does encephalopathy manifesting between 5 and 15 days following administration of the vaccine appear as a side-effect not only of pertussis vaccine but also of MMR (Health Resources and Service Administration 1997). Compensation is paid to parents in the USA if this is proved. It is difficult to believe that compensation would be paid out without sound empirical evidence. Is there any validity in Wakefield's (1998) claim that multicomponent vaccines overload the immature immune system? Multicomponent vaccines are popular with health officials because they require fewer clinic visits (Day 1998), thus saving costs. But if multicomponent vaccines increase the risk of side-effects, then, in the long term, separate vaccinations may be more cost-effective by reducing side-effects and encouraging increased immunisation rates. What none of the debates in the literature seem to address is that measles vaccine was given on its own for many years before the MMR vaccine was developed. There was no public outcry about adverse reaction to immunisation against measles before the triple vaccine was introduced. The other suspect vaccine, pertussis, is also given as part of a multicomponent vaccine. Might Wakefield et al (1998) be right?

Pilgrim & Rogers (1995) consider that immunisation policies are driven by propaganda that reviews advantages and disadvantages of vaccination or non-vaccination, and that this is deceitful and simplistic. Natural acquired immunity is better than artificially acquired immunity. How effective are these vaccines? How long will the protection last? If a child gets the disease as a young adult will the effects be worse? Will a vaccine-resistant strain develop? These are all questions that need to be addressed before full information can be given to parents. Seedhouse (1988) considers that creating and respecting autonomy is the core rationale behind health work and conveys the richest notion of health. A component of autonomy is the need for full information. How can autonomy be created or respected and a fully autonomous decision be made if some information is withheld? As Easy (1995) pointed out, since parents are asked to give consent to vaccination, they must also take full responsibility for the subsequent effects of that vaccination. One should not expect to take on responsibility without adequate knowledge. The current market-led health service places pressures on health professionals to pursue population targets (Pilgrim & Rogers 1995). This pressure on health professionals leads them into the dangerous moral minefield of failing to respect individual autonomy.

HEALTH PROMOTION VERSUS HEALTH EDUCATION

Health education and health promotion have often been taken to mean the same thing. Both are concerned with improving health status. However, health education is a term that has fallen out of favour, since it has gained the reputation of didactic instruction rather than the sharing of knowledge, thus empowering the individual to make more informed choices about their lifestyle. Although the words have changed, has this resulted in a change in the way the health professional approaches clients?

The recent emphasis on health promotion and teaching constantly raises questions about justifiable parentalism (Benjamin & Curtis 1992). Thomas & Wainwright (1996) suggest that the approach of many nurses to health promotion has tended to be either somewhat naive or authoritarian and didactic, and that there has been little discussion in the nursing literature of ethical aspects of health promotion. Thomas & Wainwright also suggest that community nurses fall into two distinct groups in terms of their health promotion interventions: health visitors take a deontological stance whereas district nurses tend to be utilitarian in their approach. This does not mean that health visitors are more parentalistic than district nurses, for both the main ethical theories have fostered this approach. Deontologists would maintain that it is your duty to behave in a certain manner –'you ought to do this' (Tschudin & Marks-Maran 1993), whereas teleologists would consider that you should consider the consequences of your actions. How many health visitors can honestly state that they have never used the phrases 'you ought to' or 'you should not'? How far should one go

in trying to alter a client's way of living in the name of better health? What form should it take? Are exaggerated threats acceptable if nothing else proves effective? When information and advice are given, it is easy to imply that dire consequences will result if that advice is not followed. Because of the experience and knowledge held by the health professional, it is extremely difficult not to behave in a parentalist manner.

Benjamin & Curtis (1992) maintain that, in order to respect the client's personhood, health professionals must allow the client to express their views. They refer to this process as rational persuasion, i.e. appealing to another person's rational capacities in order to influence them into changing their behaviour, providing reasons and information for or against certain courses of action with a view to changing the person's beliefs without indulging in scare tactics. It is important that the person attempting to persuade recognises that the person they are debating with is their equal as a person. It is extremely frustrating to observe clients indulging in risk-taking behaviour after advising them of the potential ill-health effects, but it is better by far to respect their autonomy than explicitly or implicitly to show disapproval of their behaviour, however subtly this is done.

Traditionally, health promotion aims at changing individual behaviour by increasing knowledge: this implies that people have a free choice and does not take into account socio-economic factors. The previous government produced the document *The Health of the Nation* (Department of Health 1992) to prove their commitment to preventative medicine and promoting good health. In it they identified several areas of concern and recommended reduction of the incidence of these conditions by a certain period of time. They emphasised that health was the responsibility of the individual. This is classical victim blaming, taking the assumption that people are always responsible for their actions. Clarke (1999) warns that health professionals need to be critical of their approach to health promotion, especially with relation to the emphasis on individual responsibility. *The Health of the Nation* placed the onus on health professionals to meet these targets laid down by the government. How feasible was this?

Smoking is a good example of typical victim-blaming and a perpetual bone of contention. Smokers are denigrated by society generally. Fears of the effects of passive smoking on non-smokers has increased intolerance of smokers. Although there are conflicts as to whether passive smoke is carcinogenic or not, cigarette smoke is unpleasant and irritant to others. Employers are liable under the Health and Safety at Work Act 1974 (HSC 1974) to provide a safe environment. This includes eliminating atmospheric pollutants, which includes cigarette smoke. Many employers are imposing non-smoking policies and places of entertainment are increasing the areas where smoking is not allowed. For non-smokers this is excellent and is a good example of when overruling the autonomy of individuals (the smokers) is justified under the principle of beneficence and utilitarian principles of the greatest good for the greatest number. What it does result in, however, is an increase in victim-blaming. Smokers are perceived as weak-willed, self-indulgent and feckless; after all, the effects of smoking have been well documented since the 1950s, haven't they? There have been instances of smokers being refused cardiovascular surgery. Whereas this can be justified on clinical and utilitarian grounds, the smoker feels victimised. There is a feeling that blame is being attributed to the individual. Health-promotion activity is targeted at the smoker. Smoking is a pleasurable experience for those who smoke. Of course it is – nicotine is an addictive substance. Smokers do not want to know about the ill-health effects. Smoking is associated with social activity, naughty but nice and, in the case of under age smokers, there is the illicit thrill of indulging in a forbidden activity. Even those smokers who want to give up experience the greatest difficulty because they are addicted to the nicotine content. There is an acceptance that alcoholics are not to blame for their addiction, that drug addicts have been led astray by unscrupulous drug pushers, but it is not accepted that smokers are equally helpless in the throes of their particular addiction.

Health education campaigns have failed to affect the numbers of obese people in our society. There are ethical dilemmas in giving dietary advice, as in any aspect of health-promoting activity – that of coercion and manipulation by a parentalistic approach. A stock answer that is given time after time is that the health visitor should empower the client by providing knowledge and information. Sounds wonderful, does it not? But beware that the word 'empower' does not become a weasel word, overuse of which renders it meaningless.

The health visitor is ideally placed to encourage mothers to feed their children healthy choices, since they are available for advice on infant feeding very shortly after the mother comes home. If the advice given is successful and the baby thrives, then why are unhealthy choices given once the child is weaned? Why is the advice of the health visitor, so sought after when the child was an infant, ignored once solid foods are introduced? The lure of sweet, fatty convenience foods is too great, it would appear. Perhaps health visitors would be better advised to start a campaign to ban food advertising on television. Advice to individuals may be seen as interfering with individual autonomy, but reducing the number of advertisements could have a considerable impact on consumption of fattening goodies. Campaigning against food advertising would be the most beneficial outcome for society even if it were not the most beneficial outcome for a particular group (the food manufacturer). It would minimise harm by cutting down on obesity and do the most positive good by removing the temptation to snack between meals.

Much advice given regarding exercise is well-founded and research-based, but how ethical is it? Walking at least 15 minutes a day is commonly advocated as a way to keep healthy, lose weight and stay fit. In inner city areas, how ethical is it to encourage the daily walk, let alone jogging? The exercise may be beneficial but exercise increases the heart-rate, which increases respiration and results in more air intake. Within cities and towns the air is contaminated by many pollutants. Fresh air has always been perceived as beneficial: grandmothers may talk their daughters into believing that the baby should spend part of every day in the open air. That's fine if you live in the comparative peace of a rural area or a nice suburb with large gardens and very little traffic pollution. If, on the other hand you happen to live within 500 metres of Spaghetti Junction in Birmingham, putting the baby outside is more likely to result in lead poisoning. Basic advice, such as the daily walk, is only ethically sound advice if you live in a pollution-free area.

CONCLUSION

There is a basic assumption made by health professionals that individuals have a choice about choosing a healthy or an unhealthy lifestyle. This assumption does not consider the political and social context in which we live and, without this consideration, health promotion goals may be unrealistic and thus unethical. Social scientists highlight social inequalities in health (Townsend & Davidson 1982) as having a major effect on the efficacy of health-promoting activities. However, little has been achieved in terms of redressing the balance. Achieving change is never easy, but is not helped if there is no support from central government other than the paper exercise of *The Health of the Nation* (Department of Health 1992). Currently, achieving improved health goals is left to health professionals. There are ethical dilemmas in attempting to promote health by improving activities without changing the socio-political climate. People do not always have a choice about where they live or where they work. Access to education is restricted for certain groups within our society. Empowering clients through health promotion should consider the ability of the client to benefit from that knowledge.

13

Violence and health visiting

Anne Robotham

INTRODUCTION

Definitions of violence can be multiple, ranging from shouting to physical attack, from ostracism to cynical criticism, and victims can be of all ages and from all walks of society.

Most health visitors at one time or another have been party to acts of violence within the community in which they work. However, there is probably little education or emphasis on working within a violent society other than in relation to child abuse. Many health visitors have had dealings with women who have become 'battered wives' but most of their experience has been gained 'on the job' rather than from any form of education.

This chapter will deal specifically with health visitors undertaking a public health role in relation to violence and will explore issues relating to violence and the support that health visitors can give to both victims and (occasionally) perpetrators. This is not advocating a specific role for health visitors but helping to recognise that they are in a unique position through their work in homes and schools to detect and if possible prevent violence occurring. To do this the health visitor will use primarily the skills of providing a quiet environment in which to listen to the client, ask direct but nonthreatening questions to establish the position, give advice about support and services available and, finally, carefully document with permission.

There are variations around the country in the types of service available, but the organisation

Women's Aid covers the whole country and many inner city areas have hostels for women and children fleeing domestic violence. The housing department also has a statutory duty to house women who are made homeless by fleeing violent partners.

HISTORICAL OVERVIEW

In the early days of recorded history violence was accepted as the everyday life of the Roman citizen. Roman historians recorded about crowds of supporters at chariot races spilling into the streets and fighting, and Pliny the Younger (a commentator of the time) talks about the streets of Rome and Constantinople where gangs of 'fans' were able to 'control' areas of the cities, similarly to the way modern gangs of football supporters hold on to areas of the terraces. In addition, Roman history is full of the violence of incessant wars and the subjugation of conquered peoples (Owens & Ashcroft 1985).

The recorded history of Europe is littered with examples of extreme violence that appeared to have no political or economic purpose. There is also much evidence concerning the violence of chivalrous ritual. Ritual combat was rife during the Middle Ages and usually one or both of the combatants was killed. In France, between 1589 and 1608, no less than 8000 people were killed by sword-fighting (Owens & Ashcroft 1985).

British history records the history of government, the history of the English criminal and to some extent the history of civil law, which is the story of government's attempt to control violence between disputing individuals. In earlier times the law was used by citizens to avenge the wrong on the wrongdoer or to gain compensation for injury, whether physical or material. Today these same laws, albeit updated, are brought into play irrespective of whether the injured party wishes to use them or not, i.e. they seem to have become the means whereby society is the litigant and not the individual.

Today, illegal violence is seen as a breach of the peace rather than a crime against the individual. Since the 13th century the initiative for criminal law has passed to Parliament, and it is Parliament that is responsible for the definition of new crimes.

As Europe set about determining the 'nation state', organisations emerged to promulgate warfare and, in order to identify and protect economic states, even the Church encouraged warfare against the infidel. The involvement of such organisations, in a sense, led to an assumption of 'legal violence' as a means of protection of the state for ideological or economic reasons. As the major cause of human suffering, death and injury throughout history, warfare must be paramount.

'Modern' violence in context

Violence is not a modern phenomenon and the violence of today has parallels in history, as described above. The football hooligan differs little from the chariot-race hooligan. Violent crime rarely produces a death rate comparable to the death rate in France in the 16th century due to duelling. Violence still can occur within the law and is common within judicious processes, e.g. sentencing to lashing, or to solitary confinement. The use of 'legal' torture still occurs within 'civilised' countries.

In terms of scale, violence *in* society cannot compete with violence committed *by* society in the form of warfare.

DIFFERING PERSPECTIVES ON VIOLENCE

As can be surmised from the above the causes of violence were rationalised in the light of the potential outcomes of the episodes, whether in terms of formal Roman platoons, legitimate duels or simply bare-knuckled peasant sports. However, implicit within these is the question of root cause. History suggests that the root cause can be political, religious, physical or sociological. Modern anthropology suggests that to these must theoretically be added psychology and pathology. The following sections will explore the more relevant factors.

Hormonal influences

Considerable biological research has been undertaken on the body's hormone levels and violent behaviour. Most of this research (Rose et al 1971, Doering et al 1974) has been done in relation to the male sex hormones, or androgens. Some work has been done in relation to testosterone but it has not been conclusive. In relation to androgens animal studies (rats) have shown that castrated rats appear to be less aggressive than their unaffected peers. Injections of testosterone to raise levels significantly have shown the development of aggressive behaviour in other animals, while in humans similar studies have been inconclusive – the development of aggressive behaviour in one study was not sustained in others. Studies on premenstrual syndrome in affected women have shown a clear relationship in some women between progesterone levels and aggressive behaviour, to the extent that it has now been accepted in legal judgements that women diagnosed as suffering from premenstrual syndrome are capable of extremely aggressive acts (Owens & Ashcroft 1985)

Genetic factors

It is possible that certain abnormal chromosome patterns are responsible for aggressive behaviour. Studies on Down's syndrome children have shown that sufferers are particularly characterised by lack of aggressiveness and there may be other anomalies that show the reverse – a characterisation of aggressiveness in other chromosomal abnormalities. Owens & Ashcroft (1985) cite several studies that have concentrated on abnormalities in the pairing of the sex chromosomes; in inmates of secure mental hospitals, males with 47 chromosomes (XYY) instead of the normal 46 (XY) occur with something like 30 times the frequency of the incidence in the general population. Further studies on the male inmates of prisons have found that the XYY men are more likely to offend against property than individuals.

Studies of breeding in animals have shown that in the case of larger mammals – cows, horses, dogs – it is possible to breed for docility or aggression and similar potential may exist in humans.

Anthropological studies

Early 19th century anthropological studies on Tahitians showed the people to be very gentle and peaceable who not only disapproved of violent acts but also considered it shameful to have violent thoughts. However, Western contact changed the culture so that the same people became much more warlike. This was also observed in New Guinea with a change from the hunter-gatherer society to a settled form of food production. At an opposite extreme, some societies have been noted to have extremely warlike and aggressive tendencies. In a study of the Yanomano Indians of northern Brazil it was noted that violent behaviour could be used to express affection. A Yanomano woman, for example, would not believe that a man really loved her unless he left her scarred or bruised.

Attempts have been made to explain the violent behaviour of various groups as adaptive in terms of their individual circumstances but it is important to note that cultural factors do not provide a complete account of violence. Thus within a culture, some individuals may act in a way quite different from most of the culture's members. The existence of violent subcultures in larger societies may be a cause for concern if it is accepted that such cultures act as 'breeding grounds' for violent acts. The anthropological evidence provides some support for the notion that action should be taken to avoid the formation of such subcultures, in particular by eliminating contributory factors, e.g. poor housing, overcrowding.

In terms of a more general understanding of violence, the sociological and anthropological work provides strong evidence that a purely biological explanation is inadequate. Reactive aggression has been demonstrated in the laboratory with rats, inducing fighting in otherwise peaceful animals by exposing them to an electric current. Certain drugs appear to affect the probability of fighting in response to aversive stimulation. Seligman (1975) has also pointed out that a person who hits his/her head on a car door on entering may become furious, yelling at the passengers! The process of reactive aggression provides the beginning of a framework within which to consider the psychological aspects of violence.

The psychological perspective

Freud attempted to show that energy in some humans was directed towards a drive for death and destruction rather than the pleasures of the 'id' factor of the human personality. However, he found it impossible to validate this theory and few of his contemporaries supported him. Most of the early psychology work was directed more towards attempting to define an aggressive personality. Eysenck (1983) tried to show that a person with an extrovert personality was more likely to indulge in delinquent behaviour but he could make little distinction between crime in general and violent crime. Another researcher (Megargee 1966) came somewhat closer to explaining violence when he postulated personal 'control' He suggested that there were individuals who were 'undercontrolled', who make little or no attempt at self-control when in an aggression-induced situation. In this case these individuals would present with a history of a number of violent episodes and would be characterised by the ease with which violent behaviour could be elicited.

The second type of individual that Megargee (1966) described was the 'overcontrolled' individual, who held aggression in check in situations where most individuals would react violently. Certain individuals, it would appear, are normally nonviolent but suddenly and unexpectedly may commit an act of extreme violence, often disproportionate to the provocation. Because of their suppressed response to mild aggression, the overcontrolled individual would be more likely than the rest of us to be exposed to extended or intense provocation. Eventually, such provocation may reach a point where even the overcontrolled person's degree of self-control is inadequate and violence results. An additional

factor is introduced by the fact that the overcontrolled individual, unlike others, has little 'practice' at being violent. Most people, as a result of some practice, become quite skilled at matching their aggressive responses to the demands of the situation (violent blow to an attacking mugger but only a mild reprimand to a whinging child). Smacking children has long been an acceptable means of controlling undesirable behaviour in all cultures and social classes. Mothers have learnt from their mothers that physical punishment is an appropriate means of correcting one's child. However, there is a fine line between a corrective smack and an escalation into physical abuse. Mention has been made in Chapter 5 of recent work by End Physical Punishment of Children (EPOCH; Cook et al 1991) in raising awareness of smacking escalation and health visitors are now concerned to help mothers by offering alternative strategies for behaviour modification (see Chapter 10).

There are a number of problems with accepting the above theory because it is impossible to explain the relationship between situations and human responses in terms of overcontrol or undercontrol. Early experimental research showed that experimentally induced frustration could greatly increase aggressive behaviour (Bandura 1973). However, this does not explain how when aggression occurs it is not always possible to identify any accompanying frustration factor. Bandura (1973) showed that an alternative consequence to frustration in children was not aggression but regression.

Learned behaviour may play a part in reactive aggression, in that such aggression may be elicited by a stimulus whose aversive properties have been induced by the conditioning process. Much aggressive behaviour appears not to be elicited by any particular prior stimulus but rather to represent an attempt to obtain some subsequent goal, i.e. the behaviour appears to be more under the control of consequences than antecedents. This was seen as an operant conditioning response in Skinner's (1938) work on rats' and pigeons' responses to the need for food. Several behaviourist psychologists in the 1960s were able to show that behaviour could be shaped into more aggressive responses and that children who were victimised at nursery school could be guided into producing more aggressive responses to their attackers, thus changing their behaviour. Similarly, attacking a victim and producing responses of crying, defensiveness and submission may serve as a reinforcing stimulus for maintenance of this type of behaviour in the attacker.

Modelling, as a factor in producing new or altering old behaviours, was demonstrated by Bandura in the 1970s. He showed with the Bobo doll how children would adopt aggressive behaviour in the experimental situation and that this was transferred into real-life situations as a result. Thus it was possible, using this approach to see that adolescent boys who were non-aggressive had parents who had used no physical punishment in their upbringing, unlike aggressive boys, whose parents had used physical punishment on which the boy then modelled his subsequent behaviour. Thus, imitation as a reason for aggressive behaviour has generated considerable research interest from educationalists and psychologists alike. Detailed research studies into the effect of violent scenes on TV and video on the subsequent behaviour of viewers have shown that in certain individuals it leads to violent behavioural responses (Brody 1977).

Nevertheless, this does not explain why some viewers of violent film scenes do not subsequently act violently. It may have something to do with the argument put forward by TV and video producers that the audience does not see screen violence as part of the 'real' world and thus distinguishes between reality and drama. It is therefore a possibility that individuals in whom it does produce a violent response are those who cannot distinguish between 'reality' and 'drama'. It is also important to consider whether it is a combination of previously learned behaviour and the effect of viewed violence that results in aggression.

Studies of aggressive behaviour and the presence of weapons in the USA have shown that a weapon in the hands of an aggressor increases the aggressive behaviour but a weapon in the hands of the victim does little to produce it.

Weapons alone will not actually produce aggression but where aggression is made more likely (because the subject is made angry) the presence of weapons may increase its probability.

Experimental research has thus shown that there are two quite independent routes to aggressive behaviour. The first is through the process of operant conditioning – the violence of the armed robber or that of the boxer. The behaviour is relatively unemotional and is performed in the hope of gaining some clearly achievable end; there may be no specific prior stimulus discernible to which the aggression can be said to be a response. The second type of aggression, by contrast, is a clear response to some prior unpleasant event; here we might include the aggression of the individual whose toe is accidentally trodden upon or the person who acts violently when hearing of the death of a loved one. In many cases of aggression both processes combine and interact. Thus, ethologists have described at some length the phenomenon of 'territorial aggression'. In animals an intruder into their territory leads to the reactive response of driving away the intruder; in humans a similar response may lead to annoyance and thereby produce reactive aggression.

Implicit within the discussion above is the concept that it is in the early days of the development of the individual within the family that the seeds of potential violence are laid down. In the foreword to the paper *Supporting Families* (Home Office 1999), Jack Straw, the Home Secretary, makes an initial point: 'Family life is the foundation on which our communities, our society and our country are built'.

Vulnerable and abusing families

Many sociologists and psychologists have explored the meaning of family, the differences between families and the way family members interact, and much of the evidence put forward gives the professional an insight into the part that the family might play in relation to domestic violence. Sociologists tend to focus on the group and what makes a family unit, while psychologists explore the interactional and socioemotional

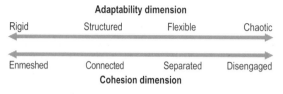

Figure 13.1 The circumplex model (reproduced with permission from Olson et al 1979)

styles within families, and what distinguishes a 'healthy family' from an 'unhealthy family'. Olson et al (1979) used the 'circumplex model' to classify types within two key dimensions of *adaptability* and *cohesion* (Fig. 13.1).

Frude (1996) discusses the extremes of these briefly and in the adaptability dimension describes *rigid families* where each member has an allotted role, the power structure is inflexible and leadership is authoritarian with little compromise. *Chaotic families* are the reverse, with no clear rules, a power structure that is unstable and support and permission-giving irregular and arbitrary. Children lack guidance and parental discipline is erratic and inconsistent. The cohesion dimension distinguishes *enmeshed families* at one end of the spectrum, which are so tightly bonded that the members have little personal identity and are suffocatingly close. At the other extreme, *disengaged families* appear to have little unity and no sense of identity.

The use of the term *dysfunctional families* is premised on the Olson et al (1979) model and these families tend to show extreme positions on one or other of the dimensions or, indeed, extreme positions on both dimensions, e.g. rigid/ disengaged or rigid/enmeshed and chaotic/ disengaged or chaotic/enmeshed. Families that are dysfunctional tend to develop problems without any outside pressures, so that the stress caused by outside pressure quickly becomes intolerable and threatens family health.

Family patterns in child abuse

Crittenden (1988) in discussing family patterns in relation to child abuse identified four definable patterns of family behaviour that she called 'abusing families', 'neglecting families', 'abusing

and neglecting families' and 'marginally maltreating families'. Using her criteria in conjunction with Olson's model, families vulnerable to child abuse would seem to show extremes of dysfunction in either or both of the adaptability and cohesion dimensions, with added criteria relating to a parent's(s') personal history of abuse, the parents' socioeconomic status and education or the child's health and behaviour.

Child abuse has a number of different categories: for example, there is physical violence, where the child is physically abused and injured. The second category is neglect – not just ignoring a child, which is not usually defined as neglect, but behaviour that may be life-threatening such as not feeding children or keeping them clean. The third category, psychological abuse, probably includes the greatest number of cases, is the most difficult to identify and may include verbal brutalisation and making the child feel inadequate, incompetent and ashamed. Finally, in sexual abuse a child can experience various degrees of interference from fondling to direct penetration.

Parton (1990), writing for the Violence Against Children Study Group, makes three important observations from the literature. Firstly, the vast majority of sexual abuse of children is committed by men, and girls are abused in greater numbers; secondly, the responsibility for physical abuse is equally distributed between men and women; and thirdly, women predominate in cases of emotional abuse and neglect. Parton highlights the role women play in the abuse of their own children, either directly or indirectly, and suggests that many writers allude to 'the abusing parent' when in reality they mean 'the abusing mother'.

In questioning why some women fail to protect their children feminists argue that the reason lies within women's relative powerlessness within the family and wider society. These women may have had a violent childhood with aggressive fathers, have low self-esteem and experience frequent abuse from their cohabitees. They continue relationships with violent men, at the expense of their children, even though they may be very frightened of them. Ong (1986) argues that coping is seen to be essential for 'successful' motherhood and when a mother neglects or abuses her children this is seen as an individual failing rather than being related to the conditions in which mothering takes place. Yet the pressures upon women to cope with the role of motherhood are powerful, both from society and from within themselves. Ong says that isolation in the home is a major factor in women's violence towards their children and is more likely to be experienced by those women who have least control over where they live and are unable to develop or maintain their links with supportive friends or family through lack of money, a car or babysitters. Thus professionals working in child abuse must move away from seeing it as an individual problem and analyse the wider context and confront the issue of violence of the institution of motherhood (Ong 1986).

The incidence and reporting of child sexual abuse is on the increase but it has taken society a long time to recognise the seriousness and scale of the problem and understand the consequences, both long-term and short-term. Child sexual abuse occurs within the family and, in a sense, the family provides psychological as well as physical resources and also sexual and affectionate needs. The family in Western society has become more isolated – away from the extended family – and thus there is greater pressure on it to cope with its needs with fewer social contacts. Thus the isolation of families may be a factor in child abuse; however, it is frequently the case that the abusing parent was themselves sexually abused. Finkelhor (1986), in the USA, found that, while physical and sexual abuse can be present in all socioeconomic levels, the poorer the family the greater the likelihood of child abuse, physical and sexual. He also made the interesting observation that child sexual abuse tended to be found in families with higher incomes, a finding confirmed by Hanks & Stratton (1988) in the UK.

Sexually abused children are put under great pressure to 'keep this as our secret' and it is only recently that as a society we have been able to believe a child who is able to share this guilty secret. There is evidence that within closed families (see *enmeshed families* above) all

the children may have been sexually abused and each child remains in silent isolation, hoping that they are protecting their siblings and at the same time, possibly, also feeling special (Frude 1996). The physical effects of child abuse may lead to bruising or more serious injuries and some children contract sexually transmitted disease, while older girls who are subjected to intercourse run the risk of pregnancy. However, much child sexual abuse takes the form of masturbation, fondling or indecent exposure and thus there is no physical damage or even forensic evidence. Psychological trauma can be very great, with children requiring long periods of counselling, often many years after the occurrence, but it must be remembered that many children do cope psychologically and appear to be healthy and adjusted. There has been concern among professionals that hunting for hidden psychological trauma may do considerable harm, a criticism levelled against the setting up of Childline by Esther Rantzen, the television personality.

Delinquency

Delinquency by young offenders can be construed as violence towards society and may be defined as involvement in activities that are normally regarded and treated as criminal offences, even if relatively minor ones, e.g. malicious damage to public property, various forms of theft, getting into fights in public and resisting arrest. There are also status offences such as smoking, gambling, under-age drinking, truancy and the increasingly prevalent drug use. These behavioural problems can be analysed in several different ways: for example, it could be argued that they are the result of a constricting society setting standards or restrictions that might be seen as repressive. On the other hand, there is much evidence to show that changes in the fabric of society, in which the family plays a less important role than earlier in the century, mean that the ground rules normally laid down through adequate to good parenting are missing. Thus attitude and personality development is skewed towards the individual and away from care of and within the group.

The bullying personality

Randall (1997) has described a number of instances when perpetrators of bullying trace the development of their behaviour back to parental violence towards them as young children. The critical stages in development of aggressive behaviour, beginning with the handling of separation from the prime care-giver (separation anxiety), through the 'terrible twos' and finally the development of skills for entry into pre-schooling or school, are those stages when it is most important that the child is exposed to steady parental handling. Parents who cannot cope with the child's normal developmental stages contribute to deficits in cognitive aspects of behavioural control. Aggression will occur when children do not learn the ability to negotiate within relationships or follow the rules set by adults. Negotiation is very dependent on the development of meaningful language. With the development of language there is a reduction in the physical aspects of aggression such as biting, throwing objects and pulling hair. Language and the ability to play alongside other children without resorting to aggressive behaviour – squabbling over possessions is an example – allows children to begin to show behaviour that relies on empathy and the acceptance of other people's perspectives that differ from their own (Randall 1997).

Parents or primary care-givers play an essential part in helping their children to channel aggressive behaviour into assertive behaviour. Social development in the form of happy social interactions, positive approaches to negative circumstances and calming attitudes and demeanours from the role model are important factors in social development. Children observe and copy the interactions of their parents and others and learn the ways in which the role model copes with their own emotions (Egeland 1988).

Baumrind's (1967) work on parenting styles has shown how the authoritarian style is not appropriate for children to learn good social interaction skills. Children who are told what to do are often not allowed to try for themselves alternative styles of behaviour or coping strategies and thus don't have the chance to explore the consequences of these.

Children quickly become aware of how parents feel about them and parents' feelings towards their children are often based on whether they perceive them as being 'easy' or 'difficult' to handle from birth. Other researchers have shown that social circumstances of material or financial poverty, poor partner relationships, maternal or paternal depression and low IQ all may create intolerably stressful situations leading to the development of aggression in the home. Conger et al (1992) showed that parents who are cold and rejecting towards their children and are inconsistent in handling them, frequently using physical punishment, are more likely to have aggressive children who, in time, develop the bullying personality.

In the past, intervention strategies have tended to focus on education and behaviour modification techniques to improve the quality of interactions between the child and its parents. Health visitors are in a good position to broaden intervention beyond these strategies, which tend to deal only with a superficial solution to the child's problems. Factors that run in parallel with aggressive behaviour, particularly in preschool children, involve emotional, social and cognitive delays in the child's development. It is therefore important that health visitors help the interaction between a previously depressed mother and her child, who have had little opportunity to develop a language-enriched relationship. Children and their parents may need to concentrate on anger/ frustration control mechanisms and carry these into the play situation. In addition, because there is evidence of loss of self-esteem in both child and parent, strategies need to be developed to improve parents' and children's personal perceptions of themselves as being 'good' or 'bad'.

Gibb & Randall (1989) comment that children who have been handled by assertive parental management need intervention strategies that focus on anger management – particularly where the adult care-giver has portrayed anger. There is also a body of opinion that suggests that not only do these children get faulty signals but their normal development is inhibited and appropriate educational approaches will be required to stimulate age-appropriate development – socially and psychologically.

The victim personality

The development of the victim personality is also centred on parenting of young children and is frequently as the result of overprotection, overindulgence and social isolation of the child from the peer group. This results in a child who is totally dependent on others and cannot relate in an independent manner to peers – either in school or later on at work. The alternative cause of victim personality can be as the result of rejection – possibly because of the inability of the parents to see that a child who does not obviously respond to their parenting efforts does, nevertheless, need as much love as the affectionate child who is much easier to love.

Overprotection of children has been seen in several studies as restriction of children's behaviour so that there is less opportunity for social learning outside the home; children are encouraged to stay close to their parents and not allowed to explore novel environments or any type of 'risk-taking' behaviour away from the parent. Studying preschool children, Hinde et al (1993) suggest that the child seeks the mother's protection frequently and that this dependency is reinforced by the mother's oversolicitous behaviour.

This results in older children in social withdrawal and can be traced back to parenting styles that set down many rules and constraints on children's psychological development, leading to reticent timid children who cannot cope in settings where there is lack of structure, such as in school playgrounds. This may lead to facial expressions of unhappiness and a capacity to cry easily, making them the likely butt of jokes and thence bullying. Often these children, especially boys, are smaller and weaker than their peers and have a tendency to behave with passivity and submission. They are loners and often seek favour with the teacher in school to get what they want; this will alienate them from their peer group. As these children grow older they attempt to become more assertive but are easily outclassed by their more competent assertive peers. As the situation continues so these children receive further rebuffs in attempts to form relationships and in due course begin to think of themselves as worthless, with poor self-perception and low self-esteem. They become more socially withdrawn and depressed and may indeed almost seek out situations where they are bullied simply to get attention from their peer group. It is hardly surprising that this continues into adulthood, when their social ineptitude makes them the victim of bullying in the workplace or neighbourhood (Randall 1997).

It is not particularly easy to identify the symptoms of victim personality and on the whole research studies have resorted to scales for identification of mental disorders to isolate characteristic behaviour of insecurity, timidity, sensitivity, anxiety and cautiousness. Many children display behaviour that is indicative of shy withdrawn children and yet do not necessarily become victims (Randall 1997). It may be necessary to observe the child over a period of time to see whether certain behaviours develop that appear to be out of character, e.g. not wanting to go to school after regular attendance – often accompanied by aches and pains and vomiting, going to school by long routes if going on their own, having relationship problems with the peer group and appearing nervous and jumpy when with peers, or stealing from home in order to pay bullies.

DOMESTIC VIOLENCE

It is argued that all violence that is perpetrated in the home is domestic violence, be it heterosexual or same-sex, involving children or adolescents, elders, whites, ethnics or within so-called religious frameworks. However, because the causes are so wide-ranging, distinctions will be made between the main types. In the UK violence between adults who are married or in a relatively stable relationship is usually considered by the media and the police to be *domestic violence*, and this may include same-sex as well as heterosexual clashes. Violence between an adult/adults and a child/children also takes place within the home but is usually called *child abuse*. Violence between children may occur within the home but also often takes place outside the home and is therefore is not considered to be domestic.

Culture, material circumstances such as bad housing and economic stresses, drug abuse, childhood relational experiences, sexual insecurities and jealousies, deep mistrust and suspicion, misogynist (woman-hating) attitudes and lack of communication are many of the frequent themes that arise from the histories of women involved in domestic violence. Eaton (1994) shows that the abuse of women in the home often takes the form of rape and that violent episodes are often precipitated by the woman becoming pregnant. This suggests that assaultive behaviour in private spaces is intricately interwoven with male subordination of women.

Housing and domestic violence

It is not suggested that housing problems are the cause of domestic violence, because relationship breakdowns occur before there are any concerns about future accommodation. Nevertheless, evidence is available that if the couple involved had some alternative accommodation to which they could resort, many failed relationships would not lead to violence. Reports abound (Amina Mama 1996) from the women concerned of the partner or cohabitant originally moving in to a house where a single mother and her children were the tenants. As it is not housing policy to house single men, if the relationship becomes violent it often has to be the woman and her children who move out to because the man refuses to go. Local authorities have a statutory obligation to house people with dependent children, but mothers and their children forced out of local authority accommodation have to join the long queues awaiting housing in hostels, reception centres and refuges.

The problems facing women who live secluded lives, as housewives or in more closed communities, and who do not have a good command of English are greater than those who have sought alternative accommodation. These women do not even know about refuges and have little idea from whom they can seek help. Many women from the Asian community do not live in local authority housing but with their in-laws or in private rented housing, often as tenants of an Asian landlord. Thus, if they do approach the local housing department they are put at the end of the queue and are possibly referred to a refuge. A 1983 study of women in hostels (Austerberry & Watson 1982) found that relationship breakdown and/or domestic violence was the biggest single cause of women's homelessness. In the case of Asian women without children they were in the desperate position of being unable to return to their families because of the shame brought to the family by their flight from violence – violence that their own families would not acknowledge (Amina Mama 1996).

In 1998 there were media reports (*The Independent*, 13 October) of young male Muslim vigilantes who had set up a business finding Muslim women who had fled from violence, often in arranged marriages, and had gone into hiding because they risked further violence if caught and returned either to their own families or to their husbands and in-laws. Many such women had been subjected to horrendous acts of violence and there were several reports of deaths in what can only be described as suspicious circumstances, reported as accidental, e.g. clothing catching fire or an unexplained fall.

Cultural factors

In 1989 a research project was commissioned by the London Race and Housing Research Unit into domestic violence in London's Black communities, particularly focusing on African, Asian and Afro-Caribbean communities (Amina Mama 1996). There was evidence that not only Black men but also Black women were being subjected to physical violence and abuse in race attacks and coercive inner-city policing. As well as this, Black women were also suffering violence at the hands of their men and the combination of these forces shows the triple oppression of the dimensions of race, class and sex. It was found that many Black women were having to leave their homes to escape from their partner's abuse and violence, taking their children with them. These women then reported extremely long periods of homelessness, with little help from the statutory agencies because of racism and sexism, as they struggled to find temporary accommodation, rehousing, financial support and legal assistance. The negative effects of these struggles on families already suffering from the trauma of repeated violence experienced often lead to permanent breakdown of the physical and mental health of the woman and her children.

As a result of the publication of the report of this research project (Amina Mama 1996), the women's movement has continued to fight to establish a network of refuges that concentrate on working towards meeting the needs of ethnic minority groups. Criticism of police responses to Black women seeking help after domestic violence has resulted in the development of response units particularly designed to be sensitive to Black women's needs. Despite the efforts put into setting up these culturally sensitive units there is still much evidence to show that Black women have more difficulty getting away from domestic violence, because of racist attitudes, than do white women.

Immigration laws also pose a threat to Black women because they allow men to threaten women of uncertain or dependent immigration status with deportation away from their British-born children. The research project found that Black women were asked more often to prove their right to welfare payments on the basis of tax and national insurance payments than white women. If they had fled without their passports they found it impossible to prove their dependent status and were excluded on the basis of 'no recourse to public funds' (Amina Mama 1996).

Black women's contacts with social service departments also varied in the effectiveness of the support offered. In some cases child-care support and temporary fostering were offered until the woman could get away from her violent husband. However, many housing departments, rather than taking the responsibility of rehousing the family, insisted that the woman should seek help from social services. Rehousing that was offered was often into extremely poor temporary accommodation where the woman and her children were herded into one room with a shared kitchen (or no kitchen) and a bathroom and toilet shared by several families. In numerous cases these women were forced to stay there for many months (on average 18 months) before they were rehoused. During this time their nutritional status deteriorated until frequently the children were ill and the woman was in a state of malnutrition (Amina Mama 1996).

The circumstances outlined above have led to the women's movement putting increasing pressure on housing departments to improve their access to public housing stock, but it is usually the bottom end of the stock that is available for emergency housing. There was evidence that the stress of poor housing or homelessness forced many women back into the life-threatening situation of domestic violence from which they had originally fled.

Following the initial research report in 1989 the London Race and Housing Research Unit ceased to exist but, because the book served as a pioneering and ground-breaking document to Black women's struggles against domestic violence, it was reissued in its original form in 1996. A foreword to the new edition noted that there had been some improvements in the public response to violence towards Black women. The Home Office has taken the lead in the interdepartmental ministerial group dealing with domestic violence and is promoting multiagency working. A number of police forces have introduced domestic violence units, now usually supported by domestic violence officers who have been specifically trained in this work. In the multiagency initiatives there are still problems with racism, and Black workers within these agencies struggle to get a positive response in a prevailing climate of inaction. This inaction may also lead to Black women's organisations being marginalised in the development of local interagency work. In terms of resources, the housing issue remains the biggest problem, and in the light of privatisation obtaining council or housing-association housing has become more and more difficult for all women and children escaping domestic violence.

The following vignettes of violence are taken from Amina Mama (1996). Case histories extracted from women in several studies make sickening reading and the degrading circumstances that women are forced into before they gain strength to make a break leave care workers horrified by their stories.

Client A was in a council flat when a young male acquaintance, B, moved in. The relationship went well until she bore him a son, of whom B became progressively more jealous. A second son made matters worse and from accusations and locking A in and hiding her belongings B began to resort to punching and knifing her. B became possessive to the point of deploying other people to follow her. B took her money and refused to allow her to visit her friends. She began to suffer frequent nose bleeds and headaches from beatings on the head and saw her doctor for her injuries. The police were called on several occasions but A refused to leave B because she felt that the children needed a father. It was only when B nearly strangled her that he was convicted of grievous bodily harm, and she left him only to move from refuge to refuge over 3 years.

R, aged 26, had three children and moved away from her husband when he began to drink heavily and subjected her to violent attacks. Friends kept telling her husband where she was and she was constantly fleeing from one refuge to another to escape his violence. She was rehoused in a flat abandoned by a Black family who had been subjected to racial attacks by their neighbours and she was then subjected to the same racial harassment until she fled that home. Her husband found where she was and attempted to burn the flat by pouring petrol through the letter box and setting fire to it. She went back to a refuge and was still awaiting rehousing.

S, from a Pakistani Muslim family, was 16 when her family arranged a marriage with a 30-year-old settled man with a good job. The first day after the marriage he assaulted her and thereafter controlled her to such an extent that all she was allowed to do was to cook and clean. She was virtually a prisoner in her own home, allowed no friends or contact with the outside world. The violence increased and when she was about 6 months pregnant she was pushed down the stairs. When the baby was born she was in fear of it crying because of his anger. She suffered depression and long periods of amnesia, being subjected to physical and psychological abuse until she finally ended up in a psychiatric hospital with a nervous breakdown. On discharge from hospital she was forced to go home as her family considered that her illness was a stigma and did not want to help her. When she finally got away from her husband because of his repeated violence the court awarded custody of their son to his father because he was financially well able to provide a better home. She is still fighting custody battles but at least now she is supported by the women's group.

In describing the effects on their health here are some of the statements made:

My whole personality changed from that violence. For 2 years I withdrew myself completely.... I became isolated and kept from everybody and everything. I was like a robot. I suffered from a lot of headaches.

I think I did actually believe time and time again that he would change when he cried and apologised. I thought about him every time, because he seemed so lost and helpless. I just didn't have the heart to tell him that I wasn't going to give him another chance when he was in such a state. He even tried to commit suicide when I really threatened to leave him once. He's driven me to several suicide attempts.

He never let me make any decisions. It was always what he wanted and he always made sure that anything I tried to do failed because he made it fail. He always told my friends that I was incapable of managing on my own. In the end I believed him and made no attempt to make any decisions on my own. I had no self-confidence whatsoever and I believed all the things that he said about me – how I was useless and could not look after the home and garden properly. It was easier to give in and just let him control me. We had endless rows and he said horrible things to me. It took me many years to realise that he was subjecting me to psychological abuse and it took me even longer to break away from him. Even then I felt that it was all my fault that our relationship was breaking down.

Statutory responses to the abuse of women

UK law in relation to the protection of women has been criticised by many groups as slow to modernise; evidence shows that there is substantial room for improvement in the interpretation and enforcement of the law by the police, courts, lawyers and society in general. Historically, both the law and its enforcement have been imbued with patriarchal values that have asserted the necessity and desirability of women's subordination to men (Dobash & Dobash 1980, Edwards 1985).

Domestic violence falls under several areas of the law. Under civil law, relevant legislation includes marital law, assault and trespass law and domestic violence acts; under criminal law there are crimes of assault and grievous bodily harm, manslaughter/culpable homicide and murder; housing law is relevant to the housing consequences of domestic violence; and, in relation to Black women, immigration law is also relevant.

VIOLENCE AS BULLYING

Modern pluralistic society with its competitiveness and tendency to violence either at the terrorist end of the continuum or the fiction of film Westerns has raised awareness of different aspects of violence, from verbal abuse and aggression to physical assaults. Harassment at work, indifference to the physical requirements of vulnerable people, rejection within friendships or marriage all lead to the knowledge that these can be interpreted as violence or bullying. The definition of bullying can be seen as a mimicry of the definition of aggression. Randall (1997) suggests that a definition of bullying is: 'the aggressive behaviour arising from the deliberate intent to cause physical or psychological distress to others' (p. 4). Randall goes on to consider various types of aggression, and particularly two: *affective aggression*, which is concerned with strong negative emotions, especially anger; and *instrumental aggression*, which is behaviour that can be very aggressive but does not have a strong emotional basis. Anger can be the cause of an emotional state that leads to aggressive behaviour and the end result is the desire to hurt somebody, either physically or psychologically. Instrumental aggression is also aimed at harming somebody but without necessarily feeling any emotion, anger or otherwise towards the victim. Instrumental aggression can simply be aimed at having power over someone, which is in effect the outcome of a bullying relationship.

Bullying carries with it the connotations of belonging only to childhood and being about teasing or taunting or sly physical attacks such as pinching or punching. However, in many instances there has only been one physical attack by the perpetrator on the victim and yet there is still a bullying relationship present. This is because fear of the bully has been instilled in the victim, which may be termed harassment if carried to extremes. The term 'harassment' is used far more in adult work and certainly has close similarities with the term 'bullying' used in children's work. Yet child bullies, if asked why they use violence against their victims, imply the need for power over their victim – power to make them cry, be subservient or gain material advantage such as pocket money or copying homework. To establish fear in a victim gives power to the perpetrator and therefore if a work boss harasses a member of staff and that member of staff fears the consequences if they do not comply, it is very closely akin to bullying and the two situations are coterminous (Randall 1997).

This argument suggests that there are two real types of bullying situation that arise in the workplace – premeditated workplace aggression and harassment, which may or may not be sexual in origin. Premeditated workplace aggression often occurs in situations where the organisation has small groups of people working on different projects under, for example, the control of a charge hand in industry. Further examples could be: a small company of men under a sergeant or NCO if in the army; a typing pool/office workers under a senior clerk in business circumstances; workers in service industries under a supervisor, or even nurses in a hospital ward under a senior staff nurse/ward sister. In all these situations and many others there are a variety of reasons why bullying takes place. Perhaps the perpetrator is a highly efficient and effective worker and to increase their effectiveness they have to drive their subordinates to support increased effort, and to do this they resort to bullying behaviour. At the alternative end of the continuum the perpetrator may use bullying tactics because of their own disaffection about the working situation or have personal problems that result in anger that spills over into the work situation. Recent concerns in the UK have arisen over the stress that teachers experience, particularly in primary schools. As a result of this there are more cases making the headlines involving senior teachers and junior staff members who are bullied to produce results that are beyond their tolerance or ability. Brady-Wilson (1991) discusses the concept of workplace trauma, in which the victim loses self-esteem and the right to security and contentment in the workplace and which, if persistent over a period of time, can grind down the victim to a state where they exhibit post-traumatic stress disorder.

Workplace aggression can be overt, but this is usually confined to situations where a small group of people are working in a close situation and the perpetrator gets other staff members to collude in his/her activities against the victim, or else the perpetrators are the entire small group of staff, who collectively bully the victim. It is probable that this macho type of bullying is most prevalent in the armed forces against new recruits or in the prison system against new inmates. Most of the available research cited by Randall (1997) indicates that premeditated aggression is insidiously covert and that the perpetrator often relies on the victim remaining quiet from fear of being disbelieved by others. The circumstances can be many and varied and are usually long-term, e.g. constantly refusing requested changes to a holiday rota or allocating the most boring or dirty jobs to the victim. Preventing opportunities for promotion or constantly demanding increased work output are other examples, as are spreading rumours or gossiping about the victim.

Bullying need not always involve individuals but can be group against group, as in teenage gang warfare, small highly penetrative groups against large populations, as in terrorism, neighbourhood against small group as with ethnic pockets in a wider population, or one particular family against a neighbourhood. Although these are very different examples they are all reasoned from similar perspectives of power and control.

Power can be pleasurable to the perpetrators and is commonly seen in neighbourhoods where small groups or gangs gain pleasure from harassing a section of the community. This pleasure can stem from either the feeling that the perpetrators have got their own back on the community, with which they are in dispute, or that they have now 'made their mark' on it. Control works on a similar basis but is more about control of resources or territory, e.g. refusing to let a family park outside its own house because the bully

next door needs space for two cars (Owens & Ashcroft 1985).

VIOLENCE IN SAME-SEX RELATIONSHIPS

The major factor evident from writing on same-sex domestic violence is that it is obviously premised on power and not gender. In heterosexual relationships it is fundamentally sexism that is at the root of abuse, whereas in homophobic incidents homophobia would appear to be the root cause. Much of the evidence available (Renzetti & Miley 1996) shows that the nature of the abuse is similar: it includes physical, emotional, psychological and sexual abuse (rape).

Physical abuse appears to be the same as in heterosexual violence, can be verbal as well as involving direct contact and can be serious enough to require medical attention. A number of studies of mysterious deaths show that there is often a sexual attack before the victim is killed, and this is common to both groups – heterosexual and homophobic.

Emotional and psychological abuse are again common to the two groups – threats to the partner's pets or children, constantly demeaning the victim, anger about the victim's friendships, manipulative lies in order to control finances. Renzetti & Miley (1996) suggest that a unique type of psychological abuse in gay or lesbian relationships is the threat of 'outing' to family, landlords, employers and others. As can be imagined, this serves to isolate the couple within the relationship to an even greater extent than women in a heterosexual abusing relationship.

Renzetti & Miley (1996) suggest that, in heterosexual abuse, there is a pattern of an abusive incident followed by a 'honeymoon period' and then another cycle of abuse to gain power or control. Similarly, in same-sex violence there is a recognisable pattern of a violent period followed by a period of calm. What is interesting is a comparable recognisable pattern of behaviour in both heterosexual and same-sex relationships, of victims moving away from one violent relationship only to fall into another. The difference is that in the same-sex repeated violent relationship the victim of one violent relationship may become the perpetrator in the next. This is one of the major reasons why support services are reluctant to support partners in violent lesbian or gay relationships – who is the victim and who the perpetrator? Indeed, if the identified abuser is counselled and supported it is not unknown for the former victim to become their abuser.

There are a number of reasons why same-sex victims stay in violent relationships, such as hope of changing the abuser, fear of reprisal, self-blame or continued love for the batterer. What is very evident is the isolation within which both partners live. To seek help would lead to revelation about the sexual orientation of the victim, very possibly resulting in job loss and exposure to family, friends and social circle.

Most of the work on same-sex violence has taken place in the USA and there has been little work on this topic published in the UK. Elliott (1996) analyses the reasons why it has taken so long to recognise same-sex domestic violence in women and has postulated several ideas. Firstly, she suggests that many battered women's refuge and service providers are themselves lesbians and that these women hide their own sexual orientation and refuse to recognise lesbian battering, although they suspect that it exists. Another reason is that, whatever their sexual orientation, women helpers have accepted the basic philosophy that patriarchy and sexism are responsible for all violence. Having adopted this philosophy it is relatively simple to ignore the issues of power and control that are the particular cause of same-sex violence and concentrate on sexist issues, in so doing failing to recognise that lesbian violence exists. It is difficult to conceptualise women as batterers and men as victims in same-sex violence. Elliott (1996) also argues that the homosexual community itself perpetrates this illusion that the root cause of violence is sexist in order not to create any further situations that might incite ridicule from the heterosexual community.

In the USA work is beginning with lesbian violence through the battered women's movement but there is little evidence of any attempt to follow suit in this country. As for violence in

relationships between gay men, the focus with the gay community appears to be on coping with AIDS and even if gay violence has been recognised there is little evidence of any interest in supporting either the victims or abusers – the attitude is that it is their own problem and they will have to resolve it.

Marrujo & Kreger (1996) undertook a survey of abusive lesbian relationships in the USA and identified particular characteristics in relation to the perpetrator (primary aggressor) and the victim (primary victim). They also recognised relationships where the situation involved fighting back, so that both partners were participants rather than primary aggressor and primary victim. However, as far as they could be identified, primary aggressors were characterised by the psychological characteristics of pathological jealousy, controlling in the relationship, highly intrusive into the partner's activities, having a sense of personal entitlement in most areas and focused on their own needs rather than on those of their partner. They also found it difficult to control their anger in circumstances outside the relationship, e.g. at work. Primary victims, on the other hand were generally depressed and felt inadequate in the relationship, were not jealous, controlling or intrusive, and tended to focus on the other's needs rather than on their own. They often tried to manipulate the environment to ensure their safety.

In finding causal explanations for same-sex domestic violence a study carried out by Farley in 1996 showed that all the men and women who were screened reported having been psychologically abused as children and a high percentage of both groups had also been physically and sexually abused as children. In addition about half of each group had been physically abused as adults and there was evidence of alcohol abuse in the family of origin of just under 50% of both men and women. This particular study also found that gay and lesbian batterers come from all segments of society and represent all ethnic and racial groups in all economic situations and from all educational and occupational backgrounds. Further work is necessary to confirm that the childhood abuse seen as the background of all the participants in the study is reflected in other studies, and also that a high incidence of substance abuse in the partners, cited as a cause in another study, is also significant.

Some work has been done to explore lesbianism in women of all racial and ethnic origins. These women are incredibly isolated by virtue of the sexism, racism and homophobia present both in society and the helping agencies. It has been suggested in the literature that abusive Black women use the threats of breaking of trust and what society will think to force the victim to remain silent. However, racism and homophobia are the prevailing concern of Black lesbian couples and this is used as a weapon by the primary aggressor in a domestic violence situation, leading to the victim maintaining a protective attitude towards them (Kivel 1996).

To accept the evidence that violence in lesbian relationships is a possibility means that health visitors may be in a position to help women trapped in such a situation. Clearly, the help available ought to be the same as for women trapped in violent heterosexual relationships, but drawing on the evidence from the USA there are attitude problems to be overcome by the helpers involved. There are probably two main ways in which health visitors can help Black lesbians in violent relationships. The first is by allowing the victim to talk about the circumstances, encouraging them to see what is happening and helping them to recognise the root cause for the violence – power. It calls for the health visitor to be aware of their own feelings about same-sex violence and for honest personal reflection to identify any racism, sexism or homophobia within themselves. Secondly, the health visitor can become an advocate for the victim with the support services available for battered women in heterosexual relations. It calls for health visitors who are working with victims to encourage the community to talk about problems and recognise the meaning of healthy relationships – especially same-sex relationships, and generally to recognise that the tip of the iceberg is hardly to be seen at this time.

If it is difficult to support and identify lesbian victims of domestic violence it is even more difficult to work with gay victims of domestic violence. The main focus of concern among gay men has been the incidence of HIV and support has involved identifying and treating infection. However, evidence from the USA indicates that HIV concerns have been used as a weapon of control between gay partners – it is the control preventing a man from leaving his violent partner. Again, research in the USA (Renzetti & Miley 1996) suggests that a sizeable minority of gay and bisexual men have to contend with both HIV and partner abuse as part of their daily lives. It is important to realise that HIV itself is not a cause of physical abuse within the relationship but may well be the cause of psychological abuse, being used either to control the victim or to prevent him from leaving his violent partner.

Merrill's (1996) work shows that the 'control' identified above works in several ways; for example, both HIV-positive and HIV-negative men report that their HIV-infected partners will feign illness in order to convince them not to leave or to entice them back once they have left. Both often have low self-esteem and tend to blame themselves for their partner's violence. In addition, the attitudes of society in general towards gay men and people with AIDS contribute towards their low self-esteem and reduce their psychological ability to escape from violent partners.

Letellier (1996) reports that there is a growing body of evidence about serious psychological problems experienced by HIV-negative men. They are prone to chronic anxiety, depression, sleep disorders, impaired concentration, feelings of shame, fear helplessness and hopelessness – a list of problems not dissimilar to those experienced by victims of domestic violence. In addition, they suffer feelings of guilt for not having contracted the condition themselves or, alternatively, for having contracted the condition and survived when those they loved have died. As the feelings outlined above can be experienced by victims as well as the guilt of either not having contracted the disease or, alternatively, having left an abuser who is affected, it is not difficult to see the overwhelming emotional and psychological stresses that leave the victim in isolation.

For HIV-positive men there are a similar set of psychological problems, compounded by the knowledge that they have little hope of any new same-sex relationship because of their HIV status. Unless their anger at being HIV-positive is such that they wish to take it out on the gay community and have no compunction about singles dating, many HIV-positive men have strong feelings of responsibility towards their community and are thus prepared to stay in an abusive relationship rather than lose the security of being in a relationship, albeit sometimes violent.

Letellier (1996) discusses the level of care that battered heterosexual women can expect from healthcare providers and suggests that these women need to be able to question healthcare workers about domestic abuse. In turn, they expect healthcare workers to respond to their questions in a caring and nonjudgmental manner. Battered gay and bisexual men deserve the same level of care and Letellier suggests that the communication can go something like: 'Some of the men I work with are hurt by their male partners. Are you in a relationship with a man? Does he hurt you? Are you afraid of him?' or 'Many gay men are hurt by their partners. Did your boyfriend/lover hurt you?'

What is very important in this type of communication exchange is that the professional/care worker concerned is fully aware of their own values and attitudes to this type of situation, and that they can cope with the responses that may come back from the abused person. Equally and on a similar level of importance is the knowledge that the professional worker can transmit to the abused person that they really care and understand.

As well as the type of communication between care worker and victim outlined above, there is also a need for exploration of feelings concerning HIV and AIDS within the victim themselves, and this includes separating out the two factors in the situation between abuser and victim, that of violence and the epidemic itself. Helping a victim to work through guilt about the situation requires considerable self-awareness on the part of the professional and appropriate courses on HIV and AIDS are very useful for professionals intending to work with domestic violence in gay and lesbian communities.

HEALTH AND ABUSE IN THE CARE OF OLDER PEOPLE

Elder abuse and neglect as a phenomenon was first described in the UK in the mid-1970s but little research work and acknowledgement was apparent until 1989, when the Department of Health recognised elder abuse and neglect as a new field of social concern. Since then the learning curve for the professionals involved has been steep but this has not been reflected in the formal education systems, which still allocate insufficient curriculum time to do more than pay lip service to family violence or elder abuse. The bulk of curriculum time is still spent on child abuse/protection matters.

Yet clearly there is a growing body of evidence illustrating the size of the problem, to the extent that it should now be recognised as a major public health issue (Eastman 1984, Bennett 1990, Biggs et al 1995).

Institutional abuse of older people has been described in history and was particularly seen in relation to practices within workhouses, none of which was ever challenged. Still today, a number of scandals reach the media, and only recently (1998) the Professional Misconduct Committee of the UKCC saw a rise in referrals, mostly cases of ill-treatment of older people in private nursing homes. It is probably accurate to say that the number of cases of elder abuse within the family that reach the ears of the media are the merest fraction of those that occur. In the majority of cases the old person will never complain from fear of losing their home and/or care. What is very interesting is the basis from which professionals view abuse: Bennett et al (1997) analyse the current approaches, showing that child abuse and elder abuse are seen as a medical problem whereas family violence is considered to be a social problem.

The increased specialisation in work with older people has stimulated the need for understanding of older people's health and social needs and the emergence of courses specific to social geronto-logy has promoted greater understanding of the sociological dimensions of aging, moving professionals away from the traditional biomedical approach of functional decline to positive agism (Blakemore & Boneham 1994, Slater 1995).

There is a paucity of good research on elder abuse in the UK and Bennett et al (1997) go to great pains to differentiate between known risk factors identified in US studies and the anecdotal research available in the UK. From the most recent work in case controlled studies undertaken between 1983 and 1994 the five risk factors most quoted are:

- the psychopathology of the abuser (intraindividual dynamics)
- the cycle of violence theory (intergenerational transmission of violence)
- dependency and exchange relationships between abuser and abused
- stress
- social isolation.

The psychopathology of the abuser (intraindividual dynamics)

In four of the six case controlled studies (above) there is clear evidence of abusers having mental health problems or alcohol misuse and abuse. However, it is not clear whether alcohol abuse arose before the elder was abused or was potentially a consequence of the stress of caring.

The cycle of violence theory (intergenerational transmission of violence)

This is seen in child abuse and domestic violence but was not evident in the case controlled studies (above). However, in two of the studies there was evidence of long-standing abusive relationships continuing into later life, with one partner stating that this was to pay back for abuse in their earlier relationship.

Dependency

Studies in the US have found for and against dependency. In some circumstances it has been suggested that the very dependence of the older person leads to their abuse. Other studies have shown that, if anything, the perpetrator was more often dependent on the older person for finance and living arrangements. In none of the case controlled studies cited by Bennett et al (1997) was the victim dependent.

Stress

Stress in the carer has been hypothesised as the most likely cause of abuse but, although one of the case controlled studies in the UK (Grafstrom et al 1992) reported that the carers stated that their health was worse than expected, they were also taking psychotropic drugs and other factors may therefore have been involved. In the 1990 study *Carers at Work* (Opportunities for Women 1990), 88% of women stated that they suffered from stress through being a carer as well as working while 44% of men stated that they felt stressed. It would appear that the prevalence of abuse is very low, between 2% and 5%, so no direct correlation can be made between stress and abuse.

Social isolation

In two of the UK case controlled studies cited above the victims and perpetrators were socially isolated but this was not so in the others. Clearly, more research needs to be done with different sample populations.

Conclusions as to risk factors

Although there is a large amount of evidence from the US about risk factors, there is less from the UK, mainly because of the paucity of research. It is clear, however, that mental health problems and alcohol abuse are risk factors in the UK and that victims are often dependent on the abuser. There is some evidence of abuse by strangers, mainly in private residential care, but the bulk of abuse would appear to occur within the family and may be a factor in family violence rather than elder abuse in isolation.

Elder abuse as part of family violence

Frude (1996) states that the family is the setting for a substantial proportion of the violence that occurs within society and suggests that family aggression is relatively common because a good deal of anger is generated in family situations and there are relatively few inhibitions to prevent this anger from being expressed as physical aggression. He makes an interesting distinction between hostile and instrumental violence. Hostile violence is driven by anger and the principal motive is to hurt the victim. Instrumental violence is driven principally by a desire for 'gain' and is used merely as a means to an end. Thus instrumental violence may be used to maintain a dominant role or to teach a family member (usually a woman) a lesson.

Family life is governed by rules, which are often related to allocation of space, duties, responsibilities, household chores, money and other resources, and anger is often preceded by the judgement that someone has broken a rule. Anger over rule-breaking is not the only reason for family violence because the fact that people have relatively few inhibitions in the home situation also plays a large part. Family members know each other's vulnerabilities and are therefore in a prime position to inflict maximum hurt, which can lead to self-blame and stigma, a lowering of self-esteem and a reduction in general coping skills. Other effects may be sleep disturbance, depression, a sense of isolation and despair and an increase in feelings of dependence. It is this latter aspect that may be a major factor in abuse of elders within the family and in many ways this reflects the situation regarding child abuse (Blakemore & Boneham 1994, Slater 1995).

Detection of elder abuse within families is difficult because elderly people do not live public lives and there is far less likelihood of contact with external agencies. In addition, there are few developmental parameters against which one can measure adult progress and thus there are problems in discerning the difference between frailty caused by age and/or illness and the effects of abuse.

Elder abuse is unlikely to arise suddenly as a new phenomenon within a family but is more likely to be a gradual deterioration of what has been a difficult relationship for many years, although it is possible that 'overload' due to other problems may suddenly change a relationship from difficult to abusive. Detection rates of elder abuse tend to be most effective in circumstances where there are other social factors such as poverty, unemployment and difficult social situations, and where they come to the attention of the authorities. Despite the previous comments, violence is not confined to families in lower social classes although rates of family violence appear to be highest in poorer urban families with high rates of unemployment (Bennett et al 1997).

Only 5% of the population aged 75–84 years enter residential care, although the figure rises to 21% for those aged 85 years and over (Department of Health 1996b). Yet despite these figures the view that institutional care is desirable for older people has been created and is perpetuated in society at large. This, however, is not the view of older people today, whose view of institutional care is coloured by images of the workhouse – although none of them is old enough to have experienced the workhouse at first hand.

Discussion still revolves around the social and financial circumstances in which older people can gain access to private residential care or care in nursing homes and as a result of community care reforms and accompanying investigative reports (the Wagner Report 1988, the Griffiths Report 1988) it has become apparent that both institutionalised care and the provision of care for people living in their own homes are expensive and complex resource issues. There are also issues concerning regulation of homes and the Department of Health (1996c) produced a White Paper about changing the requirement for residential and nursing homes to register with either the health authority (for nursing homes) or the local authority social services department (for residential homes) to registration with the health authority only. Some homes can remain registered with both bodies and arrangements are made to ensure that dual registration can be undergone with co-operation between both inspection bodies.

As with any type of institutional care, there is always the danger of neglect or abuse of inmates, but it would appear that, far from such occurrences becoming rarer, there is a steady recording of a wide range of episodes. Many of the instances of abuse take place within the context of a relationship in the institutional setting and such relationships may be between a staff member and an inmate, a volunteer and an inmate, two inmates or possibly an inmate and friends or relatives who are visiting. Such abuse can be physical, psychopathological, deliberate neglect, neglect through omission due to poor organisation, lack of basic standards, erosion of individuality of care, physical restraint, drug-induced restraint, fraud or theft, or the taking of life. This limitless catalogue of violence may be directed towards one inmate within the institution or all the inmates and may result from lack of staff training, serious staff shortages or poor management. This does not only apply to private homes but also to long-stay NHS hospitals, which are often regarded as the Cinderella of the hospital service, suffering from overcrowding, substandard furnishings, poor-quality limited-choice meals and little or no stimulation.

In the USA a number of research studies have assessed the predictors of physical abuse of older people in institutional care and found that staff burnout, patient aggression and conflict between staff and patients are the most significant predictors. Work done in the UK is further behind and limited but there is evidence from the UKCC Professional Conduct Committee of a rise in the numbers of nurses appearing before the committee who work in the nursing home sector, and that these are greater than any other area of practice (UKCC 1994b).

Ways to reduce abuse and neglect are rarely discussed openly and in fact there is evidence of the minimisation of what is an endemic problem. Clearly, much can be done in terms of education and training both of qualified and unqualified staff and better supervisory processes will also help, as will support and training for stress handling and relief. There is a need to raise staff self-esteem and morale and this may be done as a result of better and more imaginative management, particularly when taking into consideration budgets and resource costs. It is also important to recognise the need for good quality control in both the NHS and the private sector, the latter requiring better inspection and registration, the former using clinical governance and well-implemented clinical supervision.

Medical issues in older people

The percentage of the population now living to be old is rising and is a world problem. In Europe the highest proportions of older people are found in Scandinavia and the UK; on average in these countries 26% of the population are over the age of 65. In terms of the availability of medical care, older people in the UK feel marginalised and in the current market economy in healthcare are seen as expensive to treat. The emphasis on healthcare is still that we should enable frail older people to remain living in the community by successful management of their care needs in such settings. In reality, packages of care, which should be appropriate for each individual and planned before hospital discharge, tend to be care-manager-determined from a financial perspective rather than a true needs-assessed package. Patient and carer have to carry on as best they can. If the situation deteriorates into an abusive one, the same realities prevent intervention and help.

Work undertaken in the US by Jones (1990) suggests that there are a number of situations when an older person is seen in an A&E department and questions could be asked about possible abuse/neglect, for example:

- differing histories given by the patient and carer, either in explanation of injury or about its timing
- delays between injury/illness and seeking medical attention
- vague explanations for, for instance, a fracture
- frequent A&E department visits, often due to lack of medicines or their administration, despite a care plan and available resources
- a functionally impaired patient who arrives without the main carer present

- subtherapeutic drug levels on laboratory findings despite carer-reported compliance.

Two major concerns that the literature identifies (Bennett et al 1997) are: lack of knowledge on the part of both the medical and nursing professions in how to recognise abuse; and agist attitudes in such professionals, who assume that older people naturally have health deficits due to their age. Some fairly recent studies in the UK (Smith et al 1992) found that 5% of people attending A&E departments in Leicester who were 59 years and older were victims of domestic abuse. It is suggested that a 5-day study by Grunfeld et al (1994) in the US should be repeated in the UK. This study instructed all triage nurses to ask the following question: 'We know that violence is a problem for many women (or men) in their lives. Is this a problem for you in any way?' This project found that 6% of the population disclosed abuse, of whom 50% asked for help.

These aspects of the identification of abuse suggest that protocols should be produced, using questions such as: 'The injuries you have are like bruises and lacerations people get when someone hits them. Did someone hit you? Are you afraid?' or 'Sometimes patients tell me they have been hurt by someone close to them. Could this be happening to you?' (Jezierski 1992, Snyder 1994). It is also suggested that history taking should be done independently with both patient and carer where there is any suspicion of an abusive situation and that particular attention should be paid to the possibility of both overt and covert physical and psychological signs of abuse.

In attempting to increase the knowledge base of professional groups in one London borough, Zlotnick (1993) prepared an education package with the following objectives:

- to create an awareness of elder abuse/ inadequate care
- to develop a working definition of elder abuse and inadequate care
- to help members of health and social work staff to begin to tackle areas of policy and procedure in the light of the present lack of statutory policies and guidelines.

Comprehensive training packs have been developed by Phillipson & Biggs (1992) and the Royal College of Nursing (RCN 1995), which incorporate written material and videos for social work and health carers, but there is no education for medical practitioners on a regular basis and elder abuse is a low-priority topic in postgraduate medical education.

Protection of abused older people

One of the main issues in offering support to possibly abused older people is that they have every right to refuse protection and this can be frustrating for professionals concerned who feel rejected, particularly if they have worked for a long period with the person concerned. Older people often have a fierce sense of self-determination and may well feel that the possibility of abuse or danger is less important than their independence. Professionals have to accept the decision even if they do not agree with it, provided there are no grounds for suspecting mental incompetence and thus an approach under the terms of the Mental Health Act 1983. However, this does not mean that older people should be left with no provision if they wish to change their minds and professionals need to make very clear the ways in which the person can gain support and further assistance. Bennett et al (1997) make the important point that older people need to understand that abusive situations rarely consist of single acts and that as time goes on the abuse generally becomes more severe and more frequent. It is also important for the person to recognise that they are one of many older people who have experienced abusive situations and that many have managed to alter their circumstances and been able to live free from abuse and neglect.

Perceptions and attitudes in professionals who work with older people are a major factor in determining how best to intervene in potentially difficult situations. The education of professionals concerned needs to be wide-ranging, covering reflection, self-awareness and self-knowledge as well as a knowledge of systems and policies. Professionals working in these areas of practice should have developed the skills of reflection and should practise these regularly. It is also important to understand how we develop attitudes towards older people and what creates bias within cultures. Knowledge of abuse within families, particularly of a long-standing nature, is important as is the need to recognise what might be construed as positive intervention as opposed to interference. The difference between positive intervention and interference is one of concept on both sides – professional and family/client – and it is important for professionals to understand how families or victims may feel and to recognise what might be construed as overprotective or paternalistic. Phillipson (1992) argues coherently for the professional to work with the client through a process of advocacy, enablement and empowerment, particularly when the client is marginalised.

Bennett et al (1997), using a number of American studies, suggest that several generalisations can be made about professional perspectives that affect attitudes towards older people's problems. It would appear that there is greater knowledge of abuse among nurses, social workers and clergy than among doctors and lawyers, and that nurses and social workers have a greater perception that elder abuse is as common as child abuse than do the police. Social workers perceived psychological abuse and neglect as more common than physical abuse; police, lawyers and mental health workers perceived verbal abuse as more common than physical abuse; community psychiatric nurses reported more physical abuse; and social services staff reported more financial abuse. As far as the cause of abuse is concerned, lawyers and social workers thought that stress and dependency were the main causes, whereas nurses and police felt that the cycle of violence was the main cause. As a result of these factors the studies found that in approaches to intervention social workers sought to change the situation or behaviour, police sought to detect or prevent crime and nurses attended to health needs. In many instances the professionals concerned may seek to avoid or minimise difficult and painful situations and clearly professionals need help in recognising

why they may be avoiding a situation and how to combat this.

Work undertaken in Coventry by Gist (personal communication, 1996) suggested, in relation to child abuse, that where health professionals, particularly health visitors, felt they had a 'good' relationship with carers who might be abusers they were less likely to intervene and would consider the situation to be nonabusive. Similarly, there is evidence (Bennett et al 1997) that where older people were described as 'difficult', usually by virtue of possessing less desirable characteristics, there tended to be sympathy with the abuser and possible collusion against the victim. Examples like these show how necessary good clinical supervision ought to be in enabling professionals to view situations through the perspective of a colleague and at the same time to have a good knowledge of how attitudes are attained. It is thus important to recognise the need for multidisciplinary or multiagency work to allow a balance between the perspectives of the different workers and their perceived roles.

Interventions can range from the passive end of the continuum to the aggressive end, from advocacy and empowerment to the full use of the legal system. Professionals, especially health visitors and community mental health practitioners who are trained in counselling and therapy, will tend to use the passive approach, whereas the use of control may be more in keeping with the approach of a social worker. It must be recognised that neither way is all-beneficial and that there are times when the control of a problem through legal processes may be less dangerous to abused and professional alike; similarly 'using a sledge hammer to crack a nut' by employing the full force of the law may be a very short-term approach to a major problem. If the goal of intervention is for the abused to attain an abuse-free existence then it may be beneficial for the abuser and abused to be separated sooner rather than later and the skill and experience of the professional is important in determining the most appropriate time. Case conference approaches, where the perspectives of multiagency professionals come together, sound ideal but it must be remembered that professional groups can adopt a perspective of their own that may not be in the best interests of the client. Also, if legal processes are sought and not attained, the abused may be in a more dangerous situation than before.

The Department of Health and Social Services Inspectorate (1993) issued guidelines for the assessment of older people who are suspected of being victims of an abusive situation, and they strongly advocate a multidisciplinary approach individually adapted and carried out by experienced practitioners. It is necessary to take time and care in assessment, given that many older people are reluctant to discuss abuse or abusive situations.

Assessment needs to include:

- an in-depth history both of family dynamics and relationships and of the current situation
- an idea of the everyday functioning of the family or of the carer and abused
- the dependency of the abused and the stressors to the situation
- the views, beliefs and attitudes of the key players
- the ways in which the abused person has so far coped with the situation,

and the Department of Health stresses the need to assess the needs of the individuals concerned rather than needs for service provision. It may be necessary to use a needs-led assessment, but ensure that it is abuse-focused.

An aspect of protection that often causes health visitors great concern is that it can be seen as paternalistic and disempowering, but it has to be remembered that older people belong to a different generation from their carers and are often more receptive to the notion of compliance and acceptance. These attitudes themselves often create vulnerability in older people and thus protective services are necessary. In some instances, older people are not totally dependent and with appropriate support may become empowered enough to be able to avoid risk situations and, recognising the precedent factors, may be able to take avoiding action.

A holistic approach to potentially abusing situations means that a range of intervention strategies matching the differing causes of abuse

is necessary. These will extend from education and counselling to speedy access to emergency services, from safe havens for the abused older person to alternative accommodation for the abuser who cannot get out of the situation. The provision of a practical service such as a lifting aid may be as helpful, as may provision of carer relief through a sitting service. Bennett et al (1997) cite the work of Gelles (1983) in considering the value of a social exchange as a trade-off from an alteration in the abusive situation. It may mean in a sense that it would be more profitable for an abuser to accept a 'reward' than to continue in the abuser role. Likewise, it may be more profitable for the abused elder to adopt a less vulnerable subservient attitude and thus 'gain' from the acceptance of an alteration in the situation.

Practical support as an effective intervention can be material, for example the provision of finance or equipment such as a continence service or a laundry facility, respite care in an alternative situation for both the older person and their carer, or a sitting service. Finally, therapeutic interventions such as stress reduction techniques or anger management programmes.

Therapeutic interventions require an education approach and the opportunity to see an endpoint otherwise they may well be considered of little value. They may include the understanding of the difference between protection and personal liberty and how to introduce these. Other education approaches include advice and information on a wide range of issues, which may include medical information about health/illness, housing or financial benefit advice, or ways in which the employment of the carer can be maintained. Another major benefit can be gained from multi-agency support and this in itself is fraught with difficulty where there is no key worker who can act as co-ordinator to ensure a smooth service.

Violence towards older people from people outside the home is still relatively rare. However, there are regular reports in the press of older people being subjected to violence during a burglary. Much of this violence would appear to be spontaneous and greater force is often used, sometimes resulting in death either directly or as a result of the accompanying shock leading to a stroke or heart attack. Health visitors can assist in prevention of such incidents by raising awareness of the importance of not displaying signs of affluence, encouraging neighbourhood support, mounting anticrime campaigns, or attempting to reduce the social isolation of older people.

CONCLUSION

Health visitors are becoming increasingly aware of the need to increase their knowledge of many aspects of violence. James-Hanman of the Greater London Domestic Violence Project, in a conference paper (1998) accused the NHS of being very slow to respond to violence, in particular domestic violence. She particularly commented that the NHS was accident-focused rather than injury-focused, deals with consequences rather than causes, and that staff do not know of practical solutions to situations. Other factors that James-Hanman highlights are lack of education and training, embarrassment about asking direct questions and concerns about upsetting relationships.

This chapter has tried to cover the range of violent issues that health visitors may be exposed to, often as a consequence of a domiciliary or clinic intervention or other reasons, e.g. a child-health surveillance visit. Asking direct questions should not necessarily be seen as leading to intervention, but the opportunity for a victim to talk to an outsider may be more helpful than any formal response. If health visitors feel secure that they have sufficient knowledge about violence to be able to listen to victims without experiencing an overwhelming sense of powerlessness, then their response to victims is often more measured and empathetic, giving the victim a feeling of support. Health visitors should also recognise that they can be very effective in maintaining family dynamics and helping families to understand themselves, especially along the lines of the circumplex model of Olson et al (1979), providing families with insight into their own evolution.

14

Complementary therapies and health visiting

Pat Alexander

There is one thing stronger than all the armies of the world, and that is an idea whose time has come.
(Victor Hugo)

INTRODUCTION

It is my privilege in the following pages to explore the birth and growth of complementary medicine within the realms of health visiting and its integration into the NHS. We are standing on the brink of an exciting new approach to health visiting, one which will enable us to deepen further our philosophy of preventative care, of partnership with clients and of empowerment.

At the same time it is essential to acknowledge our role in the primary healthcare team where we may act as a catalyst for change, a co-ordinator and a key worker for client care.

One of our vital roles embraced under the umbrella of 'co-ordinator' will be that of a link person with the general practitioners so that complementary medicine is seen as *complementary* rather than alternative. Unfortunately, as a result of lack of consultation, discussion and mutual respect, complementary medicine continues to be regarded as 'witchcraft' with little scientific backup to support its work.

There is a long way to go and there are many obstacles to be tackled but all is possible with the right approach and positive attitudes.

Health visitors are seen as advocates for the clients they visit. They will now become advocates for complementary medicines using the basic tools learned from their training and fieldwork experience, of listening, respect, teaching and planning, both short- and long-term, based on research.

In this way they will not only assist in deepening the understanding of complementary medicine by healthcare professionals but will work towards creating a harmonious marriage between orthodox and complementary healthcare and an integrated healthcare service.

INTEGRATED HEALTHCARE – DO WE NEED IT?

Over the last 50 years there have been tremendous improvements in the treatment of illness but unfortunately this has led to increasing demands on limited resources, resulting in waiting lists and long delays for treatment. There is also growing concern regarding the potential side-effects of drugs used to combat ill health. These two major drawbacks in healthcare have spearheaded the work of the Foundation for Integrated Medicine, which believes that the integration of orthodox and complementary medicine can help to provide a solution.

How to achieve integration?

The Foundation for Integrated Medicine, a charity initiated at the suggestion of His Royal Highness the Prince of Wales in 1994, holds the vision that integration will be achieved only by 'the close working together of orthodox and complementary medical practitioners, with mutual respect and understanding'. It is hoped that this vision will be realised by the attainment of the following objectives:

* to promote awareness of the clinical and economic benefits of effective integrated health and medical practices
* to promote scientific research into complementary medicine
* to collaborate with other medical and complementary organisations
* to collect, codify and disseminate knowledge of complementary medical practices
* to promote educational programmes in integrated medicine.

The goals of the Foundation offer a holistic approach to the care of the client:

* to promote health and well-being in addition to treating illness
* to deal with people as whole individuals, obtaining their confidence and trust, building inner strength for the treatment of their illness
* to restore to people their feeling of self-worth and esteem through active participation in their own treatment, which is often essential for recovery.

The role of scientific research

The Foundation for Integrated Medicine acknowledges research as one of its important objectives. It pays special attention to cost benefit analysis and the efficacy of treatments.

It supports the following approaches to research:

* to undertake pilot research studies into new areas of integrated medicine
* to support research into the efficacy of complementary medicine for common debilitating ailments such as childhood asthma, irritable bowel syndrome, hypertension, menopausal syndromes and back pain
* to review previous research work to establish the complementary treatments that have reasonably good evidence for efficacy and to note gaps where new research might be beneficial.

The above objectives are of crucial importance as at present there is virtually no information, treatment trials or research on good integrated medical practice.

The role of education

If integration is to take place it is necessary to facilitate this through easily available study days and pertinent literature to help doctors and health professionals to become familiar with complementary therapies. As a result of an initiative stemming from the British Medical Association's 1993 publication *Complementary*

Medicine: New Approaches to Good Practice, the Research Council for Complementary Medicine is assessing the best methods of educating conventional practitioners about complementary medicine and increasing the awareness and understanding of GPs.

In a comparative study carried out by Perkin et al in 1994, which involved a random sample of 100 GPs and 100 hospital doctors in the South West Thames Regional Health Authority and 237 preclinical medical students at St George's Hospital Medical School, it was found that the majority of the respondents felt that complementary medicine should be available on the NHS and that medical students should receive some tuition about it. Some 70% of hospital doctors and 93% of GPs had on at least one occasion suggested a referral for complementary treatment, and 12% of hospital doctors and 20% of GPs were practising complementary medicine.

Research methods

On a practical level it is necessary that complementary therapists are suitably trained in research methods in order that data can be processed and analysed. The Research Council for Complementary Medicine has acknowledged that research is a complicated and technical procedure and to this end has been involved in a number of educational initiatives to teach research skills to practitioners of complementary medicine. First-time researchers gain experience in simple research designs before seeking funds for larger scale projects.

Some examples of research funded by the Research Council are:

- 'An evaluation in atopic eczema of topical treatments containing Chinese medicinal herbs'
- 'The fragrance component of aromatherapy in anxiety'
- 'Anti-nausea effect of acupuncture'
- 'Controlled trial of yoga for stress related ailments'
- 'Assessment of osteopathic manipulation for acute back pain'.

THE RELATIONSHIP BETWEEN HEALTH VISITORS, ALLOPATHIC MEDICINE AND COMPLEMENTARY MEDICINE

The greatest unifying factor of this multi-disciplinary approach is the well-being of the client. In theory, this should override any differing opinions as long as the treatment is supported by the appropriate research and all practice is evidence based.

The needs of an individual are many and complex and any imbalance in the fulfilment of these needs can cause ill health. This is symbolised in Figure 14.1.

Holistic medicine would take an overall view of the whole flower, as would a health visitor, whereas in orthodox medicine, frequently as a result of time restrictions, only one petal of the flower would be scrutinised. Both approaches are of vital importance to the client and, if combined, form a powerful force towards eliminating the causes of ill health.

Holistic care involves:

- responding to the person as a whole (body, mind and spirit) within the context of their environment (family, culture and ecology)
- a willingness to use a wide range of interventions, from drugs and surgery to meditation and diet

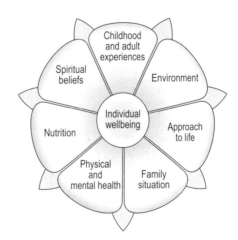

Figure 14.1 The holistic medicine flower

- an emphasis on a more participatory relationship between doctor and patient
- an awareness of the impact of the 'health' of the practitioner on the patient.

Working together

In the NHS Executive document *Primary Care: The Future* (Department of Health 1996a) it is recognised that the best services are provided when there is a spirit of collaboration and co-operation not only among professionals but also with the client and the carers if applicable. It cites the importance of understanding and appreciating the roles and skills of each member of the primary healthcare team in order to cultivate an atmosphere that is both positive and therapeutic for those involved in treatment. The document explores the option of direct self-referral plus the use of a healthcare worker to advise people on the range and types of help available.

It is a well-known fact that complementary therapies present a confusing and somewhat frightening picture to the lay person, not to mention the trial of finding a reputable and trust-worthy specialist. The specialist health visitor for complementary medicine would be sufficiently trained to fulfil this role, acting as a link between orthodox and complementary treatments and as an advisor to the client (Fig. 14.2). This would ensure an integrated health service, providing local people with access to qualified professionals in the type of complementary medicine best suited to treat their condition.

Client held records

At the moment the only documentation retained by clients in the community are:

- child-health records
- maternity records
- pilot projects in which the client records reactions to treatment.

If relationships are to be addressed seriously by professionals and clients, it is imperative that the client retains a permanent record of his general health plus details of ongoing treatment. As health visitors, key words such as 'empowerment', 'partnership', 'self-esteem' and 'shared responsibility', slip easily off our tongues and it is through the establishment of a comprehensive health record that these ideals may be achieved.

A sample of such a client held record could be as shown in Figure 14.3.

This would form a basis for partnership in care, a copy being kept by the client and another by the key health worker, who may be the health visitor or another appointed person. These details might be in the form of a small booklet, similar to the child-health records, and would ideally also contain details on:

- recommended weights, according to height
- nutritional advice on healthy diets related to weight control, heart disease, diabetes, bowel disorders and allergic conditions
- alcohol consumption, with recommended daily intakes
- the importance of exercise and types of relaxation

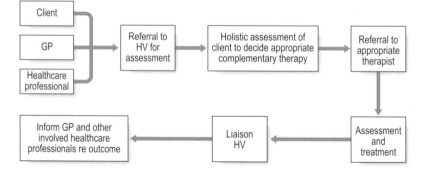

Figure 14.2   Health visitor/key worker referral/discharge procedure

Client Health Record
Name:
Address:
Telephone no:
Date of birth:
Next of kin:
GP:
Health visitor:
Key worker:

Other healthcare professionals, for example:
   1. District nurse, practice nurse
   2. Obstetrician, midwife
   3. Mental health team
   4. Complementary therapist

Date   Health concerns   Treatment   Outcome   Health care plan

Figure 14.3   An example of a client held record

- management of stress
- coping with minor illnesses (e.g. colds, flu)
- health checks for men and women
- family planning
- advice on smoking cessation.

The booklet would thus serve as a useful reference for the client regarding the maintenance of a healthy lifestyle in addition to promoting a sense of personal responsibility and involvement in the treatment of ill health. It would also contain a list of useful contact numbers where further advice and support might be accessed.

By fulfilment of the key worker role in complementary medicine the health visitor will be exploiting the four principles of practice defined by the Council for the Education and Training of Health Visitors and recognised by the UKCC – the search for health needs, the stimulation of the awareness of health, the influence of policies affecting health and the facilitation of health-enhancing activities.

It is important to remember that the most powerful way a health visitor is able to influence policies affecting health, especially in relation to the successful treatment of certain ailments through the use of complementary medicine, is through the collection of *evidence-based practice*. An integrated healthcare service will only develop through the collection of reliable and proven research-based documentation.

HEALTH MAINTENANCE BEHAVIOURS AND THE USE OF COMPLEMENTARY THERAPY

What is 'health maintenance behaviour'? Simply put, it is creating a healthy lifestyle and approach to life through the elimination of disease and negative attitudes.

It is the role of the GP to treat ill health, but the issues of maintaining good health for the local population exist in a vacuum. Health visitors adopt the role of preventative healthcare but, as mentioned in *The Scope of Professional Practice* (UKCC 1992b), there are many instances where their skills and experience are not used to their full potential. At present, in the majority of cases, health visitors concentrate on work with families of children under 5, which, although vitally important, results in other community needs being neglected. The UKCC clearly recognises this problem: 'There is merit in allowing health visitors, where they judge it to be appropriate, to use the full range of their skills in response to needs identified in the pursuit of their health visiting practice'.

In response to this innovative and encouraging statement it is clearly evident that health visiting may break free from its stereotyped 'under-5s' role to adopt a wider perspective in its approach to work within the community. A health visitor specialist in complementary medicine is just one example of how community needs may be met by assisting the client to make more informed choices and thereby create a better relationship with all those involved in optimal health. This also works towards raising the client's self-esteem and sense of responsibility to enable them to become an active member of the multidisciplinary health team.

It is important that the advice put forward to

the client by the health visitor is research-based to maintain credibility both within the medical profession and among the community. To this end the Foundation for Integrated Medicine is at present funding six research projects:

- 'Reflexology for childhood asthma'
- 'Homeopathy for childhood asthma'
- 'Osteopathy for asthma'
- 'The Alexander technique for Parkinson's disease'
- 'Marma therapy for stroke victims'
- 'A diagnostic test for lower back pain'.

Through its Research Committee the Foundation assists potential researchers in the production of sound protocols and it is the duty of the health visitor to ensure that the practitioners to whom she refers adhere to such protocols in addition to carrying out research projects.

It is important that the role of the specialist health visitor (Fig. 14.4) is far-reaching in order to create maximum awareness of the complementary therapy treatments available in both professionals and laypeople alike.

There needs also to be the backdrop of on-going research in order to guarantee evidence-based practice, which may be co-ordinated with

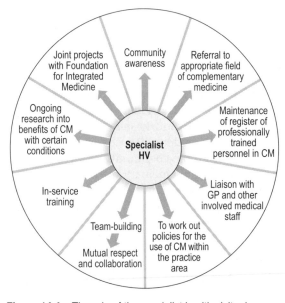

Figure 14.4 The role of the specialist health visitor in complementary medicine

the research project supported by the Research Committee of the Foundation for Integrated Medicine. The health visitor should also ensure that clear policies exist within the practice area to safeguard both the client and practitioner and to give credibility to the field of complementary therapy.

INTEGRATING COMPLEMENTARY THERAPIES WITHIN PRIMARY CARE GROUPS

The philosophy behind the setting up of primary care groups mirrors that of complementary therapies:

- to work in partnership with others
- to promote health
- to share skills.

Some of the qualities brought to the groups by health visitor specialists include:

- good communication skills
- holistic assessments
- integrated care
- resource management
- sensitivity to ethnic issues
- evidence-based practice.

The hope is that professionals will maintain mutual respect for each other's roles according to the overall plan of the White Paper (Department of Health 1997a), which is:

- to improve the health of the nation as a whole
- to improve the health of the less privileged, thus decreasing the health divide.

It is well known that at present complementary therapies remain the luxury of the privileged few, with the occasional exception where they are accessed through the NHS. The integration of orthodox medicine with complementary therapies would be instrumental in removing this divide.

In order to bring the aims of the White Paper down to grass roots level it is necessary to look at the common denominator for most people in Britain as regards health issues – the GP. It is the GP who decides, following an initial assessment, whether the client might be best suited for orthodox or complementary medicine. This ensures that any health problems requiring immediate medical or surgical intervention receive attention with the minimum delay. However, some clients may still wish to combine orthodox and complementary medicine for the treatment of life-threatening conditions and the choice is available, e.g. after cardiac surgery where the patient might also attend yoga classes to encourage relaxation and decrease stress or, alternatively, receive aromatherapy treatment to lower blood pressure and encourage a sense of well-being. Integrated medicine within primary care groups is thus able to address the health priorities listed in the national targets – heart disease, stroke, accidents, mental health and cancer.

The use of complementary therapies within the primary care group

The type of therapy used is dependent initially upon those who have been accepted by the health authority concerned. For example, South Birmingham Mental Health Trust approved the following therapies in a draft policy dated January 1996: acupuncture, the Alexander technique, aromatherapy, art therapy, auricular acupuncture, counselling, drama therapy, herbalism, homeopathy, massage, movement therapy, music therapy, reflexology, sports therapy and yoga. In order to have a brief overview we will look at four therapies and their application in practice in greater detail – aromatherapy, yoga, touch – baby stroking and nutritional medicine.

It is to be remembered that the principles behind all good primary care are those quoted by the NHS Executive in their information booklet *Primary Care: The Future* (Department of Health 1996a). These are as follows:

- *Quality*
  - Professionals should be knowledgeable about the conditions that present in primary care and skilled in their treatment
  - Professionals should be knowledgeable about the people to whom they are offering services
  - Services should be co-ordinated with professionals aware of each other's contributions (including interprofessional working) and no service gaps
  - Premises and facilities should be of a good standard and fit for their purpose, and equipment should be up to date, well maintained and safe to use
- *Fairness*
  - Services should not vary widely in range or quality in different parts of the country
  - Primary care should receive an appropriate share of overall NHS resources
- *Accessibility*
  - Services should be reasonably accessible when clinically needed
  - Necessary services should be accessible to people regardless of age, sex, ethnicity or health status
- *Responsiveness*
  - Services should reflect the needs and preferences of the individuals using them
  - Services should reflect the demographic and social needs of the area they serve
- *Efficiency*
  - Primary care services should be based on scientific evidence
  - Primary care resources should be used efficiently.

AROMATHERAPY

Aromatherapy is one of the most popular forms of complementary therapy in the UK and USA and is frequently being employed by nurses and other healthcare professionals in hospital, hospice and community settings.

Aromatherapy uses potent substances and therefore comprehensive training is essential. The therapist should be a member of a reputable professional body, e.g. the International Society of Professional Aromatherapists (ISPA), and have full insurance cover.

How essential oils work

Essential oils enter the body by inhalation plus transference to the bloodstream via the nose, lungs and skin by means of vaporisers, massage and baths. Essential oils, when inhaled, affect the brain directly by means of neurochemical messages that are picked up by the olfactory nerve endings in the nose and passed to the limbic area, which forms part of our complex brain. From there they rapidly affect our moods and emotions, giving rise to complex chemical changes in the body. The release of encephalins and endorphins, which act as the body's natural painkillers, produce sensations of well-being and calm. During respiration the molecules of oil pass into the lungs and thence by diffusion into the bloodstream with oxygen. This is facilitated by the small molecular size of essential oils and the single-cell thickness of the alveoli and blood capillaries of the lungs.

During massage oils pass by diffusion into the skin, crossing the stratum corneum, the outer layer of the skin, entering the epidermis and the dermis and thence into the capillary circulation. Essential oils can act very quickly as well as over a period of time, being released into the bloodstream and distributed around the body. They are then excreted in respiration, sweat, urine or faeces.

Application

Aromatherapy is definitely a complementary therapy in that it can be used alongside allopathic medicine and most other therapies. One exception may be homeopathy, as there is a risk of the essential oils nullifying the effect of the homeopathic remedy. Research is currently being carried out in this area.

In Appendix 2 the properties of lavender oil have been examined in detail in order to demonstrate the in-depth knowledge that is required, not only for the practice of aromatherapy but indeed for the practice of all forms of complementary therapy.

YOGA

Many people who consult an aromatherapist do so because they are under stress or because they are suffering from physical symptoms that are the result of stress and anxiety. While the aromatherapist can help to reduce stress and bring about a state of calm and relaxation in the short term, it is important to look to a long-term solution for this problem. Yoga fulfils this need by teaching the stressed person active methods to help himself.

Yoga, as aromatherapy, works on many levels. It may be viewed simply as a system of physical exercise or as a profound philosophy, and yoga teachers vary in the amount of emphasis they place on the different aspects.

Classical yoga dates back to 2000 BC when an Indian scholar called Patanjali recorded in minute detail the means of attaining 'enlightenment' or a oneness with oneself and the world. His teachings are holistic and embrace physical and mental health, aiming to create a humble, positive and sincere approach to life. Simplistically his works may be summarised in the 'eightfold path of yoga' (Fig. 14.5): *Yama* = restraints, e.g. nonviolence; *niyama* = observances, e.g. self-study; *asana* = good health through physical education; *pranayama* = regulation of bioenergy (respiratory) practices; *pratyahara* = the process of abstraction; *dharana* = concentration; *dhyana* = meditation; *samadhi* = self-realisation.

Physical benefits

Research has revealed that meditation is the most effective technique for decreasing anxiety levels, reducing alcohol, cigarette and drug intake and improving psychological health (Thomas 1997).

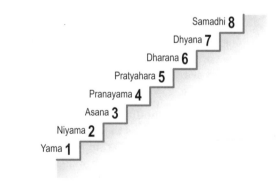

Figure 14.5   The eightfold path of yoga

Integration

From the above results it is clear that it would be of benefit to clients in the community setting to be taught the art of meditation as part of a health promotion programme either by a health visitor specialist or by a suitably trained professional. At present this is being carried out on a one-to-one basis by a health visitor trained to teach yoga in:

- postnatal and general depression affecting the client's self-esteem, confidence and ability to socialise
- stress causing anxiety attacks and insomnia.

However, meditation would also be ideal for small-group teaching, as illustrated in Figure 14.6.

It should be noted that in the teachings of classical yoga no step is taken in isolation. Clients therefore study the full eightfold path in order to reach the seventh step, meditation (dhyana). This would ensure a holistic approach to each individual covering the well-being of the person physically, mentally, psychologically and spiritually. The client would be reasssured that yoga is not a religion, as some imagine, and in no way clashes with any religious beliefs. It is a way of life that creates a positive approach to life and a sense of inner calm.

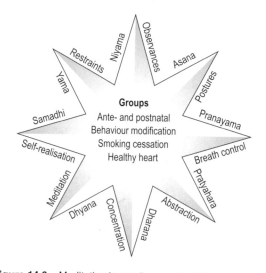

Figure 14.6   Meditation in small-group teaching

TOUCH – BABY STROKING

Anna Freud writes that being stroked, cuddled and soothed by touch helps to build up a healthy baby image and body ego cementing the intimate relationship between child and parents. It is this relationship that the health visitor works towards establishing through encouragement and support in the early months of parenthood. This may be further enhanced by teaching the parents the art of simple massage.

Additional benefits of baby massage have been recognised as:

- relaxing baby and encouraging sleep
- developing good muscle tone and suppleness
- relief of colic and constipation
- improving the appearance of the skin and assisting in the elimination of waste products and toxins
- strengthening the immune system.

If baby massage is carried out with love the end result is to create not only a feeling of security for the baby but also relaxation of body and mind for both the person giving the massage and the recipient.

Cody (1995) carried out research on the effect of infant massage on the attitudes and perceptions of mothers who massage their hospitalised premature infants. This study compared the effects of two maternal interactions, infant massage and reading, on hospitalised premature infants and their mothers. Self-report measures of maternal self-esteem, sense of well-being, perception of her infant and infant weight gain patterns were employed. A total of 19 mothers of premature infants admitted to the special care nurseries were recruited; 10 mothers massaged their babies for 10 minutes daily and nine mothers read to their babies for 10 minutes daily. The massage or reading was initiated in the hospital once the babies were medically stable. Interventions were continued at home for a total of 28 days.

The following differences were found between the two groups:

- Massaged infants had a mean weight gain of 206.5 g more than control group infants
- Massage group mothers had a greater sense of

well-being and higher self-esteem than control group mothers

- Massage group mothers demonstrated an increase in positive perception of their infants but this did not reach statistical significance
- Control group mothers changed from positive to negative perceptions of their infants from the beginning to the end of the study
- Massage group mothers remained stable on all measures, with no significant change
- Control group mothers demonstrated decreased sense of well-being, lower maternal self-esteem and a negative change in their perception of their infants from the beginning to the end of the intervention.

A discussion of future research and clinical implications was recommended.

This research, although limited, throws light on the benefits of massage not only to baby but to the mother also, affecting the total health of both and demonstrating the holistic care that massage offers to giver and receiver alike (Fig. 14.7).

Teaching baby stroking

Before baby massage or baby stroking is taught it is important that the health visitor has received adequate training. Study days or evenings are conducted by health promotion units, aromatherapy schools and other professional bodies. This ensures that instructions are safe, clear, comprehensive and are delivered in a confident and relaxed manner.

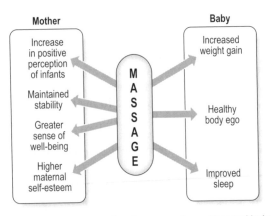

Figure 14.7   The benefits of massage for mother and baby

It is not advisable to teach baby massage directly from a book for the following reasons:

- Pressure of the hands when administering massage needs to be learned, particularly for massaging babies and children
- Comfortable positions for both the child and the person giving the massage need to be experienced at first hand
- The practitioner needs to be qualified in both the theoretical and practical aspects of massage, with particular emphasis on safety. This would also safeguard them should any complaint be voiced by a parent.

NUTRITIONAL MEDICINE

The basis of holistic healthcare is that the whole person requires attention, so it would be negligent if the aspect of dietary intake is ignored. Every practitioner therefore, whatever the therapy, should have a sound understanding of dietary therapy and its practical application in both general and specific conditions.

In cases of stress the body requires an increase in vitamins, minerals and trace elements to enable the organism to cope with the additional demands. This is because prolonged stress causes both biochemical and neurochemical imbalances within the bodily systems. Deficiency progressively leads to disease, which is the principal reason why the health practitioner needs to become aware of dietary needs.

'Contemporary foods are nutritionally deficient because of the consumption of de-nutritionalised, processed foods, imbalanced by an excess of animal fats and an underconsumption of fibres and fresh vegetables. They are unnatural because of the excessive use of additives at all levels of the food chain and all categories of food' (Bennett 1992). It is a fact well known to the health visitor that colourings and additives in the diet of some children can lead to the following problems:

- behavioural problems
- night terrors
- infantile colic
- hyperactivity.

In adults dietary deficiencies manifest themselves in numerous conditions. In the postnatal period examples are anaemia, depression, irritability and insomnia, and dietary deficiency is a contributory factor in postnatal depression. It is therefore an important role of the health visitor to create an awareness of the curative aspects of a healthy diet in order to assist clients to take responsibility for their own health. This may be done at all minimal surveillance checks arranged for the child, where the contact provides an ideal opportunity to learn about the family's health and probable manifestations of vitamin or mineral deficiency, allergy or food intolerance. This is often seen in the following conditions:

- skin disorders
- gastrointestinal disturbances
- respiratory problems
- behavioural difficulties.

The health visitor needs therefore to possess an in-depth knowledge of nutritional needs, which differs remarkably from the more basic knowledge conveyed in health promotion sessions.

INTEGRATING COMPLEMENTARY THERAPY INTO THE MEDICAL FIELD

Complementary therapies that may be considered for integration into the roles of various health professionals are illustrated in Figures 14.8 and 14.9.

An example of a complementary therapy being successfully integrated into the medical field is at the Neuropsychiatry and Seizure Clinic based at the Queen Elizabeth Psychiatric Hospital in Birmingham by Dr Tim Betts (1995), a consultant neuropsychiatrist. Dr Betts uses aromatherapy and hypnosis in the treatment of epilepsy. In one case study he writes:

Using a diary for 2 or 3 months Glynis was able to recognise that her tonic–clonic seizures were occurring in association with anxiety triggered off by problems in her relationship. She was able to recognise when she was becoming anxious (massages with camomile taught her for the first time what it was like to be relaxed and were invaluable in teaching her to discriminate between tension and relaxation). By using the smell of camomile as a countermeasure whenever she felt herself become tense she was able to completely

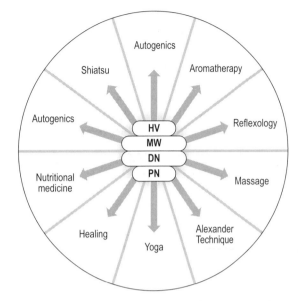

Figure 14.8   Types of complementary therapy appropriate for primary care teams (DN = district nurse; HV = health visitor; MW = midwife; PN = practice nurse)

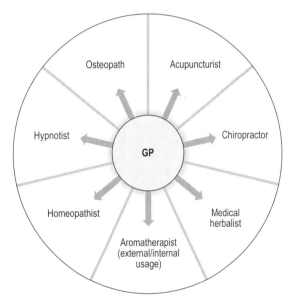

Figure 14.9   Types of complementary therapy contingent with the GP role

stop her seizures and has been seizure-free for over 3 years and has regained her driving licence.

It should be noted that the types of therapy suggested in Figures 14.8 and 14.9 are only suggestions. There are many other excellent complementary therapies, which are too numerous to mention. More details on complementary therapies may be obtained from the Research Council for Complementary Medicine, 60 Great Ormond Street, London WC1N 3JF.

For the reader's convenience a short summary of the complementary therapies mentioned in this chapter is included in Appendix 1.

HEALTH VISITING CASE STUDIES IN THE COMMUNITY SETTING

The following are case studies recently carried out, with the permission of the GP, on clients in the Hertfordshire and Essex Health Authority.

Case study 1

History

Child A was admitted to hospital in August 1997 at the age of 15 months with initially acute onset of complete flaccid paralysis of both upper limbs and respiratory embarrassment. He was transferred to the paediatric intensive care unit with the diagnosis of acute transverse myelitis; in addition he had some bladder weakness. He was discharged home 6 weeks later with the support of the GP, physiotherapist, occupational therapist, speech and language therapist, community paediatric nurses, social worker and health visitor.

Parental concerns

Mr & Mrs A highlighted the following problems since their child's discharge from hospital: muscle stiffness (there was a possibility that he would not be able to walk again); lowered resistance to infection; disturbed sleep; increased mucoid secretions with respiratory difficulties; bladder instability.

Treatment

Essential oils were selected to embrace the concerns mentioned above as follows:

- to strengthen the immune system
  - *Lavandula augustifolia* (lavender)
  - *Melaleuca alternifolia* (tea tree)
- to relax the muscle stiffness
  - *Origanum marjoram* (sweet marjoram)
  - *Lavandula augustifolia* (lavender)
- to help regulate bladder activity
  - *Cedrus atlanticus* (cedarwood)
  - *Santalum album* (sandalwood)
- to decrease mucoid secretions and assist respiration
  - *Eucalyptus smithii* (eucalyptus)
  - *Santalum album* (sandalwood)
  - *Melaleuca alternifolia* (tea tree)
  - *Cedrus atlanticus* (cedarwood).

These were mixed together in grapeseed oil to form a synergistic blend. The effect of synergy is that when two or more oils are combined a greater effect is achieved. For example, the bactericidal effect of several oils combined is greater than the effect of any of the individual oils.

A second mixture was also made to assist child A's sleep. This comprised the following oils: *Santalum album* (sandalwood) and *Cananga odorata* (ylang ylang).

Instructions were given to the parents regarding application and massage techniques for the mixtures, which were applied once daily.

Outcome

This case study is an excellent example of complementary medicine: the treatment of Child A was carried out alongside allopathic medicine. As a result of this partnership, in August 1998 Child A was beginning to take steps on his own, his breathing had greatly improved and he no longer attended the GP surgery weekly because of infections. The parents are delighted with his progress, which is attributed to a holistic health approach to the child's care whereby professionals have worked alongside each other with mutual respect.

Figure 14.10 shows a very proud little boy taking his first few steps since his illness.

Case study 2

History

Child B was admitted to hospital at the age of

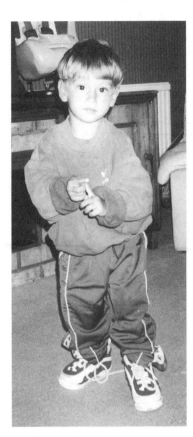

Figure 14.10   Child A after treatment

2½ years with a viral infection but, following discharge, hair loss occurred, leaving the child with very fine downy hair resembling that of patients who had undergone chemotherapy. She was seen in hospital regarding the hair loss and no cause could be diagnosed. Child B's mother was reassured that her child had no serious illness and that the hair would either grow back or fall out completely. She was advised there were good wigs available.

Parental concerns

The main concern was regarding the reaction of other children when Child B started school and the psychological damage it would cause to her personality and general self-esteem.

Treatment

With the permission of the GP a holistic assessment was carried out on Child B looking at her lifestyle, diet, personality and general health. In partnership with the parents the following was agreed:

- to massage the scalp each evening with the lotion given, rinsing this off the following morning and brushing the hair well; the lotion contained the following essential oils to help stimulate hair growth and improve the circulation:
  - *Cananga odorata* (ylang ylang)
  - *Rosmarinus officinalis* (rosemary)
  - *Cedrus atlanticus* (cedarwood)
- to ensure the diet contained foods rich in iron, zinc, vitamins B and C, and protein.

Outcome

After only 2 weeks of the above treatment the hair had started to thicken and Child B's scalp could no longer be seen through her hair. A side-effect was also that she was beginning to sleep more soundly! Figures 14.11 and 14.12 show Child B before and after treatment.

Other conditions treated by aromatherapy in the community are insomnia in children, head lice, postnatal depression and stress in adults.

Case study 3

The following includes extracts from a thesis prepared by Jean Gonella, health visitor in Harrow Community Health Trust, which looks at the effectiveness of treating stress using aromatherapy massage. 'Massage was used on a group of women where stress had become distress, who volunteered to try aromatherapy in place of or to reduce medications such as tranquillisers and analgesics.'

This pilot study was targeted at women's health and continued for a period of 6 months. It was supported by senior management and all treatment was expected to be carried out within working hours. In total, 16 clients took

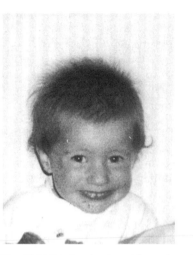

Figure 14.11 Child B before treatment (reproduced by kind permission of the child's parents)

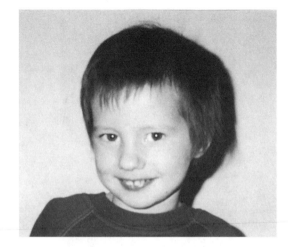

Figure 14.12 Child B after treatment

part in the study attending for 4–10 sessions each for a duration of 1–1½ hours per session.

'We would like to stress that, although a minimum of 1 hour is needed for a full body massage, it is not at all unusual for health visitors to spend an hour per visit with families with problems needing counselling and support. We see it as offering another approach to stress management, giving our clients a new dimension on their outlook and attitude towards their health.'

The criteria for selection for treatment by massage are given in Figure 14.13.

Objectives

- To alleviate stress through the use of aromatic oils with massage in order to create a sense of well-being on physical, psychological and emotional levels
- To increase self-awareness in relation to the effects of stress on the body
- To reduce GP consultation time
- To offer a more economic alternative to drug usage.

In summary, all clients reported that they felt more in control when placed in stressful situations; the quality of sleep had improved and generally they felt more confident in themselves.

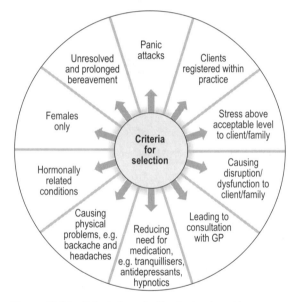

Figure 14.13 Criteria for selection for treatment by massage

All except one client had great improvement in all areas.

GP practice

The project was fully supported by the GPs. Consultations on the whole were considerably reduced – one patient had not seen her GP since commencing aromatherapy treatment, two patients took the option of massage rather than medication; one patient began to reduce her medication with her GP's permission.

Recommendations

- It might be more cost-effective if treatments were carried out on a sessional basis
- It would save both time and money if treatments were given on the clinic premises rather than in the client's home
- Oils would need to be purchased, consisting of at least 12 basic essential oils and a large bottle of grapeseed or base oil.

Conclusion

'The practical project proved 99% successful and involved 16 women over a period of 6 months. However, a much larger cohort study, using at least 100 clients and a control group, would be necessary to prove that aromatherapy could replace drug therapy.'

Such replacement would naturally be decided by the GP according to the severity of the problem at hand. It is to be remembered that, if the client's health needs are going to be fully addressed, complementary therapy can only exist in partnership with orthodox medicine.

Summary

The above case studies merely reflect the possibilities of integrated care in the community. The choice of aromatherapy as a complementary therapy is due to the author's experience in this field and is in no way intended to create a preference for a particular therapy.

In order to help demonstrate the in-depth knowledge required to practise any branch of complementary medicine a snapshot of aromatherapy is presented in Appendix 2.

THE NHS AND COMPLEMENTARY THERAPIES

At the moment there is no provision within primary legislation for patients to seek treatment from a complementary therapist under the auspices of the NHS. The only exception to this is through referral by a GP or hospital doctor to one of the five NHS homeopathic hospitals in the UK, where doctors are all conventionally trained with orthodox qualifications.

However, with changing public opinion it is likely that new legislation will be introduced. In 1991 the Consumers Association reported that one in four of their readers visited an alternative or complementary practitioner, which is double the number found in a survey in 1986. In 1990 a Medical Research Council study (Meade et al 1990) recommended that chiropractic should be available on the NHS, which has resulted in a Bill being put before Parliament for a statutory council to regulate the profession because of the demand for and use of chiropractors and osteopaths.

There have been many studies carried out by prominent medical journals such as the *British Medical Journal* over the last 10 years looking at the use of complementary therapies and doctors' attitudes to them. Attitudes have consistently been both positive and supportive. A list of these studies is included in Appendix 3.

Current opinion

In September 1992 Dr Gwen Cameron-Blackie, a senior registrar in public health medicine and Yvonne Mouncer, a health service consultant, carried out a national survey of district health authorities (DHAs), family health service authorities (FHSAs) and GP fundholders to examine purchasers' attitudes towards the availability of complementary therapies on the NHS and to establish current and future approaches to purchasing and funding such therapies. Questionnaires were sent to all DHAs and FHSAs and a sample of GP fundholders. Response rates were: 57% (110/192), 75% (74/99) and 43% respectively and a sample of the results is illustrated in Figures 14.14–14.20.

From studying these results it is apparent that homeopathy, acupuncture, osteopathy and chiropractic are viewed more favourably than aromatherapy or reflexology. However, the re-

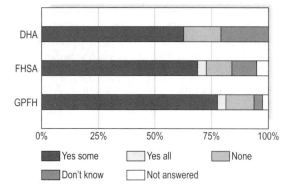

Legend:
- Yes some
- Yes all
- None
- Don't know
- Not answered

Figure 14.14 Response to the question 'Should complementary therapies be available on the NHS?' (DHA = district health authorities; FHSA = family health service authorities; GPFH = GP fundholders; reproduced with kind permission from Cameron-Blackie & Mouncer 1992)

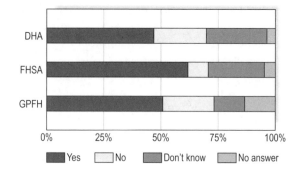

Legend:
- Yes
- No
- Don't know
- No answer

Figure 14.17 Response to the question 'Should chiropractic be available on the NHS?' (DHA = district health authorities; FHSA = family health service authorities; GPFH = GP fundholders; reproduced with kind permission from Cameron-Blackie & Mouncer 1992)

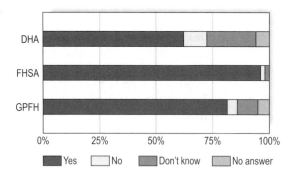

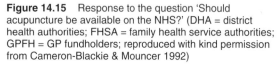

Legend:
- Yes
- No
- Don't know
- No answer

Figure 14.15 Response to the question 'Should acupuncture be available on the NHS?' (DHA = district health authorities; FHSA = family health service authorities; GPFH = GP fundholders; reproduced with kind permission from Cameron-Blackie & Mouncer 1992)

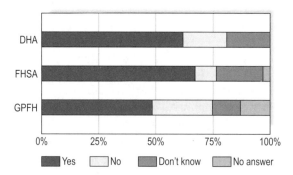

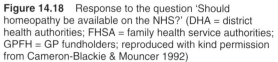

Legend:
- Yes
- No
- Don't know
- No answer

Figure 14.18 Response to the question 'Should homeopathy be available on the NHS?' (DHA = district health authorities; FHSA = family health service authorities; GPFH = GP fundholders; reproduced with kind permission from Cameron-Blackie & Mouncer 1992)

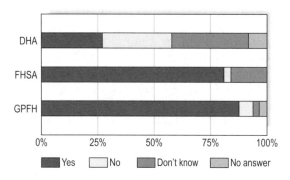

Legend:
- Yes
- No
- Don't know
- No answer

Figure 14.16 Response to the question 'Should osteopathy be available on the NHS?' (DHA = district health authorities; FHSA = family health service authorities; GPFH = GP fundholders; reproduced with kind permission from Cameron-Blackie & Mouncer 1992)

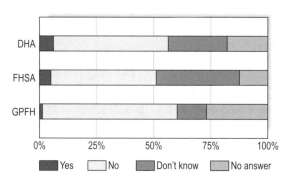

Legend:
- Yes
- No
- Don't know
- No answer

Figure 14.19 Response to the question 'Should reflexology be available on the NHS?' (DHA = district health authorities; FHSA = family health service authorities; GPFH = GP fundholders; reproduced with kind permission from Cameron-Blackie & Mouncer 1992)

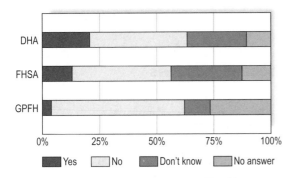

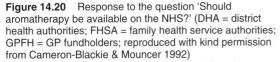

Figure 14.20   Response to the question 'Should aromatherapy be available on the NHS?' (DHA = district health authorities; FHSA = family health service authorities; GPFH = GP fundholders; reproduced with kind permission from Cameron-Blackie & Mouncer 1992)

GP fundholders: availability and appropriate uses of complementary therapies

The study revealed that complementary therapies were available in 34% of the GP fundholder practices responding to the questionnaire. Therapies being used were hypnosis, osteopathy, spinal manipulation, homeopathy, aromatherapy and counselling. The majority of these therapies were provided by a member of the primary healthcare team, which proves that integrated healthcare is already being practised, albeit in a small way, and should offer encouragement to any health visitor wishing to specialise in a complementary therapy.

Table 14.1 shows the types of therapy that GP fundholders consider could appropriately be used in the management of 10 conditions commonly encountered in general practice. Table 14.2 shows the factors said by each purchaser to be important to their decision-making on complementary therapies.

All three groups of purchasers were concerned about the lack of evidence on effectiveness, which is caused by various factors:

searchers believe this may be caused by the fact that:

- homeopathy has always been available on the NHS
- acupuncture is frequently used within the NHS
- patients are often referred by GPs privately to osteopaths and chiropractors
- reflexology and aromatherapy may be seen as relatively 'new age' therapies.

From the graphs there is also a noticeable percentage of authorities who remain unsure as to whether the therapies should or should not be available on the NHS. This is reflected by the number of 'don't knows' and 'no answers' in the results.

- there have been few randomised control trials
- the majority of the literature is on holistic studies or anecdotal evidence
- the majority of reports appear in complementary therapy journals, which are not readily available in local, medical, hospital or university libraries.

Table 14.1   The therapies GP fundholders consider could appropriately be used in the management of conditions commonly encountered in general practice (from Cameron-Blackie & Mouncer 1992)

Therapy	Acupuncture	Osteopathy	Chiropractic	Homeopathy	Reflexology	Aromatherapy	None	Don't know	No answer
Chronic back pain	59	74	41	9	3	1	8	1	2
Osteoarthritis	59	36	17	15	1	1	14	4	6
Rheumatoid arthritis	47	21	10	30	1	5	24	5	7
Hay fever	14	0	0	40	1	1	32	5	13
Anxiety	23	0	0	32	10	14	22	7	11
Insomnia	20	0	0	32	7	10	24	7	10
Obesity	18	0	0	1	0	1	41	7	20
Smoking	54	0	0	9	0	1	28	7	6
Peptic ulceration	5	0	0	12	0	0	51	9	20
Maturity-onset diabetes	2	0	1	6	1	1	61	8	18

Table 14.2 The factors stated by purchasers to be important to decision-making on complementary therapies (from Cameron-Blackie & Mouncer 1992)

Factor	%
District health authorities	
Lack of information on effectiveness	66
Lack of resources	24
Lack of demand	20
Lack of information/knowledge	14
Other priorities	14
Demand by GPs/public	10
High cost	8
Professional scepticism	8
GP fundholders	
Lack of information on effectiveness	48
Lack of information/knowledge	36
Lack of resources	31
Patient demand	16
Low priority	7
Lack of district health authority provision	7
Family health service authorities	
Lack of information on effectiveness	59
Lack of information/knowledge	25
Lack of resources	25
Public/GP opinion	20
Lack of information re quality/training	17
Lack of demand from GPs/public	13
Lack of support from GPs	13
Low priority	11

The above comments reflect the need for research as an ongoing duty for any health professional becoming involved in complementary medicine. It also highlights the importance of supplying accurate information on therapies to purchasers so that they are able to make informed decisions. The information requested covered:

- a basic understanding of what the therapy involves
- the principles/theoretical basis underlying the therapy
- the appropriate qualifications/training of therapist
- the medicolegal implications.

Funding

GP fundholders commented that funding complementary therapies would be dependent upon demonstrable cost-effectiveness and savings in other budgets, e.g. drug budgets or reductions in referrals.

Recommendations

- Additional research into the effectiveness of complementary medicines
- Evaluation of complementary therapy services currently available within the NHS
- Research into the cost/benefits of complementary therapies
- Development of standards for training and qualification
- All research findings and general information to be disseminated widely.

CONCLUSION

It is vital that complementary medicine is seen and understood as complementary: it is not alternative nor competitive but wishes to work alongside orthodox medicine. The only way forward is through mutual respect for the role each health professional plays in the prevention of disease, the maintenance of good health and the treatment of ill-health. Without this professional integrity the client will become a victim in the battleground for medical supremacy. However, there is no ideal therapy; we are all individuals reacting to the stresses and strains of the world in different ways. We need to celebrate this diversity and, at the same time, celebrate the fact that, for each unique person, there is a unique therapy that will meet their needs perfectly. 'What is required is a humble realisation that we are but partners in a healing relationship. There is no doctor alive who has ever cured anyone of anything. Only the body heals. Our part is to support the body in its cleansing and regenerative processes. We should strive to be part of the solution and not part of the problem' (Bennett 1992).

It is clear that there are many amazing possibilities ahead in the health field and it is hoped that this chapter may serve as a springboard for action for those health professionals who wish to pursue a specialism in complementary medicine. It is also clear that, while there are thousands of studies showing the efficacy of various complementary therapies, many of them are uncontrolled, involve small experimental groups or lack objective measurement criteria. The need for well-researched evidence-based practice is paramount.

Health visitors are in a privileged and exciting position in the field of preventative care and, through choosing to extend their role by specialising in an area of complementary medicine or becoming a liaison specialist, may serve as pathfinders for the profession.

Live your beliefs and you can turn the World around.
(Henry Thoreau)

APPENDIX 1: AN OVERVIEW OF COMPLEMENTARY THERAPIES

- **Acupuncture** literally means 'needle insertion'. There are two main forms of acupuncture, the first using traditional methods of needle insertion and selection of acupuncture points following traditional Chinese principles of diagnosis and disease classification based on the need to restore the balance of chi energy, which is considered essential to good health. The second form uses a modified form of acupuncture in which selection of points is based on dermatomal distributions of pain.
- **The Alexander technique** is a type of therapy that aims to prevent and treat a range of disorders using a system of postural changes. The principle is that habit influences the use of the body and that use in turn affects the way in which the body functions.
- **Aromatherapy** is most often used to describe a particular type of treatment in which essential oils or aromatic essences are massaged into the skin, inhaled or occasionally ingested.
- **Autogenics** consists of a series of easy mental exercises designed to switch off the stress 'flight or fight' responses of the body and switch on the rest, relaxation and recreation system.
- **Chiropractic**. Chiropractors specialise in the diagnosis and treatment of mechanical disorders of the joints, especially those of the spine, and their effects on the nervous system. Chiropractic is mainly used in the treatment of common musculoskeletal complaints.
- **Healing**. Most healers call themselves simply 'healers' although some add the qualification 'spiritual'. All healers believe in the existence of a healing force that can be channelled through them to patients. Some believe it to be channelled through God while others believe the force to be more natural but not yet recognised by science.
- **Homeopathy** is a system of medicine based on the principle of 'like curing like'. Homeopathic remedies are believed to assist the body's tendency to heal itself. Symptoms are believed to be the result of the body's defence mechanisms resisting attack; therefore homeopaths prescribe substances which, if used in a healthy person, would produce symptoms and signs similar to those presented by the patient. Remedies are prepared from repeatedly diluted extracts from, for example, minerals and plants. However, the effectiveness of a remedy is not directly related to its 'strength' as measured conventionally, and may in fact increase in potency with increasing dilution.
- **Hypnotherapy**. There are two main types of hypnotherapy. In the first the patient is put into a trance and the therapist suggests that their symptoms will disappear. In the second type they are put into a trance to facilitate the psychological treatment being used, e.g. to enable the therapist to explore what is going on in their subconscious mind.
- **Medical herbalism**. There are two main strands of herbal medicine – Western and Chinese. Both work from the basic principle that the symptoms of illness are a sign of underlying disharmony and are the physical manifestations of the body's attempts to heal itself. The herbs prescribed by the practitioner help this self-healing process.
- **Nutritional medicine**. Therapists believe that an unhealthy body is partly due to an

inadequate diet. They aim to restore health by altering the body's biochemistry through dietary changes. The changes are determined by pinpointing whether an individual is suffering from vitamin or mineral deficiencies and whether certain foods are acting on his body as a mild poison.

- **Osteopathy** is based on the principle that 'structure governs function'. The osteopath is concerned with identifying and treating 'osteopathic lesions', primarily by manipulating joints in order to restore them to their normal positions and mobility. Such manipulation is intended to relieve tension in muscle and ligaments and thereby alleviate dysfunction.
- **Reflexology** involves a method of treatment using massage to reflex areas found in the feet and hands – most commonly the feet are treated. It is based on the proposition that energy/life forces run through channels and that each channel relates to a zone of the body. It is believed that each organ or part of the body is mirrored on the foot and that organs that lie in the same zone are represented in the same segment of the foot. By feeling people's feet reflexologists can detect which energy channels are blocked and by massaging appropriate areas the channels can be unblocked.
- **Shiatsu** means 'finger pressure'. The therapy incorporates aspects of acupressure and, like acupuncture, is based on promoting health by stimulating chi energy using pressure on the skin at various points along meridians associated with the function of vital organs.
- **Yoga** implies perfect harmony of body, mind and spirit. On a physical level it implies glowing health attained through exercise with controlled breathing and relaxation techniques. On a mental level, it implies the harmonious integration of the personality and the corresponding elimination of psychological 'complexes'. On the soul level, yoga implies union of the little self with the greater self, of the ego with the vastness of cosmic awareness.

APPENDIX 2: THE USE OF LAVENDER OIL IN AROMATHERAPY – A SNAPSHOT

In order to highlight the complexity of essential oils, lavender has been chosen as an example because it is one of the most versatile and well-known of all essential oils. It is hoped that this will demonstrate the in-depth knowledge that is required not only for the practice of aromatherapy but indeed for the practice of all forms of complementary therapy.

Lavender, true (*Lavandula augustifolia*)

Plant family: Lamiaceae (Labiate).
Method of extraction: Essential oil by steam distillation from the fresh flowering tops.
Volatility (speed of evaporation): Middle note.
Safety data: Nontoxic, nonirritant, nonsensitising.
Principal constituents: Over 100 constituents including linalyl acetate (up to 40%), linalol, lavandulol, lavandulyl acetate, terpineol, cineol, limonene, ocimene and caryophyllene, among others. Constituents vary according to source – high altitudes generally produce more esters.

The high percentage of terpenes and alcohols make lavender a safe oil to use.

The terpenes (hydrocarbons) give a mild therapeutic effect, as do the alcohols, which are also calming, soothing and antibacterial. The additions of the esters encourages cell regeneration, which is why lavender is often used in healing wounds and burns (Table 14.3).

APPENDIX 3: RESEARCH ON COMPLEMENTARY THERAPIES AND FURTHER READING

Research on complementary therapies and doctors' attitudes to them

Aldridge D, Pietroni P 1987 Clinical assessment of acupuncture in asthma therapy: discussion paper. *J Roy Soc Med* 80: 222–224
Anderson E, Anderson P 1987 GPs and alternative medicine. *J Roy Coll Gen Pract* 37: 52–55
Fulder SJ, Munro RE 1985 Complementary

Table 14.3   The uses of lavender oil

Body system	Properties	Conditions treated	Method of use
Circulation	Hypotensive sedative and decongestant; alleviates fluid retention	Hypertension; stress	Baths, massage, application
Digestion	Cleansing and calming	Indigestion, colic, nausea, flatulence, mouth ulcers	Compresses, massage, application
Emotional/nervous system	Sedative; nerve tonic	Nervous tension, stress, insomnia, headaches, migraine, depression	Inhalations, vaporisers, baths, massage, application
Genitourinary and endocrine systems	Antispasmodic; bactericidal; antiviral	Dysmenorrhoea, labour pains, genital infections	Compresses, inhalations, vaporisers, baths, applications, douche
Immune system	Antispasmodic; antiviral	Colds, flu, infections	Compresses, inhalations, vaporisers, baths, applications
The mind	Affects memory and emotions (two olfactory nerve tracts run into the limbic system)	Dementia, epilepsy	Inhalations, vaporisers, applications
Muscles and joints	Analgesic; anti-inflammatory	Muscular sprains, aches and pains, rheumatism	Compresses, baths, application, massage
Respiratory system	Analgesic; anti-inflammatory	Colds, flu, sinusitis, throat infections	Inhalation, vaporisers, application
The skin	Analgesic; anti-inflammatory; fungicidal; regenerative	Cuts, insect bites, eczema, infected wounds, athletes foot, head lice, herpes simplex, burns	Application, massage, compresses

medicine in the United Kingdom: patients, practitioners, and consultations. *Lancet* 2: 542–545

Pietroni PM 1987 Holistic medicine: new lessons to be learned. *Practitioner* 231: 1386–1390

Reilly DT 1983 Young doctors' views on alternative medicine. *Br Med J* 287: 337–339

Steehan MP et al 1992 Efficacy of traditional Chinese herbal therapy in adult atopic dermatitis. *Lancet* 340: 13–17

Swayne J 1989 Survey of the use of homeopathic medicine in the UK health system. *J Roy Coll Gen Pract* 39: 503–506

Symposium 1990 Symposium. *Practitioner* 234: 111–125

Thomas KJ, Carr J, Westlake L, Williams BT 1991 Use of non-orthodox and conventional healthcare in Great Britain. *Br Med J* 302: 207–210

Wharton R, Lewith G 1986 Complementary medicine and the general practitioner. *Br Med J* 292: 1498–1500

FURTHER READING

Davis P 1996 Aromatherapy: an A–Z. CW Daniel, London
Davies S, Stewart A 1987 Nutritional medicine. Pan Books, London
Featherstone C, Forsyth L 1997 Medical marriage. Findhorn Press, Forres
Foundation for Integrated Medicine 1997 Integrated healthcare – the way forward for the next 5 years. Foundation for Integrated Medicine, London
Lawless J 1992 Encyclopaedia of essential oils. Element Books, Shaftesbury

Montagu A 1978 Touching. Harper & Row, London
Price S 1991 Aromatherapy for common ailments. Gaia Books, London
Price S, Price L 1995 Aromatherapy for health professionals. Churchill Livingstone, Edinburgh
Sturgess S 1997 The Yoga Book. Element Books, Shaftesbury
Wilson E, Lewith G 1997 Natural born healers. Collins & Brown, London
Yoga Sadhak Group 1975 Patanjali's yoga sutras. AH Pawaskar, Bombay

15

Pharmacological intervention – insight into prescribing for health visiting

Iain P L Coleman

INTRODUCTION

The last 15 years have witnessed considerable changes in the provision of drugs as part of a therapeutic regime. One important development is the expansion of those healthcare professional groups permitted to prescribe apart from doctors. For instance the pharmacist now has a far more advisory role and nurse prescribing is an important development for the future.

In her article on nurse prescribing, Brew (1994) states quite clearly: 'certainly nurses need some knowledge of pharmacology if they are fully to understand the implications of their prescribing and be aware of the long term effects' and later in the same article 'thorough knowledge of the item to be prescribed, its therapeutic action, side-effects, dosage and interaction'. A worthy intention, but it immediately begs the question – how much knowledge? And therein lies the difficulty for the healthcare professional. The immediate basis of pharmacological intervention lies in the interaction of a chemical agent with some component of the body's physiological system. While the effect observed may well be viewed and experienced holistically, it is fairly certain that the interaction occurs at a molecular level. The vast tract of pharmacological information is derived from a knowledge of chemistry and related molecular sciences, quantitative methods and a fairly reductionist approach to physiology. The majority of pharmacologists will have pursued a very scientific career and undergraduate teaching presumes a strong base in science. A rather different range of skills is demanded of the healthcare professional from a considerable range of disciplines and requirements. This may make a classical approach to acquiring the 'necessary' pharmacological knowledge at best tedious and at worst insurmountable.

The sheer volume of the body of pharmacological knowledge compounds the problem. A standard reference textbook will often run to nearly 2000 pages of densely composed script, heavily supported by lists of references to original articles. This knowledge does not remain unaltered. New information is derived and published at a terrifying speed, particularly via the Internet. Added to this, the pharmaceutical companies are engaged in a fiercely competitive business; the consequence of this is an ever-increasing variety and number of new compounds available for clinical use. Being confronted by this vast array of drug information can be intimidating, not least for those approaching the territory from a nonscientific background. Nevertheless, the healthcare professional has a distinct advantage over many undergraduate students of pharmacology. As a result of training and, more importantly, experience, they have had the opportunity to observe the use of drugs in a 'real-life' situation. The therapeutic consequence of drug treatment will have been observed and probably the manifestation of side-effects. They will have a familiarity with drug names. One approach to the acquisition of pharmacological knowledge for the healthcare professional is to build from this base of their experience and lead into exploration of the science of pharmacology to explain the observations of experience.

In addition to this, the healthcare professional knows that new knowledge and understanding is not merely derived from 'the standard textbook'. Useful though this may be, it is but one source that might be consulted initially. Many other sources of information on drugs are available to healthcare professionals, such as GPs or other doctors in their teams, fellow professionals, laboratory-based staff and, perhaps best of all, pharmacists. Libraries are an obvious source of information and there is no doubt that the Internet is a powerful and ever-growing tool for acquiring information on drugs. The pharmaceutical companies will offer a considerable amount of information on request and are often delighted to discuss their products with interested parties. Pharmaceutical sales representatives are another useful means of acquiring information. So, if a particular drug is used in a given situation, this presents an ideal opportunity to enhance the healthcare professional's knowledge.

'KEYS' FOR CONSIDERATION

It may be useful to find a means of organising drug information to make the most effective use of it. To this end some 'keys' for consideration are proposed, to serve as a framework around which the pharmacological knowledge that underpins a particular drug's use or a particular therapy can be developed. If you are likely to prescribe a given drug or a drug is proposed for use within your sphere of operations, it is always useful to enhance your own drug knowledge for that specific drug. The following list is by no means perfect nor indeed exhaustive but does indicate some aspects of knowledge that are useful. The order of the list may advise a process of information retrieval but should not be seen as mandatory.

- *Drug name*
  - The chemical name, e.g. 4-amino-5-chloro-*N*-(2-dimethylaminoethyl)-2-methoxybenzamine
  - The generic (or approved) name, e.g. metoclopramide
  - The brand (or trade) name, e.g. Maxolon. Clearly, the chemical name is rather unwieldy and the brand name is restricted to a single manufacturer or distributor, so the generic name tends to be the one in most frequent use.
- *Information sources*, e.g. pharmacopoeia. It may seem an obvious point, but the information that any professional seeks to elicit with regard to any given drug governs the source of information researched. Details of the molecular site of action are more likely

to be found in classical textbooks of pharmacology and appropriate journal articles. Recommended routes of administration are often provided within drug information sheets supplied by the relevant manufacturer.

- *The law, prescribing limits, protocols and responsibilities.* Drugs are highly potent entities, which can exert a powerful effect on recipients. The potential for benefit may, however, be matched by the toxicity of some compounds. In some instances, ethical issues may also be of significance, as in the prescription of oral contraceptives. To control drug use and protect both prescriber and recipient, the law governs the use of different drugs to some extent. Similarly, protocols are devised to ensure the proper use and monitoring of drugs. In terms of acquiring knowledge of a drug, such information provides a useful background context.
- *Routes of administration, dose adjustment, absorption, distribution, metabolism and excretion*
- *Drug regimen.* This is one of the key aspects of classical pharmacological knowledge. In order for any drug to produce a therapeutic effect, it must enter the system and be distributed to a site of action.
- *Site of action.* Another key point: the impact of a drug at its site (or indeed sites) of action is what gives the drug its therapeutic property. The manner in which this interaction occurs is a fundamental aspect of pharmacological knowledge and often clarifies the reaction of the recipient to the prescribed drug.
- *Confounding aspects.* Not all recipients will respond to drugs in exactly the same way. Any number of factors may compromise a particular drug's effectiveness; these may include age, gender, ethnic origin, pregnancy, lactation and diet. In sick patients, underlying chronic disease, poor nutritional status, even psychological status may well influence the effectiveness of drug use.
- *Adverse drug reactions and interactions.* Not all drugs are well tolerated by individuals within a population. A given proportion of a group of patients may well exhibit side-effects to a particular medication, often as a result of genetic predisposition. It is important to be aware of potential adverse drug reactions and their possible causes. In addition, it is vital to note whether individuals are taking other medication and check whether there is a potential interaction between different drugs.
- *Related health education.* Healthcare professionals recognise very well the importance of this aspect of their role. Drug therapy is of scant value without additional advice to support therapy. In considering the use of any medication, it is useful to include a commentary on the drug, the consequences of its use and the *modus vivendi* that should be part of a given therapeutic regimen. Perhaps an important intention should be to promote a lifestyle that can obviate the need for pharmacological intervention.
- *Sources of drugs.* While this is not a crucial key in the first instance, it is useful for the healthcare professional to have some awareness of the source of drugs used to provide therapy. Some of this may be of historical interest but future useful pharmacological products are likely to come from natural products, novel uses of existing compounds and perhaps most significantly, the efforts of pharmaceutical companies' work on drug discovery.

PHARMACOKINETICS AND PHARMACODYNAMICS

One view of the key notion of pharmacological intervention for therapy is that we need to get the right amount of the drug into the right place at the right time for the right duration of time (and, it hardly needs to be said … at the right price!). To explain this a little further, the science of pharmacology is often divided into two main aspects:

- *pharmacokinetics* – what the body does to the drug
- *pharmacodynamics* – what the drug does to the body.

While this may seem trite, it is a useful point to remember. To achieve its effect a drug interacts with a discrete component or site of action within the body (pharmacodynamics) but it cannot achieve this until the drug has moved from the outside of the body to this site of action (pharmacokinetics). This is crucial, as a number of barriers may exist between the point of administration and the target site. This will tend to reduce the amount of drug that eventually arrives at the site of action. In addition to this, drug molecules may well possess a structural resemblance to the body's own molecules. As a consequence they are likely to be metabolised by the body and again the amount of drug available (the so-called *bioavailability* of the drug) will be lessened. For these reasons, a knowledge of the means of administration and the processes of absorption, distribution, metabolism and excretion – a description of the drug's journey through the body – has a vital bearing on 'getting the right amount into the right place at the right time'.

All healthcare professionals are very familiar with the means, procedures and protocols for the administration of drugs. Table 15.1 reminds us that no orifice is ignored as a means of drug entry and, where no appropriate orifice exists, parenteral injection or infusion can be used.

Selection of the route of administration is important. Take, for example, medication administered orally for a drug that will have, ultimately, an effect upon the central nervous system. It will be absorbed by the gastrointestinal tract, probably in the jejunum, and pass via the hepatic portal vein to the liver. Most drugs are organic compounds and will have some ability to cross the cell membrane. This ability will vary from compound to compound, but the degree of lipid solubility is significant. Generally speaking, the more lipid soluble a drug the more readily it will traverse these biological barriers such as the gastrointestinal tract.

In the liver, the drug may be converted to other forms. This transformation may render the drug less active, more active, or alter its physicochemical characteristics. From the liver the drug is likely to be distributed around the body by the vascular system. Many drugs will be bound by plasma proteins, in effect retaining them, albeit on a temporary basis, so that they are not available to fulfil their function. It is the unbound or 'free' drug that is the active entity that can deliver the required pharmacological effect. Drugs may also be sequestered or held in body

Table 15.1 Routes of administration of drugs

Route of administration	Comments
Oral	A fairly safe, convenient and economic means of drug delivery, although a number of factors compromise the amount and time taken to arrive at site of action. Patient compliance may be a problem, especially with irritant drugs.
Rectal	In some ways similar to oral but avoids gastric irritation and may reduce hepatic metabolism. Useful for unconscious subjects. Irritant drugs may be a problem.
Sublingual	A safe means of delivery. Drugs absorbed here avoid 'first pass' hepatic metabolism. Repeated use may cause mouth ulcers.
Nasal/inhalation	Capable of giving a very rapid reaction as a result of potentially swift absorption characteristics. Good control of dose can be achieved. Drug needs to be presented as a gas, vapour or aerosol.
Eye drops	Direct application of (sterile) solutions. Tends to require absorption through the epithelium of the conjunctival sac.
Intravaginal, intraurethral	Specialist route of entry to target drugs, often versus infections.
Topical/transdermal	Direct application for skin conditions. Transdermal 'patches' increasingly popular for drug delivery. Good control of plasma levels possible, but drugs must be presented in a highly lipid-soluble form.
Intravenous	Gives virtually immediate effects upon administration, largely because there are virtually no barriers to absorption. However, there is a greater chance of adverse reactions. Self-medication is difficult.
Intramuscular	A good means of drug delivery for drugs that are poorly absorbed orally. Useful for administration of 'depot' drugs. Absorption can be slow in some cases. Possibility of pain immediately following injection.
Subcutaneous	As for intramuscular
Intra-arterial	Allows localisation of drugs to specific tissue or organ
Intrathecal/epidural	Means of delivering anaesthesia
Intraperitoneal	Generally used in experimental settings

compartments as a result of binding to body components or different pH conditions modifying the ability of a drug to be easily transported across cell membranes. Quite clearly, the result of liver metabolism and distribution around the body is often to decrease the amount of drug available to reach the site of action. On reaching the brain, our drug will have to cross the so-called blood–brain barrier, which is a formidable barrier to absorption of drugs. Regardless of whether or not the drug actually reaches its site of action, it will still have to be excreted from the body. Most drugs are converted during metabolism to water-soluble forms and may be removed from the body in the urine. Other drugs may pass from the body via faeces, sweat, expired breaths and a mother's milk, this last example having obvious implications for the infant receiving the milk.

Figure 15.1 indicates the general relationship between absorption, distribution, metabolism and excretion. All these factors are interrelated in a dependent but changing situation that conspires to modify the amount of drug available to reach the 'target' or site of action in sufficient quantity to achieve therapy.

The definition of 'the right place' is the key to pharmacodynamics, the impact of drugs on the body systems. A popular trend in recent times has been to refer to this as 'the drug target' and the last century has seen a progression from studies of drug action that relied on drug application to minute anatomical structures with a fine paintbrush to the precision of the molecular biologist in modifying at the level of a single amino acid. With a few exceptions, drug targets are protein molecules. Drugs will interact with these molecules, either to promote or enhance their actions or to inhibit them. In each instance, this interference brings about a biological effect, which hopefully results in a therapeutic benefit.

A drug will interfere with a system either by stimulating it or by inhibiting its function. Drugs that stimulate are often referred to as *agonist drugs*; a well-known example would be salbutamol. This drug achieves its therapeutic effect by stimulating specific proteins to bring about bronchodilation. On the other hand, drugs that

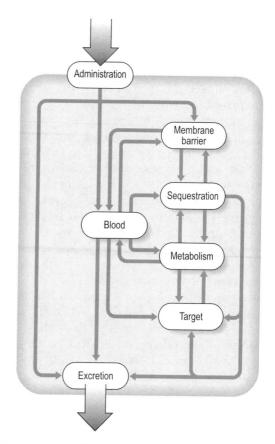

Figure 15.1 An illustration of the possible relationships between administration, absorption, distribution, metabolism and excretion of drugs

inhibit or block are often referred to as *antagonist drugs*. A considerable proportion of clinically useful drugs are antagonist drugs. Two very familiar examples are the beta-blocking drug atenolol and the H_2-blocking drug cimetidine. Conventionally we might consider that there are four 'classical' targets for drug molecules. These are specific receptors, enzymes, ion channels and transporter systems. Physiological function is dependent on the integrity of these protein mechanisms. Often, a consequence of pathology is physiological dysfunction and modifying appropriate target proteins permits some alleviation of symptoms and at best a cure for the condition.

Generally speaking we may class our target proteins into one of four types. One is the *receptor protein*, usually found on the outside of the cells.

Such proteins are involved with the process of recognition and are an essential step in the transmission of information by chemical communication. This is the 'target' hit by drugs such as those mentioned above, cimetidine and atenolol. Upon interaction with the receptor, a drug may cause an ion channel to open or, by operating through membrane and cellular transduction mechanisms, alter enzyme function, DNA transcription and modulate (rather than directly open) ion channels. Indeed ion channels themselves are an example of a *target protein*. Some drugs, e.g. the diuretic amiloride, act by directly blocking up the 'hole' that is the ion channel. In the amiloride example this would prevent the reabsorption of the sodium ion by the renal tubule cells, thus promoting diuresis.

Enzymes, the catalysts of biological reactions, are an obvious target for drug action. Physiological processes are utterly dependent on enzymes: any interference with specific enzyme activity will significantly affect many physiological phenomena. A couple of examples that we will explore later are the familiar aspirin and the relatively recent ACE (angiotensin converting enzyme) inhibitor drugs.

As humans, we are exceedingly complex structures, assembled of literally millions of cells. To achieve co-ordinated function there must be, among other attributes, communication between cells. This is not confined to exchange of information but also requires exchange of nutrients and ions across the membranes of the cells. This is often accomplished by a *carrier protein*. Such proteins, which can span the cell membrane, allow glucose and amino acids to enter the cell and arrange the balance of sodium and potassium across the membrane. Even the transport of neurotransmitters such as noradrenaline and 5-hydroxytryptamine needs these proteins. Consequently, many carrier proteins are ideal candidates for drug targets; drugs such as digitalis (inhibits the so-called 'sodium pump' or sodium–potassium-dependent ATPase) and fluoxetine (inhibits the re-uptake of 5-hydroxytryptamine) are particularly good examples of drugs that achieve a therapeutic effect by interacting with carrier proteins.

While most drug targets are protein in nature, there are some important exceptions. The infused diuretic mannitol exerts its action by an osmotic effect. Many of the drugs used in cancer chemotherapy are effective as a result of their ability to interfere directly with the DNA (deoxyribonucleic acid) molecule and thereby alter the function of some malignant cells.

In summary then:

- *Pharmacology* is the study of the preparation, use and actions of drugs
- *Pharmacokinetics* may be defined as the study of the administration, absorption, distribution, metabolism and excretion of drugs. Some authors limit this definition to embrace a mathematical description of the process.
- *Pharmacodynamics* is the study of the action of drugs, whether at the level of the entire human, organ system, tissue, cellular, subcellular or molecular levels.

A way of exploring some of the science that underlies pharmacology is by way of scenarios that give a number of clues to a drug's action. The examples illustrated allow a consideration of pharmacological action set against the context of some imaginary situations and pathological circumstances. Each scenario is followed by an explanation of the appropriate pharmacology. The purpose is twofold. One is to provide a brief résumé of some pharmacological knowledge. The second purpose is more important. It is to indicate a possible method of acquiring pharmacological knowledge starting from the position of observation in a 'real life' context and progressing along any number of lines of enquiry and achieving a working knowledge of relevant pharmacology. Needless to say, the explanation is not an exhaustive account nor indeed a unique explanation. Any healthcare professional will find a number of routes of enquiry; the intention is to encourage curiosity. A degree of licence has been exercised to contrive certain issues. Nevertheless, while each example is entirely fictional the science is not.

Our first example is a cautionary tale, taken from the pages of the Daily Enquirer (Fig. 15.2).

The Daily Enquirer   Tuesday, May 19th 1998

Shock Death of Local Builder

The sad death of Mr George Davies poses many questions for East Marcham Coroner, Dr Judith Smythe.

Mr Davies, a 57-year-old building worker, had suffered from depression for many years, which had not responded to a variety of treatments. His daughter, Michelle, in an exclusive interview with our reporter, explained the background to her father's death last March. Recently Mr Davies had been prescribed a new course of treatment which, according to his daughter, had given him a new lease of life apart from some dizziness when he stood up. The family was overjoyed that George was able to take part again in a normal family life.

Michelle did not know much about this treatment. Apparently, George had been given an information card by the doctor but unfortunately, in his confused state, had lost it on the way home. A few days before his death George had developed a nasty cough and cold which had made him

feel unwell and he was a bit down. Beryl, George's wife, had asked the practice nurse for advice when she went to the surgery for her smear test. The practice nurse was very helpful and suggested that Mr Davies should take some Actifed, which would help his cough and cold. Beryl found some in the kitchen cupboard and George took a dose before lunch.

In an effort to cheer him up Beryl had cooked his favourite meal, shepherd's pie, but since the BSE scare, George was wary of meat. Resourceful as ever, Beryl had used soya 'meat' flavoured with Marmite and George had not known the difference. He finished off with some ripe cheese and biscuits and a glass of beer. After lunch, George took one of his red tablets and sat down to watch the racing on television. Soon afterwards he began to feel unwell – with a throbbing headache, fever, rapid pulse and sweating. When Beryl took in a cup of tea she found George collapsed in the armchair. Michelle called the ambulance and George was rushed to the Stormcaws Hospital where, despite the efforts of the Casualty staff, Mr Davies died.

The Coroner will be examining the case tomorrow and will be reviewing the legal implications and liability of the professionals highlighted in this unfortunate tragedy.

Figure 15.2

A number of points arise from this article. What was the identity of the medication provided? Is there any significance in the composition of George's last meal? How would you view the practice nurse's advice on treating a cold?

George had obviously suffered for some time from depression, which may well be deep-seated and endogenous. It might be reasonable to suppose that a number of therapies had been applied in the past, with little apparent success. Generally speaking, in patients with a history of depression where tricyclic antidepressant drugs have been of scant value, *monoamine oxidase inhibitor drugs* (MAOIs) have been prescribed to good advantage. A popular and useful drug from the 1950s, the MAOIs fell into disfavour, partly because of the side-effects and partly because of adverse reactions with other drugs and certain

substances in food, particularly mature cheese and yeast extract products such as Marmite. George's sudden demise came after suffering from a throbbing headache, fever, rapid pulse and sweating. A possible conclusion is that George suffered a severe hypertensive crisis, with intracranial haemorrhage. This might be due to the infamous 'cheese reaction', a classical interaction between MAOIs and food. Orthostatic hypotension is a common side-effect of this group of drugs, which might well account for George's dizziness on standing up. Without much doubt, the medication in question was a monoamine oxidase inhibitor such as phenelzine or tranylcypromine.

Apart from depression, MAOIs have a number of other applications in treating phobic disorders, post-traumatic stress disorders, obsessive compulsive disorders and panic attacks. It is believed that they are of some value in bulimia and migraine prophylaxis. Narcoleptic attacks are reduced by MAOIs and they may also provide a useful adjunct to L-dopa therapy for Parkinson's disease. MAOIs have a good pharmacokinetic profile: they are readily absorbed from the gastro-intestinal tract and may reach a peak plasma concentration within 2–4 hours. However, the value of these drugs is compromised to some extent by their side-effects, which include ortho-static hypotension because of altered cardio-vascular reflexes, and a very marked stimulation of the central nervous system leading to tremors, excitement, disturbances in sleep patterns and a possibility of convulsions. Weight gain is not uncommon.

How does pharmacological knowledge explain these phenomena? Perhaps the starting point is the drugs' target: in essence, as the name suggests, they inhibit monoamine oxidase. So our exploration should continue by looking at the physiological role of monoamine oxidase. An immense variety of molecules are present in the central nervous system; the key group in this particular instance is a group often referred to as the biogenic amines. Some typical examples would be noradrenaline, dopamine and 5-hydroxy-tryptamine, all of which have putative neuro-transmitter roles in the central nervous system. Most neurotransmitters are synthesised, released to produce their effect and then have to be terminated, otherwise their effect would be prolonged far longer than necessary. The role of monoamine oxidase, in parallel with other biochemical mechanisms, is to contribute to the termination or dissipation of these compounds.

So, if the enzyme that breaks down these biogenic amines is inhibited, then fewer biogenic amines are broken down and they can remain in the system far longer. This increase in the levels of 5-hydroxytryptamine, noradrenaline, dopamine and other similar amines may be responsible for the antidepressant effect of the MAOIs, according to some theories of affective disorders. Other theories consider regulation of receptors or cellular signalling to be possible targets. It is in the primary mechanism of action

of MAOIs that we find the answer to George's sudden death. Tyramine is a naturally occurring amine that is a dietary component. It is also described as a *sympathomimetic*: this is a compound that is structurally similar to noradrenaline and increases its release. Generally speaking, monoamine oxidase, also present in the liver, will break down tyramine. However, if the enzyme is inhibited, excessive amounts of tyramine will appear in the circulation and in turn trigger the release of above-normal amounts of noradrenaline, which will tend to have a hypertensive effect. Most foodstuffs contain insufficient tyramine to cause a major problem. Unfortunately, George consumed several items noted for high tyramine levels: ripe cheese, yeast extract and beer. The situation has not been helped by the advice to take some Actifed, which contains ephedrine, another sympathomimetic. The combination of all these factors had inevitable consequences.

While a number of key principles emerge from this case, it is possible to investigate MAOIs a little further. The example alluded to above is rather nonspecific. Monoamine oxidase itself is not a single enzyme but exists as at least two isoenzymes, MAO-A and MAO-B. MAO-A seems predominantly to break down noradrenaline and 5-hydroxytryptamine while dopamine is broken down by both forms. Relatively specific inhibitors have been produced for both iso-enzymes. One clinically useful form is moclobe-mide, which is thought to be specific for MAO-A and seems to be less likely to have the unfortunate tyramine interaction of previous MAOI drugs. A final comment: MAOIs can also inhibit mixed function oxidase enzymes in the liver. This may lead to increased levels of a number of other drugs, such as barbiturates, aspirin, opiates and alcohol.

This idea of an enzyme as a therapeutic target is underlined even more by the second example; and again the thought that enzymes can exist in more than one form is important in our investigation.

SHEER AGONY ON THE ORIENT EXPRESS

Monsieur Befnipour sniffed as he eased his aching frame through the sliding door into his small

conductor's compartment. It was 10.15 pm as the Orient Express hurtled towards Simplon on its return from Venice. He lit a foul smelling Gitanes and counted the days to the end of the month and his retirement. It had been a bad day. He sniffed irritably as he reflected on the outrageous demands of the passengers. The unbroken stream of orders barked by Colonel Thompson (Retd) which had seen him dashing hither and thither, more often than not 'at the double, man!' had not helped the dull pain in his stomach. In fact, thanks to the Colonel, he had forgotten to take his lunchtime medication and the effect was definitely beginning to wear off. He sniffed again but – *alors* – for all the good these tablets were he might just as well have stuck to aspirin, cheaper too! His feet were absolutely killing him. Hmmm, should he take another dose?

His ears were still ringing from the bellicose shrieking of the very pregnant Madame Pratlgandison which had done nothing for his tinnitus. 'Oh, my stomach! Oh, my back aches!', complaining all the time. Her husband was wringing his hands and trying to explain that an aspirin was all that she could have in her condition. Could he, M. Befnipour, suggest anything? *Mon Dieu!*, he sniffed, what could he a simple conductor offer? was he a *pharmacien*? He only hoped that she wouldn't go into labour before the train reached Simplon.

Neither had it helped when he had stumbled over Sergeant Jerome's skis laid thoughtlessly across the opening of his sleeper compartment and stubbed his toe – painfully. The sergeant's skiing injury, acquired while on the piste on Mount Baldo, required constant attention from his companion, who was engaged in rubbing copious quantities of Ibuleve on to the afflicted parts and had commandeered several buckets of ice from the bar, much to the annoyance of those who preferred their wine well chilled.

'*Eh bien*, tomorrow's another day' he thought as he sniffed and swallowed the extra tablets. He tidied his cabin and lay down in his narrow bunk, dog-tired, but sleep would not come.

The central theme of this scenario, from a number of clues (and the odd anagram) is the action of the drug ibuprofen, one of a large group of drugs, the *NSAIDs* (nonsteroidal anti-inflammatory drugs). Our friendly conductor, Monsieur Befnipour, is probably suffering from some sort of musculoskeletal disorder, possibly even rheumatoid arthritis. The various aches and pains would indicate this sort of condition, particularly after movement. The constant sniffing may indicate rhinitis, a potential side-effect of NSAID therapy, though nasal polyps and bronchoconstriction are other possible effects. Of more significance could well be the dull pain in his stomach – a reminder of one of the more common side-effects of NSAID treatment. Gastro-intestinal effects associated with the NSAIDs can include abdominal discomfort, vomiting,

diarrhoea, bleeding and ulceration. Added to this, the man is hardly helping his cause by smoking and, perhaps through no fault of his own, omitting his medication at lunch time. Ibuprofen has a half-life of just over 2 hours and needs to be taken between two and four times per day. As for our brave Sergeant, the nature of his wound is unspecified but the suitability of NSAIDs for all aches and pains might be questioned. Interestingly, we have the comparison of rather liberal doses of ibuprofen given topically with (missed) oral doses of the drug. What of the pregnant mother suffering back and stomach pains? The instruction to avoid NSAID drugs during pregnancy offers a clue.

The NSAID drugs may cause an increase in the time for gestation of the fetus, and in addition lengthen the duration of spontaneous labour as well as promoting a delay or even an interruption in premature labour. From a fetal point of view, the patency of the *ductus arteriosus* may be compromised and in the presence of NSAID drugs there may be a premature closure of this blood vessel before parturition. Many of the usual physiological phenomena of pregnancy are modulated by the presence of certain prostaglandins, particularly those of the E and F series, and prostacyclin. The prostaglandins are an important group of autacoids or endogenous chemical mediators, which are themselves members of a much larger group of mediators called the *eicosanoids*. Other members of the eicosanoid group are the thromboxanes and the leukotrienes. The eicosanoids are an important group of very potent though short-lived autacoids, with an extensive range of biological activities. These effects are achieved by binding to quite specific cell-surface receptors, an example perhaps of one of our protein targets in pharmacology. Apart from the effects viewed in pregnancy, prostaglandins influence vascular smooth muscle, platelet aggregation, gastro-intestinal activity and respiratory function, and have a role in the onset of fever and the heightened perception of pain. Some of these influences appear to be beneficial and others tend to be associated with pathology. An apparent paradox.

Interestingly, eicosanoids are all made from the same starting molecule or precursor, arachidonic acid, which is itself synthesised from the fatty acids linoleic and linolenic acid. Neither of these acids is present in humans and must be supplied in the diet (cold-water fish such as cod are an excellent source). Arachidonic acid is converted by an enzyme, cyclo-oxygenase (COX), to prostaglandin. After production, eicosanoids are not stored in the cell. The amount available for activity is determined by the amount of precursor available and whether or not there has been a stimulation for synthesis. It is here, at the level of the COX enzyme, that we find our pharmacological target. Not the cell-surface receptor, though this may in itself offer possibilities, but the enzyme that converts the arachidonic acid to prostaglandin. We can immediately explain the value of the drug in terms of its ability to cover the symptoms of pain and inflammation, particularly for inflammatory joint disease and related musculoskeletal conditions. By reducing the amount of prostaglandin released, there is a reduction in some of the phenomena caused by prostaglandin presence in such pathological conditions and we see a useful alleviation of symptoms. Unfortunately, as the prostaglandins also fulfil many admirable physiological roles, a number of the adverse reactions reported are probably the consequence of insufficient prostaglandins at a number of sites of action. Nevertheless, provided caution is exercised, the NSAIDs represent a most valuable therapeutic tool.

In recent years, it has been discovered that there are two different types of cyclo-oxygenase, known as COX-1 and COX-2. It appears that COX-1 is a constitutive enzyme (in that it is always present), while COX-2 is an inducible enzyme (i.e. it is induced if an appropriate stimulus is applied). It is an attractive notion to design a drug with a higher selectivity for COX-2 than for COX-1 and thereby to gain therapeutically, at the same time reducing the incidence of the adverse reactions arising from COX-1 inhibition. Such a drug, meloxicam, has been demonstrated in clinical trials to offer therapeutic advantages allied to better gastrointestinal safety.

Nonetheless, such is the wide range of effects exerted by prostaglandins that, while the selective COX-2 inhibitor drug offers the potential to improve specificity of therapy, complete inhibition of COX-2 may not be without its risks in human subjects.

A PRESSURE SITUATION

It was with considerable reluctance that John found himself waiting, somewhat impatiently, in the local health centre waiting room. His wife had nagged and nagged at him to attend the 'well man' clinic until, amazingly, a letter had invited him to attend on such and such a date. Well here he was – and he had much better things to do. For a start, he was due to prosecute in a particularly unpleasant case tomorrow and he wanted to make sure that he had made certain of his brief. The practice was taking off, thanks to all the hard work, and he was determined not to let things slip. Anyway, he hadn't had a day's illness in his life and it wasn't so many years ago that he stopped playing football for quite a successful amateur side. So … what was the point?

To his surprise, at the end of the check-up he was told that his blood pressure did seem to be a bit on the high side. Would he mind coming back for a few more checks? Yes he damn well would but natural courtesy (and an impressively professional performance by the practice nurse) prevented him from giving voice to the thought and he entered some suitable dates in his diary.

Subsequent visits confirmed that he had a moderate degree of hypertension. He suffered a gentle homily on his weight. Yes, well he did spend an inordinate amount of time at a desk when he wasn't in court and yes he was a little too fond of his wife's cooking. He agreed to do something about it. What was that? Try and relax? Hah! Fat chance of that. Apart from work, his parents had announced that, after 40 years of living in Britain, they had had enough of cold wet miserable winters and were returning home to Trinidad. Apart from the hassle of actually helping them he wasn't so sure it was a good thing. They were a very close family and he was going to really miss them. Besides they were getting old and he felt that as a dutiful son he should be close if help was needed.

He hoped that the tablets would help. He didn't like the idea of the consequences of what would happen if he couldn't have his BP sorted out. He hadn't felt ill before all this started but these tablets were a nuisance. Unless he planned things carefully…. Well it didn't look too good to have to ask the judge for an adjournment 10 minutes into a hearing. He noticed the odd rash and there was something else. Not to put too fine a point on it, his wife had bluntly asked him if he was seeing somebody else….

His blood pressure wasn't really much better and he was quite pleased in a way when a change of therapy was made. He had to admit to himself that he also need to try a little harder (suffered another homily and advice and leaflets on diet!). What was that – no peanuts – he loved a quick handful (or two), especially with a couple of G&Ts before dinner.

He did try, very hard, but it was depressing to just come home and live on what he disparagingly referred to as his 'muesli diet' (it wasn't, but he was missing the usual culinary delights). He found it hard to motivate himself to work. Sometimes, as autumn drifted into winter, he occasionally imagined that he was feeling a little chesty. This distinctly worried him. Back to the doctors … again!

This time he had his tablets changed again, although his blood pressure was improved – thank heavens for small mercies. And they noticed that he had lost some weight (well done – do try to lose a bit more!). To start with these new tablets seemed a lot worse: he imagined he was having flushes and for a week or so there was a bit of a problem with headaches, although mercifully that passed. After about 3 weeks he actually felt quite good, his blood pressure seemed to be well controlled and he had continued to lose weight very gradually. Now there was just this problem of coughing to resolve.

Here we have a rather familiar scene. A man in middle age, accustomed to enjoying good health with a positive, vigorous attitude to life. Nevertheless it is easy to perceive that here is an individual exhibiting hypertension and it is fairly straightforward to pick out a number of risk factors. John is working in a reasonably stressful environment and in all probability putting a lot of pressure on himself. He is clearly anxious on behalf of his parents. A sedentary lifestyle, allied to appreciation of good food and drink, have conspired to increase his weight. There is also some evidence that salt sensitivity is present in individuals of Afro-Caribbean origin. An opportunity exists for useful health education with regard to lifestyle modification but if John's blood pressure substantially exceeds the World Health Organization guidelines of 135/85, then pharmacological intervention is needed.

Three types of medication are described within this particular scenario. Each has been administered to lower blood pressure and each has a different mechanism of action. In physiological terms, blood pressure is occasioned by two main components: resistance to flow through the vascular system (*peripheral vascular resistance*) and *cardiac output*, which is the product of heart rate and stroke volume. If either or both of these parameters is raised then blood pressure will be similarly raised. Simplistically, a rationale for therapy is to reduce either or both parameters.

If blood volume is increased, as possibly may occur in salt-sensitive subjects where the additional salt (or sodium) burden causes a retention of fluid, then blood pressure will be elevated.

Consequently, any reduction in blood volume will tend to lower blood pressure. Which is where the first choice of therapy for John exerts its action. From the description, particularly the potential request to leave the courtroom, he is receiving a diuretic, probably a thiazide diuretic such as bendrofluazide. The primary action is to increase the rate of fluid loss, which lowers blood volume, hence cardiac output and thereby blood pressure. The thiazide diuretic drugs achieve their pharmacological effect by inhibiting the action of a specific carrier protein in the distal portion of the kidney tubule. This carrier protein is responsible for the re-absorption of sodium chloride; if its activity is inhibited, both sodium chloride and by definition water cannot be re-absorbed and so will continue to flow through the tubular system and eventually out of the body. Hence the diuretic effect. They also possess a secondary effect: after a few weeks of regular therapy these drugs can produce a degree of vasodilatation. A fall in peripheral vascular resistance occurs and a consequent lowering of blood pressure. Usually such drugs can produce a lowering of about 10–15 mmHg in blood pressure, so they are possibly of limited value except in treating mild to moderate hypertension. The side-effects are relatively few despite John being unfortunate to suffer from a minor rash and implied (uxorial cross-examination) loss of libido. Indeed, the next few years are likely to see their demise as a sole means of controlling hypertension with the advent of new antihypertensive agents.

The second choice of therapy may be fairly swiftly identified as a beta-blocker. There is reasonable control of hypertension but the adverse reaction noted in the scenario is the presence of symptoms similar to asthma. The beta-blockers exert their mode of action by antagonising beta-adrenoceptors, of which there are two main groups distributed about the body, beta-1 receptors and beta-2 receptors. In terms of our pharmacological target, these are protein molecules sited on the outside of the cell membrane. As a consequence, if John were to be receiving a fairly nonselective beta-blocking drug such as propranolol, we might well observe a decrease in cardiac output as a result of blocking beta-1 receptors, which predominate in the ventricular myocardium and normally have a chronotropic and an inotropic effect. However we might also observe a possible bronchoconstriction. When beta-2 receptors in the bronchioles are stimulated they will normally cause bronchodilation but if these receptors are inhibited then the opposite effect may occur, which would be broncho-constriction. A possible explanation for John feeling a little 'chesty'? Indeed, the selection of this beta-blocker for John may also be question-able in view of his ethnic origin. It might be argued that a more selective beta-1-blocker such as atenolol would be a far better option.

Beta-blockers are, in general, a useful form of antihypertensive therapy but their mode of action is not entirely certain and is fairly com-plex. To begin with, these drugs do not produce a fall in the blood pressure of 'normal' individuals. It is only in the hypertensive subject that this decrease in blood pressure is observed. While there is no doubt that initially beta-blockers produce a fall in cardiac output, after a period of time cardiac output returns to its original value. After a similar period, a fall in total peripheral resistance is reported, although no particular evidence exists for these drugs as vasodilators. This would certainly serve to produce a decrease in blood pressure. A number of possible explana-tions are possible. Within the central nervous system, there are beta-3 receptors which, upon stimulation, may serve to decrease sympathetic drive to the cardiovascular system; again, blood pressure would fall. Another explanation suggests that the release of renin from kidney juxtaglome-rular cells following sympathetic stimulation is blocked by beta-blockers. Part of the explanation here relates in some way to the third drug offered with some measure of success to John.

When renin is released from these kidney cells it is involved in an enzyme pathway that leads to the formation of a compound called angiotensin I followed by the production of an autacoid (or endogenous compound) called angiotensin II. In terms of its chemical nature this is a very short-chain peptide. This peptide is a powerful agent for causing an increase in blood pressure, as a result of three mechanisms of action. It is a potent vasoconstrictor, it promotes the release of the hormone aldosterone (so more sodium is reabsorbed) and, in the long term, high levels of angiotensin II maintained over time will promote significant remodelling of the vascular system and cardiac hypertrophy. A good target for therapy is either to prevent the effects of angio-tensin II or prevent the formation of angiotensin II in the first place. Angiotensin II receptors exist and the drug losartan achieves its effects by blocking these receptors. However, to date a more successful approach has been to inhibit the production of angiotensin II. The final step in the enzyme pathway is the conversion of angio-tensin I to angiotensin II, and the enzyme respon-sible is called angiotensin converting enzyme. In the early 1960s it was discovered that the venom of pit vipers contained components capable of inhibiting this enzyme. Research and development of these components resulted in a very useful series of drugs, the *angiotensin converting enzyme inhibitors* (or, as they are more popularly known, *ACE inhibitors*), of which enalapril is a good example. Burdened with few side-effects, these drugs make a substantial con-tribution to the treatment of hypertension and a number of other cardiovascular conditions.

A last point here that relates to the pharmaco-kinetics of these drugs. Many of the ACE inhi-bitors are prodrugs. The form in which they are administered is not particularly active: it is only after they have been metabolised that the active form is produced by the body and is able to exert its therapeutic effect.

COLIN'S COUGH

Colin and Janet had very mixed feelings about their move to Bromwell, an industrial town in the heart of the West Midlands. True, the move represented a long deserved promotion for Colin at the bank, and yes, he relished the challenge of managing his own branch, not to mention the distinct advantage of the resultant hike in salary. Janet had been fortunate enough to find a librarian's post at the local library, so financially they were far better off than they had ever been in their lives. Still, in some ways they missed their friends and their old way of life in a small market town on the River Wye. It had been quite a wrench to leave their eccentric old cottage, which needed a lot of work to keep it up to scratch, and move into a very modern mock Tudor

residence in the suburbs of Bromwell. **Nice to have central heating at last, and no more unpleasant draughts lurking round cold corners in winter, but the stop–go drive into town was a bit of a pain and the dark evenings could be pretty depressing.**

Colin had always been 'a bit chesty' and although he had given up smoking years ago could still get 'wheezy' if he tried to walk too briskly during cold weather. Now, though, it seemed to be a lot worse and there was no sign of improvement. He had had a few checks, and it looked as if he might have mild asthma. The few respiratory function tests had shown that his peak flow was down and his total lung capacity was rather higher than might be predicted. He had an inhaler and whenever he felt breathless a quick puff had soon sorted things out. Sometimes the odd cup of coffee helped. However, as time passed the inhaler had become less effective and he suddenly realised that he was using it more and more. Not only that but Janet had noticed that sometimes his hands seemed to shake a bit. It's a busy life, being a bank manager, and under the pressure of work – dramatically exacerbated by redundancies at the branch – he laboured on in increasing discomfort, often with a tight feeling in his chest, until one dramatic episode persuaded him that it was time to return to his GP to think again.

After another round of tests, his respiratory function seemed to have declined quite significantly since the last time. To help with the investigation he underwent fibreoptic bronchoscopy and a biopsy sample was taken. The report revealed some goblet cell hyperplasia, distinct hypertrophy of airway smooth muscle and mucous gland hypertrophy. His treatment was changed to a morning inhalation of steroid and indeed after this treatment had been initiated he noted a marked improvement. Colin was quite happy to continue in this way: he no longer suffered distractions from his work. Janet, on the other hand, was not so easily convinced and had some suspicions about steroids – hadn't they stunted the growth of one of her friends' children, or something? She took full advantage of her position as librarian to read up on asthma and the drugs that were used to treat the condition. She perceived the need to change Colin's therapy but wondered if there was a little more that might be tried. There was this new drug out apparently – zafirlukast – perhaps Colin could ask about it next time he went to the doctors.

It is fairly straightforward to pick up the idea that Colin is suffering from asthma. The early clues are quite indicative, the tight chest and 'wheeze', induced by exercise and cold weather. The results from spirometry support the initial diagnosis. Clearly there is also some circumstantial evidence, a change in lifestyle, exposure to increased traffic pollution and perhaps the central heating encouraging the presence of house mites. All of these may conspire to initiate asthma.

The consequent treatment, by use of an inhaler 'on demand', may well be appropriate. The drug is likely to be salbutamol. This is a well established, short-acting drug described as a beta-2 agonist, which achieves its therapeutic effect by causing the relaxation of bronchiolar smooth muscle and thereby dilating the bronchioles – a classical example of a drug interacting with a target protein that is a cell membrane receptor. No doubt, from a pharmacokinetic point of view, inhalation allows rapid access of the drug to its physiological site of action and hence it is very useful as an 'on demand' agent.

There are, however, a number of adverse effects that can easily occur with both acute and chronic use of the drug. These are mainly due to the stimulatory effect of the drug on other beta-2 receptors distributed in other tissues throughout the body. Interaction with beta-2 receptors in both skeletal and vascular smooth muscle may well result in tremors and a reflex increase in heart rate. Increases in insulin secretion and decrease in potassium levels have also been reported. Use of short-acting beta-2 agonist drugs seems to exacerbate the asthma. It has been suggested that this may be due to a toxic effect of the drug but it is more likely that there has been a gradual worsening of the asthma.

On extensive re-examination (well beyond that usually afforded to asthma sufferers!), we gain a clearer indication of the pathology of Colin's asthma. From the description of goblet cell hyperplasia, the distinct hypertrophy of both airway smooth muscle and mucous glands, there is little doubt of the inflammatory nature of asthma. Here we have the symptoms of partial airway obstruction, airway inflammation and, in all probability, increased airway responsiveness, in which a treatment that places an increased emphasis on anti-inflammatory therapy may be more successful. There is little doubt that inhaled glucocorticosteroids to counter this inflammation have become a vital part of asthma treatment. There is somewhat greater doubt, however, about the means by which they exert their response.

Steroid molecules, including glucocorticosteroids, will penetrate the cell wall quite easily as a result of their lipid solubility and after a number of complex biochemical steps they will activate and bind to a glucocorticosteroid receptor within the cell. This combination will in turn bind to a specific sequence of DNA in the nucleus, resulting in changes in cell products in terms of the means of physiological regulation and biochemical effects downstream of the DNA molecule. One such interesting process is that these glucocorticoids can induce an increase in the number of beta-2 receptors in a variety of tissues. Whatever the mechanism, there is considerable improvement of both inflammation and bronchial hyperresponsiveness.

This effective therapy can be maintained by administration twice or four times daily, though the latter is the better regimen provided there is adequate patient compliance. (Perhaps Colin is being somewhat short-changed in this respect!) It is also possible to use the inhaled corticosteroids in conjunction with short-acting beta-2 agonist drugs. Adverse reactions may be encountered, such as adrenal suppression, growth suppression in children (so Janet need not be concerned on Colin's behalf) and osteoporosis. It should be noted that there is considerable patient variability in terms of susceptibility to these drugs' side-effects. The effects can be reduced by means of spacer devices on the metered-dose inhalers used to deliver the drug. Interestingly, this mode of administration in itself appears to reduce the potential for systemic toxicity, by virtue of the fact that the drug delivery method directs drug more effectively to the site of action. Less drug needs to be used to achieve the therapeutic response and, by definition almost, there is less drug available to cause the adverse reaction.

As to the future, in relatively recent years, longer-acting beta-2 agonists such as salmeterol have emerged as a potentially useful therapeutic approach. Salmeterol is a beta-2-selective agent that, like salbutamol, produces bronchodilation. Its advantage lies in its high degree of lipid solubility. This permits it to dissolve in the predominantly lipid membrane of smooth muscle cells, including those, obviously, of the bronchioles. In this way a slow-release depot effect is achieved, allowing a much longer-lasting effect of the drug from the dose administered. Another approach to therapy arises from investigation of mediators that can give rise to the inflammatory

disease aspect of asthma. Earlier in this chapter, during a discussion of the NSAIDs, attention was drawn to the role of prostaglandins in pathology and prostaglandin synthesis from arachidonic acid through the action of the enzyme cyclo-oxygenase. Arachidonic acid is also acted upon by another enzyme, 5-lipoxygenase, to give rise to another series of highly biologically active molecules, the *leukotrienes* (LT). At least two members of this series of molecules, leukotriene C_4 (LTC_4) and leukotriene D_4 (LTD_4), are potent bronchoconstrictors and achieve this effect by interacting with cell-surface receptors. Both these leukotrienes have been shown to be secreted in asthma. Here we have two potential targets for pharmacological intervention. Inhibit the enzyme 5-lipoxygenase and leukotriene synthesis is prevented; hence two of the mediators involved in the asthma are removed. This enzyme inhibition may be accomplished by a drug such as zileutin. Although an effective therapy has been noted, the drug is almost certainly less effective than the inhaled corticosteroid drugs. From a target receptor approach, a drug such as pranlukast or zafirlukast is an effective competitive antagonist or blocker at LTD_4 receptors and can exert a useful therapeutic effect. Again, it should be said that in comparison the inhaled corticosteroid is a more effective agent.

A more physiological intervention may be observed in our next scene and the importance of pharmacokinetics cannot be discounted.

THE STORK ALSO FLIES, BY NOWALL ROWARD

Characters in order of appearance

Anne   the Practice Nurse.

Mandy   27 years, housewife. Epileptic with complex partial seizures maintained on 300 mg phenytoin. One child aged 3 years with a cleft lip and palate.

Fiona   31 years, advertising executive. Married, no children. A fanatic for taking exercise. Enthusiastic partaker of vitamins, particularly vitamin C, which is consumed in massive doses.

Maureen   35 years, librarian. Single. Has recently been away on a discreet holiday with a long-term companion but forgot to pack her oral contraceptives as she was starting a new packet.

Felicity   36 years. Permanent relationship, six children.

Vegan, very earnest but slightly scatty. An enthusiastic advocate of whole food and a wide variety of vegetarian products.

Sam   17 years. Single. College student, but attendance is compromised by the aftermath of regular partying. Probably running to 30 units a week of alcohol.

Helen   22 years, teacher. Married, no children. Recently treated for an unpleasant bacterial throat infection.

Susie   24 years, supermarket checkout operator. Married, no children. Also under investigation for Crohn's disease.

All have been taking some form of oral contraception; however, all are in the early stages of pregnancy.

Scene 1: Gyneville Health Practice, the waiting room of the antenatal clinic

The curtain rises

In this cast list, quite simply, we have a group of subjects taking oral contraceptives who have now become pregnant. The purpose of the exercise that follows is to furnish an explanation of the fate of our cast for the benefit of the playwright. An approach here may be to consider how the effective action of an oral contraceptive drug has been compromised. Is it through a lack of activity at the target site of action or has sufficient drug even arrived at the site of action? To appreciate the mechanism of action of oral contraceptives, we need to review the basic physiology of the female reproductive cycle. In essence, the major physiological input is by the endocrine system. Initially, the hypothalamus releases gonadotrophin releasing hormone (GnRH). This passes to the anterior pituitary and stimulates the release of follicle stimulating hormone (FSH) and luteinising hormone (LH). In turn each of these hormones will, in the case of FSH, stimulate the release of oestrogen from growing follicles in the ovary and, in the case of LH, bring about the full development of the follicles and a full secretion of progesterone. LH also brings about ovulation, production of the *corpus luteum* and further secretion of oestrogen and progesterone as well as relaxin and inhibin.

The consequence of all this endocrine activity is the cyclical development of a growing follicle, through the stages of primary follicle, secondary follicle to the mature (or graafian) follicle. This is due to the FSH-stimulated release of oestrogen

from the growing follicle. At the same time there is some increase in the thickness of the endometrium. At the stage of the mature follicle, progesterone secretion is stimulated by luteinising hormone, ovulation occurs, the ovum is released into the pelvic cavity and the *corpus luteum* is formed. Under the influence of progesterone and a second surge of oestrogen release, the endometrium becomes highly vascularised and more secretory in function, with numerous blood vessels and ducts. Should the ovum be fertilised, the endometrium is now primed to provide a suitably welcoming environment. If fertilisation does not take place, the *corpus luteum* degenerates, decreasing the maintenance supply of oestrogens and progesterone that maintains the endometrium, thus provoking the onset of menstruation. How then does the oral contraceptive interfere with this cycle to prevent conception?

The means whereby oral contraceptives exert their action depends on the type of preparation administered. Usually, oral contraceptives are either combination oral contraceptives comprising a mixture of synthetic forms of oestrogen and progesterone or progestin-only contraceptive pills. The combined oral contraceptives usually exert their primary action by providing a negative feedback type of inhibition of the hypothalamus–anterior-pituitary–ovary axis. This inhibits GnRH release and consequently FSH and LH release from the anterior pituitary, thus effectively preventing ovulation. In addition, cervical mucus is thickened, which lowers sperm penetration. Endometrial receptivity is decreased as well. As is well known, medication is taken for 21 days of 28, the point of commencement usually coinciding with the end of menstruation. Progestin-only contraceptives may exert their action by thickening cervical mucus, suppressing ovulation by reducing the LH surge, disrupting follicular activity and also rendering the endometrium unfavourable to implantation. This medication is taken for 28 days of 28.

Here we may have our answer to Maureen's case. If she was about to start a new packet then this coincided with the start of a new cycle. Without inhibition of the hypothalamic–pituitary events, ovulation could take place and the risk of fertilisation would be present. It is unlikely that such a mechanism is responsible for Sam's plight. With a relatively high alcohol intake, it may be that general compliance is inadequate, so that there is insufficient maintenance of an adequate dose level of drug. An alternate piece of speculation may be lack of contraception as a result of alcohol-induced vomiting. The oral contraceptives are a most effective group of drugs: it is more likely for failure to occur as a result of inadequate drug level than failure to inhibit the GnRH system.

Our remaining characters may well have compromised absorption or metabolism in some way. A fairly obvious explanation for Susie is that if she has started to display the presence of Crohn's disease her ability to absorb the drug will be significantly lowered. Crohn's disease is a malabsorption syndrome characterised, among other things, by a flat jejunal mucosa revealed at biopsy. Diminished absorption gives a diminished pharmacological action; hence the resulting pregnancy. Fiona and Felicity might be grouped together. Both may be including items in their diet that alter the absorption of the pill. Maintenance of drug levels is also assisted by the presence of the enterohepatic circulation of these compounds. Changes in gut bacterial microflora by possible excessive use of vitamins may alter oestrogen absorption. Neither is it inconceivable that a vegan diet is high in fibre. Gastrointestinal transit time is shortened to the extent that the drug is excreted in the faeces before there has been time for adequate absorption. Helen may have been prescribed a broad-spectrum antibiotic for her infection. These antibiotics will change gut bacterial microflora to a considerable extent and severely lower absorption of the contraceptive pill. In the case of all three, there was insufficient drug present to inhibit GnRH release and ovulation, followed by fertilisation taking place.

Finally Mandy, who reminds us of the capacity of some agents to cause teratogenic effects. The cleft lip and palate of her child could have been the consequence of phenytoin presence during pregnancy. However, in the case of her second pregnancy, the problem may have been caused by phenytoin. Among its other properties, phenytoin is a very effective hepatic microsomal enzyme inducer in the smooth endoplasmic reticulum of the liver. The synthetic oestrogens and progesterones that make up oral contraceptives are metabolised by microsomal enzymes. In effect, by increasing the amount of enzyme, phenytoin is speeding up the metabolism of our contraceptive, it is broken down far more quickly and removed from the body. Under such circumstances therapeutic levels may not be attained and contraception fails.

Of course, our characters are merely fictional. Guidelines in each practice and family planning clinic are there to prevent such scenes as described above. Nevertheless, the complexity of the nature of the interaction and the variety of factors that conspire to compromise drug action are quite clearly revealed here.

THEME PARK MAYHEM

Alf Dibbs slowly eased his coach into the narrow lane and away from Bluefields Junior and Middle School, Drake Rise. The coach was absolutely heaving with its mixed cargo of schoolchildren and, thank heavens, four of their teachers who actually seemed to have some sort of control over them! The extra helpers, the granny of one of the children and one of the mums, were also comfortably settled into their seats at the front. The purpose of the trip was entirely pleasure – a visit to Packton Theme Park and a day on the rides for the children, with a picnic lunch in the middle of the day.

Most of the children were really looking forward to the day out and there was an excited hum of anticipation as the coach left the more rural roads and joined the motorway heading north. But for little Gemma Smith and Michelle Seaton, the form monitor of the top class, the journey was a matter of apprehension. Neither of them tolerated coach journeys particularly well and they had been well dosed for the outward trip before leaving home. Their caring parents had also passed over to Miss Carstairs, the Head Teacher, cellophane envelopes containing their protection for the homeward drive with strict instructions to take the tablets no later than half an hour before starting back. These were now safely installed in Miss Carstairs's voluminous handbag. The pleasant atmosphere was suddenly shattered by a volley of coughing from 4-year-old Christopher Pace, who had been suffering from a chesty cough – it had been touch and go whether he would be fit for the trip. Fortunately, Tony Bright, the middle-aged sports teacher, was suffering from a similar complaint and had brought his bottle of Benylin Chesty Cough Mixture. A quick swig of this and Christopher was soon happily restored to the back seat of the coach.

Alf made excellent progress: a distinct shortage of cones and light traffic had the coach pulling in through the garishly advertised opening of the Theme Park accompanied by excited shouts and gasps from the schoolchildren. Gerald Plover was the first off and with an astonishing turn of speed for one of his years raced towards the Gents followed by a coterie of boys, intent upon a similar mission of relief. The girls were more decorously organised by Miss Carstairs. Ten minutes later the boys had all rejoined the main party but Mr Plover took some time to re-emerge. 'Sorry, Isabel,' he apologised to his Head, 'Usual problem'. In the meantime, Jennifer Morgan and her two helpers had purchased the group's wristbands and the party was neatly divided into small groups each with their own adult in charge. The smaller children made a beeline for the animal roundabout and were soon happily enjoying the ride.

Time passed only too quickly and lunchtime arrived. All the children and staff met on a pleasant area of grass overlooking one of several scenic lakes. As an extra treat, once the packed lunches had been consumed, Granny Roberts bought all the children an ice cream. Sadly, this encouraged the arrival of a large squadron of wasps and a great flapping and waving of hands. The inevitable happened and poor Kevin James was stung quite badly. From the depths of her bag, Miss Carstairs produced a tube of sting cream and liberally smeared it on Kevin's arm. For good measure, Granny Roberts, who had some pills for her itching, thought that these would help and slipped him a couple of Dr Martyn's One a Day antihistamine tablets when no-one was looking. 'Thanks' he whispered 'That sting really hurt!'.

General good humour was restored in the party and the children persuaded the adults that rather than just watching them enjoy themselves they should join in the rides as well. Gerald Plover was attracted to the Pirate Ship; after all it bore a fleeting resemblance to the swing boats he recalled from his youth. Initially the ride was enormous fun, until the 'Ship' started to reach the apogee of its swing and he could actually view the mechanism of the swing below. Suddenly he felt extremely unwell and regretted his impulse. After what seemed like an eternity the ride ended and he walked unsteadily in the direction of Isabel Carstairs to see if she had anything to stop him feeling quite so queasy. Sure enough, she was her usual brisk and helpful self. 'Here, a couple of these Kwells will soon sort you out.' Unlike the luckless Gerald, the children were becoming accustomed to the sensations of speed and general hurling around that was taking place and soon the fearsome 'Python' was again attracting their attention. That is, apart from Christopher Pace, who must have had a tiring morning and was discovered sound asleep on a nearby bench.

All too soon it was time to go home. Isabel Carstairs efficiently dosed her two travelsick pupils, counted heads, ensured that all children and adults were safely aboard. Gemma was very sleepy and drowsy, kept complaining of a headache and said that things looked fuzzy through the window. Things were a little messier at the back of the coach: poor Michelle was engaged in periodic bouts of violent sickness and was feeling decidedly unwell. Isabel Carstairs decided that next year they would visit a local museum.

Mayhem – of the pharmaceutical variety – is about right here! We have a number of subjects receiving medication, for the most part for motion sickness, and, rather more disturbingly, a lot of dispensers and amateur prescribers. In the course of the day out we encounter a couple of clear opportunities for motion sickness to occur: one is the journey by motor vehicle while the other is the 'ride' offered by the theme park. One theory of motion sickness is that it is thought to be caused by a conflict between the sensory information passed to the central nervous system from the eyes and information transmitted from the vestibular apparatus of the ears and perhaps other forms of proprioception. A popular example of this may be the difference between being a front seat passenger in a car, able to view the passage of the journey, compared to being asked to scan for some time the detail of a map. It is possible after a time to suffer a conflict between the sensation of movement detected through the vestibular apparatus of the ear and the visual perception, which is fixed on a particular image. It seems that this conflict gives rise to an imbalance of cholinergic or parasympathetic activity over the sympathetic activity within the medulla of the brain. If this balance continues unchecked without respite in the causative sensation of motion, the inevitable consequences of nausea, often accompanied by quite violent vomiting will occur. Indeed, many of the symptoms that precede vomiting can be attributed to a greater activity of the parasympathetic nervous system, such as pallor (vasoconstriction), excessive salivation and sweating.

Therapy for this particular condition is aimed at a correction of the imbalance, either by antagonising these parasympathetic or cholinergic effects or by promoting sympathetic activity by use of so-called sympathomimetic drugs. The latter are generally less popular and tend to be used in combination with cholinergic antagonists. To emphasise the unlikely use of a combination approach, the main example of its use would be for service personnel in an invasion situation, in landing craft. To combat the seasickness often observed under such circumstances, an anticholinergic drug such as scopolamine (hyoscine) would be used to treat the sickness but would leave the subject somewhat drowsy, hardly an ideal state of readiness for combat. The side-effect of the scopolamine could be counteracted by a concomitant dose of dexamphetamine, a well-known sympathomimetic drug. The clear potential for drug abuse mitigates against a more widespread use of the combination.

In general, most anticholinergic drugs achieve their effect by antagonising the actions of the so-called *muscarinic receptors*. These receptors are sited at the point where the parasympathetic nerve fibre encounters the tissue or organ that it innervates. By definition, antagonism or blockade of these receptors will inhibit or curtail parasympathetic activity at these tissues. Consequently, as well as resolving the parasympathetic–sympathetic conflict in the medulla, these anticholinergic (or strictly antimuscarinic) drugs will bring about a decrease in the secretion of saliva, tears and sweat. It should also be noted that hyoscine penetrates the blood–brain barrier rapidly and is able to exert its effects at the level of the medulla in order to achieve some control of the initial conflict between parasympathetic and sympathetic effects. Possible side-effects are likely to arise from CNS depression, with responses such as drowsiness, amnesia, fatigue and dreamless sleep. In the eye, the pupil will be dilated and relaxation of the ciliary muscle may bring about paralysis of accommodation which will impair near vision – hence Gemma's vision problems and sleepiness. It may be interesting to speculate that Gemma and Michelle were dosed in haste and received each other's medication! Michelle shows every sign of an inadequate dose of anti-emetic whereas Gemma displays sufficient side-effects to suggest a much higher dose than necessary. A reminder, perhaps, of the importance of subject age, for example, in determining the size of dose. Other effects will be an increase in heart rate and a decrease in gastrointestinal activity. These drugs are also likely to promote urinary retention in elderly men with prostatic enlargement. Miss Carstairs has done poor Gerald Plover no favours by administering 'a couple of Kwells': these tablets contain hyoscine and are likely to exacerbate his urinary problem. Furthermore, such medication is far more effective used prophylactically than after the onset of sickness.

Apart from the antimuscarinic drugs, it would appear from our story that antihistamines have seen some use during the course of the day. Indeed, it may be that they have been employed as anti-emetic agents as well. Histamine is another example of an autacoid with a significant range of physiological influences. Often released in response to mechanical trauma or in allergic reactions, histamine will cause effects such as increase in capillary permeability, bronchoconstriction and gastric secretion. To initiate these effects, histamine can interact with a variety of receptors or protein targets. Of relatively recent interest has been the successful use of H_2-receptor blocking drugs, such as ranitidine, to control gastric secretion and hence the problem of gastric ulcers. However, our interest in this scenario concerns H_1-receptor blocking drugs. Such drugs may be present in the 'sting cream' for topical treatment of the itch, redness and flare (Lewis triple response to histamine at the site of, say, a puncture wound). Granny Roberts, no doubt with the best of intentions, has offered Kevin James an antihistamine tablet. The cream may be sufficient; there is no real need for the tablet, and in any event, pharmacokinetic principles will decree some delay before the drug reaches its target.

Elsewhere, Tony Bright has been most generous in sharing his Benylin with Christopher Pace. Reference to a *pharmacopoeia* will reveal that two constituents of Benylin are dextromethorphan (an analogue of codeine) and diphenhydramine (an antihistamine). Dextromethorphan is an effective antitussive that tends to act by elevating the threshold for coughing to occur. It suffers the drawback, in some subjects, of causing CNS depression. Diphenhydramine is a fairly typical H_1 antagonist drug and will antagonise many of the H_1-receptor-mediated effects of histamine. Therapeutically useful effects include the blockade of histamine-induced capillary permeability, though diphenhydramine will be of little advantage to treat bronchoconstriction. The major side-effect of these antihistamines is sedation and subjects taking them should be warned as to their impact on daytime activities. An additive effect has been noted if such antihistamines are taken with alcohol or other CNS depressants, in which case, side-effects can include dizziness, tinnitus, lassitude, fatigue, blurred vision, possible lack of co-ordination and tremors. Given that Tony Bright is middle-aged and Christopher Pace is only 4, noting the adverse reactions and potential interaction of the drugs in Benylin allied to differences in the quantity given to adults compared to infants, it should come as no surprise that Christopher has such a restful day!

The use of these H_1 antihistamines as anti-emetic drugs is interesting. Diphenhydramine is described as a first generation antihistamine; one of its characteristics is a high level of lipid solubility, which permits passage across the blood–brain barrier. Conversely, the newer or second-generation antihistamines, such as terfenadine, do not possess this degree of solubility and will not penetrate the brain. Consequently, CNS effects are not observed and neither do these antihistamines possess anti-emetic properties. The first generation antihistamine's ability to effect motion sickness, then, is probably a central nervous system action and is almost certainly due to the fact that these drugs possess anti-muscarinic properties as well as antihistaminic properties. Despite our desire that drugs should be aimed at specific targets, here is an example of a therapy that suffers the drawback of a number of side-effects and possibly the drug is likely to impact more on a secondary target.

This brief selection of examples will hopefully serve to stimulate, in part, an interest in aspects of pharmacological knowledge but more importantly will foster a spirit of enquiry. A given drug may not be used for ever and a day. The information provided above is subject to constant change and will become dated very soon. It is important to progress and have a better understanding of the disease process and its context. If we are to employ a pharmacological intervention, the better we are at achieving our desideratum of the right drug at the right amount of the drug in the right place at the right time for the right length of time (and in these days – at the right price!), then so much the better for the recipients of therapy. It is perhaps fitting to close by looking to the future and emphasising the importance of frequent review of pharmacology, such will be the pace of change and the advent

of novel and hopefully highly specific agents of therapy.

There is much emphasis on evidence-based medicine. In turn this will lead to a greater expectation of the qualities of medicines made available for therapy. It will not be considered sufficient to achieve a palliative effect. Safe, preventative and curative compounds will be required: not only should morbidity and mortality be reduced but also a maintenance of the quality of life and productivity of an individual may be enhanced. How might this be achieved? In terms of pharmacological intervention, by improving the selection of drug targets, which itself will come by investigating and identifying the genetic nature of disease and discovering the potential molecular targets for drugs. This will be of advantage in multigene diseases such as asthma or heart disease. An example of this might be through the investigation of susceptibility genes. These may reveal that a given pathological condition is not a single disease but a combination of several different lesions. Potentially, each of these may need a different treatment. Another instance could be routine genotyping to select individuals whose inherent physiology and metabolism might give rise to side-effects.

Pharmaceutical companies need to focus on targets that are worth the high level of investment needed these days. One way in which this may be achieved is by integrating aspects such as molecular physiology, human genetics, bioinformatics and functional genomics. Genomics is defined as the collection, codifying and data handling of DNA clones, their sequences, variations and screening. Bioinformatics supports this integration by providing information systems for identifying genes and mapping them, linking them to their proteins and biological function so that worthwhile, relevant and effective targets are discovered. Allied to this process, the key pharmaceutical companies have developed combinatorial chemistry techniques, a means of modelling and building chemical libraries of compounds that might be drug molecules.

Following on from such integration is a process of phenomenally rapid screening of several millions of compounds. Clearly this increases the chances of discovering a medicinally useful molecule. The speed of screening is markedly enhanced by refinement of the techniques used and the use of advanced robotics. Rapid-throughput screening is not the only means of making the search for the medicines of the future more effective and efficient. As was observed at the beginning of this chapter, not only should a drug exhibit useful pharmacodynamic properties (biological activity) but its pharmacokinetic properties also need to be considered. Preclinical tests include, among other tests, administration of multiple compounds (cassette dosing) to retrieve pharmacokinetic data. This accelerates the process of data acquisition and, very importantly, allows a very substantial lowering of the numbers of animals used in pharmaceutical testing. All this research is supported by extensive use of powerful computing facilities that allow a range of activities from 3D modelling of a potential drug molecule (pharmacophore) to control of automated process and collating and comparing the vast tract of knowledge that emanates from the research of the disease process and its resolution.

A study of the history of pharmacology reveals a concern to focus on accurate targeting of drug molecules. From Paul Ehrlich's magic bullets to the very sophisticated molecular sciences used today, there has been an endeavour (not always successful) to produce compounds that can cure and alleviate rather than induce illness. The effective delivery of medicinal compounds requires the right drug to be available, with minimal (no?) side-effects but appropriate biological activity that takes into consideration both pharmacokinetic and pharmacodynamic principles. It should be readily available and easily administered. Perhaps it should not be particularly expensive. However, none of this will be of any value unless the patient actually takes the drug and appropriate compliance is observed. The role, then, of the healthcare professional in this area of health education and pharmaceutical delivery is one of immense significance and should be strongly emphasised.

FURTHER READING

In this approach to pharmacology, to encourage a freedom of source discovery it is something of a contradiction to provide a list of texts. The sources 'trawled' include leaflets provided with medication, ingredients on labels, conversation with drug representatives, information sheets from pharmaceutical companies, specialist journals in a variety of disciplines, encyclopaedias, other professionals, pages on web-sites and some textbooks.

As a guide, a few 'classical' texts are listed here as well as some interesting current web-site pages.

Burley S, Mitchell E E, Welling K, Smith M, Chilton S, Crumplin C 1997 Contemporary community nursing. Edward Arnold, London

Brody TM, Larner J, Minneman KP, Neu HC 1998 Human pharmacology: molecular to clinical, 3rd edn. Mosby, London

Feldman RS, Meyer JS, Quenzer LF 1997 Principles of neuropsychopharmacology. Sinauer Associates, Sunderland, MA

Hardman JG, Limbird LE, Molinoff PB et al (ed) 1996

Goodman and Gilman's the pharmacological basis of therapeutics, 9th edn. McGraw-Hill, New York

Herfindal ET, Gourley DR 1996 Textbook of therapeutics: drug and disease management, 6th edn. Williams & Wilkins, Baltimore, MD

Katzung BG 1998 Basic and clinical pharmacology. Appleton & Lange, Stamford, CT

Lodish H, Baltimore D, Berk A et al 1995 Molecular cell biology, 3rd edn. WH Freeman, New York

Martini FH 1998 Fundamentals of anatomy and physiology, 4th edn. Prentice Hall International, London

Munson PL (ed) 1995 Principles of pharmacology: basic concepts and applications. Chapman & Hall, London

Rang HP, Dale MM, Ritter JM 1995 Pharmacology, 3rd edn. Churchill Livingstone, Edinburgh

Rowland M, Tozer TN 1995 Clinical pharmacokinetics: concepts and applications, 3rd edn. Williams & Wilkins, Baltimore, MD

Zubay GL 1998 Biochemistry, 4th edn. Wm C Brown, London

Useful web-sites

http://www.glaxowellcome.co.uk
http://www.oup.co.uk/drugsj/contents/
http://www.virtual drugstore.com
http://www.zeneca.com
http://www.pitt.edu/~nursing
http://www.md.huji.ac.il/mirrors/netpharm/dlmaster.htm

16

Public health needs of south Asians in Britain

Shobha Gogna and Tejinder Hari

INTRODUCTION

South Asians are defined in this chapter as people who originate from the Indian subcontinent, e.g. Indians, Pakistanis and Bangladeshis, and the term south Asians will be used interchangeably with Asians. In addition, this section of the book will look critically at the part professionals/organisations play in supporting the identified needs and analysis of the health and social needs identified within this group.

Since public health, and how it relates to south Asians, is our main concern in this chapter we need to examine whether the definition of public health in fact relates to the needs of this group. The following statement in *Healthy Public Policy* in the Adelaide Charter (WHO 1988) is seen to be universal and encompasses the needs of all people including south Asians, although it does exclude reference to race, culture and ethnicity: 'Healthy public policy is characterised by an explicit concern for the health and equity in all areas of policy and by an accountability for health impact'.

The main aim of Healthy Public Policy is to create a supportive environment to enable people to lead healthy lives. Such a policy makes healthy choices possible or easier for citizens and makes social and physical environments health enhancing. In the pursuit of Healthy Public Policy, government sectors need to take account of health as an essential factor when formulating policy.

Cruickshank & Beevers (1994) state that 'utilisation of health will vary according to whether the individual has been socialised only at home in a rural or urban area – the first generation, at home as well as in the new environment for those who migrate in the early adolescence – the second generation; or in new environment only – subsequent generation'. Health needs are often tailored to third-generation Asians because they speak English and thus can articulate their needs better; for example, it is assumed that health education material printed in English will also cater for the needs of first- and second-generation families who do not speak English.

This chapter is being written in the light of the present Labour government's health policy contained in *The New NHS – Modern, Dependable* (Department of Health 1997a) and *Our Healthier Nation* (Department of Health 1998a). One of the key emphases in *Our Healthier Nation* is the development of primary care groups in the community so that the health needs of the population residing within the primary care group's area could be easily targeted in terms of public health, with emphasis on meeting health needs at local level. Moreover, as the primary care groups develop, targeting health and social needs to south Asians living in their areas is going to be difficult, as there is no collated comprehensive data on these groups of people. These data are essential to target resources in the Asian community.

Given that south Asians have been settled in the UK since the 1960s, and have relatively stable populations in various towns and cities, data on these populations have been collated in an ad hoc fashion, e.g. from census figures, health education lifestyle studies, focus groups within various districts or sometimes from health education departments. Therefore the data used to inform policy, if there is a policy concerning health delivery to south Asians, are often misinformed, patchy and whenever target projects are identified they are usually short-term. As soon as the allocated funds are finished the service needs are marginalised because they no longer form part of the long-term health strategy of the organisation. It is not surprising, therefore, that the health/social needs specific to the relevant ethnic group become lost in the mainstream delivery of care. Since no data are used as part of the assessment

to plan for the health/social needs of south Asians, organisations do not have to justify services sensitive to the needs of those groups that might be identified by the data.

There are arguments that collection of 'ethnic data' might be seen as 'race data', with its negative implications. Cruickshank & Beevers (1994) have compared this with the USA, where a breakdown of racial and ethnic data has allowed the development of specific preventive health programmes for minority health problems. They believe that the lack of such data in the UK has in fact perpetuated health and social problems for ethnic minorities rather than alleviated them. Along the same lines, Sheldon & Parke (1992) take a more rigid stance and state that ethnic data collection will be the 'minimum data sets which all provider units in the National Health Service will have to generate for each patient'. This will also elicit personal details and health-related information and 'ethnicity will be recorded using the same categories as in the census'. Although Sheldon & Parke (1992) state that no socio-economic data will be collected, it is argued that to give a more holistic view of the communities both quantitative and qualitative data are necessary.

Generalisation of national health information to the local ethnic population has failed to recognise that Asians are not a homogenous group but heterogeneous, with each group likely to be influenced by different lifestyle factors, e.g. religion and diet, that affect their health/social needs and behaviour. Lack of data and effectiveness of measurable outcomes of healthcare delivered and accessed to this group also raises concerns. The document *Good Practice and Quality Indicators in Primary Health Care* (NHS Ethnic Health Unit 1996) found that, although 36 health authorities had set targets in terms of service delivery to their minority population, only six (and four family health service authorities) could specify these and few proposed measurable objectives and levels. Perception of delivery of care in some cases was just in terms of translating health-promotion materials, acknowledging 're-spect for culture and spiritual beliefs', and agreeing that translation or interpreter services should be provided. This type of apathetic attitude among service planners may persist unless a more concrete, substantial tool, such as community profile data, is used to identify the health needs of south Asian people.

Community profiling here includes not just the quantitative data (e.g. age, sex, religion, ethnic group) but also more qualitative data (e.g. at family/individual level, social needs, family structure, support within the family). Further qualitative information gained from, for instance, focus groups, community activities, e.g. urban regeneration programmes, and local pressure groups would also help to identify local needs. Data collection, however, does raise the issue of terms that are used interchangeably – race, ethnicity, culture and lifestyle. How the terms are used in data collection needs to be clearly defined in the context in which the data are being collected. Ethnicity, for example, is not easy to define; as Senior & Bhopal (1994) state, 'ethnic boundaries are imprecise and fluid' and according to them ethnicity implies 'shared origins in social background, shared culture and traditions that are distinctive, maintained between generations and lead to a sense of identity and group, and a common language or religious tradition'.

Race, on the other hand, has a more biological base. According to Senior & Bhopal (1994), race is 'differentiated by physical characteristics'. In comparison, Husband (1982) and Bhat et al (1988) see race as a socially constructed phenomenon that cannot be analysed in medical research 'in isolation from a wider discussion of racial oppression and its historical context'. Ahmad (1993), on the other hand, argues that 'race, as a term, has legitimated exploitation on the basis of "scientific" and "natural" superiority of some over others'. Culture, according to Cruickshank & Beevers (1994), describes a far wider influence on the individual, where 'learned behaviour is affected by home, religion, ethnic group, language, neighbourhood, school and age-group'.

The explanations of the above terms may seem simplistic but it is felt that they do at least raise awareness of how they are used in data collection. Obviously, the terms will have to be subjected to greater rigor of definition, especially when epidemiological data are collected.

This chapter will examine the lives and health of south Asians – particularly focusing on those aspects that are critical to healthcare. It is likely that at times health professionals may be working with assumptions about aspects of Asian life and it is important for health visitors to recognise the less well publicised aspects of these people. The following topic areas will be discussed: religion; perception of health from religious perspectives; diets and infant feeding; health promotion; family roles; homosexuality and sexually transmitted diseases; mental health; and finally death.

RELIGIONS

It is important to realise that it is difficult to make broad generalisations about any religion. Here, we shall examine Hinduism, Sikhism, Islam and some other sects and their cultures. After all, no culture is, or ever has been, entirely homogenous. Just as differences exist between Christian faiths, variations exist in many other religions. While there are no variations in the teachings and principles for followers of each faith in different parts of the world, slight differences may be found in customs and practice. These often reflect the influence of the host country. Although the chapter offers basic information, there may be differences even within the UK. For example, customs, practices and even the languages used by Gujarati Hindus from the north of India differ from those of Hindus from the south. Similar variations can be found in Islam and Sikhism and often depend on an individual's origins. This might be due to differences within a country (for example a Sikh from north India may have different practices from a Sikh from south India) or differences from one country to another; variations in Islamic faith can be seen in this context.

Hinduism

Hindus have been present in the UK in small numbers for many centuries; the majority arrived in the 1950s and 1960s. While some came directly from India, others came from east Africa, particularly from Uganda, as they sought safety from Idi Amin's regime. Hindus have also come from Fiji and Guyana. It is thought that there may be 400 000 Hindus in the UK but the figure could be higher. Most live in large towns and cities – particularly in Coventry, Leicester, London (especially in Wembley and Harrow) and Manchester (Weller 1991).

Hindu religious practice varies a great deal, depending on the caste and area of origin, because of the significance of local deities. Hinduism is a social system as well as a set of beliefs. Customs and religious practices are therefore closely interwoven. Caste, or social status, is determined by individual *karma*, meaning reward for good deeds and punishment for wickedness. The belief in reincarnation is strong; the status, condition and caste of each life is determined by behaviour in the last life, making each person responsible for who s/he is and what s/he does. The fundamental belief of Hinduism is that the truth is with all of us. Hindus believe in God as a universal force pervading everything. If the 'universal force' pervades everything, then it follows that this must include human beings and they, like everything else in this world – both animate and inanimate – are material expressions of an abstract force. This means that God exists both inside and outside each individual. Therefore the important belief of Hinduism is that the energy within each person is the same energy that drives the universe. Hinduism has much in common with other religions such as Buddhism and Sikhism, which are often described as variants of Hinduism rather than contradictions.

Hinduism encompasses a great tolerance of belief and practices. Different Hindu communities have different ways of expressing their faith, and usually have their own local temple. Religious values and social values are intertwined, so that a Hindu who follows the social customs laid down for him/her is also fulfilling a religious duty.

Fasting

Some Hindus fast on several days a year. The particular day depends on the religious sect to which someone belongs or the deity that they worship. Many fast on Mondays, the day of Lord Shiva, while others fast on Tuesdays, the day of Lord Hunaman (the Monkey God). Men may fast on Saturdays.

Individuals may abstain from certain foods for long periods for a special reason, e.g. during pregnancy to ensure a successful outcome, or to aid recovery from an illness. But a Hindu fast does not necessarily involve abstaining from all foods. Most people will eat one meal a day, eating foods such as fruits or yoghurt, nuts or potatoes, which are considered pure. Very few Hindus would insist on fasting while in hospital.

While fasting, prayers to the appropriate deity are said either first thing in the morning or in the evening. There is normally a shrine in each home; it may be in a separate room, if space is available, or in a corner. The shrine will dictate the kind of prayers and general ethos of the household. Often, food is presented to the gods in the family shrine before consumption.

It is also customary to fast during certain days of festivals. The following festivals are of most significance:

- *Shivratri* (March), a celebration of Lord Shiva
- *Holi* (March), associated with Lord Krishna. It is a festival of colour: people sprinkle coloured dyes and water over participants to welcome spring
- *Ramnaumi* (April), a celebration of the birth of Lord Rama
- *Rakshabandan* (August), a celebration when sisters tie a raakhi (a band of coloured thread) on the wrist of their brother, who then promises to protect and help them. Brothers also give gifts to their sisters
- *Navratri* (October – lasts 9 days), a festival of dancing to honour all the goddesses
- *Dussehra* (October) commemorates the time when Lord Rama fought King Ravana and was victorious. Celebrations take place over 10 days, during which the story of Ramayana is enacted in dramatic form. On the 10th day, an image of King Ravana is burned
- *Durga Puja* (October) involves 4 days of worship, after which images of the warrior

goddess Durga are immersed in lakes and rivers

- *Diwali* (November), the Festival of Lights, commemorates Lord Rama's return from banishment to his kingdom of Ayodhya. Welcoming lights are displayed around houses and public buildings and there are firework displays.

The holy book, *Bhagavad-Gita* (*Gita*), 'the song of the Lord', should be kept in a cover cloth. It is important to be purified by being physically clean in preparation for worship. Most people will bathe first thing in the morning before they pray and will not eat anything until they have completed the *puja*. Hindus feel strongly about purity and pollution, especially when they are ill. People who are bed-bound may seek help with a wash at certain times before they pray.

Sikhism

Religious and cultural background

The majority of Sikhs in the UK originate directly from the Punjab; however, a significant minority arrived here from former British colonies (in east Africa), where the families had originally migrated. During the First and Second World Wars, many Sikhs fought in the British Indian armies and some of these ex-servicemen later settled in the UK.

There are approximately 400 000 Sikhs in the UK, mostly in large towns and cities, particularly in Birmingham, Bradford, Cardiff, Coventry, Glasgow, Leeds, Leicester, London (Southall, Hayes) and Wolverhampton.

The Sikh religion is the youngest of the major world religions (1469 AD). It was founded by Guru Nanak Dev Ji (*guru* means 'teacher'); the word *sikh* means 'disciple'. Throughout its 530 years of history it has won a reputation for dynamism, socialistic outlook and progressive thinking. According to the Sikh faith, 'there is but one God'. He is the supreme truth, the creator, without fear, without hate, omnipresent, immortal, unborn, self-existent and the enlightened.

The teachings of Guru Nanak Dev Ji flourished and grew in the care of nine successive spiritual masters who expounded, propagated and gave practical shape to the principles and doctrines of the founder prophet. Guru Gobind Singh Ji, the 10th and final guru, ordained the Guru Granth Sahib Ji (the holy Sikh scriptures) as the manifest body of all the gurus, for guidance of the Sikhs. Guru Nanak Dev Ji's emphasis was on the worship of one God, earning livelihood by earnest means, sharing your possessions, love, service, humility, equality and fellowship. Guru Nanak Dev Ji's teachings do not belong to one race, sect, community or clan but to all human beings.

Further to these beliefs, a Sikh can serve his God best by serving His creatures and meditating on His name. A Sikh must constantly aim for the beauty of life, which can be achieved through killing the five dragons: jealousy/envy, anger, sexual lust, greed and false pride. Fasts, pilgrimages and donations are not substitutes for good deeds.

There should be no caste system, and women are equal to men in every walk of life. Guru Gobind Singh Ji (the 10th Guru) added a new dimension to Sikhs after the martyrdom of two gurus before him. Like St George, he decided that when affairs are past all peaceful remedy, it is then justifiable to unsheathe the sword in defence of religion and righteousness. Guru Gobind Singh Ji also created the Khalsa, a group of individuals who are free from prejudice of caste, colour and social status. Guru Gobind Singh Ji baptised these individuals himself and was then baptised by them, so he was Guru and a disciple in one, and gave them the five Ks. These are:

- *kesh*, uncut hair – signifies a spiritual element
- *kangha*, a small comb – for pride in one's own appearance
- *kara*, a steel bracelet on the wrist – signifies that the wearer is bound both morally and spiritually to the teachings of the Gurus
- *kaccha*, a special underwear – for chastity and self-respect
- *kirpan*, a sword – a sign of strength (only to be used in self-defence or in defence of the weak).

Apart from the five Ks, the Guru also gave them the turban, another symbol of dignity and self-respect usually worn by men. Although Sikhs in the UK vary how strictly they adhere to the five Ks, many devout Sikhs wear them all the time, and will never remove them completely, even when they are ill in bed, or washing. It is important for practitioners to understand the significance of these religious symbols. If any of the symbols have to be removed for carrying out procedures, a full explanation and discussion should take place with the clients and their families at the start.

Most Sikh homes display the Guru's photographs. Some may have a room reserved for Guru Granth Sahib Ji in the house. As special care and respect is required, no one can use this room for any other purpose. Family members and guests will use it for prayers and meditation. Before prayers are said, individuals will wash or have a shower as an act of purification. A devout Sikh may follow the principle of giving 'one-tithe'. This means one-tenth of time is spent in prayers daily and one-tenth of earnings spent on the needy or other charitable causes.

Many events are celebrated throughout the year, e.g. festivals of birthdays, accessions, anniversaries of the Gurus and martyrdom anniversaries. However, some of these are shared with Hindu festivals and are celebrated all over the world. The main events celebrated are:

- *Baisakhi* (April 13th), the birthday of Khalsa
- *Rakshabandha* (August), shared with Hindus
- *Guru Nanak Dev Ji's birthday* (October/ November)
- *Diwali* (October/November), shared with Hindus. Sikhs celebrate this because the sixth guru, Guru Har Gobind Ji, came to Amritsar in 1620 after his release from Gawalior jail
- *Guru Gobind Singh Ji's birthday* (December).
- Martyrdom of Guru Teg Bahadar Ji (the ninth Guru; December).

These events are celebrated in all *gurudwaras* (Sikh temples) and last for 3 days. The scriptures (Guru Granth Sahib Ji) are continuously read for 48 hours by relays of readers and are followed by *kirtan* (singing hymns) and *katha* (discourse).

Langer (food) is available to all during this period, regardless of caste or religion. All people sit and eat as equals. The 48 hours of unbroken reading of the Guru Granth Sahib Ji is called an *Akand Path*.

An *Akand Path* or a *Sahaj Path* (lasting from a week to a month) can also be held in the homes during special occasions, e.g. when moving into a new home, the birth of a new child, birthday celebrations, before a marriage and following a death.

Guru Granth Sahib Ji (the Adi Granth), should be kept in an elevated position, opened, read and closed reverently.

Sikh religion strictly demands that Sikhs do not eat Halal meat, cut their hair, gamble, steal, commit adultery, smoke or use any intoxicants i.e. alcohol and drugs (recreational).

Sikh women do not wear a veil. Sikhs do not worship idols or sacred animals.

Islam

There have been a significant number of Muslims in the UK since the early 1800s, when Middle Eastern Muslim seamen and traders settled around several major ports like South Shields, Liverpool and Cardiff. About two-thirds of the UK's Muslims originate from the Indian subcontinent, having arrived here either directly or indirectly through east Africa or the Caribbean. The remainder of UK Muslims have a variety of ethnic/national origins, e.g. the Arab world, Cyprus and Malaysia. There are about 1.5 million Muslims in the UK, found in most towns and cities, particularly in the West Midlands, Lancashire, West Yorkshire, Greater London and Glasgow. Although some settlement occurred following the First World War, in the 1950s and 1960s Muslims sought employment in textile mills and factories. More recent arrivals have come from Somalia and Bosnia, and from African countries.

The Islamic religion began approximately in 500 AD. Islam means 'submission to the will of God' and is based on the teachings of the Al-Qu'ran (Koran). The five pillars of Islam are:

- *Shahadat*: the declaration of faith that there is

only one God (Allah) and that Mohammed is his prophet

- *Salat*: the prayers that are said five times a day facing Mecca, before sunrise (*faju*), at noon (*zuhr*), mid/late afternoon (*asr*), late evening (*maghrib*) and at night (*isha*)
- *Zakat*: the giving of alms to the poor
- *Sawan*: fasting during the month of Ramadan (pronounced as Ramazan), known as *Roza*
- *Hajj*: making a pilgrimage to Mecca at least once during a lifetime.

Prayers are also said before and after meals, with clean hands. A clean space is required for praying; a piece of clean material or a special rug can be used to pray on.

During the month of Ramadan, Muslims must abstain from food and liquids between dawn and dusk. Each day the family will eat before they begin the fast, a couple of hours before sunrise, and again after sunset, when the fast has ended. The routine of most families, particularly the women, is completely altered. As they rise very early, and stay up very late, cooking and cleaning after the family has eaten, many women require a rest during the middle of the day, which may affect attendance at clinics. It is also advisable to check when a woman may be ready to receive home visits during the month of Ramadan.

Fasting is excused after a recent childbirth and during menstruation. Although Muslims are not required to fast when they are ill, most devout Muslims will not take any medication orally or nasally between dawn and sunset. Some may even object to suppositories and injections. Fasting should be taken into account when prescribing medication.

Schools need to pay extra attention to the young who are fasting. Especially in the afternoons, children may need to be excused from games and sport and other energy-expending activities.

Eid-al-fitr marks the end of the month of fasting. It is celebrated joyously by wearing new clothes, praying and being with extended family and friends to exchange goodwill. *Eid-al-Adha* symbolises the submission and commitment of each Muslim to the will of God (Allah). It is the feast of animal sacrifice (a sheep, goat, cow or camel). There are no fixed dates for these festivals, as they are based on a lunar calendar.

Friday is a holy day. Most men will go to the Mosque for prayers; women pray at home.

Muslims believe in four prophets: Abraham (Ibrihim/Ibraheem), Moses (Musa/Moosa), Jesus (Isa/Eesa) and Mohammed, who was born 600 years after Jesus and was the last of God's prophets.

The Qu'ran should be kept wrapped up in a cloth cover and should only be unwrapped by a follower of the faith. Muslims will wish to wash their hands and feet before taking the Qu'ran in their hands. Muslim women cannot pray, fast or touch the Qu'ran during menstruation. The position of men and women in the holy Qu'ran is defined as equal in marriage, education, social, economic and political aspects of life.

Muslims do not eat pork and prefer Halal or Kosher meat (meat that has been prepared according to religious custom). Muslim women should wear clothes that cover them from head to ankles, but some are adopting Western styles.

Buddhism

Buddhism started in north-east India and spread to central and south-east Asia (Japan, China), Tibet and more recently the West. It was founded by Siddhartha Gautama, also known as Shakyamuni, more popularly known as the Buddha. The word *buddha* means 'the enlightened one' and is not a proper name – it describes a state of life. Buddhist faith centres on:

- *Buddha*, who is revered not as a God but as an example of a way of life
- *Dharma*: the teachings. Buddhists believe in reincarnation and so accept responsibility for the ways in which they exercise their freedom in life, since the consequences of their actions may be seen in subsequent lives. It is therefore important that the individual behaves properly and this includes not killing. Buddhist traditions condemn abortion and active euthanasia
- The *Sangha*, the religious community.

As there is no 'God', there is no actual worship, but the act of *puja* ('to respect') is the Buddhist way of acknowledging an ideal.

Serious interest in Buddhism in the UK began in the middle of the 19th century and today there are an estimated 130 000 Buddhists in Britain out of an estimated world Buddhist population of 327 000 000. Many have come to the UK as refugees from Tibet and Vietnam, but most are native converts. There are three main traditions of Buddhism:

- *Theravada*, 'the way of elders', is the predominant form of Buddhism in Sri Lanka, Burma and Thailand
- *Mahayan*, 'the great way', is the most widespread of the Buddhist schools, in Nepal, China, Korea and Japan
- *Hanayana*, 'the lesser vehicle'; many different sects of Buddhism emerge from these traditions.

Many Buddhists are vegetarians and Buddhism emphasises the avoidance of intentional killing.

All three schools refer to the same scripture, the Tipitaka, and various *sutras* (i.e. narratives and texts) may be followed. Private meditation is undertaken daily with a chant or mantra. Main religious festivals are celebrated by different sects on different days. Most sects celebrate the new year. The calendar is lunar, so the festival dates vary from year to year. There is no one specific holy day. Languages used are those of the country of origin, and English.

RELIGIOUS OBSERVANCE

The first part of this section described the different types of religion practised within the same racial group. It is also assumed that as south Asians become more settled in Britain and 'integrated' with the British way of life, the significance of their religion in their lives may decrease. Literature on different religions practised often states the standard and established norm of the relevant religions. However, variations within the religious practices may occur, e.g. some Hindus eat meat and others do not, some Sikh men do not have long hair and wear a turban, and some Muslim women wear a burkha while others do not, and yet these people may be very devout and would perceive themselves as distinguished by belonging to a particularly religious group. Especially when collecting data, these qualitative differences should be highlighted and assumptions should not be made from standard, stereotypical understanding of a religious group. As William (1995) states, religion is 'made up of among other things a moral vision, a sense of individual and group identity, and a practice designed to symbolise and reaffirm all of these elements'. In fact the retention of religious identity can be very strong. William found in his study of religious identity retention into middle age in Clydeside 35-year olds and in Glasgow south Asians aged 30–40 that religious identity was 'actually OK, virtually complete in the case of Sikhs, Muslims and Hindus'. The qualitative variation in the extent to which the religion is practical must be identified by professionals, so that appropriate advice regarding, for example, diet can be given.

PERCEPTION OF HEALTH FROM DIFFERENT RELIGIOUS PERSPECTIVES

South Asian religions see health as totally interlinked to their religious practices and beliefs, with emphasis on 'holistic health', i.e. interaction between the spiritual, mental, physical and external (environmental) dimensions. Therefore, during interviews and health assessment an ethnocentric stance that sees health and disease being rooted in 'mind' and 'body' will be in conflict with Asian religious beliefs. It is now well accepted that some south Asians 'somatize' their symptoms when experiencing health problems. Similarly, terms indicating the inevitability of their illness, i.e. *karma*, might be used by Hindu and Sikh clients. Underlying this concept is the law of *karma*, which means that the type of action that an individual performs will result in the person experiencing the consequences of their actions. Hence in health terms a disease is experienced as a result of the individual's actions in a past or the present life. This process of *karma* is also seen as purifying the soul before it can merge with the Supreme God. Within the same belief structure is the concept of life as a continuous cycle of birth and death. When patients therefore 'refuse care', e.g. when suffering from cancer, this may raise professional, moral and ethical dilemmas as to whether healthcare should be maintained or not, especially if the patient feels it is his/her *karma* to experience the disease.

Religion, on the other hand, is not just seen as an experience unique to an individual: positive health experience can also be found in group activities. Gogna's unpublished research on Punjabi Sikh women (1991) revealed that for 95% of this group participation in congregational singing called *satsang* contributed to their physical, social and spiritual well-being. Such types of cultural/religious variation need to be understood when planning group work in communities. Professionals using their own models for community health promotion programmes where spirituality is not in congruence with a biomedical model of, for instance, health education, may ignore 'spiritual approaches'. This type of ignorance is typified by a nurse academic, who was informed of spiritual approaches and *satsang* and the sense of well-being experienced by Sikh women. Her explanation was that singing led to a greater intake of oxygen in the body, which gave the sense of well-being, rather than the *satsang*.

DIET

Diet in south Asian society is viewed from many aspects, including culture, religion and family eating practices. This section will also examine diet and health.

Cultural diet

In terms of religious beliefs, Muslims are given strict instructions on diet by the Qu'ran. Only animals with cloven feet can be eaten, and then only those that have been slaughtered in a particular way to make it 'Halal'. The dietary habits of Hindus are largely dependent on caste and region of origin. However, in general, beef is not eaten, and often no meat or fish is consumed and they are in effect vegetarians. Ghee (clarified butter) is used widely and is highly prized by Hindus and Sikhs. It is considered a sign of wealth and is used in religious ceremonies, about which Sikhs are given guidelines in Guru Granth Sahib Ji.

In terms of region of family origin, those originating from Pakistan and north-west India – Punjabis – will tend to use wheat as their staple food and have a chapatti-based diet. Ghee is also widely used in cooking by Punjabis. Gujaratis, from the area around Bombay, who traditionally used millet as a staple for chapattis, tend to use wheat instead in the UK. The staple food of the Bangladeshi community is rice, and they tend to use relatively large amounts of fish in their diet. For cooking purposes they tend to use oil rather than ghee. South Asian diets in general consist of rice, fish and vegetables (Sheikh & Thomas 1994).

Hindus believe that all living things are sacred and therefore many Hindus are vegetarians and do not eat meat, fish, eggs and anything made with them. The cow is particularly sacred and therefore beef and its products are strictly forbidden. Some Hindus will not touch pork, as pigs are scavenging animals in India. Strict vegetarians do not eat eggs, as they are a potential source of life, or cheese if it is made with animal rennet. Some may avoid onions and garlic as they are believed to be stimulants like tea and coffee. Alcohol is officially frowned upon.

As there is a lot of variation when following dietary restrictions, the most devout are likely to be careful about what they eat. It is also important to remember that strict vegetarians will be unhappy about eating vegetarian food if it is served from the plate or with the same utensils as meat. As diet has a strong religious aspect, it is important to ascertain such matters when dealing with Hindus so as not to give offence. Apart from practices based on religious belief, some Hindus may have strongly held traditional ideas about taking certain foods at particular times, e.g. during and after pregnancy. The beliefs vary and need to be discussed with the individual. Some women may become vegetarian during

Table 16.1 Hot foods and cold foods

Hot foods	Cold foods
Most pulses	Cereal
Garlic	Rice
Ginger	Wheat
Eggs	Fruit
Nuts	Potatoes
Lamb	White sugar
Honey	Chick peas
Chilli	Mung beans
Onions	Green leaf vegetables
Dates	Milk/milk products
Aubergines	Salad
Tea/coffee	

pregnancy and observe the customs of 'hot' and 'cold' foods. This relates to the perceived priorities and strengths of the foods and has nothing to do with temperature or spicy qualities (Table 16.1).

Dietary discipline

Foods are broken into six types: sweet, sour, salty, pungent, bitter and astringent. Ayurvedic medicine, an Indian healing tradition that treats the patient and not the disease, is a blend of yoga, meditation, herbal medicine and dietary advice. Medicinal remedies are designed to heal patients. These are made from natural substances such as herbs, vegetables and minerals. Each remedy is custom-blended to create the right balance of ingredients for the individual. A patient is also prescribed different types of food according to his or her individual needs. Food is also prepared and consumed in accordance with external factors, such as the time of year, time of day and weather conditions. It is also important that food is fully savoured, well chewed and swallowed in a relaxed, contented state of mind.

Diet and disease

Rickets, a childhood disease causing softening and deformation of the bones due to a deficiency of vitamin D and calcium, was reported in the south Asian community in the 1960s. In the following period to the mid-1980s, evidence indicated that the incidence was in decline and it was at a low level in 1985. Although there have been many studies into the causes of rickets among Asians, and much is now known, further work is needed. A number of risk factors appear to be related to susceptibility to rickets; the most important is diet. The risk is high in the UK for this reason.

Vitamin D deficiency and osteomalacia (a bone disorder in adults resulting from vitamin D and calcium deficiency) first aroused concern in the early 1960s following a report in Glasgow. Subsequent studies have estimated its prevalence. It ranges from 3.5% to 38%. A steady, small number of cases of osteomalacia in Asian women continues to be reported.

Evidence associated these conditions with diets rich in phytate (a substance found in whole grain cereals that binds with minerals so that they cannot be absorbed) and fibre, with little or no food of animal origin. Such a diet is likely to increase the need for calcium and vitamin D. Foods of animal origin are considered to be protective. Other risk factors are a low exposure to sunlight, poor housing and living conditions, customs relating to clothing and seclusion and having pigmented skin.

Comparison of the vitamin D status of a sample of the healthy Asian population with a control group indicated that 22% of Asians had low serum vitamin D levels. There was no relationship with vegetarian diet or length of residence in the UK, suggesting that low vitamin D levels are found in all Asians, irrespective of geographical origin or socioeconomic group (COMA 1980).

Between 1979 and 1983 in England and Wales, mortality from coronary heart disease (CHD) among Asian men and women was higher than the national average. Rates of CHD are also high among Asian communities in other parts of the world (Coronary Prevention Group 1986).

Analysis of conventional risk factors suggests that, while hypertension, diet, serum cholesterol and stress are important, they do not completely explain the high incidence of CHD; however, a high rate of non-insulin-dependent diabetes makes a significant contribution (Marmot & McKeigue 1988, Simmons et al 1989). The role of stress remains largely unexplored as yet, although there is a belief that endurable stress is caused by extra pressures from family commitments and the responsibilities of extended family, which has an effect on an individual's health.

Patterns of change in diet

Some Asian communities have maintained their traditions more strongly than others. At the more nontraditional end of the spectrum are those who came from East Africa. Punjabi Sikhs and Gujarati Hindus show more adherence to tradition, while Pakistanis and Bangladeshis are less likely to have maintained their traditions. Clearly, this is a broad generalisation and within each community there are individuals who follow traditional patterns more or less strictly.

This diversity is also seen in eating patterns. Those who are socially isolated from the majority white population are more likely to eat traditional foods. This group includes the old, people with poor language skills and women whose activities outside the home are restricted by cultural tradition. Among Hindus, more women than men maintain a vegetarian diet, while those following a mixed diet tend to be younger and to consume only small quantities of meat.

The person responsible for food shopping can also affect the types of food available within the household. Among Moslems, the task is often carried out by men, who are more inclined to purchase only what is familiar to them, e.g. imported vegetables from Asian-owned shops. In less traditional households, women are generally responsible for food purchases and make a more varied choice. However, frozen and canned foods are rarely consumed.

Some evidence suggests a loss of confidence in the nutritional value of a traditional diet as a result of negative attitudes in the wider community. Unfortunately, changes in food habits that do occur may in fact reduce the quality of the diet. For example, younger people appear to be increasing their consumption of fizzy drinks, confectionery and fast foods. The extent of this trend, however, has not been thoroughly investigated.

Infant feeding practices

It is difficult to make generalisations about breast- and bottle-feeding or to identify trends. Pakistani women tend to breast-feed for longer periods. A variety of reasons for Bangladeshi women not wanting to breast-feed are:

- observation of the high levels of bottle-feeding in the host community
- the prestige value attached to bottle-feeding as a Western practice
- lack of privacy due to overcrowding; unsuitable housing conditions
- difficulties in communicating with health professionals
- a desire for an early return to work situations where there are no opportunities for breast-feeding.

Reports are frequently made of both early and late weaning and prolonged feeding of cow's milk. It is common for Asian women to change from infant formula to 'doorstep' milk at about 6 months of age. Late weaning seems to be more common among children born in the Indian subcontinent, or born to mothers who have only been in the UK for a short time. Children who are born in Britain are more likely to be weaned early. Investigation has revealed prolonged bottle-feeding of Asian children. Most were still using a bottle at the age of 2 years, and two-thirds of the milk feeds were sweetened.

Excessive and inappropriate use of commercially prepared baby foods has also aroused concern, since Moslem mothers will not introduce savoury weaning foods that contain non-Halal meat and vegetarian households avoid varieties containing meat altogether.

Although there are many customs and practices that spring from religious beliefs and so differ from one religious group to another, other practices are common to all communities. Infant care is one such practice. In Asia the tradition generally is for women to breast-feed their babies (particularly in rural areas). The mother will usually breast-feed on demand until the baby is 1 year old, and possibly until the age of 2. They may not breast-feed during the colostrum stage as they believe that colostrum is bad or dirty and may harm the baby. The baby is normally given sugared water until the colostrum stage is over.

Women new to Britain may have problems with bottle-feeding if it is unfamiliar to them. Procedures for mixing milk powder and sterilising equipment must be fully understood. As with breast-feeding, weaning customs will be different, depending on the tradition of that particular area the mother has come from, but in general Asian families wean their babies much later than their counterparts. As there is no traditional diet between milk and adult food, it is customary to wean when baby is able to tolerate more adult foods. Weaning is done suddenly, often by putting some unpleasant-tasting substance on the nipple. The food then given to the infant is the same as that of the rest of the family, except that fewer spices are used.

Many mothers do not use proprietary baby foods in case the ingredients break religious dietary rules. For example, many proprietary baby foods are unsuitable for Muslims and vegetarians. Therefore it is generally more useful to find out what is eaten by the adult members of the family and to base nutritional advice on this. There is a tendency to rely heavily on sweet, dessert-type baby foods, often low in protein and iron. However, when giving advice it must be remembered that, in an extended Asian family, a young mother does not have sole responsibility for decisions about her child's diet. Older female relatives often play a major role and should be included in any consultations.

HEALTH PROMOTION

Most current health promotion activities tend to be based on epidemiological investigation of medical problems, e.g. heart disease. This type of approach gives an 'externalised' view of the disease in which the person feels they have no say and the approach has been conceptualised from outside. More participatory and qualitative approaches take into account the needs of clients/communities, their perception of disease and contributory social factors. Externalising the

problem alienates the client from it, so qualitative information on clients' lifestyle becomes very important if the health promotion messages are going to be effective.

The participatory approach also means empowerment of the client and community. When literature presented is 'inappropriate', showing lack of cultural understanding, or is simply unavailable, clients cannot be expected to make independent informed choices. For example, the Royal Society for the Prevention of Accidents (ROSPA 1993) found in their study of safety and minority ethnic communities that health messages regarding safety would only be effective if they were created in 'Asian, Chinese or Vietnamese languages as well as in English', and translations should include consultations with members of the community at whom the information was aimed.

The study further states that the material presented should not be 'academic' in style and that its presentation should have relevance to the target group. The community in the study also found that they were more concerned about lack of information than about the quality of the material itself.

How health messages are promoted also needs to be considered. Most health promotion material tends to be in written form (bear in mind that some Asians are not literate in their own language); more innovative methods of transmitting health messages have not been explored, e.g. in a popular soap opera, where health messages could become a theme, or on Asian radio channels, which are fast becoming popular with all generations of Asians. There is no reason why radio cannot be used as a mode of transmission, e.g. chat shows discussing health issues. That health messages are imparted in relevant languages is important and also that those messages are clear and simple and not too theoretical.

The relevance of material and how it is presented has also been supported by Johnson (1996), who states that material used should be for 'specific audiences in appropriate languages (not translated directly), and presented in bilingual formats. Their illustration needs to match the target group culture'.

How organisations have dealt with health issues and health promotion also causes concern. There appears to be a lack of commitment: the Department of Health (1996d) reported that even managers from areas with large ethnic minorities did not have 'specific organisational focus, such as explicit value statement, policy, priority or staff appointments, on minority ethnic issues'. It was expected that existing resources would meet the needs of ethnic minorities, but this did not take into account that some of the services were 'inappropriate, underused or inaccessible', and that the service provision needed to be assessed. In the same study, some managers argued that ethnic minority health policy and service developments were not formulated because of 'paucity of information' about local minority populations. This marginalising of ethnic minority health issues was also evident when some managers argued that specific ethnic needs policies had not been developed because dealing with organisational change took priority over other needs. This argument questions whether ethnic minority health policy is part of organisational strategy in the first place. As to dealing with 'organisational changes', the changes themselves within the NHS have been constant and not a new phenomenon, which does not justify the argument.

Even where organisations have been supportive in initiating specific ethnic minority projects, e.g. the Stop Rickets campaign, once the focus of the project is dealt with and the problems are solved it does not become part of the organisation. According to Silvera & Kapasi (1996), even when the project remit has been widened and recommendations are made that could affect the whole organisation, they are not supported.

One of the key issues about health promotion and ethnic minorities is that there is a lack of a strategic approach to the whole issue, which appears to be fragmented. Given the current climate in the NHS and scarce resources, the targets of health promotion need to be clearly defined and evidence-based, so that the necessary resources can be allocated. Managers might argue about pressure to meet other organisational agendas, but there is also apathy and

the belief that ethnic minorities will eventually integrate into mainstream host society, and that this justifies them not having to implement any health policies especially for them. On the other hand, collecting data or formulating strategies that would highlight the needs of south Asians is deliberately avoided – lack of this information justifies not implementing any health provisions for ethnic minorities. Organisations must therefore have clear, well-formulated health promotion strategies that are evidence-based and have achievable targets.

Collaboration with target groups and communities is essential so that strategies can be negotiated. This middle approach is important and maintains a power balance between the service providers and users. Often familiar, vociferous members of the community are used to represent a community/target group who might not be familiar with the health issues at hand. Service providers here have been poor at using consultation strategies; an easy way out has been what Chandra (1995) describes as the 'take me to your leader' syndrome. Somehow, these leaders are vested with tremendous power and knowledge on every issue. This might be true in certain instances, such as religious matters, but health issues, for example, require a far broader representation. It is interesting to note that very few women from ethnic groups are asked to be representatives. On the surface, this tokenistic approach fulfils the political agenda of consulting ethnic minorities, but the reality is that the quality of consultation remains superficial, fragmented, poorly informed and defeats the whole object of consultation. Therefore, suggesting representatives who have a sound knowledge base on health issues is important. Community groups also need to indicate who they want as their representatives and since south Asians are such a heterogeneous group, different sections of the community might require different representatives. Monitoring how strategies are implemented, the process of consultation, needs assessment and evaluation of outcomes should be carried out so that the effectiveness of the whole process can be assessed.

'Outreach' programmes run in Sparkbrook

aim to provide young women with a culturally sensitive health visiting service offering the information they need to care appropriately for their children and themselves. This is targeted at first-time mothers, who have often come to Britain for arranged marriages with little knowledge of English or of the culture of their adopted country. These young mothers have little awareness of the services available or how to access them and may also feel inhibited from seeking help.

Women are visited at home before giving birth to be informed about the project. They are also invited to a monthly antenatal support group at a local health clinic. Women have the opportunity to discuss topics with professionals. The availability of link workers offers encouragement for women to use the information to decide for themselves how to bring up their children. After birth they are visited each week to establish feeding patterns, and then monthly until baby's first birthday.

The programme encourages mothers to breast-feed and then to wean their babies on to 'family' food rather than commercial baby foods, to help them establish healthier eating habits.

One woman explained how she was able to compare her own 'new' education on child-rearing with the childcare practices within her extended family. She gave her child 'proper meals' rather than snacks or bottle feeds and had experienced no problems with establishing 'good' feeding habits and sleeping routines, whereas her relatives automatically responded to their baby's cry with a bottle and the eldest child, who was fussy about foods, was taking longer to be weaned on to family foods. Women also came to the clinic for other reasons, such as 'just to talk to someone', 'to exchange ideas', 'to get information' and 'to learn English'. Women feel it is a culturally safe place to go to and husbands are happy to accompany them. Many have become recruits for new community parents projects, enabling them to help other women and also to pursue their own learning and development. This all goes towards initiatives in accordance with the government's family policy and the setting up of 'Sure Start' centres (Department for Education and Employment 1999).

Strategies

Health education departments have recognised the need to improve communications and ensure access for those who are not comfortable with the English language. Their communications strategies of interpretation and translation have been used by many health-related agencies. It is important to understand the differences between the two processes.

The Health Education Authority's document *Many Voices, One Message* (Health Education Authority 1997b) recognises a 'binocular' approach. Most research and evaluation shows that people generally prefer bilingual (target language and English) presentation. This may be because most people are bilingual, although one language may dominate over the other. Reading messages bilingually, therefore, gives a 'binocular' focus. This approach checks the nuances of meaning in both languages and readers are able to mediate when reading it aloud or during discussion with target language speakers. The readers can be satisfied about the message and that, by the language used, culture and traditions are respected and taken into account by sensitive providers. A bilingual approach also allows monolingual people to be sure of the information that is being provided.

The translation process should take account of the following points:

- *Clarity*: the original version of the text needs to be in clear and plain language
- *Mistranslation*: not all words can be translated
- *Readability*: it is useful to involve someone who is familiar with language and can read the translation aloud to check naturalness and appropriate use of language, as too much emphasis on linguistic accuracy and keeping to the original text can lead to an unreadable translation
- *Consultation* will ensure that the basic message is not unduly influenced and that the interests of the target group remain the guiding principle.

Most agencies and groups of people are adopting a 'free translation' approach. Here the original text is used more as a trigger than as something that must be followed rigidly. This approach requires collaboration with the translator, who may or may not be familiar with the technical aspects of the topic. The main advantage is that the final product is more 'natural' and authentic. The text is comprehensible and is more likely to be accepted and read widely, as it makes sense. For example, a project to produce an alcohol leaflet for the south Asian community was led by a bilingual health promotion officer with local knowledge and contact with target communities (Health Education Authority 1997b).

THE FAMILY

Asian families are often seen to be supportive, nurturing and self-sufficient. While this is a positive impression about such families, the reality is that conflict can also be present. This issue is highlighted because professionals and policy makers alike often seize quickly on the idea that where extended families exist no support input is required from professionals. Government policy recognises healthcare delivery as coming from central policy, local policy and the individual. Therefore, professionals working in partnership with patients/clients to plan, assess and deliver care need to be aware of possible tensions within extended families and should carefully assess relationships between family members. The term 'extended family' and its perceived associated support systems could be a misnomer in itself.

Overall, the three main ethnic groups share very similar extended family kinship within the home. However, in Muslim families there is a greater degree of biological kinship: married couples may well be cousins. This usually involves a deeper and extended responsibility to the family for both women and men. So, for example, if a woman wants to leave her husband the implications involving her own family, who are also related to him, must be carefully considered. In all three groups family 'honour' is paramount and professionals who work with these families need to be aware of this. In stress situations, if professionals are not aware of how to deal with situations, hasty decisions might

be made, e.g. to remove a child or woman to a safe haven instead of using other skills in trying to solve family problems. Obviously, in life-threatening situations and child protection issues, clients will have to be removed to a place of safety. While this course of action might protect the professional, the long-term damage caused by the break-up or separation of the family can be immense. What is lacking, of course, is knowledge about cross-cultural ways of working with families that might involve, for example, negotiating skills specific to certain cultural situations. It is not a surprise, however, that Asian professionals who themselves lack such skills and work using Western approaches are perceived to be 'Westernised' and 'colluding with the white establishment'.

Another source of conflict that might occur in such families is that, because they are seen as a great source of 'support' and 'cohesiveness', they are often expected to take on the caring roles. Gogna (1991) showed that elderly women always live with their sons (this is common to all three ethnic groups). It is a cultural norm that women do not live with their daughters, as daughters leave their natal homes and become part of their husband's home. On the other hand, their daughters-in-law have left their own natal homes and become daughters-in-law to the elderly women. The cultural expectation is that daughters should not have the same degree of affection or ties to their natal homes, so daughters must subdue their feelings and emotions, as they are not supposed to display the same degree of care towards their own mother. This also affects the way in which daughters are viewed by these cultures; the term used in Punjabi is *paraya dhan*. English cannot really conceptualise this term, but the nearest translation is 'daughters are not yours to keep, daughters are being kept for someone else' and 'they are on short loan to you'. It might be argued that this might cause psychological and emotional distancing from daughters but in reality the bonds can be very strong and a lot of families compensate for their expected future 'loss' of their daughter through marriage by giving her a lot of love and nurturing.

The reality is that, although daughters might

be married and living considerable distances away from their mothers, their psychological and emotional ties to them are usually very strong. The study also found that elderly women expected their daughters to be established in their husband's household, because any stress on the daughter's marriage would also cause stress to the mother. Therefore the daughter's help was supplementary to other family support and depended on how 'permissive' her husband and his family were. This raises some key questions regarding support services within this group of people. Assumptions are often made that daughters will provide care. Service managers need to be aware that, even when daughters are living near, their support of their own elderly parents or extended family is not automatic and cultural issues that influence this must be understood. The quality of care given within these families should also be assessed carefully. Gogna (1991) found that, although there was a lot of emotional, psychological and physical support given by family members, the daughter-in-law's support was not 'permissive', but given to establish her own status and gain acceptance within the family. This is supported by Gilligan (1982), who points out that obligations are 'situationally and contextually based'. Finch (1989) also supports the argument that, rather than being purely supportive, daughters-in-law are helping their spouses to meet their obligations. Daughters-in-law often feel a sense of emotional and psychological distance from their extended families, especially where they feel they are 'manipulated' or 'coerced' into giving care. On the surface it might appear the whole family are carers and provide supportive roles; the reality is that one family member, usually the daughter-in-law, bears the major responsibility. If these cultural issues are not understood, no support is given to the carers within the family, who silently carry the burden of stress until some breakdown occurs. Because of this 'veneer of support', professionals often do not feel they even have to assess by whom and how the support is given. The fact is that, superficially, it meets the 'support criterion'; in reality the quality of care is never assessed. Independent interpreters are not used very often

and English-speaking family members become the substitute interpreters. Often they do not highlight the stress within the family because of the respect/*izzat* of the family.

An extended family system is central to all Eastern cultures. Its values remain central to most Asians in Britain. Traditions remain strong and are influenced by certain outlooks, beliefs and influences in the changing culture. Because of housing and mobility considerations, families may live in split households, but the bonds and mutual obligations between the family members remain strong. The group of people that is described by Western culture as 'the extended family' is merely the normal family for an Eastern culture.

In traditional households, gender roles are still often observed, with defined areas of responsibility. For example, men are the breadwinners and involved in public responsibilities and women's responsibilities lie in the day-to-day care of family members, observing religious and moral obligations when having children and staying in the background. Every member of the family has a defined status; often a hierarchical system operates, which may well be an authoritarian one, where respect is demanded rather than earned, and in many cases this aspect has a considerable influence on behaviour and a family's decision-making processes.

Money coming into a household could be considered as belonging to the whole family. Strong obligations are often felt by senior members of the family to support others financially, and money is lent or given to whoever needs it. Often families and households who are in need may be supported by other more distant members. When faced by the strong system of mutual responsibilities and obligations, each member is likely to consider him/herself as part of the family rather than as an individual.

Important decisions like marriage need to be considered carefully, as in an Eastern culture a girl will be entering into a very different partnership from a girl in a Western culture. It is vital that the bride should be the kind of person who will fit into a large, close-knit household and be happy there for the rest of her life. Her affections, loyalty and obligations to other members are as important as those to her partner. Although the marital relationship is important and needs to be considered, the husband's family is taking on a new permanent member and the choice of that new member must therefore be a family decision. This can often cause major rifts and conflicts within the family unit.

From the girl's point of view, her natal family is committing her for the rest of her life to the care and protection of a new family, upon whom she will depend for all her emotional, physical and perhaps her financial needs. After the marriage the two families will be firmly linked and will have certain mutual responsibilities.

Some elders may feel that such an important decision as marriage is a matter that cannot be trusted to an inexperienced couple, who may be easily swayed by chargeable emotions and irrational feelings. The strong belief is that if the two families choose wisely they will unite a young couple who will develop a close and loving relationship, and hence their partnership will enrich the family.

However, the traditional pattern of arranged marriage is changing. Couples are marrying at a later age; there is a greater potential for choice; and there is also an opportunity to 'cry off' before a commitment is made, with younger people having more opportunities to meet prior to any formal agreement and to choose their own partners. Asian parents still believe that arranged or assisted introductory marriages are the only sensible way for couples. It appears that Muslim families remain conservative about the traditional system compared to other groups.

Although 'love marriages' are becoming more common, they are regarded by many with fear and suspicion. There are more repercussions in an extended family, and the girl may be landed with the blame, since traditionally it is her duty to adapt and fit in.

In Hindu and Sikh communities, marriage is regarded as an indissoluble sacrament. Divorce is permitted by law, but it is rare. Under Islamic law, marriage is a contract, not a sacrament, and divorce is more frequent. Islamic law makes provision for the support of a divorced wife;

at marriage the bridegroom's family provides a sum of money to the bride which will be given to her if the marriage breaks up.

The stigma of divorce can be felt acutely by women who have marital problems and a sense of isolation, rejection and depression can be seen. In some households, the husband may be supporting his ex-wife and their children, as well as his new wife. This is often an alien concept for those providing care, e.g. in relation to social security rules or housing debts. Where the man has obtained a blessing from his ex-wife, the system seems to work satisfactorily for all.

There is little or no stigma if a widow remarries. Often, young widows may be married to younger brothers-in-law (their dead husband's brother). In Hindu and Sikh cultures, widows often withdraw from community life. They may decide to wear white, have no jewellery or make up and perform religious duties, thus earning them respect from the family and community. There are no social burdens for Muslim widows, as long as they have observed the mourning period of 3–4 months. They will then resume their place in the community and be encouraged to remarry. Remarriage is not always a solution but for a man it can be considered inevitable, as who is going to look after him? He is seen as obviously needing somebody to cook, clean and keep him company.

In Britain, Asian attitudes are changing. Girls have more opportunities in the field of education and to go out to work, and hence are gaining more independence than their mothers and grandmothers. They are taking a leading role in making decisions about their choice of partner, where to live and how much contact is maintained with extended families. Social attitudes are also changing because of changes in the law regarding inheritance, maintenance and supposedly the change in the dowry system.

South Asian marriages are lavish and ultra expensive affairs in Britain. Parents often run up large debts if they have more than one daughter. Pressures are felt from within the society to conform and keep up standards. If and when the marriage fails and the girl returns to her parents' house, the family has to face more stresses and difficulties in finding a new partner, as the girl's name has become tainted with dishonour. Making arrangements and settlements for children's future can become extremely difficult.

Children

There is an unspoken rule (great expectation) that a married couple will eventually have many children. There is no choice in the matter. Children are essential and are included in all festivities. Most children will be pampered, especially boys, to the extent that they are carried about and everything is done for them. Around the age of 5, when they enter school, discipline becomes increasingly important; in fact some Asian parents believe that loving children means disciplining them and may use corporal punishment. Children then learn what they can and cannot do. This contrasts greatly with Western families, where the emphasis is on self-discipline.

The problems associated with adolescence in Western society are thought not to exist in traditional Eastern cultures. Young people are expected to move from childhood to adulthood. This may have been the case when marriage took place in the teenage years. Nowadays, young people are influenced by education and are becoming independent from some of the constraints and have thus found a voice and are looking for a way out. In many cases, those who have found the courage to speak up face isolation from the family and community.

Asian parents in Britain judge Western-style 'love marriages' and sexual permissiveness with great suspicion. Their impressions of such values are often picked up from the media and their suspicions are confirmed by reports of rates of divorce, illegitimacy and the sexual freedom of the young. As parents may fear for their children's happiness and their own status within the community, they may try to arrange a marriage contract before the young people are ready. The thinking behind this arrangement is that at least the couple knows there is a suitable partner with whom they can start a relationship from afar. Asian parents may demand higher standards of behaviour and decorum from their children.

There is a fear that if a couple has entered into a 'love marriage' without considering other factors affecting the extended family members, there will be a break up and no chance for the elders to be cared for at a later stage. Parents may feel their children are in moral danger if they are allowed to go through a process of living together in temporary relationships.

Conflicts between different cultures are becoming serious and pose difficulties on both sides – for parents because they wish their competent and independent children to find a suitable partner within the confines of caste and society system; for children because they are anxious to find somebody who is acceptable to their parents. If there is no compromise, do they accept the partner their parents have chosen or do they refuse and risk cutting themselves off from their family and community? Further problems occur if the young person becomes 'too choosy'. Suspicions are raised. Is s/he not agreeing because s/he has somebody else in mind? Can s/he not communicate this information to the parent?

Roles

Although an ideology of shared parenting belies the continuing separation of the mother's and father's domestic roles within the family, an increasing number of fathers have become more involved in the everyday activities of housework and particularly in childcare. This has also been influenced by a changing labour market, including increasing employment of women (mainly part time), male unemployment and a shift in working patterns to working at home. If the father is not working a traditional day, for reasons of shift work, unemployment, flexible working hours or self-employment, this can also lead to changes in family roles. A role reversal in one family, for example, has led to more and closer communication between father and children.

In a two-parent family, the division of concern and responsibility for issues such as health still tend to fall in a traditional way. But while male unemployment can have a positive spin-off with regard to involvement with children, it may also have negative health consequences by suppressing men's self-esteem and self-image and ultimately affect their physical health. This is related to the threat to male identity from changes in traditional gender relations and male roles.

Lack of understanding of women's position in family roles can also cause conflict with Western approaches; for example, white and Asian professionals and neofeminists propose 'assertiveness training' for the women who seek their help. Assertiveness might work in situations outside the family context but, because of cultural and family obligations, using 'assertiveness' within the family would make the existing situation worse. What these women need are family negotiating skills and knowledge about how to get professional help to deal with volatile and aggressive situations. Many Asian women who have moved into powerful professional jobs and would have the choice of moving out of the marital home give the external impression of being successful, Westernised and independent, in order to maintain their 'personhood' they stay with their family despite any tension that might be experienced within it.

Traditional Asian women's roles in society and the ideologies that govern their roles are not understood by professionals. South Asian women are often perceived as 'the silent figures in the background', 'suppressed' or 'dominated' by men. Contrary to this belief, women in Hinduism, according to Nanda (1986) are seen as more sexually voracious than men. As the purpose of birth is for everyone to attain a higher spiritual level by performing spiritual duties, it is perceived that women, with their superior sexual powers, can distract men from performing their spiritual duties. Hence, to prevent this, women must be 'controlled' by men. This control forms the basis of how women should behave, so as not to overpower or excite male sexuality. This is seen, for example, as women's subjugation within the society and the suppressive social roles created for them. Male and female sexuality is further divided in humoral terms, i.e. women are categorised as being 'hot' and 'erotic' and men being 'cold', 'more intense' and 'ascetic'.

Although according to humoral principles 'hot' and 'cold' must interact to maintain a balance – which, in human relationships would mean equal relationships between men and women – the political and social strictures keep women in their 'inferior' roles, maintaining inequality in male and female relationships. Nanda further states the concept of 'personhood' within these relationships. The personal identity of a person (male or female) depends on whether s/he is accepted by his/her kinship and society at large, according to how the person participates and interacts within caste and kinship. The person's dependency, control by others and relationships within the caste define their personal identity and identity within society. Therefore, acceptance and respect within one's own caste is important to have any meaningful position in society as a whole. The notion of personal identity transcends into the concept of 'personhood'. Personhood, according to Nanda, means the totality of being 'human', having a strong personal identity and achieving the final fulfilment of 'personhood' where certain criteria must be met. One of the most important criteria that must be met is marriage.

Marriage is seen as an important rite whereby men and women fulfil their family and cultural obligations, where sexual fertility for both sexes is proved and higher status is given to women who produce sons. This questions the position of single women, e.g. those who are widowed. A woman's position and power are maintained only while her husband is alive. Upon his death her position in society becomes weaker, unless she has sons who replace their father's power; if they are seen to be vulnerable she remains weak. Nanda further explains that men and women who die without getting married, men who are impotent and women who do not have children are not considered to have achieved full personhood. This type of personal identity, so closely linked to gender identity and its social acceptance within the larger social group, is clearly defined. Those individuals who cannot reproduce or do not wish to get married can 'adopt' a more 'meaningful role' by taking on the role of an ascetic or 'renouncer'. In accepting the ascetic role the notion of incomplete personhood could be transformed into a transcendent one. This attitude questions the position of single men and women, who may be homosexuals or lesbians and do not conform to these categories; it is assumed that they do not reach their full personhood.

HOMOSEXUALITY

An issue that has been developing within these ethnic groups is this question of homosexuality. Very little British literature is available on homosexuality within south Asians. Figures for suicide or parasuicide rates resulting from being forced into heterosexual relationships through marriage or from coming to terms with their own sexuality have not been found. Given the social construct of *izzat*/respect of families, where one partner is homosexual the reason for the break-up of the marriage is usually camouflaged as 'they did not get on'. Professionals need to recognise that, where their input regarding family support is required, if homosexuality is present it will require family counselling and support systems for the homosexual, to contact organisations who can help them meet their own needs. The cultural context of homosexuality has been well described by Shivananda Khan (1995): 'heterosexuality is clearly defined as being associated with procreativity and is seen as the norm'. In comparison, homosexuals in India do not have a direct equivalent in Indian community languages but some set behaviours do exist. In Britain it appears that the issue is not the 'difficulties' about what constitutes homosexuality but Asian society's denial that it exists. The greater social acceptance and openness of homosexuality by the host society has helped to support Asian homosexuals, who are slowly beginning to become open about their sexuality where it is felt to be 'safe'. Khan (1995) also explains that what matters with these ethnic groups is that 'gender roles' are strictly defined: the status of an adult male and man is given to a boy upon his marriage; a girl becomes a woman through marriage and children. Where gender status depends on marital status marriage becomes essential and the norm. Unmarried people do not have the same social status. As Khan

explains, it is only conferred on men who are married and women who produce children.

The three main ethnic groups also share similar cultural attitudes (Khan 1995), about arranged marriages, and family respect and honour (*izzat*). Extended families and the personal sense of self being subsumed into a family sense of self exert their influence on the sexual behaviour of the individual.

Given this type of cultural background, with its distinct parameters of sexual behaviour – i.e. the importance of heterosexual behaviour – any behaviour that does not conform to this definition will be denied. Khan (1995) points out that homosexual 'deviant' sexuality is 'invisibilised' and not discussed. This would also include lesbian relationships. To make such behaviour visible would be to bring shame and dishonour to the family. Regardless of the person's sexuality, the family's identity is paramount. The homosexual's individual needs, 'personal desire, choice and privacy are lost and the individual becomes subsumed within the family'. According to Khan (1995), honour is a 'possession not a quality' and 'shame arises from honour being lost'. These cultural aspects still influence ethnic minorities in Britain, where visible behaviours influence the status of the family in 'social acceptance, duty, obligations and honour'. One of the most important aspects of family honour and identity is to be 'visible' about the obligations of the family. Homosexuals in this country often enter into heterosexual marriage so as to be accepted by society; the family is saved from dishonour and shame as they have fulfilled their social and family obligations. These people suffer in silence and as Khan (1995) puts it: 'the person tries to assimilate into society through marriage and having children, yet expressing alternate sexual desires in purdah, in darkness, shame and in silence'.

If denial occurs in families, Asian professionals themselves often feel uncomfortable, are in denial themselves or, when being confronted with these issues, lack knowledge about different sexual behaviours and how to deal with them. It has been observed that professionals need training in how to deal with these issues themselves.

Public health issues such as human immuno-deficiency virus (HIV)/AIDS and sexually trans-mitted diseases (STD) also need to be considered in homosexuals and heterosexuals alike. The culture of shame and denial become paramount when considering appropriate services for homo-sexuals. Khan (1995) suggests in order to pre-serve 'community honour' and 'cultural necessity', significant numbers of men who have sex with men are married. Condom use is very low, so women partners of these men are at risk of contracting HIV/STD.

Underpresentation of infected south Asians is likely because HIV testing is not 'systematically identified with ethnicity' and is voluntary. HIV testing services are not easily accessed by south Asians for sociocultural reasons and because of the fear of revealing their sexuality to services that are not culture-specific (Khan 1995).

Planning services for identifying sexually transmitted diseases would normally be under-taken in discussion with community leaders. However, religious leaders often deny the exis-tence of such problems, as they stem from sexual behaviour that does not conform to the social, religious and moral code of the community. Their concerns are more about preserving the 'right' moral image of their communities than acknowl-edging that such problems exist. 'Community honour' and sanctity must be maintained. Their lack of knowledge of such issues means that service planners need to be cautious about who is consulted regarding service needs in this area.

Educating people about HIV and explaining about different sexualities may also cause prob-lems. Terms like 'heterosexual', 'homosexual' and 'bisexual', and the related lifestyles and iden-tities, have little significance to south Asians. Translation of this terminology for use in health promotion work could itself cause confusion and problems and some terminology has a different meaning in different communities which can sometimes be abusive and negative. This may increase stigmatisation for certain people and their psychosocial needs, therefore, cannot be denied (Khan 1995).

Service planners need to take into account the cultural diversity of individuals who suffer from HIV/STD or are homosexuals. The needs of white gay men cannot be generalised to gay men from the south Asian community because of cultural influences and demands, community conformity, racism and religious codes of prac-tice. Counselling services must therefore have counsellors who are well informed about the religious, cultural and language influences of the homosexuals and equipped with knowledge to counsel them.

Implicit within this discussion of sexuality and sexually transmitted diseases is the likelihood that the considerable stress experienced by people who are affected could lead to a breakdown in mental health. Mental health problems belong to all societies and the concerns of south Asians will now be discussed.

MENTAL HEALTH

The area of mental health has not been without its share of problems caused by perception and assessment of the public health needs of Asian people, which may be stereotyped. One of the major problems of delivery of care by profes-sionals and planners is the ethnocentricity of their approach to mental health. Unless the senior planners have communication skills to respond to the demands of culture and language, client groups are going to get substandard, inadequate care. Cruickshank & Beevers (1994) consider that 'psychiatry should seek to enrich its communi-cation skills by training in a general approach to culture'. This might be one of the approaches used, but it could also lead to a more generalist approach in which the cultural depth of the mental health experience of the patient/client can be lost. For example, in counselling work such close therapeutic relationships are formed that rapport and communication cannot occur if the service is not specific to the client's language and cultural background. Johnson (1996) also suggests that there can be no reliance on physical signs in mental health work: 'normal behaviour' and expression of mental state are very likely to be culturally determined. Unless there is clear communication between practitioner and client, assessment of mental health needs cannot be made. It is not therefore surprising that, with such communication difficulties, hospital appointment attendance is poor and noncompliance with medication occurs.

Mental health problems are also stereotyped or culture-specific: certain behaviours are seen as occurring because of 'their culture'. For example, Balarajan & Raleigh (1993) found that suicide in women aged between 20–49 born in the Indian subcontinent is 21% higher than that of the general female population. Merrill (1989) argues that this could be due to the 'cultural conflict' surrounding traditional or Western style marriage and an inability to cope with marital problems when they join their husbands in this country. This might be seen as a typical cultural justification of why the suicide rate is higher among south Asian women. In fairness, Merrill, rather than just blaming the culture, also argues that suicide in this case might be a Western 'culture-bound syndrome' that young south Asian women emulate to solve their 'intergenerational conflict'. So not all explanations are culture bound; other influences outside the culture are also likely to have an influence.

Using standardised methods and measures to evaluate mental problems is likely to cause problems in any cultural group. At least there is some awareness that such instruments based on white indigenous populations cannot be generalised to south Asian people. The major issue involves cultural interpretation, nuances and language; not much evidence of culture-specific measures has been observed in practice, although its importance is highlighted in the literature. Sensitive assessment tools for mental health might be one issue, but lack of culture-specific tools can also cause underreporting of mental illness. As Bal (1986) reported, there was 'poor recognition of psychiatric disorders among Asian patients by GPs, including Asian GPs'.

The emphasis on cultural knowledge and language is not just specific to patients, as stress is also reported by staff who work with Asian patients. Hingham (1988) found that various problems were reported by nursing staff that stemmed from awareness of lack of knowledge about cultural differences, as much as language,

without which, according to Murphy & Clark (1993), they could not form therapeutic relationships with their clients, and this caused them stress. Lack of cultural awareness by professionals could lead to a totally wrong assessment of a situation. For example, Thompson (1997), in her short study about detecting postnatal depression in Asian women, found that one woman refused to take medication for postnatal depression, fearing that it would reduce the chances of her daughter getting married if the community found out. The concept of mental illness and how it can socially affect the individual and community at large are poorly understood by professionals, particularly how mental illness affects individuals who have been living in Britain for a long time. Thompson (1997) suggests that professionals use a few key phrases, but in reality this is unhelpful and can be seen as patronising.

Another stereotype evident in mental health work is that most Asians somatise their symptoms. According to Rack (1982) south Asian patients present psychological distress in terms of physical symptoms and culture-bound syndromes such as 'sinking heart' among Punjabis (Krause 1989). This might imply that somatisation is a culture-specific phenomenon unique to Asian patents, yet Hamilton (1989) reports that indigenous British patients are also likely to somatise their symptoms of 'depression and anxiety'. However, third-generation Asians might not show similar patterns of somatisation. Culturalisation of behaviour, in mental illness and in illness in general, often produces culturalised pathologies that are marginalised as 'ethnic need', with the implication of being subjected to all the inequalities of service provision and access.

There is evidence that social and family support systems also contribute to the well-being of patients. Birchwood et al (1992) found considerable evidence suggesting that the relapse rate of mental illness was lower among Asians, which could be attributed to support given by extended families. Although this gives a positive impression of support systems within the family, as discussed earlier, 'extended families' should not be used to justify not supplying professional support services where necessary. Often, these families report a lack of respite care and many families refuse to divulge the extent of the pressure they are under in providing care for mentally ill family members. Some even have refused to let a family member attend a day centre in case the community found out about the mental illness. In the cases of adolescents, the extent of their problems might be hidden to avoid stigma from the community that would jeopardise their chances of marriage. Halford (1994) discusses family intervention strategies to support these families, in terms of education, stress management and goal setting. However, these interventions must be culture-sensitive. For instance, in the concept of stress management, the Western client-centred approach whereby clients are encouraged to explore their own feelings and make changes in their behaviour would be inappropriate. These approaches might well be meaningless to clients, as the stress and its causes are seen to be external to themselves. Hence the 'counsellors' would be expected to have a more practical approach to the problem by using a more directive rather than a reflective approach, which would also mean understanding the client's culture and his 'cultural mode'. This also raises the issue of transcultural counselling, especially as white ethnocentric approaches are not effective.

Zastowny et al (1992) also found that 'communicative skills' in family intervention work was the most important determinant of positive outcome. In issues of mental health work one of the most common problems is communication and unless this issue is addressed south Asians' mental health needs will continue to be marginalised and underrepresented and needs will be unmet.

Group work or therapy appears to be very popular in mental health work. The authors' experience with some groups has shown that, although initially there was very positive response to group work, the numbers attending very quickly dwindled despite the fact that the counsellor was Asian and was fully conversant with the clients' language and culture. What the

clients and patients identified in these groups was that they were expected to 'bare themselves' emotionally; this was an infringement of their privacy. Group sessions also meant discussing stresses that involved their families and this was felt to be 'disloyal'; clients felt that their own credibility as a family member was reduced in front of other group members by disclosing information about their families. This also involved losing 'respect/*izzat*' of their family and their constant fear that what was discussed in groups was not confidential. Group work might be seen by service planners as being a cheaper option and meeting the quantity criterion, where more clients can be seen in the same time. However, most clients requested individual contact with the practitioner.

DEATH

In Western culture, mourning is usually a private matter. Grieving publicly and crying openly is embarrassing; a certain code of behaviour is admired and expected. This is in complete contrast to Eastern and Middle Eastern cultures, where a display of open grief is considered essential, normal, praiseworthy and healthy. The whole family, however scattered around the globe, will come together to show its grief, talk openly and freely about the deceased and concentrate on the loss. Periods of unconcealed sorrow are allowed and are considered necessary to heal the grief. A newly bereaved person is not expected to be 'brave' and control their feelings. All relatives and friends have a binding obligation to visit, share in the mourning process, attend the funeral and offer moral support. All rites and duties are organised and performed by the family, according to religious codes, although the deceased may not have been a true believer.

In the Hindu religion the elder son has to perform certain rites at the funeral; hence the importance of having a son. Days of mourning may differ in each religious order and culture. Most women will wear white clothes as a sign of mourning. The family says special prayers and eats simple meals during the period of mourning.

CONCLUSION

Access to services and how this is facilitated becomes very important given that ethnic groups are not homogenous but have different religions and cultural backgrounds and the services need to be appropriate and sensitive if there is going to be equity in access to them. Balarajan & Raleigh (1993) argue that access to healthcare is further disadvantaged by known excess mortality and morbidity rates in certain diseases, e.g. coronary heart disease and diabetes. In order to alleviate this, service providers need to make the issue of access to healthcare central to their strategies of health planning, so that these issues have high profile and are not just marginalised.

Access to GPs of similar ethnic background and using their services also needs to be questioned. The cultural perception of illness is that health is highly valued and any symptom, whether somatised or not, may be seen to cause ill health and will mean seeking medical care. Health as a priority also means that illness should be attended to quickly. Thus the perception of a need for immediate treatment means that the patient will seek a system that does not include appointments, with days of delay. 'Culture-blaming' is also used by professions to cover poor communication, lack of information and access difficulties and sometimes there is total lack of knowledge about ethnic groups.

USEFUL ADDRESSES

Hindu Cultural Society
321 Colney Hatch Lane
London N11

The Buddhist Society
58 Eccleston Square
London SW1

Islamic Cultural Centre
London Central Mosque
46 Park Road
London NW8

Sikh Art and Cultural Centre
21 Montague Road
Hounslow
Middlesex

RESOURCES
Islam

Islamic Cultural Centre
London Central Mosque
146 Park Road
London NW8
0207 724 3362

Hinduism

The Hindu Centre (London)
39 Grafton Terrace
off Malden Road
London NW5
0207 485 8200

Buddhism

The Buddhist Hospice Trust
PO Box 51
Herne Bay
Kent CT6 6TP
01580 891 650

Sikhism

The Sikh Missionary Society
10 Featherstone Road
Southall
Middlesex UB2 5AA
0208 574 1902

FURTHER READING

Ahmad WIU, Baker M, Kernohan E 1991 General practitioners' perceptions of Asian and non-Asian patients. Family Practice 1: 52–56

Baxter C 1993 The communication needs of Black and ethnic minority pregnant women in Salford. Health and Race Constancy, Salford

Bhopal DS 1988 Health care for Asians: conflict in need, demand and provision. In: Equity: a prerequisite for health. Proceedings of the 1987 Summer Scientific Conference of the Facility of Community Medicine and World Health Organization

Brannen J, Dodd N, Oakley A, Storey P 1994 Young people – health and family life. Open University Press, Buckingham

Brown I 1991 Singing in tune. Health Service Journal 101: 24

Clarkson L, Barter MJ, Marshall T, Wharton BA 1982 Secular changes in birthweight of Asian babies born in Birmingham. Archives of Disease in Childhood 57

D'Souza SW, Lakan P, Waters HM et al 1987 Iron deficiency in ethnic minorities: association with dietary fibre and phytate. Early Human Development 15

Eaton PM 1982 What do Asian women in Birmingham eat during pregnancy? Proceedings of the Nutrition Society 4

Flaskerud JH, Liu PY 1990 Influence of therapist ethnicity and language on therapy outcomes of South East Asian clients. International Journal of Social Psychiatry 36(1): 18–29

Freimuth VS, Mettger W 1990 Is there a hard to teach audience? Public Health Reports 105(3): 232–238

Healey MA, Aslam M 1990 The Asian community: medicines and traditions. Silver Link Publishing, Nottingham

Henley A (1979) Asian patients in hospital and at home. King's Fund. Pitman Medical, London

Henley A (1982) Asians in Britain. Caring for Muslims and their families: religious aspects of care. DHSS King Edward's Hospital Fund. National Extension College, London

Henley A (1983a) Asians in Britain. Caring for Sikhs and their families: religious aspects of care. DHSS King Edward's Hospital Fund. National Extension College, London

Henley A (1983b) Asians in Britain. Caring for Hindus and their families. DHSS King Edward's Hospital Fund.

National Extension College, London

Holland J, Mellthner M, Sharpe S 1996 Family matters: communicating health messages in the family. Health Education Authority, London

Hume JC 1977 Rival traditions: Western medicine and unan-i-tibb in the Punjab 1849–89. Bulletin of the History of Medicine 51: 214–231

Jones E 1993 Family systems therapy: developments in the Milan systemic therapy. John Wiley, Chichester

Jones VM 1987 Current infant weaning practices within the Bangladeshi community in the London Borough of Tower Hamlets. Human Nutrition: Applied Nutrition 41A

Kleinman A 1988 The illness narratives: stuttering, healing and the human condition. Basic Books, New York

Landy D (ed) Culture, disease and healing: studies in medical anthropology. Macmillan, New York

Madhok R, Bhopal RS, Ramaiah RS 1992 Quality of hospital services: a study comparing Asian and non-Asian patients in Middlesborough. Journal of Public Health Medicine 14(3): 271–279

Pilgrum S et al 1993 The Bristol Black and ethnic minorities health survey report. Bristol University, Bristol

Shah A, Piracha AH 1993 Hello, can you hear me?: A study of the communication experiences of the Asian community with Health Services in Blackburn, Hyndburn and Ribble Valley Health Authority Health Promotion Unit. Blackburn Health Authority, Blackburn

Tunon C 1986 When in Rome. Health Education Journal 45: 103–104

Warrington S, Storey DM 1988 Comparative studies of Asian and Caucasian children. 1. Growth. European Journal of Clinical Nutrition 42

Warrington S, Storey DM 1989 Comparative studies of Asian and Caucasian children. 2. Nutrition, feeding practices and health. European Journal of Clinical Nutrition 42

Wilson E, Wardle EV, Chandel P, Walford S 1993 Diabetes education – an Asian perspective. Diabetic Medicine 10(2): 177–180

17

Afro-Caribbean and Travelling families' health needs

Joy Jeffrey, Joanne Davis and

Helen Hoult

INTRODUCTION

This chapter explores two very different cultures living in Britain today and examines the role of health visiting with each group. As will be seen as the chapter progresses, the macro-term 'Afro-Caribbean culture' embraces a number of different groups with this origin. Similarly the macro-term 'Travelling Families' embraces at least two distinct groups within the culture, with different origins.

The writers of this chapter have been working within these cultural groups for several years and have built up the knowledge, understanding and skills to enable effective health visiting practice to be undertaken.

AFRO-CARIBBEAN CULTURE AND HEALTH VISITING PRACTICE

Joy Jeffrey

The aim of this section is to describe the role of health visitors in working with Afro-Caribbean families. Initially, aspects of ethnicity, race and health are discussed, followed by a discussion of some cultural practices and beliefs and their relevance to health visiting practice. The section concludes with a discussion of the possible way forward for health visitors working with the Afro-Caribbean and minority ethnic community.

The importance of clarifying terminology and using terms sensitively when writing about issues involving ethnicity and race can never be overemphasised. The terms immigrant, ethnic minority, West Indian, Afro-Caribbean and Black British have all been used to classify people whose origin, or that of their parents, was the Caribbean. The term Black has also been used more recently to refer to people of Afro-Caribbean and Asian descent and reflects the unity of experience of racism in society.

There are many people from minority communities in Britain who do not identify themselves as Black but who, because of their ethnic origin, language, culture or religion are often referred to in the literature as 'minority ethnic'.

For the purposes of this chapter, the term Black and minority ethnic will be used to reflect references in the literature and, where necessary, specific use of the term Afro-Caribbean will be used in discussions.

BACKGROUND .

Britain is a multicultural society, with approximately 6% of the total population (about 3 million people) representing Black and minority ethnic groups in England and Wales (Balarajan & Raleigh, 1993).

Defining the Afro-Caribbean group however, is not straightforward: previous statistics were based on 'country of birth', later the 1991 census used the category 'ethnic group' and more recently the 1997 Policy Studies Institute survey included an additional category of 'family origin' (Modood et al 1997). The Afro-Caribbean community is the second largest ethnic minority group in Britain, with approximately 40% of the total Afro-Caribbean population actually born in the UK.

There is an uneven distribution of ethnic minority groups throughout Britain: the greater proportion live in areas where the original immigrants settled, together with suburban areas to which some families from inner city areas moved over a period of time. Most of the larger Afro-Caribbean communities were established in metropolitan areas where there was a high demand for labour – London, Greater Manchester, West Yorkshire and the West Midlands (Balarajan & Raleigh, 1993).

Caribbean migrants to Britain came from many different countries of the English-speaking Caribbean – Jamaica, Trinidad, Barbados, Antigua – from English-speaking countries on the South American coast – Guyana – and from the eastern Caribbean, which includes Cuba and the Virgin Islands. It is important to note, that as well as the diverse countries of origin of the Afro-Caribbean population in Britain, there is also diversity in terms of ethnicity. The main ethnic groups are African, Indian, Amerindian, Chinese and Portuguese.

ETHNICITY, CULTURE AND RACE

As noted previously, information on ethnic minorities has tended to rely upon ethnicity, although the definitions used were unclear. Therefore, much of the data on ethnic minorities, which was based on crude categories, do not reflect the diversity of the group. More recent research takes the concept of ethnicity more seriously and acknowledges that ethnic minorities are a heterogeneous group with a diverse cultural identity.

The concept of ethnicity is a multifaceted phenomenon based on identity, cultural practices and outlooks that characterise a given group of people and distinguish them from other groups. The population group is seen to be different by virtue of language, ancestry, religion, a common history and other shared cultural practices such as food and diet and style of dress (Modood 1994).

Race, on the other hand, is defined as the physical and biological characteristics of individuals: their skin tone, hair colour and texture. However, race as a term has acquired a social and cultural meaning and is often used to express much more than physical characteristics (Jones 1994). Many researchers support the view that the prejudice and discrimination felt by the Black and minority population are based on the social meaning attached to race and ethnicity.

It appears that a stronger Caribbean identity has been developed in Britain among the children of Caribbean migrants; women in particular have developed an ethnic distinctiveness through

Black churches, the use of Patois/Creole, their hair and dress (Carter 1986).

It is important to note the growing number of mixed partnerships; the recent population statistical information (PSI) survey indicated that approximately 20% of Caribbean heads of household with partners had a mixed relationship (Modood et al 1997). This number represents an increase on previous figures, and was consistent with the increase in numbers of young adults of Caribbean origin born in Britain. It may in the future have implications for the definition and concept of ethnic identity.

The importance of race, cultural and ethnic differences, however, runs much deeper and is relevant to the discussions taking place about the healthcare needs of Afro-Caribbean and other minority ethnic groups.

It is not within the scope of this section to debate the highly complex issues related to race, ethnicity and identity. However, in any discussion on the health- and social-care needs of Black and minority ethnic groups, these issues as well as the important influences of gender, class, period of residence and socioeconomic status cannot be ignored (Douglas 1998).

REVIEW OF THE LITERATURE

Recent literature supports the view that history, culture and personal circumstances all have an impact on health. An understanding of some of the cultural differences between the Black and minority ethnic groups means that professional practice can be closely matched to need. At the same time, being aware that attributing health problems entirely to cultural difference diverts attention from the real causes (Mares et al 1985). The review of the literature that follows discusses some of the key themes that present related to culture – religion, food and diet, the use of home remedies, children and families, health and social needs – in the Afro-Caribbean community.

Religion

The belief in a mainly Christian doctrine is a powerful force within the Afro-Caribbean com-

munity. The largest groups are from the traditional doctrines – Methodist, Anglicans, Roman Catholics and Seventh-Day Adventist. A growing number of Afro-Caribbeans join what is known as 'a Black Church' – Pentecostal churches, mainly in inner-city areas. Although there is variation within belief in the different doctrines, principles such as compassion, responsibility and faith guide the daily lives and choices that are made (Schreiber et al 1998). A strong belief that health and wellness 'is in the hands of the Lord' may prevent some of them from valuing the effectiveness of health promotion or healthcare interventions, while others believe their faith gave them strength to deal with 'stresses of life'.

In addition to spiritual guidance, the church is an important resource for social support, especially among older Afro-Caribbeans. It also provides the religious context for bringing up children, with an emphasis on grandparents taking children to Sunday school.

There is some representation of minority faiths such as Rastafarianism and Shango, as well as the Muslim and Hindu faiths.

Food and diet

There are very strong, widely held beliefs about food and health in Afro-Caribbean communities and in general a traditional Caribbean diet is high in fibre and low in fat (Douglas 1987, 1990). Food also has social and cultural significance. The preparation, cooking and serving of food is an important aspect of Afro-Caribbean family life – part of the experience of the food being the communion in savouring it, the conversation and the gathering of family and guests, whatever the occasion.

Dietary practices vary immensely among Afro-Caribbeans because of the influence of the different countries that make up the Caribbean, but there are similar types of food and cooking methods common to most of the population. Cleanliness is a prime requirement for the preparation of all foods, particularly meat dishes, and this often adds to the time required to cook and serve food.

The diet consists mainly of foods with a high

starch content, e.g. rice, yams, sweet potatoes and green bananas, and this is usually served with green vegetables, fish or meat. Many traditional foods are not always easily available and may be more expensive than other foods. Low income and lack of access to reasonably priced Caribbean foods are particularly significant to the elderly population as these affect their health and nutritional choices.

In the past assumptions have been made about high levels of breast-feeding by Afro-Caribbean mothers, but surveys conducted in the Caribbean and in the UK appear to suggest that the period of exclusive breast-feeding is very short (Douglas 1987). A survey carried out in Birmingham in 1986 among Afro-Caribbean mothers supported this finding and also suggested that many mothers were influenced by both Caribbean and UK beliefs and practices when weaning their children. In general, Afro-Caribbean mothers sought dietary advice from their families rather than health visitors (Douglas 1987). Most Afro-Caribbean mothers have no problems weaning their children; choices are often influenced by traditional beliefs and practices as well as some British feeding practices.

Religion and food restrictions

A variety of religious faiths are represented in the Afro-Caribbean community and some have strict dietary practices. Seventh-Day Adventists, for example, do not eat pork, or fish without scales and fins, and may be vegetarian. Rastafarians have similar dietary restrictions, but they also avoid food containing additives such as salt and may be vegetarian.

Home remedies

Self-care as a concept is not unknown in most societies. Most people seek various forms of help for problems, ranging from family or friends, alternative remedies to more formal services. There is a paucity of research in the use of home remedies by Afro-Caribbeans (Donovan 1986), but anecdotal evidence suggests that home remedies traditionally used in the Caribbean, many

derived from an African heritage, are often used with the belief and faith that the remedy works.

The purpose in using home remedies is to prevent illness, alleviate symptoms or effect a cure before a doctor is consulted. The knowledge of medicinal properties of certain bushes and plants has been passed on from one generation to the next or shared with friends and relatives. Women as well as men are often proficient in selecting the right remedy for a particular complaint. The regular use of remedies based on ingredients or preparations available in Britain includes teas such as cerecy, ginger, clove and periwinkle for headaches, tummy aches or to 'purify the blood' – most of these teas are harmless and may in fact cure minor ailments (Douglas 1990).

Some home remedies are related to food, e.g. using food as a healing agent to cure a cold, taking hot toddies or drinking castor oil with orange to cure flu symptoms. One of the most commonly used home remedies is cod liver oil capsules or liquid. It is often given to children of all ages 'to maintain health' and 'strengthen their bones' and used by the elderly Afro-Caribbean population 'to preserve health'.

Healthcare practitioners must accept that self-care in many instances is an effective therapy. However, as with any self-care treatments, problems may arise when information about the treatment is not shared so that positive choices can be reinforced and unsafe choices discouraged.

Children and families

Families have been changing rapidly over the last 30 years and the traditional structures that upheld family life have been greatly influenced by many factors (Jones 1994). It is only in the last 20 years that researchers have begun to try to distinguish between myths, stereotypes and facts related to Afro-Caribbean families, and to look at the effects of social and economic inequalities and discrimination on the family.

More recent researchers are attempting to develop a new methodology based on a cultural understanding of Afro-Caribbean families and more accurate empirical information. Afro-

Caribbean families are heterogeneous and functional and, to varying degrees, have upheld traditional family structures and culture. Barrow (1982) suggests that Afro-Caribbean families take several different forms ranging from 'Christian marriage', based on the model of the Victorian family, through the 'common law family' of unmarried partners, to the 'mother household', in which the mother and/or grandmother is the sole head.

The concept of the nuclear family may appear to be weakly structured from an Afro-Caribbean perspective but, to compensate for this, other associations in the community are much more significant in everyday life. Mares et al (1985) suggested that single Afro-Caribbean mothers often faced real difficulties in their contacts with welfare services and professionals. However, Blackburn (1991) found that all single mothers regardless of background faced poverty, inadequate housing and unemployment.

In general, the extended family and a wide circle of 'kin' play a more active role in all aspects of parenting. The children automatically look to all the adults for comfort, guidance, treats, attention and punishment. This attitude that adults have a responsibility to children is of crucial importance whenever families separate or children move away from the community.

In some Afro-Caribbean families, children are treated more as junior members of the family, where they have a role as domestic helpers or as 'carers' for younger siblings. In some ways, it seems that they are subjected to contrary pressures and expectations – on one hand responsible 'adults' and on the other hand 'well behaved children'.

Attitudes to discipline

There are limited data on the child-care practices and experiences of Afro-Caribbean and other minority ethnic families. In society great emphasis is placed on parental responsibility, not only for caring for children or exercising of discipline but also for their wrongdoing. Parents frequently feel judged on the performance and behaviour of their children and thus have a powerful

investment in their successful development (Jones et al 1987).

Over the years, child-care specialists and professionals have debated the complex issues of different child-rearing practices, child abuse and attitudes to corporal punishment. Errors in diagnosing child abuse may cause resentment and a loss of confidence in the health services, especially if the family has limited experience and understanding of the community services and is already feeling suspicious and insecure (Jones et al 1987). It is fair to say that behaviour may be more understandable in the cultural context, but this does not resolve whether this behaviour should be treated as child abuse in society or whether a different standard should be adopted. In a wide-ranging study in the USA, Gil (1973) concluded that 'culturally determined attitudes towards the use of physical force in child-rearing seem to constitute the common core of all physical abuse in American society'. Discussion on this issue is restricted by inadequate research, deep feelings and ingrained prejudice. It is certainly dangerous to see one set of child-rearing beliefs and practices as superior to another, and yet the needs of the child must always remain paramount.

Fierce parental criticism and the threat of punishment is a strategy many Afro-Caribbean women use to assert their authority with children. Understanding the context in which this takes place is important – it is not viewed in a dominating and oppressive way, but reflects their desire to be 'good parents' beyond reproach.

One reason for this may be, as Hooks (1993) suggested, that, living in a society where mothers are often blamed for any problems that arise with children, some Black mothers feel the need to assert control over their children; the parent's desire to 'care' for the child is placed in competition with the perceived need to exercise control. Afro-Caribbean parents place great emphasis on 'good' behaviour and may be overcritical, not because they are angry with the child but because of their desire for the child to behave 'appropriately' in public settings. Since no in-depth studies have been done to analyse this aspect of the parent–child relationship, it would be easy to speculate that being a 'good parent' is synonymous with the extent to which one is able to exercise control over a child's behaviour.

Health and social needs

There are many variations in religion, ethnicity, class and gender, all of which impact on health status. There are important variations in patterns of ill-health and mortality in Black people and minority ethnic groups living in Britain as well as differences between ethnic groups within Black communities (Balarajan & Raleigh 1992). Therefore, there are many different requirements within the context of Black and minority ethnic health needs.

Most of the epidemiological research available is underpinned by a biological model and focuses on illnesses and diseases affecting the Black and minority ethnic communities. It is well established that mortality from hypertension and strokes is higher in the Afro-Caribbean population (Cruickshank et al 1980). Concern for the levels of ill-health associated with diseases such as sickle cell disease, thalassaemia and diabetes is also well documented (Davis et al 1981, Anionwu 1994). The Afro-Caribbean population has a higher admission rate to psychiatric hospitals and is more likely to be diagnosed as schizophrenic than the white population (Littlewood & Lipsedge 1988, Cochrane & Bal 1989). And although the mortality from breast and lung cancer is low in Afro-Caribbeans, there is some evidence that the incidence of mortality from cervical cancers could be rising (Balarajan & Bulusu 1990).

The problem in collecting data on health status using classifications of the subject population into categories such as 'Asian', 'African–Caribbean' and 'white' groups, is the assumptions it involves about the homogenous nature of the population (Douglas 1998). Important influences of socio-economic status, gender, country of origin and length of residence in the UK have often been ignored (Douglas 1998).

According to Donovan (1986), the opinions of Afro-Caribbean people about their own health have been largely ignored, as have the obvious links between health and the large and growing literature on race and health in Britain

PUBLIC HEALTH NEEDS
Access to services and information

Health does not exist in a vacuum; working to guarantee, for instance, access to good housing and good nutrition would have an impact on the health of Afro-Caribbean families. This includes economic and social forces such as availability of transport, and a safe working and living environment. Evidence suggests that Black and minority ethnic populations encounter particular difficulties in accessing most services at each level (Smaje 1995). At the same time many have argued that the differences in health and the use of services by Black and minority ethnic communities are to some extent attributable to lack of information about health and social services, inadequate training of health professionals in particular and the inability to communicate (Ahmad 1993).

In the NHS, inequalities in health due to racism within the system and a lack of understanding of cultural differences by some health professionals were identified as important reasons for Black and minority people not gaining access to adequate and suitable health care (Baxter 1988, McNaught 1988). There is also a growing body of evidence about the attitudes of Afro-Caribbean and minority ethnic groups towards take-up of health services. For example, Patel (1993) found that although minority ethnic elders identified a range of felt needs for community services, community nurses did not endorse them because they assumed that the extended family would provide sufficient care and support. Service managers have misconceptions that all patients from Afro-Caribbean and other minority ethnic groups are cared for by relatives (Norman 1985) but they fail to appreciate that many either do not have children or they live in another country.

Communication

The official language of most of the Caribbean is English, but many Afro-Caribbean people use a Patois/Creole dialect with its own vocabulary, pronunciation, proverbs and manner of expression to communicate with each other. The most recent PSI survey reported that more Afro-Caribbean women than men understood and regularly used Patois/Creole (Modood et al 1997).

There is an general lack of knowledge about available services, especially among older people, even though the need for more information about health and social services has been well documented (Donovan 1986). Lack of information about health services can present a barrier to Black and minority ethnic families. The reasons for this may be varied, but often assumptions are made about the necessity to communicate with the Afro-Caribbean population. Class, race, gender and culture all influence our ability to communicate and the lack of a common use of the English language makes it more difficult. This can result in inappropriate care, foster racism, waste resources and is dangerous (Ahmad 1993).

Health visitors have a responsibility to ensure that they can communicate effectively. Research suggests that the quality of nurse–client interaction plays a significant role in the effectiveness of the outcome of health advice (Macleod-Clark 1993). Eye contact from health professionals is considered important by Afro-Caribbeans before they perceive the interaction to be positive. This is particularly important to older Afro-Caribbeans, who also see it as a mark of respect and may refuse to go to particular doctors or health professionals because of their nondirectional gaze (Donovan 1986). It is widely known and supported by researchers that Afro-Caribbeans use private GPs in parallel with the NHS GPs. As well as the desire to obtain a second opinion and a full physical examination, the main reason offered for these additional consultations is often that payment for the service is equated with a better standard of communication. (Donovan 1986, Douglas 1990).

PRINCIPLES FOR GOOD PRACTICE

There is a recognition within the nursing profession of the need to deliver culturally sensitive care. This is reflected in the *Code of Professional Conduct* for nurses, midwives and health visitors which states that each practitioner must 'recognise and respect the uniqueness and dignity of each patient and client, and respond to their need for care, irrespective of their ethnic origin, religious beliefs, personal attributes, nature of their health problems or any other health factors' (UKCC 1992a).

Until recently, major government documents failed to address specifically issues of culture, ethnicity and health. The White Paper *The New NHS – Modern, Dependable* (Department of Health 1997a), the *Report of the Independent Inquiry into Inequalities in Health* (Department of Health 1998e) and the recent Green Paper *Our Healthier Nation* (Department of Health 1998a) have acknowledged that inequalities in health exist and indicated the government's commitment to tackling it. In the Acheson review consideration was given to several areas for future policy development including poverty, ethnicity, gender and socioeconomic status (Department of Health 1998e). Criticism has also been made of the inadequacy of nurse education programmes, which in the past have concentrated on informing nurses on 'cultural aspects of care' while excluding issues of discrimination and disadvantage.

The nursing and health visiting curriculum needs to change to take account of the limitations of this culturalist approach to a broader perspective (Culley 1996). A survey carried out by the Training Health and Race Project (Higham 1988) indicated considerable gaps in the knowledge of health workers about the needs of Black and minority communities. These findings were again highlighted in a recent research document on nurse education (Baxter 1997). Unless nurse, midwifery and health visiting education can address these issues, it is questionable to what extent culturally sensitive practitioners can be produced (Burrows 1983, Tullman 1992, Alleyne & Thomas 1994).

Several authors have also argued that, although there is a need to explore and examine cultural beliefs and practices, this should be done in a positive manner, without prejudice or attributing blame (Mares et al 1985, Tullman 1992).

THE CHALLENGE FOR HEALTH VISITING

Reducing inequalities is one of the two main aims of the government's new health strategy and its shared priority for health and local authorities. Local action involving public agencies, voluntary organisations and community groups and the private sector has been identified as the vehicle to drive these policies (Department of Health 1998a). There are several opportunities and challenges for all health visitors emanating from the present shift in emphasis to community-based primary care. The White Paper *The NHS – Modern, Dependable* (Department of Health 1997a), clearly identifies health promotion and community health as top priorities in the nation's health objectives.

The relative autonomy of the health visiting role and the scope of responsibility for individual clients throughout their lifespan creates a climate of opportunity for contact with the Black and minority ethnic population. It is essential, therefore, that a truly holistic approach, one that explores the complex issues of ethnicity, race and health, disadvantage and discrimination, should be used when working with Black and minority ethnic families.

Health visitors must be prepared to work with the population and not for the population; this may require the profession to 'leave some things behind' and look outwardly at the context within which health visiting is practised in order to adopt initiatives that may be unfamiliar (Jeyasingham 1992). Nurses, including health visitors, need but often lack a broad understanding of the vast range of social, cultural, economic, political and racial factors that influence and affect the health of Black and minority ethnic communities (Culley 1996).

Considering the challenges of today's practitioners, such as increasing social deprivation and poverty, inequalities in health and growing morbidity and mortality from conditions that particularly affect Afro-Caribbean people, such as strokes, coronary heart disease and diabetes, the principles of health visiting are as relevant today as they were in the 1970s (Blaxter 1990).

The way forward

It is essential for health visiting as a discipline to avoid the trap of focusing only on providing culturally sensitive care as a response to ethnic diversity. Public health nursing approaches demand attention to the socioeconomic and political context in which health visiting is practised (Billingham 1997). This may provide a starting point for health visitors working with Black and minority populations.

Community participation, collaboration and a multiagency approach are the cornerstones of public health nursing and must become part of the health visiting service for the future. The traditional fragmented policy and service approach cannot address such complex issues as inequalities in health for the Black and minority ethnic community (Benzeval et al 1995).

As important as it is to have in place policies that increase cultural awareness, these only address part of the agenda of meeting the health needs of ethnic communities (Douglas 1998). If all the critical factors associated with health are ignored and only one part of the agenda is delivered, the opportunities to reduce inequality and develop healthier communities in which policies and action work in tandem to promote health and prevent disease will be lost.

In working with families from any minority ethnic background, practitioners must recognise that they will become 'students' again. To date, the importance of language and culture has been acknowledged by providers of care, but to learn about how the client sees the world – a world in which race is among the most fundamental of social divisions – networking with agencies and individuals from that community is essential. Health visitors and health visitor education need to contextualise the health of minority groups and, through research, explore the dynamics of discriminatory practices that structure many aspects of everyday life (Culley 1996).

This means practitioners with allocated time, working at an advanced level, who must have the necessary skills to work with various communities to identify and address community health problems. Practitioners need a firm grounding in ways to bring people together, in coalition building, in political advocacy and other community related skills, if they are to be effective in advancing the health of the community (Leininger 1997).

This approach has the potential to avoid the use of an exclusive, single-faceted model that fails to address the complex situations influencing the health of Afro-Caribbean and other minority ethnic individuals and families.

INITIATIVES TO IMPROVE THE HEALTH OF BLACK AND MINORITY ETHNIC PEOPLE

Voluntary sector initiatives usually focus on providing an advocacy service as well as interpreting. The use of advocates, particularly with the elderly Afro-Caribbean population, is a way forward in addressing the power imbalances faced by this group in the community. The difference between interpreting and advocacy is seen as a difference in both purpose and perspective, with the interpreter playing a reactive role on behalf of health professionals while the proactive, client centred role of the advocate enables them to put forward the client's perspective (Cornwell & Gordon 1984).

Opportunities for health visitors to work with agencies establishing initiatives such as food co-operatives, community transport and community cafes in disadvantaged communities can help families cope with the effects of poverty and isolation. One such initiative, involving a food co-operative, the local residents, a housing association, the health authority and health visitors has been set up in Sandwell in the West Midlands and has provided many staple Caribbean foods at a reduced cost to local families.

Self-help groups as an initiative

Playgroups, mother and toddler groups and other self-help groups such as postnatal groups are an important feature of present-day support offered by health visitors and other professionals to parents in the community. Concern is often

expressed that these services are underused by Black and other minority ethnic children and their parents. The reasons for poor uptake are varied. Afro-Caribbean parents make important use of family and friends to provide their children's day care and Afro-Caribbean lone parents are more likely to be in work (often in part-time and low-paid jobs) than other lone parents (Modood et al 1997). Research also suggests that Afro-Caribbean parents place more emphasis on the importance of formal learning, as distinct from play, and may not see playgroups as an important part of their child's development. This view was supported by a survey carried out by Barnardos Under 8's Project into the daycare needs of Black and minority families in a West Midlands borough. It found that Afro-Caribbean families made significantly greater use of education nursery schools than services such as playgroups (Bekenn 1995).

Black and minority organisations have a more generic approach to meeting the needs of the community (Baxter 1997). Churches, law societies and community centres often provide a variety of services, reflecting the reality of life in the society. Support tends to be holistic, dealing with health, social, emotional and financial needs and issues of racial harassment and housing, all of which impact on the health of the individual.

Better links need to be made by health visitors with the growing network of emerging minority ethnic individuals, groups and communities who are committed to and already working in various self-help initiatives.

EVALUATING OUTCOMES

Issues about the complexity of assessing the needs of Afro-Caribbean and other minority ethnic populations have already been discussed. However, the identification of their health- and social-care needs is essential if health visitors are to demonstrate the effectiveness of their care. Without this information, health visitors often resort to their own perceptions of health need. These perceptions may not only be inaccurate in reflecting the needs of Afro-Caribbean individuals and communities but will also create a situation where it is difficult to assess the extent to which those needs have been met.

Information about Black and minority communities, the nature of their housing, employment and the numbers of homeless, can help ensure that services better reflect needs and form the basis from which the effectiveness of care can be monitored.

CONCLUSION

Health visiting practice must reflect the ability to facilitate change that leads to positive health outcomes, rather than work from an 'expert knows best' perspective. The skills and approaches needed to help Black and minority ethnic families make informed choices and achieve optimum health are complex; efforts must be made to build on the strengths and knowledge of the community with other agencies. Keeping the client foremost, making the health system accessible and feel seamless are among the challenges that health visitors face in working with diverse communities.

WORKING WITH TRAVELLERS AND GYPSIES

Joanne Davis and Helen Hoult

DEFINITION OF TRAVELLERS/ GYPSIES

The definition of Travellers, under the 1968 Caravan Sites Act, is: 'Persons of nomadic habit or lifestyle, whatever their race or origins'. The recent Criminal Justice and Public Order Act 1994 that replaced the 1968 Caravan Sites Act adds the concept of: 'purposeful travel for economic independence and to a degree a tradition of travelling'. Okely (1983) described Travellers as: 'a self-reproducing ethnic group based on a principle of descent, with an ideology of travelling, a preference for self-employment and a wide range of economic activities'.

The Travelling community see themselves and are regarded by others as a separate ethnic group by virtue of the following characteristics:

- a long shared history, which, even though largely unresearched, can be traced back for many centuries
- a shared set of values, customs, lifestyle and traditions associated with nomadism
- a shared language
- endogamy (marrying within the group). Travellers come from a small number of ancestors. Different families are associated with different parts of the country. One becomes a Traveller not by choice but by birth
- self-ascription as Travellers (Irish College of General Practitioners 1995).

Travellers and Gypsies see themselves as two distinct groups in society; however, to the outsider it can be hard to distinguish them. Travellers are Irish in origin and have come to live in the UK over the centuries, mainly for personal economic improvement. They are often wrongly called 'tinkers', which, apart from being derogatory to them, is in fact a highly skilled trade and not a descriptive label of a group of people. Gypsies are English and Welsh in origin and some of the families acknowledge Romany ancestors. These Romany Gypsies can ascribe their roots directly to nomadic tribes deriving from the Indian subcontinent. However some of the English and Welsh Gypsies one meets have also become nomadic for usually economic reasons and have intermarried with Romany Gypsy families. Over the past few years it has become commonplace too for English/Welsh and Irish to marry, thus blurring the boundaries further.

HISTORICAL OVERVIEW OF TRAVELLERS' AND GYPSIES' CULTURE AND BELIEFS

There are documented records of Gypsies living and working in Britain since the 15th century. However, the Travelling population is a very complex one and to consider Gypsies as a single group of people is wrong. Today's Traveller may be descended from one of a variety of groups once important to this country's economy. Their former vital economic role protected them to an extent from the discrimination they now face.

Despite this economic importance, during the reign of Henry VIII and subsequently, the Gypsies' nomadic lifestyle has been viewed with suspicion by the settled population. Gypsies were seen to use local resources such as land and food without the responsibility of local taxation and duties. This has a familiar ring to it, as it is this nonpayment of tax that is commonly used in accusations of criminality today. Legislation under Henry VIII banished them under pain of death, thus confirming local suspicion.

This persecution, when it has suited the settled population, has continued through the centuries. In the 20th century, under the Nazis in Germany, 300 000 Gypsies were killed in concentration camps and the plight of eastern European Gypsies is in the news today. In this country, although supposedly protected by the 1976 Race Relations Act, it was not until 1988 (Commission for Racial Equality v Dutton) that it was clarified that Travellers were not to be discriminated against either directly or indirectly. Despite these judgments, prejudice is inherent in our society.

Gypsies see this discrimination as part of everyday life. This resignation, alongside poor education, allows the media – particularly newspapers – to publish and broadcast offensive and discriminatory views. This covert and insidious discrimination is all the more dangerous because it is constantly reinforced by the State's criminalisation of Traveller lifestyle and work opportunities, thus serving to convince the general population that their views are justified.

The Traveller population of Britain is impossible to assess accurately, but it is thought that there are at least 12 000 caravans inhabited by about 60 000 people. Families in Britain tend to be either Irish Travellers or English and Welsh Gypsies. Although these two groups have some cultural similarities, they also have fundamental differences and share a mutual antagonism; these occur through perceived attitudes to each other's racial grouping. As already stated, English and Welsh Gypsies can trace their heritage back to

Indian nomadic tribes and will indicate that their traditions of travelling are descended from centuries of nomadism. They criticise Irish Travellers as having less of a tradition of travelling and also as being less economically self-sufficient and often dependent on state benefits.

Naturally it goes without saying these beliefs and antagonisms are usually founded in misunderstanding and unreliable information and as a consequence Travellers do not have a common voice and are not a united community. As society has marginalised and now criminalised their lifestyle, they suffer discrimination and prejudice at the hands of most statutory services and so have unequal access to everything we take for granted.

The recent legislation (the Criminal Justice and Public Order Act 1994) withdrew the statutory duty of local authorities to provide site facilities for them (although they still can if they want to) and allows for eviction of camps every 24 hours, with powers to enter and remove vehicles from land. Penalties can be imposed of up to £1000 if Travellers do not leave land as soon as possible, or reoccupy it in less than 3 months. Under this legislation, penalties, if found guilty of an offence, can be a fine of up to £2500.

Traveller and Gypsy Culture

It is said that you cannot become a Traveller, you have to be born one. A culture is essentially a series of beliefs that are shared by a group of people and give those people a sense of belonging. A culture also distinguishes those members who share it from others.

As with all cultures, there are the old-fashioned ways and beliefs held by older members of society, while young people may have different attitudes. Naturally, with television and video Travellers are not immune to the changes in our society and some of these have become adopted into theirs.

Much has been written about the Gypsies' hygiene and pollution beliefs (Okely 1975, 1983, Miller 1975, Sutherland 1987), and this is an area of academic dispute. These beliefs are based on a view held by Gypsies of there being an inner-self denoting cleanliness and the secret ethnic self, and the outer self, which is public and the one presented to the outsider or *gauga*. These beliefs are held to be the basis of the rules about separate bowls for washing people, clothes and food. This is an area where it is easy to fall foul as a health professional: inadvertently using the wrong bowl to wash hands can cause great offence. Most families adhere to the use of different bowls for different uses. When this is discussed with them, they all say it is for preventing germs spreading or to 'be clean', are amazed to be asked and even more amazed that these rules do not apply within the settled population. None has ever mentioned views about the outer world being polluted and polluting them, and certainly none has mentioned this as being a reason for refusing immunisation. It is probable that the use of different bowls is a pragmatic response to a lack of clean water and of there being many people in a small space.

The more elaborate concepts of hygiene proposed by Okely, among others, have been used to explain poor uptake of childhood immunisation among Travellers. Travellers are said to see the immunisation of a child as polluting the inner-self with something from the outer world. In our experience, the most frequently voiced reason for refusing immunisation is a commonly held, but mistaken, belief that the whooping cough vaccine causes brain damage. This is a view shared by a significant minority of the settled community. Travellers also have a marked reluctance to 'hurt' their child with the needle.

Family life is the mainstay of their culture, children being the centre of their world. The rearing of Traveller children is a curious combination of extreme indulgence in the form of material things like sweets, clothes, money, gold jewellery and lack of discipline, coupled with an acceptance of the responsibility of young children for jobs around the site, e.g. working with their father (boys) and care of and responsibility for their younger siblings (girls). It is not uncommon for girls as young as 6 or 7 to look after the baby, being responsible for feeding, clothing and changing and also playing with and comforting the child. Such types of responsi-

bility, along with cleaning the trailer and making men and boys meals and drinks, make many child care specialists and professionals from outside the community uncomfortable, feeling that the children's own childhood is being denied. What they fail to see is the difference between Traveller/Gypsy culture and their own. The expectation of Traveller parents of their children is firmly set in the gender rules by which they themselves have been reared and accept, i.e. that boys particularly are adults by 11–12 years old and, as such, can contribute to the family economy. They thus reject education beyond that age in favour of learning their 'trade', be it tarmacking, garden labouring, tree-felling, scrap, stripping old cars or hawking. Most now accept, however, that their complete illiteracy is a handicap to modern life and want their children to be able to read and write a little. For girls their 'trade' is to be able to look after a home, cook, clean and look after children.

Much academic discussion has focused on these strongly defined gender roles (Acton 1974, Okely 1983) within the community, where the taboos about acknowledging and voicing issues of sexuality, sex education and associated issues are often talked of by health professionals as vital to both understanding and working with the community. The discussion centres on issues of social control (Acton 1994). This gender role of differentiation has been linked with the hygiene taboos previously discussed as an attempt to keep women suppressed and not a threat to men. Thus anthropological studies (Thompson 1929) talked of the 'uncleanness of women' while discussing the pollution of childbirth and menstruation. These views are probably not widely held now. It is more likely that this gender differentiation, avoidance of sexuality and the maintenance of the 'private nature of female sexuality' (Pahl & Vaile 1986) is to do with the very close and un-private nature of their lifestyle and the diminished economic role for the women outside the home. Work for Traveller men has declined on the whole with the advent of industrialisation, recycling and our disposable, throw-away society, so a strengthening of the home role for women is the probable result (Okely 1983). However, both Okely and Acton indicate that this preservation of gender roles is essentially cultural and almost reinforces Gypsy culture.

This clear boundary of men's work and women's work is broadly adhered to among the community, but as with all populations there are greater and lesser degrees. We have been from trailers where 'baby' dolls have nappies firmly Sellotaped to their nappy area to prevent the boys of the family seeing the doll naked, through trailers where pregnancy and childbirth have been openly discussed in front of adolescent girls, to a young couple where the father was present at the birth of his second child.

REVIEW OF LITERATURE

There is little published research about Traveller Gypsies, especially with regard to their health and healthcare. The literature available on the subject is divided into four main areas: culture and folklore, accounts of intervention by health service personnel and epidemiological studies, reports of activity by pressure groups and charities, and discussions about the problems of undertaking research with Travellers.

There are many books about traditional Gypsy life (Sampson 1930, Kendrick & Bakewell 1995). These explore traditional gypsy culture and the folklore that surrounds it. The majority of published literature comprises descriptive accounts written by health visitors and associated health personnel. They usually give evidence of methods and actions taken to offer healthcare and service access to Travellers. The accounts give details of custom and practice among Travellers with regard to health issues.

There is little epidemiological research evidence available. The best-known study is by Pahl & Vaile (1986), who looked at a group of Kent Gypsies. The study dealt mainly with women's and children's health and concluded that prenatal mortality, stillbirth and infant mortality were considerably higher than in the general population and the incidence of low-birthweight babies was also higher. The study looked at child and adult health and morbidity and concluded that the health status of Travellers is worse than

that of social class V (Registrar General's classification). The causes identified were:

- poor sites and environmental conditions
- enforced nomadism
- poor access to primary healthcare services and preventive health measures.

Other studies have looked at the impact of mobility on health (Durward 1990). Further studies have tried to look at child health in particular but all suffer from a lack of reliable collected data, e.g. immunisation uptake (Simpson & Stockford 1979) and growth (Carroll et al 1974, Creedon et al 1975). Also, the studies are smallscale and it is difficult to draw reliable conclusions from them. The same problems occur for studies of adult Travellers' health – some have looked at lifestyle factors (Wilson 1987, Crout 1988) and others at chronic disease (Thomas 1985, Thomas et al 1987). However, again these are small studies that draw few reliable or widely applicable conclusions.

Reasons for the problems with research about Travellers – which makes up a large body of literature by itself (Feder 1990) – include the fact that the population is highly mobile and is not an ideal research population. The absence of medical records and poor memory recall of illness render retrospective studies of health inaccurate and impossible to check for reliability. This makes it difficult to formally reference views about Travellers and their health and so most of the evidence given to support argument is experiential or anecdotal.

Finally, there exists a large amount of literature in the form of reports, mission statements and conference proceedings. These explore issues of relevance to Travellers' health (e.g. service provision, site conditions and provision) and make local and national recommendations about conditions that affect Traveller health.

SETTING THE SCENE

Traveller Gypsies live in Britain in a variety of settings – on local-authority-provided sites and on privately-owned sites, on both of which payment is made for rent and utilities. Others live on unauthorised encampments in fields, road sides, parks and derelict land, where they are subject to regular eviction under the terms of the Criminal Justice and Public Order Act 1994. Others live in houses, both privately owned and rented, where they maintain the culture and lifestyle of being Travellers.

Generalisations have had to be made in this section because the experience of both authors has in the main been of mobile Travellers who resort to urban areas to live. We are aware of differences in culture among urban groups and also that Travellers who live in settled rural communities and the health workers who work with them may have different experiences of healthcare provision.

THE RANGE OF HEALTH VISITING WITH TRAVELLERS

All generic health visitors possess and use a range of skills that enable them to successfully achieve their remit within their client group. For a health visitor working with Travellers these skills must be further complemented, refined and their presentation made appropriate so that the community is able to uptake services successfully.

Networks

The overriding difficulty of working with Traveller Gypsies is the one from which their name derives – they travel. This nomadism poses many problems for the health visitor (and this is true not only of permanently mobile families but also of those who are sited or live in houses, most of whom spend some part of the year in other areas of the country where they have connections). Firstly, it becomes an impossible task to successfully profile the caseload – although individual families can be profiled. However it is not possible to accurately state which families are resident in the specialist's area on any particular day. Actual caseload numbers can fluctuate enormously, particularly when large groups, sometimes of over 100 trailers, move into an

area for a short time, increasing the specialist's workload dramatically.

These problems are further compounded by the difficulty of rigid health authority boundaries. Unknown to themselves, Travellers cross these boundaries daily and often have no idea which local authority's jurisdiction they are in until an eviction officer arrives. Health visitors are in general unable routinely to cross boundaries. When working with the Traveller community, particularly if neighbouring authorities have no provision for health visiting Travellers, it may be necessary to cross boundaries for follow-up care.

Other difficulties faced when families cross from one health authority to another is that the authority they have left has no obligation to continue supplying services. For potentially lengthy service input such as speech therapy or physiotherapy the transfer of care to another authority would be inappropriate, families usually having moved on before further input could be arranged. This bureaucratic nightmare makes it necessary for the health visitor to be somewhat vague when asked about the actual location of the client's trailer. Individuals are usually happy to travel many miles to an appointment with a practitioner they know rather than recommence treatment elsewhere where their reception may be less positive.

Many families have no contact address and, for those that have, the address may be used by up to 100 individuals or more. The likelihood of one individual receiving their post is minimal, given that a large percentage of the community are illiterate or have very poor literacy skills, and have very similar names. It is common within Traveller culture to name children after relatives, therefore large numbers of family members of varying ages often have identical names. It is particularly important when visiting Travellers that both parents' forenames and dates of birth if possible are taken to avoid confusion.

With mobile Travellers not having a postal address, many use the health worker's address for the receipt of medical appointments. It is a particular quality of specialist working to acquire knowledge about family networks, and so the worker will know mobile phone numbers or relatives' contact points through which messages can be passed.

Using the specialist's address has another advantage. Travellers do not generally have tools such as diaries and calendars that are used by literate society. They have to rely upon their memories to remember forthcoming events such as appointments. If these appointments are far in advance, without any further prompt it is highly likely that they will forget to attend. Most specialists keep a record of forthcoming appointments for families and remind them, using a variety of methods, nearer to the time. It is worth noting here that some families genuinely have little idea of months of the year and sometimes even days of the week. It is not uncommon to be asked 'Which month comes before September, love?' and they almost always refer to December as Christmas month. Older individuals often do not know their own date of birth and many forget to celebrate their children's birthdays or their own – their mental calendar is very different from ours.

Healthcare

Families' expectations of healthcare is generally low as often their positive experiences have been few. They are often refused access to services the general public take for granted such as GP services and the preventive services allied to them. Travellers tend to be led by curative rather than preventive medicine. They would not see, without input, the importance of preventive clinics but would attend for medical treatment once ill and experiencing symptoms. They very quickly attend, particularly to the Accident and Emergency Department (A&E) if children are unwell or suffer accidents. Travellers tend to prefer the 'drop in' nature of A&E care as they are never refused treatment and seem to believe that hospital doctors and hospital premises, with their banks of machinery and facilities for various investigations, are much more thorough than any GP. Travellers often use the A&E department inappropriately for illnesses that would generally be treated by a GP, but because of registration difficulties they are often unable to access GP services, particularly in the evening or at weekends.

Outcomes

Audit and outcomes are phrases routinely used in many aspects of primary care, but in preventive work quantifiable outcomes are difficult to determine.

Immunisation rates are the most commonly recorded outcome for health visiting activity. Health visitors with Travellers give many home immunisations; however mobile families often move on before immunisation courses can be completed – it is therefore unknown whether a child has completed the course elsewhere or not. This inaccuracy results in poor immunisation statistics for Travellers, but experience shows that many families who decide to have immunisations ensure that their children receive the full course wherever they happen to be staying.

Parent-held records have become invaluable for health visitors working with this community as many Travellers are very poor historians and often, in common with many members of the settled community, have no idea what previous injections any of their offspring have received or when or where the last one was given.

A study undertaken in Glasgow in 1985 by Riding found that of 109 Travellers aged 5–61 years, who had no previous recollection of ever being immunised, over 80% had antibodies to polio and diphtheria and over 50% had antibodies to tetanus.

Parent-held records

Travellers in the Black Country region have had purpose-produced parent-held records since 1990 and for new births Travellers are now given the national record. This up-to-date information allows health visitors to immunise children on first contact and complete the record appropriately for any injection or developmental assessment undertaken. The record also allows accurate chronological information to pass between professionals as many families ensure that they take the record with them to all hospital or GP appointments. Further information can also be gained easily if necessary from professionals who have previously seen an individual, using the contact numbers in the book.

Advocacy

Health visitors in this field need also to be knowledgeable regarding housing and benefits. Travellers are often discriminated against by staff in these departments and health visitors acting as an advocate for the client often find themselves in the same situation, at times being dealt with with cynicism and rudeness.

Travellers often find themselves in a 'trap' with regard to housing. In most areas it is local authority policy that persons applying for housing must have been resident within the borough while their application is being processed and until accommodation is offered. Mobile Travellers are constantly evicted by the local authority who try to ensure that families move out of *their* borough at each eviction. Therefore Travellers who need to stay within the borough to qualify for housing with the local authority are being moved on by a branch of the very organisation that insists they must reside there to qualify. Many therefore apply but fail to remain long enough to be successfully housed.

Another common problem arises when local authority housing departments cannot decide through which channel Travellers should apply for housing. Some insist Travellers apply via homeless services, others that they apply via the standard route as they are not literally homeless. However in a letter to all chief planning officers in England (Ref: PDC 34/2/7 dated May 1998) Richard Jones, Head of the Developmental Control Policy Division of the Department of Environment, Transport and the Regions stated that 'a person is regarded as being homeless if he or she has a caravan but no place where they may legally put it and reside in it'. This may go some way in ensuring that Travellers no longer fall into such gaps in housing policy.

The health visitor's role with Travellers is very varied. Travellers are a demanding group to work with whose culture must constantly be considered prior to every contact.

HEALTH NEEDS OF TRAVELLERS

This section will look at the health needs of Travellers both in a private sense and in the area of public health. It will give details of some of the problems and barriers faced by Travellers concerning their health and try to show why health visitors are well placed to work with this group of people. One of the fundamental roles of the health visitor is to seek out health needs and address them. To do this she must be able to use and give information and secondly to empower people to use this knowledge in their own situation in a constructive way.

Travellers as a group, with some notable exceptions, are disadvantaged in today's society. Socially they are marginalised and criminalised by legislation. Their culture reinforces this in that their first loyalty is to their family and so Travellers are not a cohesive co-operative group and therefore are not organised to work together to improve their social standing within the wider society.

Economically they are also disadvantaged. Many traditional occupations for men have disappeared or become less financially viable (e.g. scrap dealing, labouring on railways and road systems) and many Travellers now are dependent on benefit at least for part of the year.

Educationally Travellers are disadvantaged. The vast majority of Travellers have patchy educational careers and are thus illiterate. As a group they place little reliance on written information, preferring to rely on passing information around verbally. However, illiteracy poses many problems for them when they come into contact with the settled society where documents are regarded as evidence of existence and forms are used to access many different services.

Having demonstrated that Travellers are a disadvantaged group we can turn our attention to their health needs. Fundamentally they have the same health needs as everyone else in society. As with other groups, young families and the elderly are high consumers of healthcare and

Travellers are no exception; however unlike the settled community, which has an aging population, the Traveller community is dominated by the young. Services needed range from the care of the healthy (e.g. contraception and pregnancy) through preventive healthcare measures (e.g. immunisation and health screening) and the needs of the ill (e.g. care of minor illness in children) to the care of the chronically sick. Other commentators have attempted to quantify their needs in terms of morbidity but statistical evidence is very limited. It is thought that Travellers suffer from raised levels of morbidity related to lifestyle and inherited factors as a result of consanguineous marriages and have a significantly shorter life expectancy than the settled population. If asked about their health needs Travellers almost universally respond that their main health need is not based on what medical task needs completing but about how access to healthcare is achieved. This leads us on to a discussion of the public health needs of Travellers.

Public health issues

The most important need Travellers have is somewhere to live. This for many would be a small permanent site where they could live with members of their extended family. Many would choose only to move off for a few weeks of each year – for work, for family reasons or just for a change of scene.

Many would not like to settle at all but pursue a mobile way of life. This involves living for short periods of time in one place while looking for work or dealing with family matters and then moving on. The most suitable accommodation for these families are transit sites or short-term stopping places.

The advantages of sites to Travellers are that they are legitimate places to camp so that:

- they are not continually evicted
- they have a permanent address from which to gain access to services
- they have access to proper sanitation facilities and clean water.

Sites also reduce the amount of discrimination and abuse suffered by Travellers from the general public when they stop in unauthorised areas. Naturally, on the other hand they reduce the nuisance experienced by the local population. Temporary roadside sites have neither of these and so pose a health risk to Travellers and the settled population alike. For professionals working with Travellers, site facilities mean that relationships can be built up with local service providers, e.g. health centres, schools, play facilities and DSS/Social Services. Co-operation and communication can be improved and cross-cultural training can be given to improve understanding on both sides. It also allows resources to be targeted and used effectively. Campaigning to increase the numbers of sites is part of the political role taken on by specialist health visitors.

Activity is usually undertaken in three ways. Firstly, there is the development of interagency groups working together at a local level. These usually comprise representatives from public health, local council officers responsible for eviction, education for Travellers, health (usually the health visitor) and housing. Sometimes representatives from police and social services attend. The group seeks to influence policy changes within the local council with regard to site provision and planning.

Secondly, health visitors play a significant role in raising the awareness of individuals from many organisations with which Travellers often need to liaise. Many individuals working with statutory organisations discriminate against people whose lifestyle they judge as meaningless and it is the role of those who work with and know the community to challenge this behaviour and attempt to resolve it. Thirdly, there is a National Association for Health Workers with Travellers (NAHWT), which seeks to influence national policy towards Travellers, particularly with regard to discriminatory legislation concerning lifestyle, and planning and site provision. This group acts as a consultative body commenting on any new policy documents concerning Traveller issues.

From a public health perspective sites for Travellers would allow campaigns such as home, road and play safety to have a focus and also ensure that campaigns targeted at the wider literate population could be directed at Travellers, e.g. folic acid, meningitis awareness.

Finally, with regard to benefits, contrary to popular belief Travellers often do not receive benefits to which they are entitled, such as child benefit, attendance allowance and disability living allowance. Many benefits to which families are entitled can be sent only to a private address, i.e. not a post office or PO box, and post is not delivered to mobile illegal stopping places. Some families use the address of a relative to receive post, but for some it may be necessary to use the health visitor base as a secure address through which to receive mail.

Problems with benefits are usually concerned with verification of people's identity and postal addresses; sites that have correct postal addresses would go some way to solve these problems.

BARRIERS TO HEALTHCARE

Access

Having discussed the health needs of Travellers in depth, what are the problems that create barriers to health? Access to healthcare is regularly denied to Travellers on the grounds of having no permanent address. Primary healthcare is organised (usually) on the basis of GP practices covering geographical addresses and remuneration is received per head of population. After this, remuneration is given on items of service. Although temporary registration is available this may also depend on postal address. Commonly Travellers are denied access on these grounds alone. However, our experience is that there is a commonly held belief that Travellers do not accept preventative health measures such as immunisation, health screening, etc.; this mistaken view discourages GPs from registering Travellers even on a temporary basis, as they believe that this will prevent them meeting targets and consequently affect their remuneration.

These difficulties with registration lead the health visitor to be frequently in contact with the local health authority requesting GP allocation forms and completing these on the client's behalf. However when clients are allocated in this way GPs are obliged only to offer care for a minimum of 3 months, in the same way as temporary registration, and can then remove them from their list. The whole procedure then begins again.

It may be difficult for health visitors to influence this situation greatly. It is possible to visit GPs local to the newly arrived site and discuss the situation and this can often be useful for both Travellers and GP practice alike. However, Travellers often find GPs who are sympathetic to their situation and where they receive a positive experience. They will then contact them again as will their families and other members of their community. This usually only involves one or two practices. Consequently the health visitor is able to liaise closely and ensure that relationships are maintained and any intervention considered necessary by the GP is properly communicated to the Travellers. It is possible to maintain quite a high level of care in this way.

The major problem for many Travellers with regard to healthcare is their inability to register permanently with a GP. People with no permanent address are unable to register permanently with a GP, and if an individual has no permanent GP they are not issued with a medical card. Many Travellers do not realise that without a medical card they still have a right to be seen by a GP (in Ireland this is not the case, which often leads to confusion).

Mobile Travellers are generally registered temporarily with GPs for a period not exceeding 3 months. This type of registration leads to difficulties for the client as many GPs are unwilling to refer temporarily registered patients for consultant appointments and many preventative services such as cervical cytology and breast screening are regulated via the health authority, whose listings are of permanently registered patients only, thereby further denying access to services.

Traveller Gypsies are often viewed by GPs and society in general as demanding and difficult. Practices become concerned that if Travellers are accepted on to their caseload permanently, immunisation and health screening targets will not be achieved, thus affecting the practice budgets, although in our experience if Travellers can gain access to these services the uptake rate is good.

It is too early yet to give any opinion on whether primary care groups will go some way to change this problem of difficulty of access for Travellers.

CULTURE

Within the primary care relationship, culture plays a great part and where cultures meet misunderstandings and discrimination can occur on both sides. Work with Travellers is defined by their own agenda and there are both positive and negative aspects of their cultural attitude to health. It is here that health visitors try to bridge the gap. A health visitor is the most common response by health authorities or trusts to work with Travellers. Some work specifically with Travellers and others have some dedicated time for Travellers alongside the demands of their own caseload. What all health visitors for Travellers deal with is that they are from an outside culture working within another. It is vitally important not to lose sight of the positive aspects of Traveller culture when trying to help them access healthcare designed for a different culture – and in circumstances in which Traveller culture is not viewed positively by wider society.

Positive aspects of Traveller culture are based on their many strong family relationships. Most families help support each other with care of children, the elderly and the ill and would not expect statutory services to take over that role. Also, family life is the mainstay of their lives, with children being regarded as central to this. Children are thus cared for and protected by the whole community, with all members taking responsibility. Occasionally the NHS culture clashes when Travellers are not aware of the structure and functioning of health services, e.g. specific appointment times and appointments that only cater for one person, *not* the whole family. Travellers also have high expectations of what primary care can offer or achieve and so are regarded as demanding of services. Health visitors

are fundamental in advising Travellers of the limitations of what is possible or available and have to try to work in partnership with them concerning their health.

PARTNERSHIP AND EMPOWERMENT

These two areas of a health visitor's work – to empower clients to act independently and make their own choices about health and also to work in partnership with clients – are not easy to achieve with Travellers. Their lack of knowledge and the barriers to services that exist preclude them exercising choices at the moment, although with continuous health visiting intervention future generations will hopefully develop these skills.

Specialist health visitors for Travellers form relationships with all members of large extended families and often find themselves working with clients in different parts of the country – especially where there is no health visitor provision. In this way influence filters through several generations and they in turn learn how to use health services appropriately and for their benefit.

As for working in partnership together, this is difficult where clients have limited skills and where the structure of services and society generally seeks to prevent it. Generic health visitors can only create limited partnerships because their contact with Travellers is usually only brief, while the camp is in their area. In this situation the health visitor usually has to deal immediately with any needs the Travellers may express.

As a specialist covering a wider area the health visitor will probably have contact with a group over a longer period. In this situation it is easier to facilitate Travellers to deal with their own health needs by giving them the information they need, paving the way with relationships and prompting them to act. As Travellers learn to function independently they carry this information and skills with them as they travel to different places.

Already discussed have been rules and regulations surrounding access to GP care, and problems when clients cross trust boundaries when they move camp – particularly when being referred to secondary or paramedical care. These issues have both organisational and financial implications for health authorities and trusts.

ETHICAL ISSUES

Finally, health visitors will face some ethical dilemmas when working with Traveller families. Certainly, many members of society would say that if Travellers settled on sites or in housing their difficulties with access to services would cease. Certainly with some families with multiple needs and difficulties health visitors would agree. This can create dilemmas when needs are apparent and cannot be met simply because of the mobile nature of their lifestyle. In this situation solutions are found by working flexibly across all agencies and also, with regard to health, across community and acute health trusts. Individual solutions are tailored to each different situation. However only by educating other professionals across the country to respect the family's choice of lifestyle and seeking to work with them to confront these difficulties can any progress be made.

Other issues that can be equally problematic are the interrupted education of children due to mobility and the very limited play opportunities for preschool children. Many Travellers now acknowledge that education is of benefit to their children but it is unusual, though not unknown, for children to attend school after the age of 11–12 years. Travellers tend to see the benefit of literacy rather than education in its wider sense, and Travellers alerted by visual media fear that if their offspring attend secondary education they may become involved in substance abuse, sexual abuse and other reported problems, which they view as inherent in general society. Traveller children, however, are educated for life and work from a very early age, and their knowledge of what would be deemed adult skills such as extended child care (girls) and the value and subsequent selling of scrap metal (boys) are far in advance of the average non-Traveller house-dwelling child. By nature of the limited space available in caravans and the poor environ-

mental conditions outside many toddlers spend considerable amounts of time confined in caravans or strapped into car seats. As a health visitor it is difficult not to acknowledge parental concerns of safety and a pragmatic approach to protecting their children but also difficult to see the curbing of a toddler's natural desire to learn by investigating his environment.

These issues of a safe place to play are hard to address. However, many permanent sites, particularly small, privately owned family ones, do make play areas available. On temporary roadside sites the situation is impossible to alter, as it would only be by the provision of transit sites for mobile Travellers where safe play facilities could be provided that any difference could be made.

SPECIALIST HEALTH VISITORS WITH TRAVELLER FAMILIES

Health visitors working solely with Traveller Families are not an extravagance: it has been found that they represent value for money, for the following reasons:

- they are knowledgeable about Traveller lifestyle and culture and therefore will not offend families by asking unacceptable questions or giving inappropriate responses; in short they give appropriate care acceptable to Traveller culture
- they become known to families, who often have had very negative experience of authority, including healthcare workers – they become known to be trustworthy and stand or fall by their reputation among large extended family networks
- they act as a resource for peer groups and other professions within and outside the health service
- they are able to carry out cross-boundary work to encourage continuity of care – they often act as a link between services that may otherwise find it difficult to locate families
- they have national knowledge and connections with other health visitors for Travellers around the country, enabling networking and further continuity of care

- there is evidence that if it were not for health visitors' work, Travellers would not receive preventative care such as immunisation, family planning and antenatal care
- the health visitor's role can ensure investigation and follow-up for families with specific difficulties
- the community is receptive to health promotional ideas and again health visitors are at the forefront in disseminating this information
- the advocacy role of health visitors is another success and applies equally to dealing with other agencies such as the Department of Social Security and housing departments, as discussed in previous sections.

At a local level health visitors take a major role in ensuring that health needs are considered before eviction of camps, particularly with regard to the access of women about to give birth to hospitals and follow-on midwifery care. Circular 18/94, *Gypsy Sites Policy and Unauthorised Camping*, issued by the Department of the Environment in November 1994, reminded local authorities of their obligations to Traveller families under other legislation such as the Children Act 1989, the Housing Act 1985 and various circulars from the Department of Education. Circular 18/94 suggests that, prior to eviction of unlawful encampments, local authority officers should liaise with other relevant statutory agencies who may be involved in these families' welfare, prior to a decision being made regarding eviction.

For example, families who have a newly delivered woman among them should not be evicted until such time as the statutory services have fulfilled their obligations. In practice, local authorities may request information from professionals involved with the families' care but then evict all the families in trailers other than the trailer in which the newly delivered woman is living – it is highly unlikely that this action would result in the woman staying: as the local authority is aware, she will move off to be with the rest of her extended family. This 'consideration' of health needs also applies to families

with a member suffering from severe illness or in hospital or requiring other community health services, e.g. district nursing.

There are many successes at a local level that are due to health visitor intervention. Two points need to be made. Firstly, successes are local and due to personal activity; change in national policy is far harder to achieve and this will be discussed more fully in the next section. Secondly, and contributory to this lack of national success, health visitors are not well placed nor supported to collect data or evaluate their activity to provide any statistical or proven evidence of the effects of their interventions nor of the health needs they encounter. Although the number of families/individuals may be fewer than those seen by the generic health visitor the actual input per capita is much higher, resulting in little quantitative data, only qualitative. This makes it difficult to present the case of Travellers as a supported argument rather than as a statement of what workers know to be true.

NATIONAL POLICY CHANGE
Current problems

There has been no national policy change to improve the position of Travellers in society. Indeed, current legislation in the form of the 1994 Criminal Justice and Public Order Act serves to criminalise their lifestyle further and allows harsher penalties. Legislation combined with discrimination and the cultural inability of Travellers to organise into cohesive pressure groups has prevented social change from occurring despite activity by those who work with them and seek to represent them.

Politically, mobile Travellers have no voice in that they have no vote and Traveller issues are regarded as vote losers for local councillors seeking to represent residents. It is also appropriate to mention that Travellers are not included in the national census. There is thus no information available to highlight government policy changes that may be necessary.

Travellers themselves have little expectation of wider society and feel powerless to influence what happens to them as a community. This can mean that they lack motivation to meet the demands made of them and so misunderstandings can occur with the rest of society, e.g. assistance with taking their children to school.

Attempts to influence or alter policy are usually made by partnerships between health, education, environment, public health and civil rights groups. It is hard for Travellers to join these partnerships because of their lack of experience of the democratic procedure and because of their illiteracy.

Possible solutions

Policy needs to be altered nationally in terms of site facilities and the availability of transit sites and an attempt should be made to combat the prejudice and discrimination experienced by this group of people. The position of GPs and primary care has already been discussed, as has the value of specialist health visitors to work with Travellers.

Policy makers should be made aware of the way reform of the NHS has increased the inflexibility of services, thus preventing access to secondary care by marginalised groups with no named GP. It is now difficult to achieve direct access to maternity units and other services because of financial barriers. This has removed one of the major ways in which health visitors worked to allow Travellers increased access to care, with the result that much time is wasted finding a GP who is willing to refer people to hospital.

It is clear that health visitors are the main deliverers of services to Travellers. Notwithstanding the previous discussions of how national policy towards Travellers needs to be altered in order to offer them equality of access to healthcare and meet their health needs, it is worth considering how health visitors alone can improve their service to Travellers.

Over the years a common response has been to take the service to them, i.e. to use mobile facilities. Although the advantage of this is that once on a site the Travellers are able to seek a service spontaneously and do not have to travel anywhere else, the disadvantages are that a full range of services cannot be offered and as a result Travellers are again not treated equally. It is not usual for these services to have a GP with them and so problems with access to primary care still exist. The other disadvantage is that often funding is removed from these facilities, particularly if there is a wide fluctuation in uptake, which naturally occurs with mobile groups.

Other changes that would improve the situation greatly would be the development of salaried GP/primary healthcare teams specifically employed to work with 'difficult' inner-city populations. These may of course be nurse-led with the advent of advanced practitioners and/or nurse prescribing. However, it may be that these teams/sessions are also intended for use by the homeless, mentally ill and substance-dependent. It is difficult to envisage how appropriate this setting would be for Travellers, whose health needs have already been described as the needs experienced by young families with children.

Health visitor services are already improved for the highly mobile by the use of parent-held records for child-health activity, and women also carry their own antenatal records. It would be ideal if Travellers could carry their own primary care records, particularly those members of the community who suffer from chronic conditions requiring follow-up and regular medication.

WIDEN THE SCOPE OF HEALTH VISITOR PRACTICE

The extended role of the health visitor to include advanced practitioner roles has already been mentioned in this chapter. Within the health visitor for Travellers network this is seen as probably the most likely practical way to improve Traveller health in the short term, notwithstanding the need to keep up political pressure for policy change. Although most health visitors have other practical skills, e.g. midwifery and family planning, it is in the area of diagnosis and treatment of minor illness that an extended role would be so useful with Travellers. This also introduces the subject of nurse prescribing.

As has already been discussed, access to health care is the overriding problem Travellers have to face and health visitors are usually their most positive and regular health contact. It is very frustrating to be able to tell a parent that their child is suffering from a minor skin condition, e.g. thrush, eczema, ringworm, impetigo, and then to have to advise them to find a GP to prescribe for them as you cannot do it yourself. It is true that issues of funding would have to be solved and decisions made over prescription of over-the-counter medicines, e.g. paracetamol, nappy rash creams and head lice treatments.

CONCLUSIONS

Much has been written about the effectiveness of health visitors and how that effectiveness can be measured. It is extremely difficult to assess the impact of the intervention of a health visitor on parenting. As described in the section on partnership and empowerment, it is possible to be positive about the impact of health visiting on Travellers' lives and its influence across generations, with regard to health. As Travellers have more contact with health visitors influence can be brought to bear on their cultural patterns of child-rearing.

In the wider population, evidence can be shown of the health visitor's impact on public health, e.g. the nutritional requirements of babies, children and their mothers, hygiene and sanitation issues, the use of family planning to space children and reduce the size of families, and most recently the campaign to reduce cot deaths. Health visitors may not have been the instigators of these campaigns and may well have not done the research but it is they who carry these messages day after day into people's homes.

It may be possible to audit a health visitor's day-to-day work with Travellers by looking at issues raised by Travellers and assessing the amount of time spent by the health visitor in dealing with problems raised by her clients. Although not designed to evaluate the effectiveness of the role, it will demonstrate the breadth of needs met by the health visitor and highlight those issues where the health visitor is not in

a position to help. It is hoped that this will show how the service is used by Travellers and what if any extra resources would improve it.

Services could further be monitored using the already existing data collection models based on ethnicity. Certainly this would demonstrate birth rates, death rates and use of secondary care services. However, Travellers are well aware of the settled population's dislike of them as a group and would understandably be reluctant to describe themselves as Traveller/Gypsy on official forms or to figures in authority. It would be unwise to expect those who complete forms with clients to decide a person's ethnicity merely on appearance or accent. In Birmingham consideration has been given to using a particular post code (e.g. B99) or even to using one nationally to encompass anyone giving a caravan site address (whether official or unauthorised), but this would exclude all those Traveller/Gypsies who use a relative's or spurious address when asked in an attempt to make services more accessible for themselves.

It is clear that health visiting practice, as with all professional practice should be evidence-based and grounded in research. It is not always possible to research or prove as fact all aspects of health visiting. As already indicated earlier in these conclusions, the impact on health and parenting of health visiting is hard to assess but should not be underestimated.

Research with Travellers has many practical problems to overcome. Briefly these are a lack of verifiable records due to problems with accurate names and dates of birth, and little opportunity for longitudinal data collection due to Travellers' high mobility. This is combined with generally poor history/life events recall by Travellers. Because of the use of family names within extended families, the possibilities for duplication of data are endless. Lastly, Traveller illiteracy at such a high rate does not allow any questionnaire-style surveys.

As already indicated, systematically collected data would give epidemiological evidence of morbidity and mortality. If these data were available then a true health needs assessment would be achievable.

Finally, further qualitative research could investigate Traveller health beliefs, potentially around their attitudes to preventative health measures, e.g. antenatal care and uptake of immunisation. If preventative care beliefs were investigated there would be an achievable outcome of possibly an ethnic/community attitude to these measures, which would better inform practice and service delivery. If a more comprehensive interview of health beliefs was undertaken, such as beliefs about illness, medical treatment and personal attitudes to and responsibilities for health, it might be possible to assess a community attitude to health that would render the need for epidemiological data collection superfluous.

FURTHER READING

Bedford HE, Jenkins SM, Shove C, Kenny PA 1992 Use of an East End children's Accident and Emergency Department for infants: a failure of primary health care. Quality in Health Care.

Birmingham FHSA 1993 Public Health Report, ch 3 Traveller families' health

Bliss HA 1982 Primary care in the emergency room: high in costs and low in quality. New Engl J Med 306: 998

Cohen J 1987 Accident and emergency services and general practice – conflict of co-operation. Fam Practit 4: 81–83

Dale J 1992 Primary care: the old bugbear of accident and emergency services. Br J Gen Pract 42: 90–91

Green J, Dale J 1992 Primary Care in Accident and Emergency and general practice – a comparison. Soc Sci Med 35: 987–995

Morgan W, Walker JH, Holohan AM, Russell IT 1974 Casual attenders: a socio medical study of patients attending accident and emergency departments in the Newcastle upon Tyne area. Hosp Health Serv Rev 70: 180–194

Myers P 1982 Management of minor medical problems and trauma: general practice or hospital. J Roy Soc Med 75: 875–883

National Audit Office 1992 Report of the Comptroller and Auditor General: NHS Accident and Emergency Departments in England. HMSO, London

Safe Childbirth for Travellers, June 1992 Joint action to stop eviction of Traveller mothers and babies. Information Pack

Save the Children Fund 1993 Bringing up children in a Traveller community. Leeds Traveller Project, Leeds

Watson P 1994 The Organisation and Delivery of Health Care Services for Gypsy and Traveller Families in the West Midlands. Report for the Association of West Midlands Community Health Councils Surveys and Information Committee

18

Choice and opportunity in health visiting

Karen Reeves Attwood

INTRODUCTION

Choice and opportunity is the vista that opens up for the practitioner as s/he moves beyond the baseline of training and first development in integrating skills to a wider level of practice. Making the right choices at this level can only follow once the opportunities are fully understood. In this chapter there will be discussion of four key areas that have determined these openings for health visitors, with particular interest in the changes in public health and primary healthcare delivery that have taken place in the last 9 years.

Overall, it is the ability to effectively analyse the context in which practitioners find themselves that clarifies the opportunities for each person and their team. Higher level practice demands the ability to take informed choice through to the wider context. It is the key tenet of this author that examining choices for the best option we can find entails considerable effort that reflects contextually specific opportunities. The issue of values and consequent priorities is important, and appreciating that this is the case is the assumed point of departure. As higher level practitioners it is not sufficient to 'care' and let others decide how or even if that care is available. What is involved in work that has traditionally sought the improvement of people's health is the recognition that this is a value in itself. There is nothing to be ashamed of in this. As Titmuss explains: 'There is no escape from values in welfare systems.... Not only is "policy" all about values but those who discuss problems of policy have their own values (some would call them prejudices)' (Titmuss 1974, p. 132).

These values that drive choices are seen here as influenced by three factors – history, culture, and social power. These three themes are critical to problem definition when examined as the basis of social research. It is the influence of these factors that will be used as reference in the examination of the sections outlined above. Historically, a new epoch has been announced by the current government in recent legislation and other documents, yet the trends are apparent in earlier events. The cultural shifts of health visiting and primary care work are perhaps more easily seen as spanning decades rather than single years. Social power is examined in terms of feminist thinking.

All these strands of this overview of the choices and opportunities for health visiting come together over the practitioner's ability to deliver, whatever the context limitations or openings may be. This chapter therefore seeks to outline some of the missed opportunities and to offer suggestions where choice may still be fruitfully exercised. Using the diversity of practice available, choice and opportunity are there for the taking if practitioners have the determination to channel this into coherent and cogent work.

The response of the health visiting profession in practice can be understood in terms of its principles of practice with the emphasis on the role of searching and stimulating awareness for health needs, influencing health policies, preventative work and facilitation of health-enhancing activities (CETHV 1977, p. 9, Robinson 1982).

SEARCHING AND STIMULATING

Kathy has worked for 4 years to set up a well-validated women's resource centre of which there are 16 up and running in the country. 'Getting funded' is the big issue, and the bad news is that her presentation failed at the second stage of the bid round. Later she hears that, despite having a good approach, there was 'not enough pathology in the presentation'. She has to return to the local women's group, who are frustrated since they had worked jointly on the bid. One of them astutely remarks that going up to the Council house was a bad move, they should have made the funders come to them. Sadly

Kathy reflects on her failure to see this opportunity. She hears from her local social worker colleague who has a Council contact: 'Sorry, there's not the political will. They'd rather fund the Smileymum project, its cheaper'. Kathy thinks now that she needed to understand these issues better; perhaps this failure in the funding round was in fact about not being political enough. Or would the support of the local GP (who hadn't come to any meetings, although invited) have helped?

INFLUENCING HEALTH POLICIES

Julie has really enjoyed the work of the specialist play and support group she has run with community physios and the help of the speech therapy service, incorporating a linkworker and learning disability nurse together with a nursery nurse student, for the last 2 years. The group is targeted towards a small but significant minority ethnic group in the area whose children, aged up to 3 years, have an identified special need. The mothers come for a brief time each week to break their social isolation and the burden of stigma that handicap has proved to be for them, from experiences shared in the group, which are informally recorded and written up with the women's permission. She is delighted to be invited to a specialist conference and jointly present the model of collaborative working that has been developed. Later the Health Authority invites a further presentation for a visitor from the Department of Health, and an article is requested for a journal. Julie reflects that the outcomes of the group are much more wide-ranging than she had expected.

PREVENTATIVE WORK

Pamela is the new health visitor attached to the practice of Dr Reyhat. The practice has a clinicians' meeting every week, something new to Pamela, who has considerable health visiting experience. She attends each week but takes little notice when mention of the local mosque is made since she assumes that this is probably a private religious matter. She passes the mosque each week but has little idea of what it is all about, but eventually she becomes curious and so starts asking questions of the other practice staff. The practice nurse looks blank at first, and then explains that a small team of staff visit the mosque regularly. For the past 3 years the practice has been working with the people who go to this mosque about the difficult issue of intercousin marriage and related high levels of congenital defect and incidence of other hereditary disorders, e.g. beta-thalassaemia. Dr Reyhat and the small team give advice and medical care; there has been some indications of real impact recently. Dr Reyhat has been asked to share his work with managers from the Health Authority. Pamela is embarrassed. How come she did not know about this? The practice nurse sees her discomfort and says, in an attempt to comfort her, 'Don't worry, we were going to talk to you about it but you seemed busy with that project of yours'. Now Pamela is really distressed since 'the project' was the profile she had proudly presented to her trust manager only that very morning (Bundey & Alam 1993).

FACILITATION OF HEALTH-ADVANCING ACTIVITIES

The practitioner of the future? What is your response? ... So many others telling how it should be.... As we near the end of this text perhaps it is time to put ourselves centre stage ... the change agent is you.... Like all good fairy tales or fables the hero/ine has to discover his/her own skills. Where are the limits to my higher-level practice? What are the resource restraints? Do I understand the politics of health as they impact on my clients in my local situation? What goodies do I have to sell and where are my allies to be found? Whatever my personal style, am I ready to develop practice appropriate to the needs of the most vulnerable of the population? Could that higher level practitioner they keep talking about be me? If not, how do I get to that stage?

INFLUENCE OF ECONOMIC RESTRAINTS ON THE DEVELOPMENT OF PUBLIC HEALTH IN HEALTH VISITING

Higher level and specialist practice can only develop where there is recognition by policy makers, those implementing and applying policies in practice, of some of the wider issues that may determine what work will be undertaken, otherwise there is the question whether existing commitments will be allowed to continue. Availability of and allocation of resources to fund public health work in health visiting to date have been on an informal basis, with varying levels of recognition of this professional expertise. Work in teams has given the clearest expression of a delineated public health role, as in the former work of the Strelley team in Nottingham (Boyd et al 1993). Where managers decide budgets, this variability and uncertainty forms a key factor in the continuation of a trend such that actual public health strategies are often project-based, without using and investing in the available expert skills of staff already working in health visiting. Erosion of the public health role is, however, also the responsibility of the professional. It is the author's opinion that it is these factors, together with unexamined historical patterns of funding of the health visiting service and public health needs, that have created the current situation. The skill-mix/grade-mix debate may be proved on the hospital ward, but it appears

that health visiting has not commanded sufficient respect to allow one of its key aspects to have become truly established or develop. The Black Report, produced now some 20 years ago, identified what has become known as 'the inverse care law', and the consequences of the failure to tackle public health issues at the resource level remains (Townsend & Davidson 1988, Weaver 1996).

This section covers economic restraints in the context of the history of health visiting and social trends that influence such economic decisions. In this sense it covers a partly historic and cultural perspective of public health work within health visiting. It also prepares the ground for consideration of what factors underlie some of the very real choices that will be taken about the health visiting services in primary care groups and eventually primary care trusts throughout England. There will also be some discussion of the social power debate, but here in terms of feminism, a theme that the author considers key to understanding why these restraints have come into place and partly why they may well continue.

The need for interventions for the poorest and most vulnerable people in society is the key work for any profession that seeks to deliver on public health. Awareness of the impact of poverty on health has been well researched and directed towards health visitors as a prime target for their work (Blackburn 1991). Development in this work to appreciate the impact of inequalities on various groups such as ethnic minorities (Ahmad 1993, Birmingham Health Authority 1997) only serves to accentuate the urgency with which these issues must be addressed. Health visiting, if it has failed in the arena of public health, may only be reflecting an economic and social understanding that assumed that a wealthy Western economy need not concern itself with the marginalised. In recent years understanding of the issues of relative poverty and social exclusion has grown (Lister 1996).

In terms of health services in the Western hemisphere, compared to many European economies and certainly compared to that of the USA, health visitors' existence and continued funding could lead to the opposite view, namely that there has not been so much restraint as good resourcing of the service. However, recent severe cuts in the funding to health visiting suggest a different picture, with these cuts as the culmination of a long period of restraint in public health work, particularly at fieldwork level (Gloucester Health Authority in 1998 and Cambridge, see below).

If there has been any shortfall in delivering on the public health agenda by health visitors, it could be argued that they only have themselves to blame. However, this would be a severe criticism of the profession as a whole since it would suggest a break with its identity as a profession committed to public health work. However, where resources are allocated may determine what services are delivered, and the link to the primary care team and the GP may be a particularly important issue. This will be further explored below. The last section of the chapter will progress the discussion by examining the impact of policy on health visiting practice in the broadest sense, taking the view that developments are punctuated by policy changes and not always as a result of these high-level decisions.

Health economics is a growing discipline in its own right. This section seeks not to analyse the economics of public health finance but to appreciate the context about what 'opportunity cost' choices have been taken and to discuss some of the factors contributing to these choices. The term 'opportunity cost' is being used here as key, in the central issue of economics that addresses the challenge of scarce resources, where: 'resources used by an intervention could always be put to other uses' (Øvretveit 1998, p. 110).

The concern is that health visiting practice may not be advancing towards a fuller expression of public health work but rather repeating its past failure to develop. It is this that may lead to a severe contraction of the service. The opportunities lost in the past could be the restraints that continue into the future, where health visiting and public health do not flourish. This came into sharp focus with the harsh choice of Cambridge Health Authority to severely cut their health visiting service in 1997 (*Health Visitor* 1997a). These cuts led to a situation which as far as

public health is concerned has virtually ended the health visiting service. (*Community Practitioner* 1998). In other areas, but less well publicised, there have been attempts to increase the number of health visitors where the service was deemed the most suitable for client need (Littley 1996 – East Thelbridge, Sarah Taylor, personal communication 1996 – Coventry).

The significance of the Cambridge decision is that it was taken across a whole county service and has set a precedent, while similar decisions are still being planned (*Community Practitioner* 1998). The concern is that the entire role was weighed against other services – particularly to children, and was found wanting. Health visitors now find themselves working in the health setting with a mixed remit that can develop in a variety of ways, as suggested in other chapters. Where does this leave health visitors who are ready to advance practice and have concerns for the public health role? They can be clear that it was identification with the less exciting and apparently less dynamic choice of general practice and health over local authority and community development that left them out of the running to influence the public healthcare agenda. The only choice economically was to 'follow the money' to the general practice setting in order to be able to retain preventative care at all, albeit in its largely individual form. Further, because of the increasing trend to follow the medical, individualised model of healthcare, health visitors, who need to give more time to needy clients, became themselves identified with 'the poor'. This meant developing an understanding of the dilemmas that face the poorest and most vulnerable in society but also the loss of power that is often associated with such commitment. A sense of invisibility is a feature of this situation and so health visitors come not to be identified with public health at all. Ashton & Seymour, writing in 1988 about the 'new public health' make no significant mention of health visitors. The King's Fund seminal text *The Nation's Health* subtitled *A Strategy for the 1990s*, mentions health visiting only in relation to health surveillance for children and briefly in relation to elderly care (Smith & Jacobsen 1989, p. 319). It is hardly surprising if health visiting's public health role is under threat when their work is not even recognised.

To recover and develop the public health task it is important to grasp that addressing questions of budget allocation is now a task for any practitioner who seeks to influence the allocation of resources. In England the previous fundholding contracts are changed for GPs and awards of contracts with community health trusts into a unified Budget that is allocated to each primary care group, delineated by the level of responsibility taken on by each primary care group or, as many will soon be, trust. Unless history is to repeat itself, it is important for professionals to effectively brief their boards, including the nurse representative. This needs to include awareness that the assertions made by health visitors about their role are not necessarily widely accepted. The opportunity is present for practitioners to recognise and face the challenges that have at times been avoided, since the locus of control and the means of influencing this are nearer to field level, and budgetary management and information in many services are now held at this level.

Public health in England today finds itself suddenly centre stage within the focus on primary care, and with a minister devoted to its development (Birt, 1997, p. 1). Recognition of public health as more than investment in clean water and effective sewage works has been brought into sharper focus with the health improvement plans now required for each primary care group in England (Department of Health 1997a, p. 5.9). Its neglect mirrors other economic blind spots of the past, such as the significance of ecology and environmental issues, and thus offers a hopeful sign for health visitors. Positively, this could lead to an evaluation and recognition of the often hidden skills that health visitors can offer in turning public health aims into deliverable objectives. The wider context that determines economic decisions is particularly relevant here. The serious effect that this would have on the whole of British society and the issue of this as a public concern has only recently been acknowledged: 'until recently, few would have predicted

the extent of the devastating social effects of a widening income distribution' (Wilkinson 1994).

Just as the understanding of the impact of relative poverty on all members of society was lost to decision-makers for a significant period of time, its burden on health professionals (and colleagues in social services and education) has had a part to play in the poor showing that health visiting made in public health work. Appreciation of the effects of the increase in relative poverty as outlined, for example, by Trowler (1996, p. 17–18) are keenly felt by fieldworkers. In many ways the failure within health visiting to address this issue of poverty in practice has to be accepted as one of the costs paid for professional survival. Blackburn's work, quoted earlier, continues to have significance for practice development in this area. However such excuses are of little comfort when some of the struggles of clients are understood as directly resulting from economic and resource allocation decisions. It will be interesting to see if the primary care groups develop a wider social perspective, e.g. in concern for the housing of their patients, that do have social services/the local authority represented on the primary care group board. Initiatives within the Housing Association movement suggest that the health issues of their population seriously concern them (*Housing Today* 1998, p. 2). Engagement in public health issues in the future may require a strategic approach that seeks broader alliances and it may be this feature of work that offers health visiting the most hope for its public health remit.

An analysis of the economic context informs decisions made about how public health has been limited in health visiting. The nature of what constitutes healthcare is the signal factor. This has been largely in support of the medical model of symptom management rather than a holistic approach that sees the symptom largely as coming from within a whole-person perspective. This view, discussed in Chapter 2, links to the Western capitalist individual perspective that eschews social models of health. The Welfare State in Britain has certainly modified the impact of this, but issues of prevention have not been addressed.

In terms of culture the public perception of what the service is there for is also of significance here. Nursing, largely committed to hospital care, developed its role and health visitors continued to hold the public health remit but in an increasingly individualised form. There was from the first an inherent tension for health visitors as they moved between treating medical difficulties and preventing ill health while also promoting good health. This is reflected in the official definition of 'medico-social worker' of the Jameson Committee, Ministry of Health Report of 1956. Linked into the primary care setting, public health has suffered by association, since the position primary care occupies vis-à-vis secondary care was not considered as significant for healthcare in the UK, as until recently acute or secondary care was always the main focus. As Barnes (1998), writing in response to the Labour government initiatives in 1997, reminds us: 'The popularity of the NHS in the eyes of the people of the UK, the strength of the medical lobbies and the size of resources devoted to it have enabled the health service to dominate thinking about health as well as illness'.

Cultural norms are often confirmed or even perpetuated by the images, as in the British media coverage of the nurse in a hospital setting as the prime image for 'pressures in the NHS' stories. The considerable difficulties experienced by all community nursing disciplines regarding workload stress are just not deemed newsworthy. This decision is held to by media, no matter what the impact on the service or its patients. Here the hospital takes precedence over the community every time, with acute treatment as key rather than the primary care service. That economics for public health will reflect prejudices of popular thinking should not be any surprise since the government is affected by public opinion, as recent controversy about work and single parents has indicated (Denny 1997).

Further, if the evidence is that health visitors' work has become increasingly distanced from public health, it has to be accepted that preventative work in this country has always tended to be on a macroeconomic scale, with interventions of a microeconomic nature only recently being considered. If health visitors' prime role identifier is public health, to take the contrary view could it be that there was a lack of development in public health itself that has led to stasis? In a world of rapidly changing healthcare, health visiting appears out of date, possibly because public health has also lost impact. The development of public health work in health visiting viewed over history is sometimes talked of as though it was a golden era of exciting innovations. This rosy picture may not be the case, as Symonds (1993) has suggested.

The history of health visiting itself illustrates some of the essential features of the failure to deliver on public health. Allocation of resources to public health started under the aegis of the (usually male) doctor in the direction of the first fieldworkers, with hygiene and sanitation work in the slums of the new industrial cities in the 19th century (Ashton & Seymour 1988, p. 23). This early work, its origins and development have been more fully discussed elsewhere in this text. From these first days the work progressed via the need for fit soldiers for the Boer War so that health and defending the economy were clearly linked and resources were allocated in response to this need. Doctors also progressed to becoming general practitioners but largely on an individual basis (see below). Meanwhile, public health medicine became increasingly specialised, formalised and remote from communities, located more recently in the public health sections of health authorities.

Therefore, at the economic level, high-technology intervention still wins its way over simpler and often cheaper options for improving health – e.g. heart bypass operations versus stop-smoking campaigns. Considerations of the consequences of long-term investment in secondary as opposed to primary care are appropriate in examining situations where choice for initial resource commitment is being made. That these decisions are consequent to prior commitments, e.g. to a wing of a hospital or funding for a medical/surgical infrastructure, are issues that may now enter the area of discussion with the future influence of primary care groups in secondary care. In the West, the medical precedent has been established, so it still appears easier to consider funding intensive hospital care than to address, for example, reduction of smoking in pregnancy that might prevent premature deliveries and other sequelae. Such issues of resource allocation are complicated by difficulties in measuring outcomes (see below), and perpetuated in historical resource allocation that funds secondary care far beyond primary care. This is definitely the case for the Western world where the hidden assumption determining budgetary commitment is that preventive care, as Shenkin puts it, 'doesn't work for the purpose of saving money' (Shenkin 1996, p. 22). This author, examining the issue of rationing in healthcare from an American perspective, expresses well one of the assumptions underlying the culture of economic restraint in resourcing public health work.

An unsophisticated approach counting opportunity cost in ways that exclude the factor of time is of particular relevance to this argument. Health visiting is a service whose benefits are perhaps not discernible in the short term. Inputs need, quite often, to be considered over a lengthy period of time, possibly even over the span of a generation. With greater experience, the use of longitudinal studies and a realisation of the limitations of high-tech medicine, particularly in terms of quality of life, has come a revisiting of preventive and public health strategies. Babies born to mothers who smoke can be treated for their asthma and their glue ear, but it is now clear that it would improve life quality and has actually been proved to be more cost-effective to put in a smoking cessation programme than to pay for the problems that result from smoking in pregnancy (Buck et al 1997).

Rather, it is priority setting in the healthcare agenda's key area of choice and opportunity for health visitors that needs to be understood when seeking to move on an appreciation of factors that have determined the place that public health/health visiting has been given over the years. The argument for the redirection of resources is now strengthened precisely because acute medicine is so expensive. There is very little prospect in saving money, with soaring costs for Western-style healthcare. There is an increased demand for more expensive treatments and the medical market could expand exponentially. Action taken over a number of years to curb prescribing costs in the UK indicate a trend that will spread (Ferguson 1997). Basically, as summarised by Bruce & Jonsson (1996, p. 105) the traditional approach is not 'cost containing, efficient or effective enough'.

The development of primary groups and trusts, as units covering populations of 100 000 or so, much smaller than many community trusts and possibly losing through economies of scale, will face tough budgetary challenges. In a community health budget, staff costs form the largest part. Bed closures, as in the acute sector, are not an option. Each service in community health must, sooner or later, prove its worth. The choice for health visiting is to prove its case or be cut as an 'opportunity for savings' in primary care budgets.

The influences that limited public health work, economic priorities of a short-term nature and the powerful medical focus supported by popular conception, are all there, as well as the significant male/female divide, which will be considered below. The gender issue affects priority setting in the economic field and possibly most interestingly affects the actual public health/health visiting role. It is the social power issue that affects priority setting in the field of health economics and is, in the opinion of the author, key to appreciation of why these difficulties persist. The historian and social policy analyst Titmuss outlined the changes for women in particular that gave them a possible 36 more years of active life after child-bearing was ended. The 'new and fundamental problems' that this would present for 'makers of social policy', i.e. men, is an indication of the very real threat that greater economic freedom represented to policy makers of that time – women would want to work (Titmuss 1952).

The struggles that feminists from Beatrice Webb, Amelia Earhart, Betty Friedan, Kate Millett and others to Germaine Greer have stood for are continued by women today still trying to break through the 'glass ceiling made of lead' (Caulkin 1999). Even for 'postfeminists' the 'small detail' of equal pay is agreed to be an outstanding issue

(*Today* 1999). Paying attention to what money goes where is important and the author agrees with polemical writers like Kathy Letts who see the feminist issue as still very much alive. It only serves to confirm that the 'economic restraints' on something women consider important may relate as much to the role of women as to any other issue. To allow women to develop independently as a profession might be possible, to give them power, i.e. resources to undertake change, would be another issue. The impact of these difficulties in professional practice is further considered elsewhere (Davies 1995).

The gender issue becomes therefore a double-bind: the female health visitor was left 'in role' to work closely with the largely female clientele, including children, female parents and possibly the elderly. This oversimplification picks up on the issue of gender identification and feminism as vital to seeing why health visitors were unable to direct resources, possibly even their own work time, that could have funded wider public health. The tendency to become stuck in unhealthy patterns and to see, for example, smoking while pregnant as a private matter may be frighteningly close to the health visitor's choice to concentrate on her caseload and individual clients rather than drawing together the strands for public health interventions. Reflection on the work on women, smoking and health that Blackburn & Graham undertook indicates that under extreme pressure to care yet without the resources to provide what was needed came a reinforcement of the trend of behaviours that the women themselves knew were not beneficial (1992, p. 5). Working with vulnerable clients themselves, health visitors, not surprisingly, can find themselves mirroring their clients' struggles, finding it too hard to develop healthy strategies in their work. Difficulties in priority setting, short-termism, historical patterns of care, have all been considered, but do not explain the strong sense of a power struggle that lies behind much of what has and has not happened in health visiting. Should this feminist focus seem overstated the question has to be asked: what are the other factors that could so prevent an entire profession from fulfilling one of its core tasks?

This limiting of female involvement in the activity that governs resources is confirmed in recent events. It is part of the explanation of the balance of practitioners on boards for primary care groups. These bodies, with a key role in provision of primary care, health promotion and public health, came to be seen as of great significance by the medical establishment. It is deemed essential that GPs once again take the lead role. The White Paper (Department of Health 1997a), denotes both doctors and nurses as leading primary care groups but by the time the guidance on this is received, lobbying by the British Medical Association has reduced this to one or two nurses with four to seven doctors, with the GPs to choose a GP chair. It is the contention of the author that public health work for health visitors has not developed since the health visitor was, albeit loosely in earlier times, linked into the medical framework and there was no political will from the government (the Treasury), colleagues, GPs or the wider public to take this aspect of the NHS forward.

Now opportunity may be presenting for the first time where economics itself, issues of primary versus secondary care, medical versus holistic treatment, the perspective of prevention and the growing expectations of the still predominantly female workforce in health visiting vis-à-vis that of a still predominantly male GP group (at least in those holding partnerships), ready to have their say, can combine to 'open the door' for a dynamic change. Exploration of some of the themes that have emerged recently, offering positive routes beyond this 'door of opportunity', are covered in the following sections of the chapter. Consideration of the need for a marketing strategy for health visiting is hardly surprising, but it forms part of these positive openings in the healthcare field that health visitors are seeking to exploit. This will be examined in the next section.

MANAGEMENT, CONTRACT CULTURE, COMMISSIONING AND MARKETING

The introduction of fundholding was the key

change that Bruce & Jonsson, writing about this new culture in 1996 likened to a 'Big Bang'. Consequent on this 'explosion' was a fundamental shift in the locus of the control of community care services. This change to delivery of medical service in primary care was outlined in the NHS and Community Care Act 1990. The formation of what is termed the 'primary-care-led NHS' was initiated here and formally set out later (NHS Executive 1995b). This did not, however, help to resolve the conflicting issues already present in priority setting, handed down with no apparent solutions; fieldworkers had to find their own . Chris Ham has written on the impact of this (Ham 1998) and elsewhere points out the 'risk of fragmentation' for services with the contract culture, often termed more softly as 'purchasing' (Ham 1996, p. 210–211). The breakthrough for health visitors was when it became clear that, in a market, knowledge of the target population for a service, its needs and ways to address them for evaluation of service delivery would be extremely useful. Thus the development of commissioning for health services opened up a unique opportunity for health visitors, although this was not at first apparent. At the time this change was largely seen as presaging a loss of autonomy, and issues around this will be discussed in the next section.

At a local level all the networks and developments for a broad-based primary care service were put under pressure, as a splintering of activities ensued. A development that was designed to give greater freedom to local practitioners did so but at the cost of emerging locally coherent strategies. Weaver, writing as a Locality Manager, saw these 'fundamental and rapid changes' at first hand: 'the introduction of GP fundholding and NHS Trusts has multiplied the difficulties involved in securing a co-ordinated local response to identified health needs' (Weaver 1996, p. 95). Cohen identifies the effect as one of fragmentation by the 'logic' of the market (1996, p. 15).

The perception of threat to health visiting staff at the fieldwork level is reflected in their relatively slow response to these critical changes. As late as 1995 *Health Visitor* has a Professional

Briefing that states: 'Many health visitors and community nurses still feel excluded from the commissioning process for community health services …' (Connolly 1995, p. 70). This exclusion not only reflected the ignorance, low level of confidence or management failure to which Connolly's article alludes but also illustrated some of the fundamental unanswered questions that health visiting faced. Twinn's analysis of health visiting highlights this well. Individual advice giving, environmental control and psychological care form three of her four part roles and paradigms model, adapted from Beattie's work on sociology of health (Twinn 1991). The fourth concept of emancipatory care is of particular interest when public health work is considered. Here knowledge and expertise is shared openly and is of particular use when 'networking with community groups', and Twinn, following Hennessy's work notes that this 'may prove to be a much more effective method of working than the traditional individualistic approach, currently employed by many practitioners' (Twinn 1991, p. 968).

The importance of selecting the appropriate paradigm is emphasised by Twinn and it is having the necessary understanding of one's own practice philosophy that must form the basis for higher level practice. Twinn's concern for this issue underlines the failure of health visitors to face the challenges and to be ready to exploit the opportunities that the new commissioning approach offered. The flexibility is required, so that, without compromising the fundamental principles of practice, work can be directed to exploit opportunities and retain choices. It develops further the self-understanding that higher-level practitioners continually develop as they are able to respond effectively to professional challenges in a cogent manner.

As previously discussed, health visiting was struggling to meet this challenge well, and serious questions continued around funding. Cuts in services appeared, hitherto unprecedented. The fundamental change that came into the NHS with the introduction of the market approach was perhaps a necessary wake-up call for health visiting. To compound matters, basically health visiting activity was not properly known or understood by decision-makers. The launch of the marketing strategy was essential, as summarised in a management consultancy report for the Department of Health: 'The Coopers and Lybrand study reveals a disturbing lack of understanding about the work of health visitors among GPs and health authorities' (Moore 1994, p. 334).

Marketing arose therefore directly out of the situation where insufficient knowledge could seriously impact on a purchaser's decision to cut a service. The expectation of a cascade throughout the country was perhaps not formally achieved but an understanding of the need to speak up and tackle the prevailing thinking has developed.

For a variety of reasons, as discussed earlier in this chapter, public health, the core task, was not mandated or adequately prioritised to develop within health visiting in this period. It is therefore not surprising that the same report 'uncovered a lack of interest in health visiting management and the wider community role of health visitors'. It has to be faced that the continuation of severe service cuts might suggest that the marketing strategy was a flop. However this assumes that a turn-around in perception would come quickly, which is not always the case. The accentuation of the nature of the general practitioner's role that came with GP fundholding was not one that would facilitate this change (see also below). Whatever support health visiting could offer to the commissioning process, clearly a public health task, was seriously compromised by a failure to see the link with this strategic level (Goodwin 1992). More recent developments in the Green Paper *Our Healthier Nation* (Department of Health 1998a) mark a move to a more integrative approach, already prefigured by commissioning. However, the very subtitle, *A Contract for Health*, suggests that there is a continuation with the contract culture – there has not been a complete break with the past and health visitors need to be aware of this. The discussion of outcome measures below follows on from this theme.

This mixed picture has been discussed mainly in terms of health visitors and GPs, yet managers' impact on the service profile needs also to be considered. Many health visitors complain that they could address the challenges more adequately. Yet it was often middle managers who developed and exploited the opportunities available, as in the marketing strategy. It could be expected that management would be readier to respond to the 'contract' culture that developed since 1991, since it was to them that negotiations often fell in fundholding practices. However, at the same time a swathe has been cut through this level of the service, leaving only senior managers and fieldworkers, with a few specialist posts in between. With few such managers remaining, it now falls to health visitors themselves to face the challenge. Today the pressures continue to save on budgets yet still deliver a quality service. The changes noted in the public health strategy of the present government have not diminished these pressures on the managers. Some managers welcome this challenge as a necessary transforming process. 'In my own trust, we have decided to move from a universal service that aims to provide the same level of support to all, regardless of need, to a more targeted service' (Rodrigues 1998, p. 39).

Where this leaves public health work is unclear, but in general, service cuts have not appeared to target public health work as a priority (see above). Significantly, some 9 years after the formal introduction of the contract culture, it is still this culture that remains a determining feature for decisions about service delivery.

The view that health visitors are a threatened service in community healthcare can miss the depth of some of the issues that face primary care as a whole and in the context of developments in fundholding itself. This context is important since the cuts in health visiting have arisen out of this situation. The inception of fundholding was a simple but radical change that resulted in a variety of unforeseen developments, chief among them being the emergence of groups of fundholders and the health authorities' own response. Significantly, health authorities, who were rather out of the government picture in the early stages, began with interested GPs to become more involved in innovative patterns of purchasing. Ham & Willis, writing in the *Health Service Journal* in 1994 noted that, with these developments, 'Each approach has its own distinctive characteristics, but all share a concern to combine the sensitivity of Fundholding with the population focus of HA purchasing' (1994, p. 27).

Over the next few years there was a rapid development that meant, for example, that in the West Midlands research could start to typify certain aspects of primary care and found a coherent pattern in service delivery, while each still retained their own distinct character. Fundholding had not penetrated throughout the region in a uniform way. This 'mosaic', as Smith et al describe it, therefore included multifunds (groups of fundholding GPs) and total purchasing projects (the same but with extended purchasing power), and a variety of commissioning groups – joint, health authority, locality and practice-sensitive. The researchers noted one particular common feature of particular relevance to the health visiting situation: 'a locality focus which was of universal importance' (Smith et al 1997, p. 30). This applied as much to the initiative arising from local need that got the particular development going as in the shift to the primary care team as 'the focus for health commissioning' (Smith et al 1997, p. 30). Some of the pressures on primary care were being experienced by GPs, for a 'primary-care-led NHS' would mean GPs having to bear a considerable burden of responsibility not experienced before. Like health visitors, GPs found themselves with an increased spread of responsibility, which at times appeared to compete and even conflict with their usual clinical focus. Coming up to the present, the new format of management in primary care groups is not without its difficulties. The GP management time required has been likened to the equivalent time for GP work with a population of a city the size of Sheffield (Lilley 1998).

The advantage for health visiting, focused on its public health remit, of this locality and health commissioning focus is clear. It is eminently a part of health visiting work to consider population needs on a locality basis (Chapter 2). The place of health visiting in this market structure, therefore, does not need to be reduced to a simple issue of cost or status. These pitfalls are ones that practitioners must avoid if the 'sales pitch' is not to be spoilt and the 'closure' – delivery of better healthcare to clients – is to be made. Higher level and specialist practice can flourish in this continuing contract culture once what is available for the market is recognised and positively 'sold'. It is a serious misconception to see health visiting as a monolith that cannot adapt. If such an image is perpetuated, it only serves to distance the service from the developments that are actually bringing community healthcare closer to some of the key principles of health visiting work. This is not to underestimate the difficulties, or to determine whether health visiting as it stands in the field of public health and nursing can overcome current constraints. How this may be achieved, with a more detailed consideration of the issue will be pursued in the next section. It is to consider the need to integrate public health into the primary healthcare team that the argument now moves.

THE NEED TO INTEGRATE PUBLIC HEALTH INTO PRIMARY CARE

This section will consider recent research that has sought to develop the basis for a model of public health within primary care. If the wider definition of primary care had always been the norm, it could be argued that there would have been little need to perform any exercise to integrate public health into primary healthcare. It might be, as Starfield (1994) defines it: 'first contact, continuous, comprehensive and co-ordinated care provided to populations undifferentiated by gender, disease or organ system'. However, a significant piece of research undertaken on behalf of the Public Health trust contradicts this view. Their first stage report highlights the difficulty that must be faced as concerns about relative poverty increase and inequalities persist (as Acheson has reported) so that 'the need for primary care to address equity issues is becoming increasingly pressing' (Peckham et al 1996, p. 1).

The authors' identification of a population

focus for initiatives that involve equity, collaboration and participation seem somewhat distant from many practitioners' perception of what primary care currently entails. These three characteristics provide a useful tool to analyse the challenges this situation presents. The term 'primary care' is often used, as their literature review for this research concludes, simply to denote the work of the general practitioner and surgery staff, without reference to wider community health workers. In this sense the move for health visitors' involvement with GPs by attachment to their practice could be seen, positively, as an early part of the opening up of primary care to public health issues.

The recent developments in primary care, with cuts to health visiting, as discussed earlier, have made many practitioners more aware that health visiting needs to argue its case in this context of primary care. Actual changes to service delivery of this nature will continue if the argument for public health in general practice is not won. This section will examine the medical and nursing roles as the two chief stakeholder groups within the primary healthcare team, looking at the GPs' historical progress, in particular with reference to the issue of the integrated nursing team. The broadening of the primary healthcare team towards a commissioning role will be discussed, with particular reference to profiling, which links with the theme of collaboration. Of all the situations for health visitors, involvement in and influence of general practice towards this goal is an opportunity that should be well within every practitioner's grasp. Participation relates to the issue of patient involvement, generally acknowledged as a hugely neglected area, particularly for the health service. Choosing not to engage with these issues is to so limit health visiting that it forms a disservice to vulnerable client groups.

The term 'general practitioner' covers a history of development that reveals some key information for understanding the difficulties of integrating public health to the primary care team and to appreciate the importance of such a move. As Walsh explains, the basic development for general practitioners over their 90-year history

is movement from a GP working alone to 'an organisation providing community based services'. These critical changes began before the founding of the NHS itself, with the Dawson Report of 1920, which stated that the role of the GP should be broadened and a network of primary healthcare centres established (Walsh 1997). As the first point of contact, the GP is recognised as offering a unique commitment to front-line healthcare, and in this sense offers a much valued service. However the criticism from a public health perspective was that this care was still too individualistic, since GPs were, until recently, operating as small businesses with only their own aims to follow, particularly since the new GP contract of 1991. Recent legislation has formally recognised the power of the GP as gatekeeper to services at secondary level (Department of Health 1997a). This will now further increase as almost all the primary care services are brought under the doctor's control. The government has stated the remit: 'Primary Care Groups will be able to take devolved responsibility for a single unified budget covering most aspects of care so that they can get the best fit between resources and need' (Department of Health 1997a, Executive Summary).

This concentration of power and control into GPs' hands is of concern when apparently ill-informed decisions are made about the health visiting service (*Health Visitor* 1997b). It is a concomitant that responsibility for public health needs are following on this for which GPs are not especially prepared. Littlejohn & Victor correctly predicted this outcome when writing on this shift of power in 1996: 'In essence a primary care-led health service will require general practitioners to take a public as well as personal health perspective'.

Equitable service delivery will then be the first challenge for primary care groups. For example, information of prescribing practice will do much to open up these issues, although it will not address why these inequities have persisted or what action the groups will be taking to tackle them. Tackling wider or more pernicious inequalities will perhaps provide a more challenging agenda.

Development of the integrated nursing team was the logical outcome of the pressure discussed above. It also raises the theme of collaboration, but one potentially limited as it includes only nursing. Formerly, practice nurses, district nurses and health visitors operated independently and were largely ignorant of each other's roles. The teamwork sense of the primary healthcare 'team' was often notional. However, worries about cuts made working more closely with GPs, who clearly had greater potential for resources, a more attractive option. The definition offered by a health visitor's professional organisation, now aptly renamed the Community Practitioners and Health Visitors Association was this: 'A team of community-based nurses from different disciplines, pooling their skills, knowledge and abilities in order to provide the most effective care for the practice population and community it covers' (CPHVA 1996).

The opportunity was there – to focus on the health rather than the illness model, introducing concepts via the team to the GP, who has a large number of clients who are currently well but potentially sick (at some time or other). Many practice nurses, frustrated by some of the early health promotion exercises, could prove to be allies. Nursing in the community, employing a holistic model, could only move towards public health. For health visitors, the choice to move nearer their nurse colleagues in practical terms was often seen as a threat, while the title 'community nurse' applied to all in the team was not deemed suitable by some 'health visitors'. The loss of specialist areas of expertise lay behind this view, since, as Forester & Kline note, the teams were often introduced as part of a skill-mix exercise (1997, p. 229). Of course, there were a variety of integrated nursing team developments with varying agendas and motivation. Still, it is important for the issue of integration of public health issues and preventive care that these moves to integration are recognised as opportunities to influence decisions made about how public health is integrated into general practice. The advantages are there, as health visitors' experience mirrors GPs in their closeness to patients, with similar high levels of direct patient contact. This area is still one that remains underdeveloped in bridging the gap between the targets of public health and fieldwork experience. Craig's work in this area, seeking to develop a public health model in health visiting, showed a typical reaction: the health visitors felt constrained by the narrow model of care that excluded community work they saw as essential to public health initiatives (Craig 1996).

While considering the issue of integrating public health into primary care, it is useful here to consider an earlier team approach, albeit within the health visiting team, that was undertaken in 1991. The Strelley team in Nottingham developed the service identifying three strands of health visiting – family health promotion and child health, high-intervention work and public health. This followed the model targeting service delivery espoused by Kate Billingham, their then professional development officer. 'We transformed a demoralised unit of individuals into a motivated team of radical health visitors' (Jackson 1994, p. 28).

Such a vision is refreshing. It reflects some of the elements of higher level practice and is still a possible signpost for future development. In Chapter 4, such models for health visiting practice have been discussed at greater length.

Using the challenge of commissioning to take on and develop the health visiting agenda for a service is always an opportunity to be grasped. National recognition for this approach, however, was not sufficient in the face of the shift of power to the GP. The push to fundholding continued and it appeared to be a missed opportunity, since health visitors required adequate numbers of staff within a team to create a post focused on public health. This confirms that one or two health visitors in isolation may not be able to adequately effect a public health initiative. The difficulty for integrated nursing teams may well centre on whether team members understand each other's concerns or share each other's commitments. The higher level practitioner should lead the team professionals' ability to see the wider view and be able to network effectively with colleagues. However, this may place too large a burden on one single team; staff in primary healthcare teams alone may not have the capacity to either generate or sustain such work.

Having a good baseline indicator of health need is an essential task for public health work. Caseload, workload, practice and population profiling have been long seen by health visitors to be their remit and acknowledgement of the contribution that a health visitor has to make here has considerably progressed in the last few years from the concerns Goodwin expressed in 1992: 'But in all this documentation there is little reference if any to the use of the mass of information about health need which is already gathered and being used by community nurses in many community units or provider trusts' (1992, p. 78). Close fieldwork experience is of particular importance in highlighting hidden pockets of deprivation or understanding key features of a community. This facility can be used for a caseload of various health workers or in the more generic view of the practice population and a community profile. This opportunity, to make the basic first step of assessment may have been threatened initially by the greater integration of health visitors into primary healthcare teams. Billings examines 18 examples of profiling, assessing each approach within the context of this task 'in collection and interpretation of health-related information', but concludes: 'it is important to remember ... It is about translating identified needs into service provision' (Billings 1996, p. 48).

It is not surprising, therefore, that the inception of health improvement plans has been hailed as significant in bridging this theory/practice gap. These offer a significant advantage over all profiles in that there are plans that will have targets built into them. To date the means of implementation are unclear. The significance here for the implementation of public health plans is that integrated nursing teams and the changes for GPs may promote a fresh approach to working practice, which is required for public health strategies to become more than beautiful annual reports. The significance of primary care groups, based on population groups rather than fundholding practices, becomes clear, for only now can the health visitor make the most of devel-

oping in practice the insights she has into public health. It remains to be seen, however, whether the new configurations will actually be enabling in this respect. Working with the general practice in population profiling work is perhaps still an essential requirement if public health issues are to be understood (see above).

Turning the phrase and therefore the notion of 'public health' around is to identify the key issues that continue to haunt many initiatives. The 'health of the public' identifies to whom the issues actually belong. There is a need for public participation in health strategies, often referred to as the user perspective. Cowley summarises this concern: 'The idea of "partnership" is stressed in the policy documents, but only in relation to general practitioners working in partnership with health authorities, primary healthcare teams and NHS Trusts, rather than with the people they serve' (Cowley 1997, p. 89).

The publication of a booklet about 'many examples' of good practice, called *Involving Patients* (CanagaRetna 1997, p. 3), does little to change this view, since the majority of the activities appear to be rather passive in nature and have not penetrated into wider usage. Therefore it is important to note that, despite the rhetoric this issue generates, from the point of view of the primary healthcare team it does remain just that. At least it is written about, and can be used as a springboard to action. Health visitors advocating community development as a means of tackling public health issues have of course, long supported user participation (Mackereth 1996, Brown 1997). Even so, their work was not widely recognised as such for reasons discussed earlier in this chapter. The scope of the need and the many difficulties clients have therefore to face do not mean it is the same task for a health visitor as a market researcher conducting a pleasant focus group organised in a hotel by a consumer survey company, for example. Many user surveys do not get to the real issues, as McIver suggests (1993).

The current focus of government on user involvement can seem exciting except that it is couched in the language of the contract. This now involves government, local players and communities and people (Department of Health 1998a, p. 40). Each has a set of responsibilities, yet once again a certain doubt persists. Who 'signs up' to these tasks and how is the 'contract' monitored? It is to the health authorities that much of this responsibility may well fall. This falls outside the area of current discussion, but in order to develop proper user-friendly involvement of local community in the health improvement plans, much more than one member on the primary care group board is required. Local authority initiatives seem to have a lot to teach the health service; the work in Stockport, a development that linked an environment-friendly initiative to walking, fitness and local knowledge and was both simple and effective, may have essential pointers for any successful strategy (Swann et al 1997). Making the links in public health in this way is most significant for users, most of whom have no incentives apart from their own personal perceptions to change behaviour.

If integration of public health into general practices is a prime goal, its mode of achievement remains somewhat unclear. The work of the public health trust referred to earlier produced a second-phase report after research was undertaken in four areas of Britain to examine some of the key features for the roles of participants in developing integration of public health into primary care. Their conclusions were critical of the drive towards giving control of this agenda to general-practice-based approaches, seeing them as ill equipped to meet the challenge that this situation demanded (Peckham et al 1998, p. 14). This is alluded to in earlier chapters, but here it is important once again to note that the experience of being disempowered was a noted feature of health visitors and other workers in their work with the general practitioner. Sadly, and all too often, it is a gender-based reinforcement of the relative power available to the stakeholders in the primary care team that is played out in such scenarios.

Thus while the broadening out of the primary healthcare agenda opened the opportunity to a local public health strategy, historical patterns of care inherited by the GP, focusing on individual patient care, continue to dominate the work of the primary healthcare team. Yet the physical proximity now more usually the case, with most health visiting and practice staff sharing premises, and with the current pressures in the NHS for change, particularly in primary care, provides some potential for a sense of commonality and possibly the development of a shared culture. Since once again in primary care groups it is the GPs who have been given the lead, it is appropriate here to be critical of their ability to deliver on the public health agenda. While there have been, at least in certain areas of England, positive moves forward in the field of collaboration, the theme of participation by users shows that a long way has yet to be travelled. Again it is necessary to remember that the exclusion of women workers, as previously discussed and also in primary care groups, can be taken as an indication of the general failure to integrate public health into the primary healthcare team. In this context it clearly relates to failure to address the challenge of inequalities of health for the wider population. The opportunities to engage therefore carry ever greater significance – getting involved in this new version of the contract culture of health will be a real test for health visitors and requires particular competencies. It is to two significant areas of these required skills that the final section of this chapter will now turn.

THE INFLUENCE OF POLICY DIRECTIVES ON HEALTH VISITING PRACTICE

There are three critical themes in the influence that health visiting at a higher level can exert and where future opportunities exist – the notion, briefly, of what policy is, followed by two areas in which greater competency is required and must be acquired by health visitors if their service is not to be marginalised: outcomes measurement and managing change.

Harris, writing about the primary-care-led NHS indicates quite forcefully that what is required is an understanding of: 'the very nature of health policy and its implementation [which] need to be understood to judge the implications for GPs and other professionals and see where it is leading' (1996, p. 3). To facilitate this he goes on to quote Michael Ignatieff: 'policy is the selection of non contradicting means to achieve non contradicting ends over the medium to long term' (in Harris 1996, p. 3). Ignatieff's view, if seen as logical, helps in understanding the dilemma that presents itself here. From the preceding sections it emerges that there are two contrasting ways to view the drivers for policy change, which this author believes affect quite significantly the expectations of policy in practice. Resources and their organisation to tackle increasing health inequalities may be contrasted with the development of managed care, where it was the lack of coherence, the strain on costs and the drive to a consumer-led service that created the initial push to a 'primary-care-led NHS'. Therefore this fundamental change in policy holds an inherent contradiction for the service that works 'in the field' on public health – health visiting – since the starting premises and even the desired outcomes are different. The irony is clear for health visitors: there seems to be so much that contradicts and, it often appears, not enough that agrees.

However, as it has been the intention of the discussion in the previous three sections to suggest, there is no simple progression of policies into practice. This was the situation that was inherited by fundholding and it may be the key issue for health visiting at present. There can, quite legitimately, be a variety of ways of putting any one policy into practice. Harris clearly holds this view and goes further, stating that 'front-line staff may change the way a policy is implemented' (1996, p. 4).

Still, one unexamined area of this chapter has been the political dimension of the development of government health policy since the change of government in May 1997. The question is what continues and what changes, and identifying themes that may override discrete policy changes in themselves. Policy statements, in seeking to prioritise means and be clear over ends, can sometimes also appear narrow and simplistic. The advent of fundholding, viewed as a simple policy change, resulted in a variety of responses, as discussed above. This perspective on commissioning itself grew up almost silently and until

research in the summer of 1998 there was little mapping of its progress. Research by the King's Fund and the Health Services Management Centre of the University of Birmingham was undertaken in all 100 English health authorities and showed that considerable developments in GP commissioning were actually well in place before the Labour government came to power (Smith et al 1998, p. 47).

By contrast, however, the very sensitivity, diversity and richness of health visiting to which this whole volume attests has often been seen as unfocused and lacking in 'bite' in the current contract culture. Health visiting practice must ask itself whether this is the case or whether, as for health authorities and GPs in the period 1990–97, there is a way forward that limits the potential loss of this broad scope of health visiting practice, which many practitioners would see as a very serious loss to clients that would severely limit the chances of developing public health initiatives from the current fieldwork base. This cannot be undertaken, of course, without reference to what policy says, and the theme that will be examined next, therefore, is that of outcomes. Quite simply this is because if any overriding change is present from policy it is the emergence of this concern that has significantly impacted on health visiting practice.

It is particularly relevant to health visiting practice to recognise the current significance of outcome measurement in all current policy and strategy. The notion of 'health gain' was the basis for the plethora of mechanisms that have now developed to measure the effectiveness and efficiency of healthcare (Office for Public Management 1997, p. 2–3). It is important to note that for health visitors the word 'health', with many sometimes apparently confusing connotations (Cowley 1997, p. 91), is a clearly qualitative term. Set against this are tools that seek a precise definition of activity to determine what will be given future priority. There is a positive industry developing evaluation techniques, and Øvretveit warns: 'Evaluation can be confusing because there are many different approaches and because evaluation reports often assume a background knowledge of the approach used' (1998, p. 71).

Cowley, writing for the *Journal of Nursing Management* in 1994 highlights the difficulties in evaluation that still plague the health visiting service. She roundly criticises the: 'single episode of care as the base unit of activity in a long-term continuing service' (Cowley 1994b, p. 273).

As noted earlier, this type of measure effectively misrepresents health visiting work. It is often on such distorted data that decisions about the level of service commitment are made.

The news is not all bad, for, particularly in project work, outcome measurement has been identified by health visitors themselves. The Strelley project, mentioned earlier, is only one of several pieces of work where this need has been understood and integrated into the project management. This and other such evidence-based practice is listed by Pearson in her paper on this topic – Drennan in Kensington, Turner at the Riverside project, Evans at the Cowgate project, and Cope Street in Nottingham. A clutch of key features are evinced, which include the fact that it is important to impact time as well as number, that some contexts do render 'hard' outcomes, the complexity of community development and that 'consumers are a major source of evidence' (Pearson 1996, p. 3).

Today, with the primary care groups in the first stage from April 1999, the opportunity for health visitors to affect and develop their service evaluation by lobbying for a more suitable evaluation tool has arrived. National debates about such tools will take place but the visibility in what health visitors do usefully can only come if the appropriate tools are found and researched on a national basis. A critical search for such tools was undertaken by a trio of senior health visitors/researchers in 1995; the document, aptly entitled *Weights and Measures*, identified the complexity of the task and signalled the pressing need for work that could help develop the appropriate evaluation tools. The emergence of two categories from the material examined are a useful clarification of some of the dilemmas that arise as they pick up on topics for health visitors throughout this chapter. The authors stated: 'a clearer way forward has been identified, using the dimensions of "predictable/unpredictable"

and "disputed/undisputed"' (Campbell et al 1995, p. 32).

This could prove the break in the deadlock that besets evaluation of all health visiting work; it is a large qualitative activity in a contract culture environment that offers and usually accepts largely quantitative tools for measurement. Yet the difficulties are not only felt in health visiting. The new policy initiative is often given the umbrella title of 'performance measures', with a recognition that quality issues have not been properly included (Wooley 1998, p. 3). The opening here for higher level practitioners is to become more confident of the health gain and added value their service offers, challenge current measurement tools, be sympathetic to past failures that community health colleagues outside health visiting may have been party to, and to use the evidence available to their advantage. All stakeholders have a responsibility – managers and health visitors, PCG boards and user groups draw on these perspectives and use skills of practitioners to develop local delivery of preventative strategies.

A further key task is to be alert for opportunities for influence. The National Casemix Office started working on grouping for community services, largely from the perspective of the need for greater efficiency and effectiveness. The view of the Casemix group was that information needs for purchasers and the small-scale commissioning work of fundholders would differ. There would be only a small overlap, an interface between seeing the work in whole-time equivalents and as an overall service. Although out of this has developed packages of care, the simplistic nature of this view has since been abandoned with the advent of the 'new' primary care. Now further developments are assumed once a 'new, national minimum dataset' is available. What will this look like, and what is the health visiting contribution to its shape (National Casemix Office 1997)? It is most encouraging to see the conference advertisement for March 1999 openly acknowledging that much information gathered 'appears contradictory and meaningless'; to GPs, nurses, and social workers, the opportunity is wide open, the chance is there, for primary care groups are seen as: 'the perfect vehicle to move this debate forward and to eventually put Primary, Community and Social Care information into a national arena which reflects a focus on health and social improvements' (National Casemix Office 1999).

The policy directives now coming through have an imperative to tackle the shortfall in health inequality (Department of Health 1998a). Therefore it is possible to determine that the struggle of health visiting, while as great as ever in the face of those GPs who only think in terms of individual staff, may now be moving into a new phase for recognition of a service that can effectively deliver on the public health agenda. Clearly, thinking within the National Casemix Office is also moving, and gaining a voice at this level is essential if primary care and public health are to find a way forward together. The power struggles of the past do not disappear, but the maturity that higher-level practitioners offer seeks the best use of resources and is ready, as Brown puts it, to 'build a chain of evidence' (Brown 1997, p. 12). All key players, health authorities, staff of the primary care groups and NHS practitioners throughout the service have thus to face what is becoming broadly known as clinical governance, which, according to the British Association of Medical Managers 'demands a fundamental change in attitude and culture within the NHS' (1998, p. 2).

For health visitors this also requires a readiness to change. For the higher level practitioner, the clinical leader, this may involve supporting the change for others. This is critical, since the government's increased expectations of all in clinical governance may well require it. The ability to tackle this task when there has been so much change is not easy. As Walsh & Beenstock point out: 'PCGs are an external change, so to create them managers and health care professionals must go through an internal process of transition' (1998, p. 22). Distinguishing between change and a transition is a useful concept, which is expanded upon by these writers from work by Bridges on the nature of transition. The internal work that health visiting must undertake if it is to be ready for the new changes and consequent

opportunities is perhaps the task of higher-level practitioners at this very time. Bridges asks the fundamental question: 'If people feel that change has robbed them of control over their futures, can we find some way to give them back a feeling of control?' (Walsh & Beenstock 1998, p. 23).

It would be the author's suggestion that this dilemma is one familiar to health visitors, in their work at the very least. Clients often suffer such feelings and the transitional stages of life are often behind much of the neediness of the current major client group, i.e. parents and young families. This is not to minimise the mind-numbing and stultifying effects of poverty, deprivation and social need that face many clients, but to recognise that skills gathered from work may be of use to health visitors in the challenges faced in this era of the profession. At this point a sense of the huge expectations of the work, the demands of clients and the challenges from health colleagues and managers who want to think in whole-time equivalents rather than population health or service needs, can feel very daunting. This fatigue referred to above is a natural expression of such stress. Higher level practitioners, however, have learned to use new insights to reduce this stress, so that real change can take place and they are not overwhelmed by the transition.

As noted earlier, the role of middle management has currently diminished. It will perhaps be significant as to where health visitors and other community health workers find the support to tackle these issues. If success is to be found a new approach needs consideration. The 'burned-out' practitioner with an added burden of salesmen's 'target-led' anxiety is not an attractive image. However, as Edmonstone notes, empowerment of nursing staff involved in oncology can be real, and more than 'empty rhetoric'. 'Provided that those aspects of commitment, permission, opportunity and support are addressed from the perspective of those being empowered, and not just from the perspective of managers' (Edmonstone 1996, p. 386).

Stress levels in working with patients who have cancer would be expected to be high, and therefore serious consideration must be given to approaches that are really successful with such a client group. If commitment to change for the service is serious, future managers and service directors need to consider these issues. Work by some 160 district nurses, practice nurses and health visitors in the Leaders in Nursing for the Community development programme led to the discovery of key themes that affected the likelihood of a positive outcome for practitioners. These were isolation, lack of confidence in the ability to shape the future, strong pressure and influence of the GP, appropriate management, greater ability to handle business cases than realised and an overemphasis on research and academic qualifications that discounted good knowledge already to hand. It was discovered by the majority of participants that the resources needed for transformation were available to support changes in the work that they undertook: 'As the development centres progressed, group members began to express the sense that they, as a collection of professionals involved in community services, might have more power and influence than they thought' (Office for Public Management 1996, p. 7).

The earlier part of this chapter picked up on the disempowerment experienced by women workers in the face of a male establishment profession: nurses versus doctors. Interpreting this as a feminist issue is not to reinforce a division but to critically appreciate and to foster that approach toward some of the dynamics involved. Underestimation of difficulties will not empower anyone. On the other hand, polarisation of the parties involved within the primary care setting is no real solution either. It is clear that the shifts in primary care are creating pressures on doctors too as more responsibilities accrue to them for a wider primary care agenda. The healthcare agenda now has a potential that health visitors can exploit. Therefore it is important to recognise the choice for all healthcare workers to overcome these barriers and find support for their own and the service's development. The local nurses forum is, perhaps unbeknown to some community practitioners, one of the most exciting innovations, offering health visitors, community nurses and midwives a place to share, learn and grow towards the future of their work in primary care.

Policy changes do not proceed in a linear fashion but pick up on previous changes and are interpreted by fieldwork staff. Outcome measures may now be reaching a point in their development when they are the health visitor's ally and not the 'enemy', since understanding of outcome measurement is coming increasingly to appreciate quality issues and to promote empowerment as a part of change process (Pritchard 1996, p. 1). Paying attention to the inner aspects of transition is a valid strategy for health professionals, who may well have considerable resources to offer each other in this period of change.

CONCLUSION

Health visitors are commonly undervalued, yet as the breadth and depth of the work described in the chapters of this book shows, they are key workers in the task of delivering on public health. It is for them now, individually, in their local teams and at a national level, to assess their situation to determine the appropriate plan of action. The choice that has already been made by practitioners is the fundamental one to enter the field of health visiting and public health work. Perhaps now practitioners can dare to stand up and be counted as advocates for this choice to be one open for health workers of the future, since at long last the places where the work – and sometimes the worker – was 'buried' have become a positive focus for social and governmental concern. It is perhaps only now that it can be seen that the very vulnerability of being drawn into the experiences of people's lives, yet maintaining an awareness that these difficulties are not simply individual in origin, gives the reach to encompass solutions that bridge such gaps. Delivery on the health agenda for the country is no longer seen as a specialist or isolated activity and health visitors should be able to respond to that new freedom. It may now be possible to recognise that the difficulty of being identified with clients' needs is the price that many if not all health visitors have paid, for tackling the difficulty of working preventively in a society that saw such activity as dispensable. The recent recognition of the impact of relative poverty on a society's health and general prosperity is a key indicator that health visiting has actually only failed where it has colluded with an exclusively medical model of health. The resourcing issue could be resolved if this evidence is understood and accepted, as now seems possible.

As higher level or specialist practitioners the choice is already made, therefore, of practice that will combine the best preventive strategy available at individual, network and wider community level. This must also involve practical steps that offer users and clients/patients significant involvement in services to deliver the best health outcomes possible. Opportunity does now exist for practitioners to move with other community colleagues – including GPs, local authorities and service users – to deliver on these aspirations. Can we find good models of practice to use that can be widely shared to develop such hopes? There is evidence from this volume that combining the current base of ability with evidence-based and audited care and strategy plans offers a whole menu of possibilities. This mirrors the spread of development in the general area of commissioning for health. The development of Care Pathways and Casemix, to name but two recent developments, could provide the strategic link for this purpose. Research on data of this nature still requires development and wide dissemination so that the correct tools can be chosen for local situations. Higher level practitioners need to combine their clinical skills in the wider market-place of competing health approaches in a consistent and concise way, and seize the opportunity of a shift in the balance of power, where it occurs.

Thus it is possible to see the development of a truly higher level practice that takes basic understanding of our principles and moves them out into the NHS as a challenge and a pointer to where it needs to focus in its second 50 years. Practitioners, by better understanding the contribution they can make, must ensure that their activities further public health at the cutting edge

since any attempt to merely maintain the status quo will lead to stasis that is incompatible not only with our principles of practice but also with our history as a profession. The particular contribution of health visiting could be to root work in more realistic time frames, rather than quick-fix approaches that smooth over the depth of need or preclude solutions that can be usefully applied. This cultural shift could then be the proper choice of all higher-level practice in primary care.

As a profession, health visiting is uniquely placed to move between the competing demands of health and healthcare needs. This is not to ignore the apparent dichotomy between elements of policy directives and the drives to achieve them but to see it as part of an understood working tension. Where it seems that preventive approaches have low priority, compromises that violate health visiting principles must now be faced and this, despite many difficulties, gives practitioners the chance to affect health at a fundamental level. The economic power that has often eluded the profession may only have been brought within its grasp incidentally and may still only involve influencing the healthcare agenda, but this is the best opportunity yet, for three reasons. First, our long history on the healthcare scene and our depth and penetration of the healthcare activity of the NHS, as this volume attests, is gaining increasing recognition. Second, the continuing pressures on health expenditure mean that preventive strategies are becoming more attractive to the NHS, especially where they use current resources. Thirdly, a government agenda that values partnership and emphasises public health, for whatever reason, opens the door to the contribution that health visiting can and should offer, albeit within the community nursing remit. The only real choice for health visiting, as one of the key change agents within the health service, is to grasp the opportunity to take forward this agenda, on behalf of the pioneering sisters of its history, the health needs of its current clients and the profession's entire future.

References

Acheson Report 1988 Public health in England: the Report of the Committee of Inquiry into the Future Development of the Public Health Function. Cmnd 289 HMSO, London

Acton T 1974 Gypsy politics and social change. Routledge & Kegan Paul, London

Acton T 1994 Gender issues in accounts of gypsy health and hygiene as discourses of social control. Medical Sociology Group Paper 24.10.94

Adams P, Conway M, Owens N 1992 The strategic use of information systems and technology: an overview for NHS chief executives and senior managers of the management in the 90s research programme. NHS Training Directorate, London

Ahmad WIU (ed) 1993 Race and health in contemporary Britain. Open University Press, Buckingham

Ainsworth M 1965 Further research into the adverse effects of maternal deprivation. In: Bowlby J (ed) Child care and the growth of love, 2nd edn. Penguin Books, St Ives

Akinsanya J, Cox G, Crouch C, Fletcher L 1994 The Roy adaptation model in action. Macmillan, Basingstoke

Alleyne J, Thomas V 1994 The management of sickle cell as experienced by patients and their carers. J Adv Nurs 19: 725–732

Allmark P 1992 The ethical enterprise of nursing. J Adv Nurs 17: 16–20

Amina Mama 1996 The hidden struggle – statutory and voluntary sector responses to violence against black women in the home. Whiting & Birch, London

Anionwu E 1994 Women and sickle cell disorders. In: Wilson M (ed) Healthy and wise. Virago, London

Appleton J 1994 The concept of vulnerability in relation to child protection: health visitors' perceptions. J Adv Nurs 20: 1132–1140

Argyris C 1982 Reasoning, learning and action: individual and organisational. Jossey Bass, San Francisco, CA

Argyris C, Schön DA 1974 Theory into practice, increasing professional effectiveness. Jossey Bass, San Francisco, CA

Ashby HT 1922 Infant mortality. Cambridge University Press, Cambridge

Ashton J, Seymour H 1988 The new public health: the Liverpool experience. Open University Press, Milton Keynes

Audit Commission 1997 Comparing notes: a study of information management in Community Trusts. Audit Commission, London

Aukett A 1990 The Schedule of Growing Skills. Recorded interview at Carnegie Institute of Child Health, Birmingham

Austerberry H, Watson S 1982 Women on the margins. City University Housing Research Group, London

Bal S 1986 Psychological symptomatology and health beliefs of Asian patients. In: Dent M (ed) Clinical psychology: research and developments. Croom Helm, London, p 101–110

Balarajan R, Bulusu L 1990 Mortality among immigrants in England and Wales, 1979–83. In: Britton M (ed) Mortality and geography: a review in the mid-1980s, England and Wales. OPCS Series DS no 8. HMSO, London, p 103–121

Balarajan R, Raleigh VS 1992 The ethnic populations of England and Wales: the 1991 census. Health Trends 24: 113–116

Balarajan R, Raleigh VS 1993 The health of the nation: ethnicity and health: a guide for the NHS. Department of Health, London

Baldry M, Cheal C, Fisher B et al 1985 Giving patients their own records in general practice. Br Med J 292: 595–598

Bandura A 1973 Aggression: a social learning analysis. Prentice Hall, Englewood Cliffs, NJ

Bandura A 1977a Self-efficacy: toward a unifying theory of behaviour change. Psychol Rev 84: 191–215

Bandura A 1977b Social learning theory. Prentice-Hall, Englewood Cliffs, NJ

Bandura A 1986 Social foundations of thought and action: a social cognitive theory. Prentice-Hall, Englewood Cliffs, NJ

Bandura A, Taylor CB, Williams SL et al 1985 Catecholamine secretion as a function of perceived coping self-efficacy. J Consult Clin Psychol 53: 406–414

Baraclough J, Damant M, Metcalfe D, Strehlow M 1983 Statement on the interprofessional education and training for members of Primary Health Care Teams. Central Council for Education and Training in Social Works/Panel of Assessors for District Nurse Training/Royal College of General Practitioners/Council for the Education and Training of Health Visitors, London

Barker W 1984 Child development programme. Early Childhood Development Unit, University of Bristol, Bristol

Barker W 1985 The Körner Community Report: medical or prevention model? Evidence to Körner Working Group D.

Barker W 1988 The use of E H D Monitor to assess young children's health and development and to evaluate effectiveness of Health Visiting. University of Bristol Early Childhood Development Unit, Bristol

Barker W 1991 Is Monitor worth the time and effort? University of Bristol Early Childhood Development Unit, Bristol

Barlow J 1997 The effectiveness of parenting training programmes in improving behaviour problems in children aged 3–10 years. In: National Screening Committee/Royal College of Paediatrics and Child Health Proceedings: evolution or revolution? Systematic reviews of screening in child health, 17 December 1997 and 18 January 1998. Conference Organiser (c/o Child Growth Foundation), London, p 19

Barna D 1995 Working with young men. Health Visitor 68: 185–187

Barnes M 1998 Health Services Management Newsletter 3(3) 1997: 2

Barrie-Foy G 1997 The health of children in temporary accommodation. Health Visitor 70: 144–145

Barrow J 1982 West Indian families: an insider's perspective. In: Rapport N (ed) Families in Britain. RKP, London

Bassuk EL, Weinreb LF, Ree Dawson S et al 1997 Determinants of behaviour in homeless and low-income housed pre-school children. Paediatrics 100

Baumrind D 1967 Current patterns of parental authority. Devel Psychol Monogr 4: 1–103

Bax M, Hart H, Jenkins S 1990 Child development and child health. Blackwell Scientific, Oxford

Baxter C 1988 The Black nurse: an endangered species. A case for equal opportunities in nursing. Training in Health and Race, London

Baxter C 1997 Race equality in health care and education. Baillière Tindall, London

Bayley N 1933 Mental growth during the first three years. A developmental study of sixty-one children by repeated tests. Genet Psychol Monogr 14: 1–92

Bayley N 1940 Mental growth in young children. Year-book Nat Soc Stud Educ 39: 11–47

Beattie A 1979 Social policy and health education: the prospects for a radical practice. Paper for the National Deviancy Conference, Edgehill College

Beattie A 1984 The price of political awareness. Paper for the Challenge of Choice. Conference, St Bartholomew's Hospital, London

Beattie A 1991 Knowledge and control in health promotion: a test case for social policy and social theory. In: Gabe J, Calnam M, Bury M (ed) The sociology of the health service. Routledge, London

Beattie A 1993 Sociopolitical philosophy of dimensions of conflict. In: Beattie A, Gott M, Jones L, Sidell M (ed) Health and wellbeing: a reader. CB Slack, London

Beattie A 1996 Knowledge and control in health promotion: a case study in social policy and social theory. In: Calman M, Gabe J (ed) The sociology of the Health Service. Routledge, London

Beauchamp T, Childress J 1989 Principles of biomedical ethics. Oxford University Press, Oxford

Becker M 1974 The Health Belief Model and personal health behaviour. Charles B Slack, NJ

Becker MH, Drachman RH, Kirscht JP 1974 A new approach to explaining sick role behaviour in low income populations. Am J Pub Health 64: 205–216

Becker MH, Maiman LA, Kirscht JP et al 1977 The Health Belief Model and prediction of dietary compliance: a field experiment. J Health Soc Behav 18: 348–366

Begg N, Ramsey M, White J, Bozoky Z 1998 Media dents confidence in MMR vaccine. Br Med J 316: 561

Beitler B, Tkachuck B, Aamodt A 1980 The Neuman model applied to mental health, community health and medical-surgical nursing. In: Riehl JP, Roy C (ed) Conceptual models for nursing practice, 2nd edn. Appleton-Century-Crofts, New York

Bekenn A 1995 Black and minority ethnic group and day care for under 8's 1995: research findings. Dudley Social Services/Barnardos Under 8's Project, Dudley

Belbin RM 1993 Team roles at work. Butterworth-Heinemann/BMJ

Bellman MH 1984 Serious acute neurological diseases of childhood. A clinical and epidemiological study with special reference to whooping cough disease and immunization. Unpublished MD thesis, University of London

Bellman M, Cash J 1987 The Schedule of Growing Skills in practice. NFER-Nelson, Chippenham

Bellman M, Lingam S, Aukett A 1996 Schedule of Growing Skills II. NFER-Nelson, Windsor

Benedict MM, Behringer Sproles J 1982 Application of the Neuman model to public health nursing practice. In: Neuman B (ed) Neuman Systems Model. Application to nursing education and practice. Appleton-Century-Crofts, Norwalk, CT

Benjamin M, Curtis J 1992 Ethics in nursing. Oxford University Press, Oxford

Benner P 1984 From novice to expert: excellence and power in clinical nursing practice. Addison-Wesley, Menlo Park, CA

Bennett G 1990 Action on elder abuse in the '90s: a new definition will help. Geriatr Med April: 53–54

Bennett GD 1992 Handbook of clinical dietetics. Price Publishing, London

Bennett G, Kingston P, Penhale B 1997 The dimensions of elder abuse: perspectives for practitioners. Macmillan, Basingstoke

Benzeval MK, Judge K, Whitehead M 1995 Tackling inequalities in health: an agenda for action. King's Fund Institute, London

Bergman R 1981 Accountability – definition and dimensions. Int Nurs Rev 28 Feb: 53–59

Bernice J 1986 Evaluation of a developmental screening system for use by child health nurses. Arch Dis Childh 61: 340–341

Beske EJ, Garvis MS 1982 Important factors in breastfeeding success. Matern Child Nurs 7: 174–179

Betts T 1995 How we use aromatherapy. University of Birmingham, Birmingham

Bhat A, Carr-Hill R, Ohriz S 1988 Britain's Black population, 2nd edn. Gower Radical Statistics Groups, Aldershot

Biggs S, Phillipson C, Kingston P 1995 Elder abuse in perspective. Open University Press, Buckingham

Billingham K 1991 Public health and the community. Health Visitor 64: 371–372

Billingham K 1997 Public health nursing in primary care. Br J Commun Health Nurs 2(6)

Billings J 1996 Profiling for health: the process and practice. Health Visitors Association, London

Binet A, Simon T 1915 A method of measuring the development of intelligence in young children. Medical Book Co, Chicago, IL

Birchall E, Hallett C 1995 Working together in child protection. HMSO, London

Birchwood M, McMillan F, Smith J 1992 Early signs of relapse in schizophrenia - maintaining methodology. In: Kavanagh D (ed) Schizophrenia – an interdisciplinary handbook. Chapman & Hall, London

Birmingham Health Authority 1990 Child health surveillance policy. Birmingham Health Authority, Birmingham

Birmingham Health Authority 1997 Action plan for Black and minority ethnic health. Birmingham Health Authority, Birmingham

Birt C 1997 Public health into the new century. Health Services Management Centre Newsletter 3(3)

Black D 1980 Inequalities in health: report of a research working group. Department of Health, London

Blackburn C 1991 Poverty and Health, working with families. Open University Press, Milton Keynes

Blackburn C 1993 Gender, class and smoking cessation work. Health Visitor 66: 83–85

Blackburn C, Graham H 1992 Smoking among working class mothers. Information pack. University of Warwick, Warwick

Blakemore K, Boneham M 1994 Age, race and ethnicity. Open University Press, Buckingham

Blau PM 1964 Exchange and power in social life. John Wiley, New York

Blaxter M 1990 Health and lifestyles. Tavistock, London

Blumer H 1969 Symbolic interactionism: perspective and method. Prentice-Hall, Englewood Cliffs, NJ

Bolton P 1986 Developmental screening for children aged two. Health Visitor 59: 149–151

Bond M, Holland S 1998 Skills of clinical supervision for nurses. Open University Press, Buckingham

Boston M 1997 Preventing teenage pregnancies. Community Nurse 3: 18–20

Bowlby J 1953 Child care and the growth of love, 2nd edn. Penguin Books, St Ives

Bowling A 1991 Measuring Health – a review of quality of life measuring scales. Open University Press, Buckingham

Boyd E, Fales AW 1983 Reflective learning. J Hum Psychol 23: 99–117

Boyd M, Brummell K, Billington K, Perkins E 1993 The public health post at Strelley: an interim report. Nottingham Community Health Trust, Nottingham

Bradshaw JR 1972 A taxonomy of social need. In: MacLachlan G (ed) Problems and progress in medical care. Nuffield Provincial Hospital Trust, Oxford

Bradshaw JR 1994 The conceptualisation and measurement of need. In: Popay J, Williams G (ed) Researching the people's health. Routledge, London

Brady-Wilson C 1991 US businesses suffer from workplace trauma. Personnel J July: 47–50

Brew M 1994 Nurse prescribing – what nurses need to know. Nurs Times 90: 21

British Association of Medical Managers 1998 Clinical governance in the new NHS. BAMM, Cheshire

British Medical Association 1993 Complementary medicine: new approaches to good practice. Oxford University Press, Oxford

Britt DW 1997 A conceptual introduction to modeling: qualitative and quantitative perspectives. Lawrence Erlbaum Associates, Mahwah, NJ

Brocklehurst N 1998 Clinical supervision. West Midlands Clinical Supervision Learning Set, Birmingham

Brody S 1977 Screen violence and film censorship. Home Office Research Unit Report No. 40. HMSO, London

Brookfield S 1990 Using critical incidents to explore learners' assumptions. In: Mezirow J et al (ed) Fostering critical reflection in adulthood. Jossey Bass, San Francisco

Broome A 1989 Health psychology processes and applications. Chapman & Hall, London

Brotherston J 1988 Health Services Journal 7509: 759

Broudy HS, Smith BD, Burnett J 1964 Democracy and excellence in American secondary education. Cited in Eraut M 1985 Knowledge creation and knowledge use in professional contexts. Stud Higher Educ 10: 117–133

Brown I 1997 A skill mix parent support initiative in health visiting: an evaluation study. Health Visitor 70: 339–343

Brown J 1992 Screening infants for hearing loss – an economic evaluation. J Epidemiol Commun Health 46: 350–356

Browne K, Davies C, Stratton P 1988 Early prediction and prevention of child abuse. John Wiley, Chichester

Bruce A, Jonsson E 1996 Competition in the provision of health care. Arena, London

Buck D, Godfrey C, Parrot S, Raw M 1997 Cost effectiveness of smoking cessation interventions. Centre for Health Economics, University of York and Health Education Authority, London

Buhler C, Hetzer H 1935 Testing children's development from birth to school age. Allen & Unwin, London

Bundey S, Alam H 1993 A five-year prospective study of the health of children in different ethnic groups. Eur J Hum Genet 1: 206–209

Bunton R, Macdonald G 1992 Health promotion–disciplines and diversity. Routledge, London

Burridge R 1988 The role of the health visitor with the elderly. Health Visitor 61: 20–21

Burrows A 1983 Patient-centred nursing care in a multi-racial society: the relevance of ethnographic approaches in nursing curricula. J Adv Nurs 8: 477–485

Burrows DE, McLeish J 1995 A model for research-based practice. J Clin Nurs 4: 243–247

Butler J 1989 Child health surveillance in primary care: a critical review. HMSO, London

Butterworth T 1988 Breaking the boundaries. Cited in Cain P, Hyde V, Howkins E 1995 Community nursing: dimensions and dilemmas. Edward Arnold, London

Butterworth T, Faugier J 1992 Clinical supervision and mentorship in nursing. Chapman & Hall, London

Cainey L 1995 Recorded interview with former Senior Health and Social Care Specialist. NFER-Nelson, Windsor

Caldwell P 1998 Re. MMR revisited hastily! http: /www.mailbase.ac.uk/liss-f/gp-uk/1998

Calman K 1998 Government declares MMR triple vaccine safe. www.itn.co.uk/Britain/brit0312/031206.htm

Cameron-Blackie G, Mouncer Y 1992 Complementary therapies in the NHS. NHS Confederation, London

Campbell F, Cowley S, Buttigieg M 1995 Weights and measures: outcomes and evaluation in health visiting. Health Visitors Association, London

CanagaRetna A 1997 Primary health care teams involving patients: examples of good practice. NHS Executive, London

Caplan G 1966 Principles of preventive psychiatry. Basic Books, New York

Carboni JT 1990 Homelessness amongst the institutionalised elderly. J Gerontol Nurs 16: 32–37

Carnwell R 1998 Conceptual models for practice. In: Blackie C (ed) Community health care nursing. Churchill Livingstone, Edinburgh

Carpenter RG, Gardner A, Jepson-Taylor EM et al 1983 Prevention of unexpected infant death. Lancet 1: 723–727

Carper B 1978 Fundamental patterns of knowing in nursing. Adv Nurs Sci 11: 13–23

Carroll I, Coll T, Underhill D 1974 Retarded brain growth in Irish itinerants. J Ir Med Assoc 67: 33–36

Carter T 1986 Shattering illusions: West Indians in British politics. Lawrence & Wishart, London

Carter YH, Bannon MJ, Jones PW 1992 Health visitors and child accident prevention. Health Visitor 65: 115–127

Cash J 1991 Recorded interview, Birmingham Children's Hospital

Cattell P 1940 The measurement of intelligence of infants and young children. Psychological Corporation, New York

Caulkin S 1999 A glass ceiling made of lead. Observer 3 Jan

Centers for Disease Control 1999 Mumps, measles and rubella vaccine (MMR): about the diseases. Internet

CETHV 1977 An investigation into the principles of health visiting. Council for the Education and Training of Health Visitors, London, 6

Chalmers KI 1992 Giving and receiving: an empirically derived theory on health visiting practice. J Adv Nurs 17: 1317–1325

Chalmers K, Kristajanson L 1989 The theoretical basis for nursing at the community level: a comparison of three models. J Adv Nurs 14: 569–574

Chandra J 1995 Locating the goal posts – health promotion and purchasing for black and minority health. A report of the Health Education Authority Conference on improving health provision for black and minority ethnic communities. Health Education Authority, London

Charles RP 1994 An evaluation of parent-held child health records. Health Visitor 67: 270–272

Charles RP 1996 Reforming health visitor records. Health Visitor 69: 101–102

CHE News 1998 A research update. No.5. University of York, York

Child Accident Prevention Trust 1989 Preventing accidents to children. A training resource for health visitors. Health Education Authority, London

Churchman CW 1971 The design of inquiring systems: basic concepts of systems and organisations. Cited in Kitchener KS, King PM 1990 The reflective judgement model: transforming assumptions about knowing. In: Mezirow J et al (ed) Fostering critical reflection in adulthood. Jossey-Bass, San Francisco

Clark J 1973 A family visitor: a descriptive analysis of health visiting in Berkshire. Royal College of Nursing, London

Clark P 1994 Parent held records: legal implications in child protection. In: Saffin K (ed) Where now? What next? The personal child health record. Oxfordshire Community Health Trust, Oxford

Clarke C 1999 Low self-esteem: a barrier to health promoting behaviour. J Commun Nurs 13(1)

Clement S 1995 Listening visits in pregnancy: a strategy for preventing postnatal depression? Midwifery 11: 75–80

Cochrane R, Bal S 1989 Mental hospital admission rates of immigrants to England: a comparison of 1971 and 1981. Soc Psychiat Epidemiol 24: 1108

Cochrane AL, Holland WW 1971 Validation of screening procedures. Br Med Bull 27: 3–8

Cody AL 1995 The effect of infant massage on hospitalised premature infants. Dissertation. Abstracts Int 56/05: 2858

Cody A 1999 Health visiting as therapy: a phenomenological perspective. J Adv Nurs 29: 119–127

Cohen DR, Henderson JB 1988 Health prevention and economics. Oxford Medical, Oxford

Cohen F, Lazarus RS 1979 Coping with the stresses of illness. Cited in Sarafino EP 1994 Health psychology. John Wiley, New York

Cohen P 1996 Market logic fragments health visiting service. Health Visitor 69: 15–16

Colver A 1983 Home is where the damage lies. Health Soc Service J 2 June: 662–663

COMA 1980 Rickets and osteomalacia. DHSS Report on Health and Social Subjects 19. HMSO, London

Community Practitioner 1998 Ministers to investigate cuts in health visiting (news). Commun Practit 71: 235

Coney S 1995 The menopause industry. Women's Press, London

Conger RD, Conger KJ, Elder GH et al 1992 A family process model of economic hardship and adjustment of early adolescent boys. Child Devel 63: 526–541

Connolly M 1995 Commissioning community services. Health Visitor 68(2)

Cook A, James J, Leach P 1991 Positively no smacking. In Twinn S, Cowley S (ed) 1992 The principles of health visiting: a re-examination. HVA/UKSC, London

Cornwell J, Gordon P 1984 An experiment in advocacy: the Hackney multi-ethnic women's health project. King's Fund, London

Coronary Prevention Group 1986 Coronary heart disease and Asians in Britain. Confederation of Indian Organisations, London

Cotton P, Fraser I, Hill WY 1997 Primary health care in a stakeholder society. National Auditing Conference Paper

Court SDM 1976 Fit for the future. Report of the Committee on Child Health Services. Cmnd 6680. HMSO, London

Cowley S 1991 A grounded theory on situation and process in health visiting. Unpublished PhD Thesis, Brighton Polytechnic

Cowley S 1994a Collaboration in health care: the education link. Cited in Cain P, Hyde V, Howkins E 1995 Community nursing: dimensions and dilemmas. Edward Arnold, London

Cowley S 1994b Counting practice: impact of information systems on community nursing. J Nurs Manag 1: 273–278

Cowley S 1997 Public health values in practice; the case of health visiting. Critical Pub Health 7: 1–2

Cox J, Holden J (ed) 1994 Perinatal psychiatry, use and misuse of the Edinburgh Postnatal Depression Scale. Gaskell, London

Cox JL, Holden JM, Sagovsky R 1987 Detection of postnatal depression: development of the 10-item Edinburgh Postnatal Depression Scale. Br J Psychiat 150: 782–786

CPHVA 1996 Integrated nursing teams. Professional briefing paper CS/96/15. Community Practitioners and Health Visitors Association, London

CPHVA 1997 Professional Briefing 9: Integrated nursing teams. Health Visitor 70: 229–231

Craig N, Parkin D, Gerard K 1995 Clearing the fog on the Tyne: programme budgeting in Newcastle and North Tyneside Health Authority. Health Policy 33: 107–125

Craig P 1996 Drumming up health in Drumchapel: community development and health visiting. Health Visitor Dec

Creedon T, Corbay A, Keveney J 1975 Growth and development in travelling families. J Ir Med Assoc 68: 473–477

Crittenden P 1988 Family and dyadic patterns of functioning in maltreating families. In: Browne K, Davies C, Stratton P (ed) Early prediction and prevention of child abuse. John Wiley, Chichester

Crout E 1988 Have health care will travel. Health Serv J 98: 48–49

Cruickshank JK, Beevers DG 1994 Ethnic factors in health and disease. John Wright, Bristol

Cruickshank JK, Beevers DG, Osbourne VL et al 1980 Heart attack, stroke, diabetes and hypertension in West Indians, Asians, and whites in Birmingham, England. Br Med J 281: 1108

Culley L 1996 A critique of multiculturalism in health care: the challenge for nurse education. J Adv Nurs 23: 564–570

Curtis H 1993 The schedule of growing skills in child protection work. In: NFER-Nelson (ed) The schedule of growing skills. Facilitating child surveillance. NFER-Nelson, Windsor, p 5

Curtis H 1995 Letter to researcher (Reynolds M)

Daly WM 1998 Critical thinking as an outcome of nursing education. What is it? Why is it important to nursing practice? J Adv Nurs 28: 323–331

Darwin C 1877 A biographical sketch of an infant. Mind 2: 285

Davies C 1995 Gender and the Professional predicament in Nursing. Open University Press, Buckingham

Davies JK, Kelly MP 1993 Healthy cities: research and practice. Routledge, London

Davis A, Bamford J, Wilson I et al 1997 A critical review of the role of neonatal hearing screening in the detection of congenital hearing impairment. Health Technol Assess 1(10)

Davis C et al 1981 Survey of sickle cell disease in England and Wales. Br Med J 283: 1519–1521

Day M 1998 This won't hurt…. New Sci 7 March

De la Cuesta C 1994 Marketing: a process in health visiting. J Adv Nurs 19: 347–353

Deaves DM 1993 An assessment of the value of health education in the prevention of childhood asthma. J Adv Nurs 18: 354–363

Dennett L 1998 A sense of security. Granta, Cambridge

Denny C 1997 Lone mothers 'must learn then earn'. Guardian 17 Dec

Department for Education and Employment 1999 Sure Start, a guide for trailblazers. DofEE Publications, Sudbury

Department of Environment, Transport and the Regions 1998 A new deal for transport: better for everyone. Stationery Office, London

Department of Health 1986 Contraceptive advice and treatment for young people. Health circular HC(86)1. HMSO, London

Department of Health 1987 Promoting better health. The Government's programme for improving primary health care. Cmnd 249. HMSO, London

Department of Health 1988 Community Care, Agenda for Action. A Report to the Secretary of State for Social Services by Sir Roy Griffiths. HMSO, London

Department of Health 1989a Caring for people. HMSO, London

Department of Health 1989b Working for patients. Cmnd 555. HMSO, London

Department of Health 1989c Working for people. HMSO, London

Department of Health 1991 The patient's charter. HMSO, London

Department of Health 1992 The health of the nation: a strategy for health in England. HMSO, London

Department of Health 1993a The health of the nation. HIV/AIDS and sexual health. HMSO, London

Department of Health 1993b The health of the nation: targeting practice. The contribution of nurses, midwives and health visitors. HMSO, London

Department of Health 1995a Making it happen. Public health – the contribution, role and development of nurses, midwives and health visitors. Report of the Standing Nursing and Midwifery Advisory Committee. BAPS, London

Department of Health 1995b The challenge of partnership in child protection: practice guide. HMSO, London

Department of Health 1995c Health of the young nation: your contribution counts. HMSO, London

Department of Health 1995d Weaning and the weaning diet: report of the Working Group on the Weaning Diet of the Committee on Medical Aspects of Food Policy. HMSO, London

Department of Health 1996a Choice and opportunity. Primary care: the future. Stationery Office, London

Department of Health 1996b A new partnership for care in old age. Cmnd 3242. HMSO, London

Department of Health 1996c Regulation of nursing homes and independent hospitals. HSG(95)41. HMSO, London

Department of Health 1996d A study of commissioning issues and good practice in purchasing minority ethnic health. Responding to diversity. Office of Public Management. HMSO, London

Department of Health 1997a The new NHS – modern, dependable. Cmnd 3807. Stationery Office, London

Department of Health 1997b Shared contributions, shared benefits: the report of the working group on Public Health and Primary Care. Stationery Office, London

Department of Health 1998a Our healthier nation: a contract for health. Cmnd 3852. Stationery Office, London

Department of Health 1998b A first class service – quality in the new NHS. Stationery Office, London

Department of Health 1998c Modernising social services, promoting independence, improving protection, raising standards. Stationery Office, London

Department of Health 1998d Partnership in action (new opportunities for joint working between health and social services). Stationery Office, London

Department of Health 1998e Report of the independent inquiry into inequalities in health. Stationery Office, London

Department of Health and Social Security 1986 Neighbourhood nursing – a focus for care. Report of the Community Nursing Review (Cumberlege Report). HMSO, London

Department of Health and Social Security 1994 Inquiry into the death of Paul. HMSO, London

Department of Health and Social Services Inspectorate 1993 No longer afraid: the safeguard of older people in domestic settings. HMSO, London

Department of Health Specialist Clinical Services Division 1996 Child health in the community: a guide to good practice. HMSO, London

Department of Health/Department of Education and Science/Welsh Office 1991 Working together under the Children Act 1989: A guide to arrangements for inter-agency co-operation for the protection of children from abuse. HMSO, London

Department of Health/Welsh Office 1995 Child protection: clarification of arrangements between the NHS and other agencies. HMSO, London

Department of the Environment 1994 Gypsy sites policy and unauthorised camping. Circulars 18/94 and 76/94. HMSO, London

Deshler D 1990a Metaphor analysis: exorcising social ghosts. In: Mezirow J et al (ed) 1990 Fostering critical reflection in adulthood. Jossey Bass, San Francisco

Deshler D 1990b Conceptual mapping: drawing charts of the mind. In Mezirow J et al (ed) 1990 Fostering critical reflection in adulthood. Jossey Bass, San Francisco

Dewey J 1933 How we think. Cited in Palmer et al (ed) 1994

Reflective practice in nursing: the growth of the professional practitioner. Blackwell Science, Oxford

Dezateux C et al 1997 Screening for congenital dislocation of the hip: a cost effective analysis. In: National Screening Committee/Royal College of Paediatrics and Child Health Proceedings: evolution or revolution? Systematic reviews of screening in child health, 17 December 1997 and 8 January 1998. Conference Organiser (c/o Child Growth Foundation), London, p 22–23

Dezateux C, Brown J, Godward S et al 1998 Systematic reviews in child health. Royal College of Paediatrics and Child Health, London

Diment Y 1991 Routine health visiting of a family based upon Becker's health belief model. In: While A (ed) Caring for children: towards partnership with families. Edward Arnold, Sevenoaks

Dingwall R 1989 Some problems about predicting child abuse and neglect. In: Stevenson O (ed) Child abuse: public policy and professional practice. Wheatsheaf, London

Dixon J, Welch HG 1991 Priority setting: lessons from Oregon. Lancet 337: 891–894

Dobash RE, Dobash R 1980 Violence against wives. Open Books, London

Dobby J 1986 The development and testing of a method for measuring the need for, and the value of, routine health visiting within a District Health Authority. Health Promotion Research Trust, London

Doering CH, Brodie HKH, Kraemer HC et al 1974 Plasma testosterone levels and psychologic measures in men over a two month period. Cited in Owens RG, Ashcroft JB 1985 Violence, a guide for the caring professions. Croom Helm, London

Donabedian A 1980 Explorations in quality assessment and monitoring: 1. The definition of quality and approaches to its assessment. Health Administration Press, Ann Arbor, MI

Donabedian A 1988 Quality assessment and assurance: the unity of purpose, diversity of means. Inquiry 25: 173–192

Donaldson C, Farrar S 1991 Needs assessment: developing an economic approach. Discussion Paper 12, Health Economics Research Unit, University of Aberdeen, Aberdeen

Donovan J 1986 We don't buy sickness; it just comes. Health and illness and health care in the lives of Black people in London. Gower, Aldershot

Douglas J 1987 Caribbean food and diet. Training in health and race. National Extension College, Cambridge

Douglas J 1990 Black women's health matters. In: Roberts H (ed) Women's health counts. HMSO, London

Douglas J 1998 Meeting the health needs of women from black and minority ethnic communities. In: Doyal L (ed) Women and health services. Open University Press, Buckingham

Downey G, Coyne JC 1990 Children of depressed parents. Psychological Bulletin 108: 50–76

Downie RS, Calman KC 1989 Healthy respect: ethics in health care. Faber & Faber, London

Drennan V 1985 Working in a different way. Paddington and North Kensington Health Authority, London

Drillien C, Drummond D 1983 Developmental screening and the child with special needs. Heinemann, London

Drummond MF, O'Brien B, Stoddart G, Torrance G 1997 Methods for the economic evaluation of health care programmes, 2nd edn. Oxford Medical Publications, Oxford

Dudley J 1994 The stage model of reflection. Unpublished paper, University of Wolverhampton

Duncan P 1990 To screen or not to screen? Health Educ J 49: 120–222

Dunn RB, Lewis PA, Vetter NJ et al 1994 Health visitor intervention to reduce days of unplanned hospital re-admission in patients recently discharged from geriatric wards: the results of a randomised controlled study. Arch Gerontol Geriatr 18: 15–23

Dunn WR, Hamilton DD 1986 The Critical Incident Technique – a brief guide. Med Teach 8(3)

Durward L 1990 Traveller mothers and babies: who cares for their health? Maternity Alliance

Dwivedi K, Varma V 1996 Meeting the needs of ethnic minority children. Jessica Kingsley, London

Dyson S 1995 Whooping cough vaccine: historical, social and political controversies. J Clin Nurs 4: 125–131

Eastman M 1984 Old age abuse. Age Concern, Mitcham

Easy F 1995 Vaccine debate inflames reaction (letter). Health Matters 23

Eaton M 1994 Abuse by any other name: feminism, difference and intralesbian violence. In: Fineman MA, Mykitiuk R (ed) The public nature of private violence. Routledge, New York

Edet EE 1991 The role of sex education in adolescent pregnancy. J Roy Soc Health Feb: 17–18

Edmonstone J 1996 Strengthening cancer care: a practical approach to the empowerment of nurses. NT Res 1(5)

Edwards S 1985 A socio-legal evaluation of gender ideologies in domestic violence, assault and spousal homicides. Victimology 10: 186–205

Egan G 1982 The skilled helper, 2nd edn. Brooks/Cole, CA

Egan G 1986 The skilled helper, 3rd edn. Brooks/Cole, CA

Egeland B 1988 Breaking the cycle of abuse: implications for prediction and intervention. In: Browne K, Davies C, Stratton P (ed) Early prediction and prevention of child abuse. John Wiley, Chichester

Elliott P 1996 Shattering illusions: same-sex domestic violence. In: Renzetti CM, Miley CH (ed) Violence in gay and lesbian domestic partnerships. Harrington Park Press, New York

Enabling People Programme 1997 Information for caring. NHS Management Executive, London

Eraut M 1985 Knowledge creation and knowledge use in professional contexts. Stud Higher Educ 10: 117–133

Eriksen W, Sorum K, Bruusgaard D 1996 Effects of information on smoking behaviour in families with preschool children. Acta Paediatr 85: 209–212

Ewles L, Simnett I 1992 Promoting health: a practical guide. Scutari Press, London

Eysenck HJ 1983 Current theories of crime. In: Karas E (ed) Current issues in clinical psychology, vol 1. Plenum Press, New York

Fagan J 1997 Clients' views of health visitors and child health surveillance. Health Visitor 70: 146–147

Farley N 1996 A survey of factors contributing to gay and lesbian domestic violence. In: Renzetti CM, Miley CH (ed) Violence in gay and lesbian domestic partnerships. Harrington Park Press, New York

Fawcett J 1985 Analysis and evaluation of conceptual models of nursing. FA Davis, Philadelphia, PA

Fawcett J 1992 Conceptual models and nursing practice: the reciprocal relationship. J Adv Nurs 17: 224–228

Feather NT (ed) 1982 Expectations and actions – expectancy-value models in psychology. Lawrence Erlbaum Associates, Hillsdale, NJ

Feder G 1990 The politics of Traveller health research. Crit Publ Health 3

Ferguson J 1997 Managing prescribing: a view from the prescription pricing authority. Lecture, Primary Care Week, Health Services Management Centre, University of Birmingham 19 Dec

Fiedler FE 1967 A contingency theory of leadership and effectiveness. Cited in Girvan J 1998 Leadership and nursing. Macmillan, Basingstoke

Fielder A 1997 Pre-school vision screening: discussion. In: National Screening Committee/Royal College of Paediatrics and Child Health Proceedings: evolution or revolution? Systematic reviews of screening in child health, 17 December 1997 and 8 January 1998. Conference Organiser (c/o Child Growth Foundation), London, p 11–12

Finch J 1989 Family obligations and social change. Polit Press, London

Finkelhor D 1984 Child sexual abuse: new theory and research. Sage, London

Finkelhor D 1986 A sourcebook on child sexual abuse. Sage, Beverly Hills, CA

Fischbach FT 1991 Documenting care. FA Davis, Philadelphia, PA

Flanagan JC 1947 Cited in Dunn WR, Hamilton DD 1986 The Critical Incident Technique – a brief guide. Med Teach 8(3)

Flanagan JC 1954 The Critical Incident Technique. Cited in Dunn WR, Hamilton DD 1986 The Critical Incident Technique – a brief guide. Med Teach 8(3)

Flanagan JC 1963 Cited in Dunn WR, Hamilton DD 1986 The Critical Incident Technique – a brief guide. Med Teach 8(3)

Forester S, Kline R 1997 Integrated nursing teams. Professional Briefing. Health Visitor 70(6)

Frankenburg W, Dodds J 1967 The Denver Developmental Screening Test. J Paediatr 71: 181–191

Frankenburg W, Dodds J, Fandal A 1973 Denver Developmental Screening Test. Test Agency, High Wycombe

Frank-Stromborg M, Pender NJ, Walker SN 1990 Determinants of health-promoting lifestyles in ambulatory cancer patients. Soc Sci Med 31: 1159–1168

Frazer W 1950 A history of English public health 1834–1939. Baillière Tindall & Cox, London

French P 1999 The development of evidence-based nursing. J Adv Nurs 29: 72–78

Frude N 1996 Abuse within families. In: Gastrell P, Edwards J (ed) Community health nursing – frameworks for practice. Baillière Tindall, London

Fullerton R, Dickson R, Sheldon T 1997 Preventing and reducing the adverse effects of teenage pregnancy. Health Visitor 70: 197–199

Fung SF 1998 Factors associated with breast self-examination behaviour among Chinese women in Hong Kong. Patient Educ Couns 33: 233–243

Gallie WB 1955 Essentially contested concepts. Cited in Glen S 1995 Developing critical thinking in higher education. Nurse Educ Today 15: 170–176

Garcia A, Norton-Broda MA, Frenn M et al 1995 Gender and development differences in exercise beliefs among youth and prediction of their exercise behaviour. J School Health 65: 213–219

Gastrell P, Edwards J 1996 Community health nursing: frameworks for practice. Baillière Tindall, London

Gelles RJ 1983 An exchange/social control theory of intra-family violence. In: Finkelhor D, Gelles RJ, Hotaling G, Strauss MA (ed) The dark side of families: current family violence research. Sage, Beverly Hills, CA

Gephens A, Gunning-Schepers LJ 1996 Interventions to reduce socio-economic health differences: a review of the international literature. Eur J Publ Health 6: 218–226

Gesell A 1925 The mental growth of the pre-school child. Macmillan, New York

Gesell A 1948 Studies in child development. Harper, New York

Gesell A, Amatruda CS 1947 Developmental diagnosis. Hoeber, New York

Gesell A, Amatruda CS, Castner BM, Thompson H 1930 Biographies of child development. Hamish Hamilton, London

Gibb C, Randall PE 1989 Professionals and parents: managing children's behaviour. Macmillan, London

Gibbs G 1988 Learning by doing. A guide to teaching and learning methods. Further Education Unit, Oxford Polytechnic, Oxford

Gibson CH 1991 A concept analysis of empowerment. J Adv Nurs 16: 354–361

Gil D 1973 Violence against children: physical child abuse in the United States. Harvard University Press, Cambridge, MA

Gilbert A, Banks J 1997 30 degrees westward – a case study in making it happen. Ivybridge Public Health Project, unpublished report

Gilligan C 1982 In a different voice – psychological theory and women's' development. Harvard University Press, Cambridge, MA

Gillon R 1991 Philosophical medical ethics. John Wiley, Chichester

Girvan J 1998 Leadership and nursing. Macmillan, Basingstoke

Glen S 1995 Developing critical thinking in higher education. Nurse Educ Today 15: 170–176

Gogna S 1991 Extended family supportive networks towards Punjabi (Indian) elderly women. Unpublished report

Goldstone LA et al 1983 Monitor: an index of the quality of nursing care for acute medical and surgical wards. Newcastle upon Tyne Polytechnic Products, Newcastle upon Tyne

Goodman J 1984 Reflection and teacher education: a case study and theoretical analysis. Interchange 15: 9–26

Goodwin S 1983 Away with the velvet jacket brigade. Cited in Cain P, Hyde V, Howkins E 1995 Community nursing – dimensions and dilemmas. Edward Arnold, London

Goodwin S 1988 Whither health visiting? Health Visitor 61: 379–382

Goodwin S 1992 Community nursing and the new public health. Health Visitor 65: 78–80

Goudie H, Redman J 1996 Making health services more accessible to younger people. Nurs Times 92: 45–46

Grafstrom M, Nordberg A, Wimblad B 1992 Abuse is in the eye of the beholder: reports by family members about abuse of demented persons in home care: a total population based study. Scand J Soc Med 21: 247–255

Gravelle HSE, Simpson PR, Chamberlain J 1982 Breast cancer screening and health service costs. J Health Econ 1: 185–207

Green JM, Murray D 1994 The use of the Edinburgh Postnatal Depression Scale in research to explore the relationship between antenatal and postnatal dysphoria. Cited in Cox J, Holden J (ed) 1994 Perinatal psychiatry, use and misuse of the Edinburgh Postnatal Depression Scale. Gaskell, London

Green LW, Kreuter MW, Deeds SF et al 1980 Health education planning: a diagnostic approach. Mansfield Publishing, Palo Alto, CA

Greer S, Bauchner H, Zucherman B 1989 The Denver Developmental Screening Test: how good is its predictive validity? Devel Med Child Neurol 31: 774–781

Griffiths R 1954 The abilities of babies. University of London Press, London

Griffiths R 1970 The abilities of young children. Test Agency, High Wycombe

Grunfeld AF, Ritmiller S, Mackay K et al 1994 Detecting domestic violence against women in the emergency department: a nursing triage model. J Emerg Nurs 20: 271–274

Guillebaud J 1993 Contraception: hormonal and barrier methods. Martin Dunitz, London

Haggart M 1993 A critical analysis of Neuman's systems model in relation to public health nursing. J Adv Nurs 18: 1971–1922

Haggstrom WC 1970 The psychological implications of the community development process. In: Carcy LJ Community Development as a Process. University of Missouri Press, Columbia, MO.

Halford WK 1994 Familial factors in psychiatry. Curr Opin Psychiat 7: 186–191

Hall D 1986 Developmental tests and scales. Arch Dis Childh 61: 213–215

Hall D (ed) 1989 Health for all children: a programme for child health surveillance. Report of the Joint Working Party on Child Health Surveillance. Oxford University Press, Oxford

Hall D (ed) 1991 Health for all children: a programme for child health surveillance. Report of the Joint Working Party on Child Health Surveillance, 2nd edn. Oxford University Press, Oxford

Hall D (ed) 1996 Health for all children: a programme for child health surveillance. Report of the Joint Working Party on Child Health Surveillance, 3rd edn. Oxford University Press, Oxford

Ham C 1996 Tragic choices in health care. King's Fund, London

Ham C 1998 Population centred and patient-focussed purchasing – the UK experience. Millbank Q 74: 191–214

Ham C, Willis A 1994 Perspectives on purchasing. Think globally act locally. Health Service Journal 104(5385): 27–29

Hamilton M 1989 Frequency of symptoms in melancholia (depressive illness). Br J Psychiat 154: 201–206

Hamilton P 1988 A Delphi survey for the development of community health nursing theory. Cited in Cain P, Hyde V, Howkins E 1995 Community nursing: dimensions and dilemmas. Edward Arnold, London

Hanks H, Stratton P 1988 Family perspectives in early sexual abuse. In: Browne K, Davies C, Stratton P (ed) Early prediction and prevention of child abuse. John Wiley, Chichester

Harding S, Pandya N 1995 The role of health advocates in health visiting teams. Health Visitor 68: 192–193

Harris A 1996 What is a primary care-led health policy? In: Littlejohn P, Victor C (ed) Making sense of a primary care-led health service. Radcliffe Medical Press, Oxford, ch 3

Harris J 1985 The value of life. Routledge, London

Harter S 1983 Developmental perspectives on the self-system. Cited in Sarafino E 1994 Health psychology, 2nd edn. John Wiley, New York

Hatchwell PK 1992 Genetic research: implications for workplace screening. Occup Health Rev April/May: 8–11

Hatton P 1990 Measles/mumps/rubella vaccine (MMR): an audit of Leeds health professionals' knowledge of contraindications and intention to vaccinate assessed by postal questionnaire. J Publ Health Med 12: 124–130

Hawtin M, Hughes G, Percy-Smith J 1994 Community profiling – auditing social needs. Open University Press, Buckingham

Haynes R, Sackett D, Taylor D et al 1978 Increased absenteeism from work after detection and labelling of hypertensive patients. New Engl J Med 299

Health Education Authority 1995 Black and minority ethnic groups in England: health and lifestyles. HEA, London

Health Education Authority 1997a Promoting health through primary care nursing. HEA, London

Health Education Authority 1997b Many voices, one message: guidance for the development and translation of health information. HEA, London

Health Resources and Service Administration 1997 National vaccine injury compensation program: vaccine injury table. http://www.hrsa.dhhs.gov/bhpr/vic/table.htm

Health Visitor 1997a GP fundholders drop posts. Fundholding, Health News. Health Visitor 70(3)

Health Visitor 1997b Lifespan nurses discuss their next move… and the UKCC urges caution over cuts in home visits. Health News. Health Visitor 70(10)

Heath H 1998 Reflections and patterns of knowing in nursing. J Adv Nurs 27: 1054–1059

Hendriksen C, Stromgard E, Sorensen KH 1989 Cooperation concerning admission to and discharge of elderly people from the hospital. The coordinated contributions of home care personnel. Ugeskr-laeger 151: 1531–1534

Hennessy DA 1985 Mothers and health visitors. Cited in Twinn SF 1991 Conflicting paradigms of health visiting: a continuing debate for professional practice. J Adv Nurs 16: 966–973

Heron J 1986 Six category intervention analysis, 2nd edn. Human Potential Research Project. University of Surrey, Guildford

Higham M 1988 The training needs of health workers. National Extension College for Training in Health and Race, Cambridge

Hinde RA, Tamplin A, Barret J 1993 A comparative study of relationship structure. Br J Soc Psychol 32: 191–207

HMSO 1989 The Children Act – guidance and regulation. HMSO, London

Holden J 1994 Using the Edinburgh Postnatal Depression Scale in clinical practice. In Cox J, Holden J (ed) Perinatal psychiatry, use and misuse of the Edinburgh Postnatal Depression Scale. Gaskell, London

Holden JM, Sagovsky R, Cox JL 1989 Counselling in a general practice setting: controlled study of health visitor intervention in treatment of postnatal depression. Br Med J 298: 223–226

Homans G 1961 Social behaviour: its elementary forms.

Harcourt Brace Jovanovich, New York

Home Office 1999 Supporting families, a consultation document. Stationery Office, London

Hooks B 1993 Sisters of the yam. South End Press, Boston, MA

Housing Today 1998 Round up – caring and sharing. Housing Today 96

HSC 1974 The Health and Safety at Work Act. HMSO, London

Hudson R 1997 Demonstrating effectiveness: compiling the evidence. Health Visitor 70: 459–461

Hulse JA et al 1997 Population growth analysis using the Child Health Computing System: a method of assessing the value of child health surveillance. In: National Screening Committee/Royal College of Paediatrics and Child Health Proceedings: evolution or revolution? Systematic reviews of screening in child health, 17 December 1997 and 8 January 1998. Conference Organiser (c/o Child Growth Foundation), London, p 21

Hulse JA, Schilg S, Blount J et al 1998 Systematic reviews of child health. Royal College of Paediatrics and Child Health, London

Humphries E 1989 An evaluation of the developmental examination programme used in Halesowen by audit of the medical records of children statemented between January 1988 and December 1989 to determine if children with learning difficulties could have been identified before. Unpublished PGD thesis.

Hunt JM 1996 Guest editorial. J Adv Nurs 23: 423–425

Husband C (ed) 1982 Race in Britain: continuity and change. Hutchinson, London

Hutcheson JJ, Black MM, Talley M et al 1997 Risk status and home intervention among children with failure to thrive: follow-up at age 4. J Pediatr Psychol 22: 651–668

Hutchinson K, Gutteridge B 1995 Health visiting homeless families: the role of the specialist health visitor. Health Visitor 68: 372–374

HVA 1991 In their own hands. Health Visitor Association, London

Hyde V 1995 Community nursing: a unified discipline? In: Cain P, Hyde V, Howkins E (ed) 1995 Community nursing: dimensions and dilemmas. Edward Arnold, London

Hyland M, Donaldson J 1987 Hyland–Donaldson Psychological Skills Scale for health visitors. Poly Enterprises Plymouth, Plymouth

Illingworth RS 1975 The development of the infant and young child. Normal and abnormal. Churchill Livingstone, Edinburgh

Illingworth RS 1987 The development of the infant and young child, 9th edn. Churchill Livingstone, Edinburgh

Independent Review of Residential Care 1988 Residential Care: a positive choice. Report of the Independent review of residential care chaired by Gillian Wagner. HMSO, London

Ingalsbe N, Spears MC 1979 Development of an instrument to evaluate critical incident performance. Cited in Dunn WR, Hamilton DD 1986 The Critical Incident Technique – a brief guide. Med Teach 8(3)

Ingram DR, Clarke DR, Murdiq RA 1978 Distance and the decision to visit an Emergency Department. Soc Sci Med 12: 55–62

Irish College of General Practitioners 1995 Quality in practice programme. Irish College of General Practitioners, Dublin

Iyer PW, Camp NH 1991 Nursing documentation. Mosby–Year Book, Chicago, IL

Jackson C 1992 Trick or treat. Health Visitor 65: 199–201

Jackson C 1994 Strelley: teamworking for health. Health Visitor 65(1)

Jackson P, Plant Z 1996 Youngsters get an introduction to sexual health clinics. Nurs Times 92: 34–36

James-Hanman D 1998 Domestic violence: breaking the silence. Commun Practit 71: 404–407

Jarman B 1983 Identification of underprivileged areas. Br Med J 286: 1705–1709

Jarvis P 1987 Adult learning in the social context. Croom Helm, London

Jarvis P 1992 Reflective practice and nursing. Nurse Educ Today 12: 174–181

Jeffreys M 1965 An anatomy of social welfare services. Cited in Robinson J 1982 An evaluation of health visiting. Council for the Education and Training of Health Visitors, London

Jeyasingham M 1992 Acting for health: ethnic minorities and the community movement. In: Ahmad WI (ed) The politics of race and health. Race Relations Unit, University of Bradford and Ilkley Community College, Bradford

Jezierski M 1992 Guidance for intervention by ED nurses in cases of domestic violence. J Emerg Nurs 18: 28A–30A

Johns CC 1992 The Burford Nursing Development Unit holistic model of nursing practice. J Adv Nurs 16: 1090–1098

Johnson MRD 1996 Ethnic minorities, health and communication. Research paper in Ethnic Relations No. 24. NHS Executive and West Midlands Regional Health Authority Centre for Research in Ethnic relations, Birmingham

Johnson Z, Howell F, Molloy B 1993 Community mothers' programme: randomised controlled trial of non-professional intervention in parenting. Br Med J 306: 1449–1452

Jones D et al 1987 Understanding child abuse. Macmillan, Basingstoke

Jones JS 1990 Geriatric abuse and neglect. Cited in: Bennett G, Kingston P, Penhale B 1997 The dimensions of elder abuse: perspectives for practitioners. Macmillan, Basingstoke

Jones L 1994 The social context of health and health work. Macmillan Press, Basingstoke

Jones M 1996 Clients express preference for one-step sexual health shop. Nursing Times 96(21): 32–33

Jones R, Pendlebury M 1992 Public sector accounting, 3rd edn. Pitman, London

Kant I 1964 Groundwork of the metaphysics of morals, trans Paton HJ. Harper & Row, New York, p 90–91

Kendrick D, Bakewell S 1995 On the verge, the Gypsies and England. University of Hertfordshire Press

Kenny T 1993 Nursing models fail in practice. Br J Nurs 2(2)

Kerr S, Jowett S, Smith L 1997 Education to help prevent sleep problems in infants. Health Visitor 70: 224–225

Kessen W 1965 The child. John Wiley, New York

Khan S 1995 Cultural constructions: male sexualities in India. Presentation to the 12th World Congress of Sexology, 12–16 August 1995, Yokohama, Japan

Kieffer GD 1988 The strategy of meetings. Piatkus, London

Killoran A, Mays N, Griffiths R, Posnett J 1998 Growing pains. Health Serv J, 5 Nov

Kiln MR 1998 Those giving MMR vaccine had no input into it (letter). Br Med J. 316: 1824

King's Fund 1999 Briefing – what is clinical governance? King's Fund, London

Kitchener KS 1983 Educational goals and reflective thinking. Cited in Kitchener KS, King PM 1990 The reflective judgement model: transforming assumptions about knowing. In: Mezirow J et al (ed) Fostering critical reflection in adulthood. Jossey-Bass, San Francisco

Kitchener KS, King PM 1990 The reflective judgement model: transforming assumptions about knowing. In: Mezirow J et al (ed) Fostering critical reflection in adulthood. Jossey-Bass, San Francisco

Kitson A, Ahmed LB, Harvey G et al 1996 From research to practice: one organisational model for promoting research-based practice. J Adv Nurs 23: 430–440

Kivel P 1996 Uprooting racism – how white people can work for racial justice. New Society, Philadelphia, PA

Klein R, Redmayne S 1992 Patterns of priorities. A study of the purchasing and rationing policies of health authorities. NAHAT, London

Kogan M, Redfern S 1995 Making use of clinical audit – a guide to practice in the health professions. Open University Press, Buckingham

Krause IB 1989 'Sinking heart'. A Punjabi communication of distress. Soc Sci Med 29: 405–417

Laidman P 1987 Health visiting and preventing accidents to children. Research report No. 12. Child Accident Prevention Trust. Health Education Authority, London

Lalonde M 1974 A new perspective on the health of Canadians. Department of Health and Welfare, Ottawa

Lancet 1986 Developmental surveillance. Lancet, 26 April: 950–952

Larson CP 1980 Efficacy of prenatal and postpartum home visits on child health and development. Pediatrics 66: 191–197

Law J et al 1997 Child health surveillance: an evaluation of screening for speech and language delay (executive summary). In: National Screening Committee/Royal College of Paediatrics and Child Health Proceedings: evolution or revolution? Systematic reviews of screening in child health, 17 December 1997 and 8 January 1998. Conference Organiser (c/o Child Growth Foundation), London

Lawton E 1996 Leader of the pack. Health Visitor 69: 198

Leininger M 1997 Future directions in transcultural nursing in the 21st century. Int Nurs Rev 44: 19–23

Letellier P 1996 Twin epidemics: domestic violence and HIV infection among gay and bisexual men. In: Renzetti CM, Miley CH (ed) Violence in gay and lesbian domestic partnerships. Harrington Park Press, New York

Lewin K 1935 A dynamic theory of personality. McGraw-Hill, New York

Lewis M 1988 What can child development tell us about child abuse? In: Browne K, Davies C, Stratton P (ed) Early prediction and prevention of child abuse. John Wiley, Chichester

Lightfoot J 1994 Demonstrating the value of health visiting. Health Visitor 67: 19–20

Lilley R 1998 Naked truth about PCGs. Doctor 10 Dec: 31

Lindblom C 1959 The science of muddling through. Publ Admin Rev 19: 79–88

Lindblom C 1979 Still muddling, not yet through. Publ Admin Rev 39: 516–517

Lister R 1996 Strategies for change: reflections on the Commission for Social Justice Report. Lecture given at

REFERENCES

Woodbrooke College Day School on 'Social Justice in Britain – building a more just and hopeful society', Selly Oak Colleges, Birmingham, 9 March 1996.

Little L 1997 Teenage health education: a public health approach. Nursing Standard 11: 43–46

Littlejohn P, Victor C 1996 Making sense of a primary care-led health service. Radcliffe Medical Press, Oxford

Littlewood J 1987 Community nursing – an overview. Cited in Cain P, Hyde V, Howkins E 1995 Community nursing: dimensions and dilemmas. Edward Arnold, London

Littlewood R, Lipsedge M 1988 Psychiatric illness among Afro-Caribbeans. Br Med J 296: 950–951

Littley A 1996 Integrated nursing teams. Presentation to Southern Birmingham Community NHS Trust (unpublished)

Luker KA 1978 Goal attainment: a possible model for assessing the work of the health visitor. Nurs Times 75: 1488–1490

Luker K 1982 Evaluating health visiting practice: an experimental study to evaluate the effects of focused health visitor intervention on elderly women living alone at home. Royal College of Nursing, London

Luker KA 1985 Evaluating health visiting practice. In: Luker KA, Orr J (ed) Health visiting. Blackwell Scientific, Oxford

Luker K, Orr J 1992 Health visiting towards community health nursing, 2nd edn. Blackwell Scientific, Oxford

Lusk SL, Ronis D, Kerr MJ et al 1994 Test of the health promotion model as a causal model of workers' use of hearing protection. Nurs Res 43: 151–157

Lynn M 1987 Update: Denver Developmental Screening Test. J Paediatr Nurs 2: 348–351

McCallum J 1993 Elder abuse: the 'new' social problem? cited in Bennett G, Kingston P, Penhall B. Modern Medicine of Australia Sept: 74–83

McClymont M, Thomas S, Denhamm MJ 1991 Health visiting and elderly people. A health promotion challenge. Churchill Livingstone, Edinburgh

McConnaughy EA, Procaska JO, Velicer WF 1983 Stages of change in psychotherapy: measurement and sample profiles. Psychother Theor Res Pract 20: 368–375

McFarlane J 1986 The value of models for care. In: Kershaw B, Salvage J (ed) Models for nursing. John Wiley, Chichester

Macfarlane A, Sefi S, Cordeiro M 1990 Child health: the screening tests. Oxford University Press, Oxford

Macfarlene JA, Saffin K 1990 Do general practitioners and health visitors like parent held child health records? Br J Gen Pract 40: 106–108

McIver S 1993 Obtaining the views of users of primary and community health care services. King's Fund, London

Mack P, Trew K 1991 Are fathers' views important? Health Visitor 64: 257–258

McKears J 1994 Multi-agency aspects of training in child protection. Unpublished MSc dissertation, Coventry University

McKee CM, Gleadhill DNS, Watson JD 1990 Accident and Emergency attendance rates: variation among patients from different general practices. Br J Gen Pract 40: 150–153

Mackereth C 1996 What do we mean by community development? Report back from one of the workshops, Study Day Paper, April 1996. Community Development Interest Group, Community Practitioners' and Health Visitors' Association, London

Macleod-Clark J 1993 Nurse–patient communication: an analysis of conversations from surgical wards. In: Wilson-Barnett J (ed) Nursing research: ten studies in patient care. John Wiley, Chichester

McNaught A 1988 Race and health policy. Croom Helm, London

Marcé Society 1994 The emotional effects of childbirth. Distance Learning Course. H Wharton, Doncaster

Mares P et al 1985 Health care in multiracial Britain. Health Education Council/National Extension College, Cambridge

Marley L 1995 Setting up a duty health visitor rota. Health Visitor 68: 456

Marmot MG, McKeigue PM 1988 Mortality from coronary heart disease in Asian communities. Br Med J 297

Marris T 1971 The work of health visitors in London: a Department of Planning and Transportation survey, 1969. Research report 12. Greater London Council, London

Marrujo B, Kreger M 1996 Definition of roles in abusive lesbian relationships. In: Renzetti CM, Miley CH (ed) Violence in gay and lesbian domestic partnerships. Harrington Park Press, New York

Marshall A 1936 Principles of economics, 8th edn. Macmillan, London

Marteau TM 1989 Psychological costs of screening: may sometimes be bad enough to undermine the benefits of screening. Br Med J 299: 527

Marteau TM 1990 Reducing the psychological costs. Br Med J 301

Matthews E 1986 Can paternalism be modernised? J Med Ethics 12: 133–135

Maxwell R 1984 Quality assurance in health. Br Med J 12 May: 1470–1472

Mayall B, Foster CD 1989 Child health care, living with children, working for children. Heinemann Nursing, Oxford

Mead GH 1934 Mind, self, and society. University of Chicago Press, Chicago, IL

Meade TW, Dyer S, Browne W et al 1990 Low back pain of mechanical origin: randomised comparison of chiropractic and hospital outpatient treatment. Br Med J 300: 143

Meerabeau E 1992 Tacit nursing knowledge: an untapped resource or a methodological headache? J Adv Nurs 17: 108–112

Megargee EI 1966 Undercontrolled and overcontrolled personality types in extreme anti-social aggression. Cited in Owens RG, Ashcroft JB 1985 Violence, a guide for the caring professions. Croom Helm, London

Meleis AI 1985 Theoretical nursing: development and progress. JB Lippincott, Philadelphia, PA

Merrill GS 1996 Ruling the exceptions: same-sex battering and domestic violence theory. In: Renzetti CM, Miley CH (ed) Violence in gay and lesbian domestic partnerships. Harrington Park Press, New York

Merrill J 1989 Attempted suicide by deliberate self-poisoning amongst Asians. Cited in Smaje C 1995 Health, race and ethnicity: making sense of the evidence. King's Fund Institute/Share, London

Messages from Research 1995 Studies in child protection. HMSO, London

Mezirow J 1981 A critical theory of adult learning and education. Adult Educ 32(1)

Mezirow J et al 1990 Fostering critical reflection in adulthood. Jossey Bass, San Francisco

Miles M, Huberman A 1994 Qualitative data analysis, 2nd edn. Sage, London

Miller C 1975 American Rom and the ideology of defilement. In: Rehfisch F (ed) Gypsies, tinkers and other travellers. Academic Press, London

Miller D, Madge N, Diamond J, Wadsworth J, Ross E 1993 Pertussis immunisation and serious acute neurological illnesses in children. BMJ 307: 1171–1176

Ministry of Agriculture, Fisheries and Food 1989 Manual of nutrition. HMSO, London

Ministry of Health 1956 An inquiry into health visiting. Ministry of Health, Department of Health for Scotland, Ministry of Education (the Jameson Committee). HMSO, London

Minugh PA, Rice C, Young L 1998 Gender, health beliefs, health behaviours, and alcohol consumption. Am J Alcohol Abuse 24: 483–497

Mitchell JH 1969 Compliance with medical regimens: an annotated bibliography. Department of Medical Care and Hospitals, School of Hygiene and Public Health, Johns Hopkins University, Baltimore, MD

Moch S 1990 Personal knowing: evolving research and practice. Cited in Heath H 1998 Reflections and patterns of knowing in nursing. J Adv Nurs 27: 1054–1059

Modood T 1994 Political blackness and British Asians. Sociology 28: 859–876

Modood T et al 1997 Ethnic minorities in Britain: diversity and disadvantage. Policy Studies Institute, London

Mooney G, Gerard K, Donaldson C, Farrar S 1992 Purchasing and priority setting. NAHAT, London

Mooney G, Madden L, Hussey R 1993 Priority setting in purchasing – public health and economics in tandem. Paper presented at the joint meeting of the Health Economists Study Group and the Faculty of Public Health Medicine, University of York

Moore W 1994 Taking up the sales challenge. Health Visitor 67(10)

Moores Y 1991 Nursing and IT: issues and opportunities. Inf Technol Nurs 3(3)

Moores Y 1992 The nursing profession's contribution to the strategy for NHS information management and technology. Inf Technol Nurs 4(4)

Moos RH, Schaefer JA 1986 Life transitions and crises: a conceptual overview. Cited in Sarafino EP 1994 Health psychology. John Wiley, New York

Mor V, Granger CV, Sherwood CC 1983 Discharged rehabilitation patients: impact of follow-up surveillance by a friendly visitor. Arch Phys Med Rehab 64: 346–353

Murphy K, Clark JM 1993 Nurses' experiences of caring for ethnic minority clients. J Adv Nurs 18: 442–450

Naidoo J, Wills J 1994 Health promotion. Foundations for practice. Baillière Tindall, London

Naish J 1991 Access to Health Records Act 1990. Health Visitor Association Centre Circular CS. 91/31. HVA, London

Naish J, Kline R 1990 What counts can't always be counted. Health Visitor 63: 421–422

Nanda S 1986 Gender roles in India (from Hijras: an alternative sex and gender role in India)

National Casemix Office 1997 Casemix groupings for community services. A discussion paper, version 1.1. NHS Executive, London

National Casemix Office 1999 Primary care. Don't be a fish out of water – get primed! One Day conference, 1 March. NHS Executive, London

Neuman B 1989 The Neuman Systems Model. Appleton & Lange, Norwalk, CT

NHS Development Unit 1998 An organisational development resource for Primary Care Groups. NHS Development Unit, Leeds

NHS Ethnic Health Unit 1996 Good practice and quality indicators in primary health care. In: Health care for Black and minority ethnic people. NHS Ethnic Health Unit, London, p 13–14

NHS Executive 1993 New world, new opportunities: nursing in primary health care. HMSO, London

NHS Executive 1995a Planning guidelines. NHS Executive, London

NHS Executive 1995b Developing NHS purchasing and GP fundholding: towards a primary care-led NHS. HMSO, London

NHS Executive 1996 Promoting clinical effectiveness. NHS Executive, Leeds

NHS Executive 1997 Priorities and planning guidance for the NHS: 1997/98. NHS Executive, Leeds

NHS Executive 1998a Report of NHS Executive Workshop, Nurse Involvement in Primary Care Groups, Swallow Hotel, York 3 April

NHS Executive 1998b Information for health: an information strategy for the modern NHS 1998–2005. Stationery Office, London

Nicoll A, Elliman D, Ross E 1998 MMR vaccination and autism. Br Med J 316: 715–716

Nolan M 1996 The Blenheim Harding Trust: meeting the needs of young women who become pregnant. Modern Midwife 6: 22–24

Norman A 1985 Triple jeopardy, growing old in a second homeland. Centre for Policy on Aging, London

Norris C (ed) 1982 Concept clarification in nursing. Aspen Systems, Germantown, MD

North N 1997 Politics and procedures: the strategy process in a health commission. Health Soc Care Commun 5: 375–383

North Staffs Combined Healthcare Trust 1996 Promoting health visiting. North Staffs Combined Healthcare Trust, Stoke on Trent

Novak JD, Gowan DB 1984 Learning how to learn. Cambridge University Press, New York

O'Neill P 1990 State health plan for the poor stalls. Oregonian June 15

Oakeshott M 1962 Rationalism in politics: and other essays. Cited in Eraut M 1985 Knowledge creation and knowledge use in professional contexts. Stud Higher Educ 10: 117–133

Obermann K, Tolley K 1997 The state of health care priority setting and public participation. Discussion Paper 154. Centre for Health Economics, University of York, York

Oehler JM, Vileisis RA 1990 Effect of early sibling visitation in an intensive care nursery. J Devel Behav Pediatr 11: 7–12

Office for Public Management 1996 Learning from Linc. Leadership in Nursing for the Community – a development programme for nurses. Office for Public Management, London

Office for Public Management 1997 Achieving Health Gain through Health Promotion in a Primary Care-led NHS. Health Education Authority, London

Okely J 1975 Gypsy women: models in conflict. In: Ardener S (ed) Perceiving women. Malaby, London

Okely J 1983 The traveller gypsies. Cambridge University Press, Cambridge

Olson DH, Russell CS, Sprenkle DH 1979 Circumplex model of marital and family systems. II: Empirical studies and clinical intervention. Cited in Gastrell P, Edwards J 1996 Community health nursing – frameworks for practice. Baillière Tindall, London

Ong BN 1986 Women in the transition to socialism in Sub-Saharan Africa. In: Munslow B (ed) Africa's problems in the transition to socialism. Zed Books, London

Open University 1998 Clinical supervision. A development pack for nurses, K509. Open University Press, Buckingham

Opportunities for Women 1990 Carers at work. Opportunities for Women, London

Orem DE 1985 Nursing: concepts of practice, 3rd edn. McGraw Hill, New York

Orem D 1991 Nursing concepts of practice, 4th edn. Mosby-Year Book, St Louis, MO

Ormerod P 1994 The death of economics. Faber & Faber, London

Ottewill R, Wall A 1990 The growth and development of the community health services. Business Education Publishers, London

Øvretveit J 1998 Evaluating health interventions. Open University Press, Buckingham

Owens RG, Ashcroft JB 1985 Violence, a guide for the caring professions. Croom Helm, London

Padgett K 1991 Correlates of self-efficacy beliefs among patients with non-insulin dependent diabetes mellitus in Zagreb, Yugoslavia. Patient Educ Couns 139–147

Pahl J, Vaile M 1986 Health and health care among Travellers. University of Kent Health Services Research Unit, Canterbury

Parton N 1981 Child abuse, social anxiety and welfare. Br J Soc Work 11: 391–414

Parton N 1990 Taking child abuse seriously. In: The Violence against Children Study Group. Taking child abuse seriously, contemporary issues in child protection theory and practice. Unwin Hyman, London, ch 1

Patel N 1993 Healthy margins, black elders' care – models, policies and prospects. In: Ahmad W (ed) Race and health in contemporary Britain. Open University Press, Buckingham

Pearson P 1996 Looking for the evidence: research in community development. Study Day paper. Community Development Interest Group, Community Practitioners' and Health Visitors' Association, London

Pearson P, Waterson T 1992 Newcastle parent held record: report of a pilot study. Newcastle upon Tyne Health Authority, Newcastle upon Tyne

Peckham S, Macdonald J, Taylor P 1996 Primary care and public health phase 1: Project report – report to Public Health Trust Project Steering Group. Public Health Alliance, Birmingham

Peckham S, Taylor P, Turton P 1998 Public health model of primary care. Concept to reality. Public Health Alliance, Birmingham

Pender NJ 1982 Health Promotion in Nursing Practice. Appleton-Century Crofts, Norwalk, Connecticut

Pender NJ 1987 Health promotion in nursing practice, 2nd edn. Appleton & Lange, Norwalk, CT

Pender NJ 1996 Health promotion in nursing practice, 3rd edn. Appleton & Lange, Stamford, CT

Pender NJ, Walker SN, Sechrist KR et al 1990 Predicting health-promoting lifestyles in the workplace. Nurs Res 39: 326–332

Pennebaker JW 1990 Opening up: the healing power of confiding in others. Cited in Sarafino EP 1994 Health psychology. John Wiley, New York

Peplau H 1952 Interpersonal relations in nursing. GP Putman, New York

Perlin LI, Schooler C 1978 The structure of coping. Cited in Sarafino EP 1994 Health psychology. John Wiley, New York

Phillipson C 1992 Confronting elder abuse: fact and fiction. Generations Rev 2: 2–3

Phillipson C, Biggs S 1992 Understanding elder abuse: a training manual for helping professions. Longman, Harlow

Pietroni P 1996 The integrated community care practice: general practice, citizenship and community care. In: Meads G (ed) Future options for general practice. Radcliffe Medical Press, Oxford

Pilgrim D, Rogers A 1995 Mass childhood immunisation: some ethical doubts for primary health care workers. Nurs Ethics 2: 63–70

Pitts M, Phillips K 1991 The psychology of health. Routledge, London

Plant A 1992 Performance indicators. Unpublished paper, North Staffordshire Combined Healthcare NHS Trust

Polanyi M 1958 Personal knowledge: towards a post critical philosophy. Routledge & Kegan Paul, London

Polanyi M 1967 The tacit dimension. Routledge & Kegan Paul, London

Polit D, Hungler B 1995 Nursing research: principles and methods, 5th edn. JB Lippincott, Philadelphia, PA

Pollak KI, Carbonari JP, DiClemente CC et al 1998 Causal relationships of processes of change and decisional balance: stage-specific models for smoking. Addictive Behav 23: 437–448

Pollitt E 1994 Poverty and child development: relevance of research in developing countries to the United States. Child Devel 65: 283–295

Porter S, Ryan S 1996 Breaking the boundaries between nursing and sociology: a critical realist ethnography of the theory practice gap. J Adv Nurs 24: 413–420

Pound R 1992 Key issues in child protection for health visitors and nurses. In Cloke C, Naish J. John Wiley, Chichester

Pringle MK 1975 The needs of children. Cited in Straw J, Anderson J 1996 Parenting: a discussion paper. The Labour Party, November 1996

Pritchard R 1996 Measuring and improving organisational productivity. Department of Psychology, Texas A & M University, College Station, TX

Procaska J, DiClemente C 1984 The transtheoretical approach: crossing traditional boundaries of therapy. Dow Jones-Irwin, Homewood, IL

Procaska J, DiClemente C 1988 Treating addictive behaviours. Processes of change. Plenum Press, New York

Rack P 1982 Race, culture and mental disorder. Tavistock, London

Randall P 1997 Adult bullying – perpetrators and victims. Routledge, London

RCN 1990 Dynamic standard setting system. Royal College of Nursing, London

RCN 1994 Public health nursing rises to the challenge. Royal College of Nursing, London

RCN 1995 The hidden abuse. Nursing Update Series. Royal College of Nursing, London

RCN 1996 National health manifesto. Royal College of Nursing, London

RCN 1998 Caring together: clinical supervision. RCN Nursing Update 13 Learning Unit 077, issued in Nurs Stand 12(22)

Reinke BJ, Holmes DS, Denney NW 1981 Influence of a 'friendly visitor' program on the cognitive functioning and morale of elderly persons. Am J Commun Psychol 9: 491–504

Renzetti CM, Miley CH (ed) 1996 Violence in gay and lesbian domestic partnerships. Harrington Park Press, New York

Reynell J 1969 Reynell Developmental Language Scales. NFER, Windsor

Reynolds M 1992 Developmental screening: the need for change. Unpublished BSc project, University of Wolverhampton

Reynolds M 1999 A study to explore the usefulness of The Schedule of Growing Skills in enabling health visitors to fulfil their role of promoting the child's health and development in child protection work. Unfinished MPhil dissertation, University of Wolverhampton

Richardson D, Robinson V (ed) 1993 Introducing women's studies. Macmillan, Basingstoke

Riding H 1985 Serological surveillance of herd immunity to various infectious agents and the investigation of some rapid viral diagnostic techniques. Unpublished MSc thesis, University of Glasgow

Roberts J 1988 Why are some families more vulnerable to child abuse? In: Browne K, Davies C, Stratton P (ed) Early prediction and prevention of child abuse. John Wiley, Chichester

Roberts MM 1989 Breast screening: time for a rethink? Br Med J 299: 1153–1155

Roberts H 1990 Women's health counts. Routledge, London

Roberts B 1996 Health at home. In: Twinn S, Roberts B, Andrews S (ed) Community health care nursing. Butterworth-Heinemann, Oxford

Roberts K, Ludvigsen C 1998 Project management for health care professionals. Butterworth-Heinemann, Oxford

Roberts I, Kramer M, Suissa S 1996 Does home visiting prevent childhood injury: a systematic review of randomised controlled trials. Br Med J 312: 29–33

Robinson J 1982 An evaluation of health visiting. Council for the Education and Training of Health Visitors, London

Robinson J 1992 Problems with paradigms in a caring profession. J Adv Nurs 17: 632–638

Robinson J, Elkan R 1996 Health needs assessment: theory and practice. Churchill Livingstone, Edinburgh

Robinson J 1998 The effectiveness of domiciliary health visiting – a systematic review of the literature commissioned from the University of Nottingham by the NHS R & D Technology Assessment Programme. Conference paper presented to the RCN, London

Robotham EA 1998 Health visiting education: challenging present systems. Commun Practit 71: 21

Rodrigues L 1998 Survival tactics. Nurs Times 94(6)

Rogers CR 1951 Client-centred therapy. Constable, London

Rogers C 1967 On becoming a person – a therapist's view of psychotherapy. Constable, London

Rose RM, Holaday JW, Bernstein IS 1971 Plasma testosterone, dominance rank and aggressive behaviour in male Rhesus monkeys. Cited in Owens RG, Ashcroft JB 1985 Violence, a guide for the caring professions. Croom Helm, London

Rosenstock IM 1966 Why people use health services. Milbank Mem Fund Q 44: 94

Rosenstock IM 1974 Historical origins of the Health Belief Model. In: Becker MH (ed) The Health Belief Model and personal health behaviour. Charles B Slack, NJ

ROSPA 1993 Safety and minority ethnic communities. A preliminary report on the home safety information needs of the Asians, Chinese and Vietnamese communities living in the UK in the 1990s. Royal Society for the Prevention of Accidents, London

Rossman GB, Wilson BL 1991 Numbers and words revisited: being 'shamelessly eclectic'. Eval Rev 9: 627–643

Roter JB 1966 Generalised expectancies for the internal versus external control of reinforcement. Cited in Sarafino EP 1994 Health psychology. John Wiley, New York

Rotter D 1977 Patient participation in the patient–provider interaction: the effect of patient question asking on the quality of interaction, satisfaction and compliance. Health Educ Monogr 5: 281–315

Roy C 1975 A diagnostic classification system for nursing. Nurs Outlook 23: 90–94

Roy C, Andrews HA 1991 The Roy Adaptation Model, the definitive statement. Appleton & Lange, Norwalk, CT

Runciman P, Currie CT, Nicol M et al 1996 Discharge of elderly people from an accident and emergency department: evaluation of health visitor follow-up. J Adv Nurs 24: 711–718

Sackett D 1973 Periodic health examinations and multiphasic screening. Can Med Assoc J 109: 1124

Sackett DL, Rosenberg WMC, Gray JAM et al 1996 Evidence-based medicine: what it is and what it isn't. Br Med J 312: 71–72

Sackett DL, Richardson WS, Rosenberg GW et al 1997 Evidence-based medicine. How to teach and practice EBM. Churchill Livingstone, New York

Sampson J 1930 The wind on the heath – a gypsy anthology. Chatto & Windus, London

Samuelson PA 1976 Economics. McGraw-Hill, Tokyo

Sanderson D 1997 Cost analysis in child health surveillance. In: National Screening Committee/Royal College of Paediatrics and Child Health Proceedings: evolution or revolution? Systematic reviews of screening in child health, 17 December 1997 and 8 January 1998. Conference Organiser (c/o Child Growth Foundation), London, p 20–21

Sarafino EP 1994 Health psychology. John Wiley, New York

Saylor CR 1990 Reflection and professional education: art, science, and competency. Nurse Educator 15: 8–11

Schön DA 1983 The reflective practitioner. Basic Books, New York

Schön DA 1987 Educating the reflective practitioner: towards a new design for teaching and learning in the professions. Jossey-Bass, San Francisco, CA

Schreiber R et al 1998 The context for managing depression and its stigma among West Indian Canadian women. J Adv Nurs 27: 510–517

Schutz A 1972 The phenomenology of the social world. Heinemann, London

Scott-Samuel A 1984 Identification of underprivileged areas. Br Med J 287: 130

Scottish Office 1997 Designed to care: renewing the National Health Service in Scotland. Cmnd 3811. Stationery Office, London

Scottish Office 1999 Towards a healthier Scotland. Cmnd 4269. Stationery Office, London

Seedhouse D 1988 Ethics: the heart of healthcare. John Wiley, Chichester

Seligman MEP 1975 Helplessness: on depression, development and death. Freeman, San Francisco, CA

Senior PA, Bhopal R 1994 Ethnicity as a variable in epidemiological research. Br Med J 309: 327

Seyle H 1956 The stress of life. McGraw-Hill, New York

SHAC/Shelter 1988 Prescription for poor health; the crisis for homeless families. London Food Commission, London

Shaw DS, Vondra JI 1995 Infant attachment security and maternal predicators of early behaviour problems: a longitudinal study of low-income families. J Abnormal Child Psychol 23(3)

Sheikh, Thomas 1994 Factors influencing food choice among ethnic minority adolescents. Nutrit Food Sci: 4(5): 29–35

Sheldon TA, Parke H 1992 Race and ethnicity in health research. J Publ Health Med 14: 106

Sheldrake D, Sillman C, Notter J 1997 Developing partnerships in practice: using the Edinburgh Postnatal Depression Scale in health visiting. Report produced for Southern Birmingham Community Health NHS Trust. University of Central England, Birmingham

Sheldrake D, Sillman C, Notter J 1998 Developing partnerships in practice: using the Edinburgh Postnatal Depression Scale. J Commun Health Nurs 1: 50–54

Shenkin H 1996 Current dilemmas in medical-care rationing. A pragmatic approach. University Press of America, Baltimore, MD

Sheridan M 1960 The developmental progress of infants and young children. HMSO, London

Sheridan M 1975 From birth to five years: children's developmental progress, 3rd edn. NFER-Nelson, Windsor

Shickle D, Chadwick R 1994 The ethics of screening: is 'screeningitis' an incurable disease? J Med Ethics 20: 12–18

Sieghart P 1982 Professional ethics – for whose benefit? J Soc Occup Med 32: 4–14

Silvera M, Kapasi R 1996 Locating the goalposts: health promotion and purchasing for black and minority health (Report of the Health Education Authority Conference on improving health provision for black and minority ethnic communities). HEA, London

Simmons D, Williams DRR, Rowell MJ 1989 Prevalence of diabetes in a predominantly Asian community: preliminary findings of Coventry Diabetes Study. Br Med J 298

Simpson L, Stockford D 1979 Gypsy children and their health needs. Save the Children Fund, London

Skinner BF 1938 The behaviour of organisms. Appleton-Century-Crofts, New York

Skrabanek P 1990 Why is preventative medicine exempted from ethical constraints? J Med Ethics 16: 187–190

Slater R 1995 The psychology of growing old: looking forward. Open University Press, Buckingham

Smaje C 1995 Health, race and ethnicity: making sense of the evidence. King's Fund Institute/Share, London

Smith A, Jacobsen J (ed) 1988 The nation's health: a strategy for the 1990s. King's Fund, London

Smith DS, Goldenburg E, Ashburn A et al 1981 Remedial therapy after stroke: a randomised controlled trial. Br Med J Clinical Research Education 282: 517–520

Smith J, Bamford M, Ham C et al 1997 Beyond fundholding: a mosaic of primary care led commissioning and provision in the West Midlands Health Service. Management Centre, University of Birmingham, Birmingham

Smith J, Barnes M, Ham C, Martin G 1998 Mapping approaches to commissioning. Extending the mosaic, King's Fund

Smith J, Knight T, Wilson F 1999 Supra troupers. Health Serv J 14 Jan

Smith J, Ham C, Martin G 1988 Mapping Approaches and Commissioning. Extending the Mosaic. King's Fund, London

Smith S, Baker D, Buchan A, Bodiwala G 1992 Adult domestic violence. Health Trends 24: 97–99

SNMAC 1995 Making it happen: public health – the contribution, role and development of nurses, midwives and health visitors. Report of the Standing Nursing and Midwifery Advisory Committee. HMSO, London

Snowdon SK, Stewart-Brown SL 1997 Pre-school vision screening: results of a systematic review. CRD Report 9. NHS Centre for Reviews and Dissemination, York

Snowdon S, Stewart-Brown S 1998 Systematic reviews of child health. Royal College of Paediatrics and Child Health, London

Snyder JA 1994 Emergency department protocols for domestic violence. J Emerg Nurs 20: 65–68

Speller V, Learmonth A, Harrison D 1997 The search for evidence of effective health promotion. Br Med J 315: 361–363

Starfield B 1994 Primary care tomorrow: models of excellence. Lancet 344: 1129–1133

Starn JR 1992 Community health nursing visits for at risk women and infants. J Commun Health Nurs 9: 103–110

Stoate HG 1989 Can health screening damage your health? J Roy Coll Gen Practit May: 193–195

Stotts AL, DiClemente CC, Carbonari JP, Mullen PD 1996 Pregnancy smoking cessation: a case of mistaken identity. Addictive Behav 21: 459–471

Stutsman R 1931 Mental measurement of pre-school children. World Book Co, New York

Suppiah C 1994 Working in partnership with community mothers. Health Visitor 67: 51–53

Suris AM, Trapp MC, DiClemente CC, Cousins J 1998 Application of the transtheoretical model of behavior change for obesity in Mexican American women. Addictive Behav 23: 655–668

Sutherland A 1987 The body as symbol among the ROM. In: Blacking J (ed) The anthropology of the body. Academic Press, London

Sutton JC, Jagger C, Smith UK 1995 Parents' views of health surveillance. Arch Dis Childh 73: 57–61

Swann B, Wilson E, Wright L 1997 Working together in public health. Public Health Nursing Stockport's Experience conference paper. CPHVA, London

Symonds A 1993 Tracing the tradition of health visiting. Health Visitor 66(5)

Taylor P, Peckham S, Turton P 1998 A public health model of primary care – from concept to reality. Public Health Alliance, Birmingham

Tedesco D 1997 Exercise for the elderly in a rural community. Health Visitor 70: 32–33

Tejero A, Trujols J, Hernandez E et al 1997 Processes of change assessment in heroin addicts following the Procaska & DiClemente transtheoretical model. Drug Alcohol Dependence 47: 31–37

Thomas JD 1985 Gypsies and American medical care. Am Int Med 102: 842–845

Thomas J, Wainwright P 1996 Community nurses and health

promotion: ethical and political perspectives. Nurs Ethics 3: 97–107

Thomas JD, Douecette MM, Stoeckle JD 1987 Disease, lifestyle and consanguinity in 58 American gypsies. Lancet 2: 377–379

Thomason J et al 1997 Neonatal screening for inborn errors of metabolism. In: National Screening Committee/Royal College of Paediatrics and Child Health Proceedings: evolution or revolution? Systematic reviews of screening in child health, 17 December 1997 and 8 January 1998. Conference Organiser (c/o Child Growth Foundation), London, p 13–15

Thompson K 1997 Detecting post-natal depression in Asian women. Health Visitor 70: 226–228

Thompson TW 1929 The uncleanness of women among English Gypsies. JGLS Third Series 1(102): 15–43

Tiedemann 1787 Cited in Goodenough FL 1950 Mental testing. Staples, London

Titmuss R 1952 The position of women: some vital statistics. In: Black N et al (ed) 1984 Health and disease. A reader. Open University Press, Milton Keynes

Titmuss R 1974 An introduction to social policy. George Allen & Unwin, London

Today, BBC Radio 4, 25 January 1999

Tomkins CR 1987 Achieving economy, efficiency and effectiveness in the public sector. Kogan Page, Edinburgh

Tones K 1991 Health promotion, empowerment and the psychology of control. J Inst Health Educ 29: 17–26

Tones K, Tilford S 1990 Health education, effectiveness, efficiency and equity. Chapman & Hall, London

Torrington D, Weightman J, Johns K 1989 Effective management. Prentice-Hall, Englewood Cliffs, NJ

Townsend P, Davidson N (ed) 1982 Inequalities in health: the Black Report. Penguin, Harmondsworth

Townsend P, Davidson N, Whitehead M 1988 Inequalities in health and the Health Divide. Penguin, Harmondsworth

Trowler P 1996 Investigating health, welfare and poverty, 2nd edn. Collins Educational, London

Tschudin V, Marks-Maran D 1993 Ethics. Baillière Tindall, London

Tuckman B 1965 Development sequence in small groups. Psychol Bull 63: 384–399

Tullman D 1992 Cultural diversity in nursing education: does it affect racism in the nursing profession. J Nurs Educ 31: 321–324

Turner T 1998 Parenting: off to a Sure Start? Commun Practit 71: 278–280

Twinn S 1989 Change and conflict in health visiting practice: dilemma in assessing professional competency of student health visitors. Unpublished PhD thesis, University of London

Twinn SF 1991 Conflicting paradigms of health visiting: a continuing debate for professional practice. J Adv Nurs 16: 966–973

Twinn S, Cowley S (ed) 1992 The principles of health visiting: a re-examination. HVA/UKSC, London

Twinn S, Roberts B, Andrews S 1996 Community health care nursing. Butterworth-Heinemann, Oxford

UKCC 1992a Code of professional conduct for the nurse, midwife and health visitor, 3rd edn. United Kingdom Central Council for Nursing, Midwifery and Health Visiting, London

UKCC 1992b The scope of professional practice. United Kingdom Central Council for Nursing, Midwifery and Health Visiting, London

UKCC 1993 Standards for record keeping. United Kingdom Central Council for Nursing, Midwifery and Health Visiting, London

UKCC 1994a The future of professional practice – the Council's standards for education and practice following registration. United Kingdom Central Council for Nursing, Midwifery and Health Visiting, London

UKCC 1994b Professional conduct – occasional report on standards of nursing in nursing homes. United Kingdom Central Council for Nursing, Midwifery and Health Visiting, London

UKCC 1996 Guidelines for professional practice. United Kingdom Central Council for Nursing, Midwifery and Health Visiting, London

UKCC 1998 Guidelines for Records and Recordkeeping. United Kingdom Central Council for Nursing, Midwifery and Health Visiting, London

UKCC 1999 A higher level of practice, report of the consultation on the UKCC's proposals for a revised regulatory framework for post-registration clinical practice. United Kingdom Central Council for Nursing, Midwifery and Health Visiting, London

Upton DJ 1999 How can we achieve evidence-based practice if we have a theory–practice gap in nursing today? J Adv Nurs 29: 549–555

Vetter NJ, Jones DA, Victor CR 1984 Effect of health visitors working with elderly patients in general practice: a randomised controlled trial. Br Med J 288: 369–372

Vetter NJ, Lewis PA, Ford D 1992 Can health visitors prevent fractures in elderly people? Br Med J 304: 888–890

Vickers G 1984 Community medicine. Cited in Pietroni P 1996 The integrated community care practice: general practice, citizenship and community care. In: Meads G (ed) Future options for general practice. Radcliffe Medical Press, Oxford

Wakefield AJ, Murch SH, Linnell AAJ et al 1998 Ileal-lymphoid-nodular hyperplasia, non-specific colitis and pervasive developmental disorder in children. Lancet 351: 637–641

Walsh N 1997 Development of general practice and primary care in the UK 1900–1990. Lecture, Health Services Management Centre, University of Birmingham 15 December 1997

Walsh N, Beenstock J 1998 Going through the change. Health Serv J 3 Sep

Waters E, Oberklaid F 1998 Data collection in community child health. Ambul Child Health 3: 373–385

Watson G, Glaser EA 1964 Watson–Glaser critical thinking appraisal manual. Harcourt Brace & World, New York

Watt IS, Freemantle N 1994 Purchasing and public health: the state of the union. J Manage Med 81: 6–11

Watts A 1992 A tool for profiling. Unpublished paper, North Staffordshire Combined Healthcare NHS Trust

Weaver R 1996 Localities and inequalities. In: Bywaters P, McLeod E (ed) Working for equality in health. Routledge, London

Weller P (ed) 1991 Religions in the UK: a multi faith directory, 1991 census. Office of Population Censuses and Surveys, London

West Midlands Clinical Supervision Learning Set 1998 Clinical Supervision: Getting it right in your organisation. A critical guide to good practice. WMRHA, Birmingham

While A 1986 (ed) Research in preventive community

nursing care – fifteen studies in health visiting. John Wiley, Chichester

While A 1991 Health teaching in a primary school using Becker's health belief model. In: While A (ed) Caring for children: towards partnership with families. Edward Arnold, London

WHO 1988 Adelaide recommendations on healthy public policy. World Health Organization, Adelaide

Wildavsky A 1964 The politics of the budgetary process. Little, Brown, Boston, MA

Wilkie E 1979 A History of the CETHV. George Allen & Unwin, London

Wilkinson R 1994 The effects of widening income differences on the welfare of the young. Barnardos, London

William R 1995 Religion and illness. In: Radley A (ed) World of illness. Biographical and cultural perspectives on health and disease, Routledge, London, p 176

Williams EI, Greenwell J, Groom LM 1992 The care of people over 75 years old after discharge from hospital: an evaluation of timetabled visiting by health visitor assistants. J Publ Health Med 14: 138–144

Wilson G 1987 Background information (unpublished report)

Wilson J, Jungner G 1968 Principles and practice of screening for disease. Public Health Papers No. 34. World Health Organization, Geneva

Wilson J, Tingle J (ed) 1999 Clinical risk modification – a route to clinical governance? Butterworth-Heinemann, Oxford

Windsor B 1990 The Coalpool Project – health visiting, a corporate caseload. Unpublished paper, Walsall Health Authority

Wood PK 1983 Inquiring systems and problem structure: implications for cognitive development. Cited in Kitchener KS, King PM 1990 The reflective judgement model: transforming assumptions about knowing. In: Mezirow J et al (ed) Fostering critical reflection in adulthood. Jossey-Bass, San Francisco

Wooley M 1998 A new era for performance measurement in the NHS? Health Services Management Centre Newsletter 4(2)

Wright S 1998 Developing health visiting practice using action research. Commun Practit 71: 337–339

Wyatt J 1996 Medical informatics, artefacts or science? Meth Inform Med 35: 197–200

Young D 1998 Re MMR revisited hastily! http://www. mailbox.ac.uk/lists-f-j/gp-uk/1998-03/0132.Ltm.

Zastowny TR, Lehman AF, Cole RC, Kane C 1992 Family management of schizophrenia – a comparison of behavioural and supportive family treatment. Psychiat Q 63: 159–186

Zlotnick A 1993 Training strategies for elder abuse/inadequate care. J Elder Abuse Neglect 5: 55–62

Index